A Practical Atlas of Congenital Heart Disease

Springer

London
Berlin
Heidelberg
New York
Hong Kong
Milan
Paris
Tokyo

Audrey Smith and Roxane McKay

A Practical Atlas of Congenital Heart Disease

With Forewords by
John W. Kirklin and James K. Kirklin
Hajar A. Hajar Al Binali

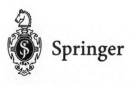

Springer

Audrey Smith PhD, FIBMS
Honorary Senior Research Fellow
The Cardiac Unit
Institute of Child Health
University College
London
United Kingdom

Roxane McKay, MD, FRCS, FRCSC
Consultant Congenital Heart Surgeon
Hamad Medical Corporation
Doha
Qatar

British Library Cataloguing in Publication Data
Smith, Audrey
    A practical atlas of congenital heart disease
    1. Congenital heart disease – Atlases
    I. Title   II. McKay, Roxane, 1944–
    616.1′2′043
    ISBN 185233729X

Library of Congress Cataloging-in-Publication Data
Smith, Audrey
    A practical atlas of congenital heart disease/Audrey Smith and Roxane McKay.
       p. ; cm
    Includes bibliographical references and index.
    ISBN 1–85233–729–X (alk. paper)
    1. Congenital heart disease–Atlases.   I. McKay, Roxane, 1944–   II Title.
    [DNLM: 1. Heart defects, Congenital–Atlases. WG 17 S642p 2003]
    RC687.S57 2003
    616.1′2043′0222–dc21   2003042417

ISBN 1–85233–729–X Springer-Verlag London Berlin Heidelberg
a member of BertelsmannSpringer Science+Business Media GmbH

Typeset by Florence Production Ltd, Stoodleigh, Devon
Printed and bound in the United States of America
28/3830–543210 Printed on acid-free paper SPIN 10910610

Foreword 1

In the current era of congenital heart surgery, with the emphasis on indications for early primary repair, methods of preserving the heart and brain during the repair process, and complex outcomes analyses following operations, the essence of the training of congenital heart surgeons seems sometimes forgotten. This book by Audrey Smith and Roxane McKay revives that essence. The beautiful photographs of heart specimens accompanied by simple but elegant line drawing diagrams rekindles memories of our interactions with Maurice Lev in the early days of cardiac surgery at the Mayo Clinic as we struggled to avoid the conduction system, and of an era at the University of Alabama when Bob Anderson would make an annual pilgrimage to UAB to share with us his latest anatomic observations on complex forms of congential heart disease. After all, the contributions of great cardiac anatomic pathologists only became truly relevant when their observations facilitated the surgical repair of complex congenital heart disease.

The authors have produced an "authored" rather than an "edited" work, a decision which promotes consistency and cohesiveness throughout the book. It also requires a great increment in effort and overall expertise. It is a decision that we heartily endorse, and in this case, the product is superior. The discussion of morphology and its relevance to surgical repair is erudite, yet practical, from the initial depiction of patent ductus arteriosus to the foray into the complexities of univentricular atrioventricular connections.

The organization of each chapter is appealing and is conveyed in the book's title. Rather than being encyclopedic, the text portion of each chapter consists of an "Introduction", which describes the anatomy of the malformation and its variants, clinical and surgical implications of these variations, and relevant surgical strategies. The succinct text is followed by a series of specimen photographs, correlated with line drawings and legends describing the anatomy and surgical repairs. At first glance, the reader may sense that the seemingly simple line drawings are an indicator of superficial coverage. Don't be deceived! The rather complete collection of photographed specimens illustrates a vast array of congenital heart malformations. The drawings and legends provide a focused and extremely useful package of information which is more instructive than the more usual stylized artist's renditions.

With access to collections of cardiac specimens almost nonexistent in most cardiac surgical training programs, the reader is treated to the gift of a permanent collection for his or her instant viewing, accompanied by a relevant, capsulized discussion of the pathologic anatomy, the goals of surgical therapy, and the logic behind specific surgical options. In an era when nearly all forms of "single ventricle" are treated with a standardized series of operations in the Fontan pathway, it is particularly enjoyable to see the extensive discussion of the cardiac morphology of the varieties of single ventricle and the inclusion of relevant morphologic and anatomic details necessary for operations such as septation of the single ventricle and intraventricular repairs associated with and leading to the Fontan operation.

The reader's pleasure and appreciation of the final product increases with each chapter, providing further evidence of the authoritative, focused, and enjoyable discussion of the morphology and surgery of complex congenital heart disease. This superb book will be a treasured resource for all serious students of congenital heart disease.

James K. Kirklin, MD
Professor of Surgery
University of Alabama at Birmingham

John W. Kirklin, MD
Professor Emeritus
University of Alabama at Birmingham

Foreword 2

The decline in infant mortality is a reflection of modernisation and progress in many areas of health care. Western countries are suffering from declining birth rates but blessed with low infant mortality. Here in most Middle Eastern countries both birth rate and infant mortality are still high. The contribution of congenital heart disease to infant mortality in the world is difficult to know precisely. D. Duff and Dan McNamara stated in *The Science and Practice of Pediatric Cardiology*[1] "congenital heart disease is the single most common major congenital anomaly, responsible for 3% to 5% of death during the first week of life and up to 33% of death during the entire neonatal period."

Pediatric cardiac surgery is a relatively new field. It started in the late 1930s with the treatment of patient ductus arteriosus, the first attempt at closure being made by John Strieder in Boston, in March 1937. This was long before the introduction of open-heart surgery. Over the last four decades, phenomenal progress has been made in the management of heart disease in general and congenital heart disease in particular.

None-the-less, knowledge of cardiovascular anatomy remains the keystone for most diagnostic and therapeutic approaches. While this is particularly true in the pediatric patient, and especially in the new-born infant, the major advances which have been made in diagnosis and treatment of congenital heart disease in children, have now resulted in patients surviving into adulthood. This, in turn, makes an understanding of complex cogenital malformations useful also for the general physician, the adult cardiologist and the adult cardiac surgeon.

This comprehensive book, divided into seven parts with a total of 30 chapters covering the major topics of congenital heart disease, is well written and very well illustrated as an atlas, and will serve as an important reference for pediatric cardio-vascular surgeons, pediatric cardiologists, pediatricians, and physicians. The meticulous and detailed drawings make the complex anatomy and the advanced plan of repair simple for us to understand, a feature which we have enjoyed in presentations from one of the authors to our departmental meetings and grand rounds at Hamad Medical Corporation in Doha, Qatar. Although progress in cardiovascular disease today is occurring so rapidly that it becomes progressively more difficult to keep up with new and evolving modalities of treatment, a book such as this helps to fill the gap in our knowledge between these recent advances in the treatment of congenital heart disease and the fundamental underlying pathologies which they address. I am pleased to include it among the achievements of our department in a young and growing country.

REFERENCE

1. Garson, A. Jr., Bricker JT, Fisher DJ, Neish SR (eds) The Science and Practice of Pediatric Cardiology
    (second edition), Vol I. Baltimore: Williams & Wilkins, 1998: 693.

His Excellency Hajar A. Hajar Al Binali, MD, FACC
Minister of Health, State of Qatar and
Chairman, Hamad Medical Corporation
Chairman, Department of Cardiology and Cardiovascular Surgery
Hamad Medical Corporation
Doha, Qatar

Preface

The inspiration for this work came during the 1980's from our surgical trainees at the Royal Liverpool Children's Hospital, Myrtle Street. Their weekly teaching sessions in cardiac morphology at the Institute of Child Health invariably translated into lively discussions over the following days, exploring the surgical application of their newly acquired knowledge. Conversely, clinical observations in the operating room were brought to the morphologist for amplification and clarification. This prompted us to try to integrate cardiac anatomy with surgical repair by presenting pictures of hearts with an anatomical description on one page, opposite to some aspect of their surgical relevance or management on the other. The format was intended to allow the reader to examine an actual heart specimen while referring to the open atlas, and hence the title of the book, "A Practical Atlas." It is not a book to be read "cover-to-cover," but rather one to be used as a reference and training tool in developing an understanding of specific cardiac malformations and technical details of their surgical management.

Simple line drawing rather than artistic illustrations have been used throughout to identify the diagnostic anatomical features and to emphasize important surgical landmarks. These are the type of sketches that any surgeon can, and indeed should, make of the hearts that are encountered, either in the pathology museum or the operating theatre. By recognizing such landmarks and understanding anatomical definitions, the pediatric cardiologist and congenital heart surgeon will become better equipped to reason through the infinitely variable morphology which is encountered in clinical practice. Furthermore, the anatomical pathologist will gain an understanding of surgical repairs which are encountered in postoperative hearts. Ample space has been left throughout the book for the reader to add comments or sketches from his or her own observations and experience.

In contrast with traditional textbooks of congenital heart surgery, this method presents neither a "typical" or "idealized" operation for a given malformation nor a comprehensive overview of any given subject. Rather, through the photograph of the heart, an actual example of a malformation is shown, followed by surgical considerations which are relevant to that particular cardiac defect. This mirrors clinical practice, where the physician is presented with a patient, for whom treatment must be individualized. Because it was based upon the hearts that were made available to us, the material is, of necessity, neither an all-inclusive atlas of congenital heart malformations nor a complete textbook of surgical management. Paradoxically, simple and common malformations tend to be illustrated less extensively than complex ones, and the length of a given chapter or section should thus in no way be seen as an indication of incidence or importance.

The detail in which the surgical techniques are presented has been scaled to the cardiac defect, more-or-less in keeping with the level of skill and experience needed for management of the malformation. Thus, closure of the persistently patent arterial duct or isolated ventricular septal defect, for example, are precisely described in considerable detail, as one might instruct a junior trainee. For more complex lesions, it is assumed that the surgeon undertaking such an operation will have mastered the necessary basic surgical skills, and considerations of technique and decision making are therefore focused at a more advanced level. Resolving complex operations into their individual components (necessitated by the layout of the material) gives the surgeon an armamentarium with which to approach any cardiac lesion; and, through the index, it is possible to identify and adapt the various parts of a complicated operative procedure to deal with atypical situations, again, much as occurs in clinical practice. The surgical techniques presented herein have all been employed successfully by many individuals and therefore should be well within the capability of any practicing congenital heart surgeon. As all of this information lies in the public domain, we have not attempted to acknowledge its source directly, nor do we claim credit for originating any of the procedures or techniques which are described.

Specimens on the anatomical page have generally been shown in the anatomical position, while the figures on the surgical page are shown as they would be seen by the surgeon in the operating room (which is usually 90° from the anatomical position). This causes the reader to practice three-dimensional mental imaging of the morphological and spatial relationships, which constitutes an integral part of congenital heart surgery. It is a skill that is necessary also to interpret echocardiograms, angiograms, and computerized axial tomography or magnetic resonance imaging in clinical practice. For easier interpretation, the photgraphs are reproduced at more than life size.

With regard to the anatomical material, line drawings have been made of each photograph to indicate the position of the picture in the heart and also allow labeling of structures separate from the picture itself. This permits the reader to "see" the details of the specimen, rather than the labels upon it. For virtually every malformation, the position of the specialized conduction tissue has been indicated, a unique feature that was made possible by our research facilities. Considerable variability exists in the terminology used to describe congenitally malformed hearts, and this remains an evolving area of controversy. Rather than embrace one nomenclature exclusively, we have tried to integrate modern, "pure" anatomical terminology with the more familiar designations which are in general clinical use, thus attempting to bridge the gap between researchers and practicing physicians. Finally, some of the illustrated hearts are, of themselves, rare and sometimes unique examples of a given malformation. If the knowledge gained from this volume prevents just one patient from life-long dependency upon a cardiac pacemaker system, our mission will have been achieved.

Over the years, a great many individuals and institutions have contributed directly or indirectly, as our friends, associates, and mentors, to the realization of this work. Without further elaboration, we gratefully acknowledge Robert H. Anderson, Robert Arnold, Donna Brownbridge, M.Gwen Connell, Albert D. Pacifico, Hamad Medical Corporation, David Hamilton, Vicki Holmes, Mark Jackson, the late Michael Jackson, John W. Kirklin, Dave McKay, Manuel F. Morales, Nick Mowat, Jeff D. Pearson, Donald N. Ross, Alan E. Smith, Springer-Verlag, Pawel Tyserowski, The University of Alabama in Birmingham, The University of Liverpool, The University of Saskatchewan, Ken Walters, and James L. Wilkinson.

Audrey Smith
Roxane McKay
May 2003

Contents

Abbreviations and Key

Ao	Aorta
AAo	Ascending aorta
ALPM	Anterolateral papillary muscle
ALSA	Aberrant left subclavian artery
AoV	Aortic valve
A-P	Aortico-pulmonary
ARSA	Aberrant right subclavian artery
ASD	Atrial septal defect
AVSD	Atrioventricular septal defect
AVV	Atrioventricular valve
CAVV	Common atrioventricular valve
CS	Coronary sinus
Cx	Circumflex coronary artery
D Ao/DescAo	Descending aorta
IA	Innominate (brachiocephalic) artery
Inf	Infundibular
IO	Infundibular orifice
IVC	Inferior vena cava (inferior caval vein)
(L)	Left sided
LA	Left atrium
LAA	Left atrial appendage
LAVV	Left atrioventricular valve
LAD	Left anterior descending (anterior interventricular) coronary artery
LBB	Left bundle branch
LBr	Left bronchus
LC/LCA	Left carotid artery
LCC	Left common carotid artery
LFT	Left fibrous trigone
LLLPV	Left lower lobe pulmonary vein
(L)LAA	Left sided left atrial appendage
LPA	Left pulmonary artery
LSV	Left pulmonary vein
LSA	Left subclavian artery
LSVC/LSCV	Left superior vena cava (Left superior caval vein)
LULPV	Left upper lobe pulmonary vein
LV	Left ventricle
LVOT	Left ventricular outflow tract
LVOTO	Left ventricular outflow tract obstruction
MPA	Main pulmonary artery
MV	Mitral valve

MPM	Medial papillary muscle
MAPCA	Major aorto-pulmonary collateral artery
NBB	Non-branching bundle
OF	Oval fossa (foramen ovale)
OS	Outlet (infundibular) septum
PA	Pulmonary artery
PDA	Patent ductus arteriosus (Persistently patent arterial duct)
POF	Patent oval fossa
PPM	Posterior papillary muscle
PTFE	Polytetraflouroethylene
PV	Pulmonary valve
PVC	Pulmonary venous confluence
(R)	Right sided
RA	Right atrium
RAA	Right atrial appendage
RAVV	Right atrioventricular valve
RBB	Right bundle branch
RC	Right coronary artery
RCA	Right carotid artery
REV	Réparational étageventriculaire
RFT	Right brous trigone
(R)LAA	Right sided left atrial appendage
RLPV	Right lower pulmonary vein
RLLPV	Right lower lobe pulmonary vein
RPA	Right pulmonary artery
RPV	Right pulmonary vein
RSA	Right subclavian artery
RSVC/RSCV	Right superior vena cava (Right superior caval vein)
RUL	Right upper lobe
RUPV	Right upper pulmonary vein
RULPV	Right upper lobe pulmonary vein
RV	Right ventricle
RVIF	Right ventriculo-infundibular fold
RVOT	Right ventricular outflow tract
SA node	Sinuatrial node
SMT	Septomarginal trabeculation
SN	Sinus node
SNA	Sinus nodal artery
SVC/SCV	Superior vena cava (Superior caval vein)

T	Trachea	TV	Tricuspid valve
TGA	Transposition of the great arteries	VIF	Ventriculo-infundibular fold
		VSD	Ventricular septal defect

Key to Tints Used in Depicting Conduction Tissue

 Edge of resected muscle

 Penetrating (non branching) bundle of specialized conduction tissue

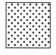 Ventriculoarterial valves

 Atrioventricular valves

Branching bundle of specialized conduction tissue

SECTION **1** ·

Extracardiac Anomalies of the Great Arteries

1 Persistently Patent Arterial Duct

Introduction

The arterial duct, which is normally patent at birth, is a vascular connection between the thoracic aorta and the central pulmonary arteries. Physiological closure by smooth muscle contraction usually begins during the first day of life, and subsequent fibrosis converts the duct into a ligament over the next two or three weeks. While the arterial duct has been found to be patent in as many as 45% of normal infants during the first five days of life, 90% of term babies who have no other cardiovascular malformation, will have complete closure by two months of age. After this time, patency of the duct is said to be "prolonged" or "persistent" and considered pathological.

Although its morphology is extremely variable as regards size and orientation, the position of the arterial duct is relatively constant. On the left side, which is the usual location, the aortic end lies a few millimetres distally to the left subclavian artery. The portion of aorta between the left subclavian artery and the arterial duct is called the "isthmus" but normally has no distinguishing histological features. The pulmonary end of the arterial duct joins either the bifurcation of the main pulmonary artery or the left pulmonary artery, just beyond its origin, and hence lies within the pericardium. Rarely, a right-sided arterial duct or bilateral ducts may occur. These are generally associated with anomalies of the aortic arch. The recurrent laryngeal branch of the vagus nerve invariably passes around the duct in the left chest and thus serves as a reliable guide to its position. In the neonate, the duct still lies in a foetal orientation as a continuation of the main pulmonary artery to the descending aorta, with a narrow angle between its upper surface and the aortic arch. Subsequent growth of these structures causes the junction between the duct and the aorta to approach a right angle in older patients.

When there is a left-to-right shunt through the arterial duct, the diameter of the descending aorta may be smaller than that of the isthmus, diminishing beyond the origin of the duct. Conversely, an aorta which enlarges distally to the arterial duct suggests the possibility of a right-to-left shunt as a result of pulmonary hypertension or more proximal aortic obstruction. Rarely, the duct becomes aneurysmal. Occasionally, the aortic end has an attachment opposite the origin of the subclavian artery such that an aortic isthmus cannot be identified.

Surgical closure of the arterial duct is carried out when pharmacological treatment with inhibitors of prostaglandin synthesis (indomethacin or ibuprofen) in the premature infant has failed, or when catheter occlusion with an intravascular device is not possible, or when the duct occurs in association with other cardiac malformations that require operation. In the latter situation, a patent arterial duct potentially allows either flooding of the lungs on cardiopulmonary by-pass or air to pass from the right side of the heart into the aorta during total circulatory arrest. Its control is therefore essential around the time when perfusion is commenced and preparation for this is done by dissection from the front via the midline sternal incision. An isolated arterial duct has otherwise been approached traditionally through a left posterolateral thoracotomy, although video-assisted techniques now also permit closure with minimal access in selected patients. The method of closure depends on the anatomy of the arterial duct and the preferences of the individual surgeon. Generally, clip closure is used when circumferential dissection would be hazardous. This would be in some preterm infants or when a limited access approach is used. Single or multiple ligation is suitable for most other situations, but division of the duct is necessary when its diameter approaches that of its length (short, wide duct) or when it is necessary to mobilize or reconstruct the pulmonary arteries (as in the arterial switch procedure). In the rare situation of a "ductal window," where there is no length to the communication between the aorta and pulmonary artery, the pericardium is opened to place a side-biting clamp on the pulmonary artery. The aortic end then is controlled either by a side-biting clamp or complete occlusion of the aorta. After separation of the vessels, the aorta is repaired with a patch and the pulmonary artery is oversewn. Because there is no development of collateral vessels in these patients, paraplegia is a risk and it is important to both maintain distal aortic flow and to minimize the period of aortic clamping. Calcification of a persistently patent arterial duct, which is unusual before the fifth decade, constitutes an indication for closure with a patch that is placed through the left pulmonary artery on cardiopulmonary bypass.

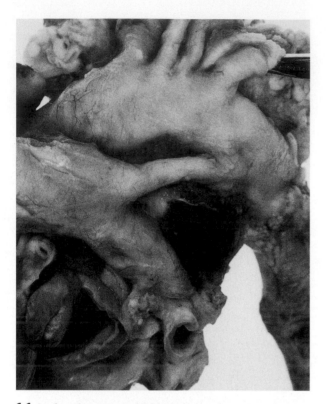

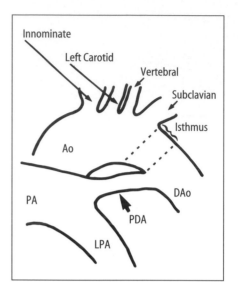

1.1 Persistently patent arterial duct. In this case, the duct is long and narrow. The transverse arch is normal in size and gives off four branch arteries. The left pulmonary artery appears as a continuation of the main pulmonary artery, after insertion of the arterial duct.

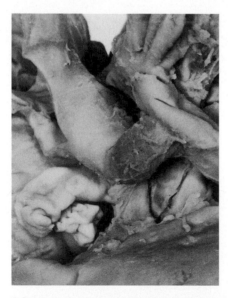

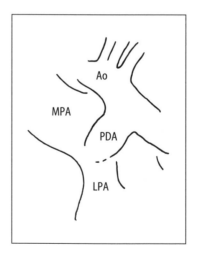

1.2 The arterial duct in this example is short and wide, its external diameter approximating that of the transverse aortic arch. The duct meets the aorta at a right-angle. This is characteristic of patients beyond the neonatal period. When the duct is of this size, it is especially important to differentiate it from the aortic arch and isthmus, as well as from the left pulmonary artery.

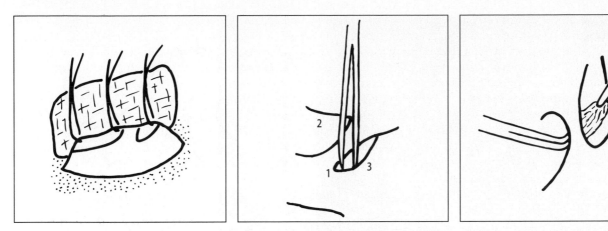

1.3 The arterial duct is approached through a standard left posterolateral thoracotomy. Retraction of the incised mediastinal pleura with stay-sutures gives access for dissection and controls the lung beneath a moist swab. The recurrent laryngeal nerve is retracted medially.

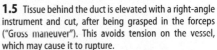

1.4 The anterior surface (1) is exposed by sharp dissection of the parietal pleura and areolar tissue, leaving the vascular adventitia intact until the pericardial extension over the pulmonary artery is identified. The inferior (2) and superior aspects (3) are then dissected. A narrow superior angle, as seen commonly in preterm babies, may be exposed by allowing the forceps to spring open between the duct and the aorta.

1.5 Tissue behind the duct is elevated with a right-angle instrument and cut, after being grasped in the forceps ("Gross maneuver"). This avoids tension on the vessel, which may cause it to rupture.

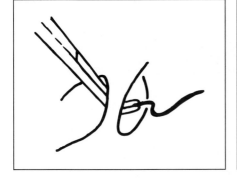

1.6 The end of a strong ligature, which has been moistened, is grasped with a right-angle instrument that passes freely behind the duct. Taking the tip of the ligature as a single strand ensures its smooth passage.

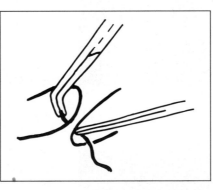

1.7 The ligature is depressed as it is retracted behind the duct to avoid trauma to the superior and posterior surfaces of the vessel.

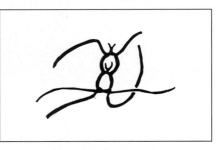

1.8 When the duct is ligated, it is necessary to obliterate its entire length with either multiple ligatures or a combination of ligatures and an intervening transfixation suture. Occlusion of the aortic end first diminishes pressure in the duct and prevents ductal tissue from being squeezed into the lumen of the aorta.

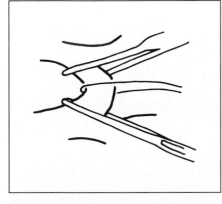

1.9 Division of the duct is necessary when its length and width are about equal and may be done electively at other times. After complete dissection, the aortic end is clamped, followed by occlusion of the pulmonary end. The clamps are placed as far apart as possible and may include part of the adjacent major vessel.

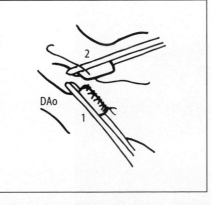

1.10 The duct is divided and each end, aortic (1) followed by pulmonary (2), is oversewn in two layers with a continuous monofilament suture.

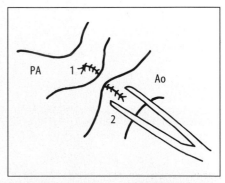

1.11 The pulmonary clamp is released and pressure applied to the suture line (1), followed by removal of the aortic clamp (2). Bleeding which does not abate after five minutes of pressure is controlled usually with adventitial sutures. Retraction of the duct prevents reapplication of clamps to the duct itself, such that any catastrophic hemorrhage would necessitate occlusion of the pulmonary artery (within the pericardium) or the aorta.

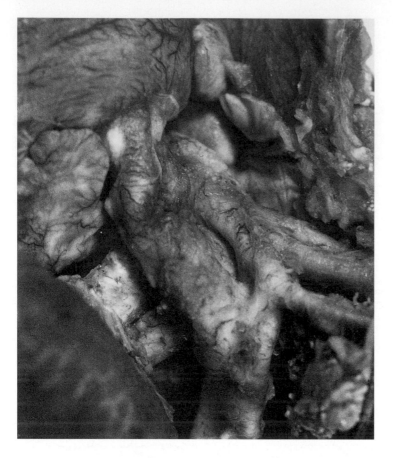

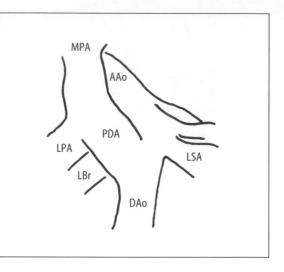

1.12 Persistently patent arterial duct. In this heart, the external diameter of the duct exceeds that of the aortic arch. There is a very short aortic isthmus between the left subclavian artery and the arterial duct. The dissection is orientated as it might be seen through a left thoracotomy.

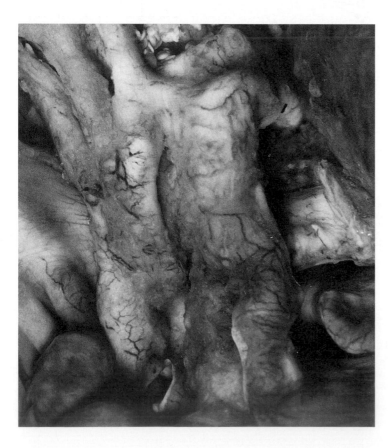

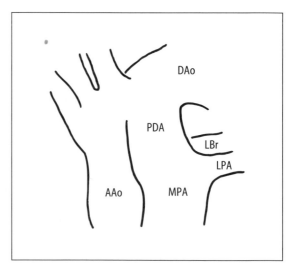

1.13 The same specimen is now orientated as the surgeon would see it through a midline sternotomy. The important landmark by which to identify the arterial duct in this dissection is the left pulmonary artery, although the recurrent laryngeal nerve also may be seen outside the pericardium. It should be appreciated that the duct in this case is larger than the ascending aorta and the transverse aortic arch.

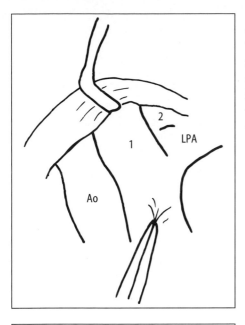

1.14 *(left)* Exposure of the arterial duct (1) from the front is facilitated by cephalad retraction of the pericardium and caudal retraction of the main pulmonary artery by grasping its adventitia with forceps or a small curved clamp. A very large arterial duct at high pressure may be more easily dissected after decompression on cardiopulmonary bypass. The anterior (1) and leftward (2) aspects are exposed until the left pulmonary artery is identified with certainty.

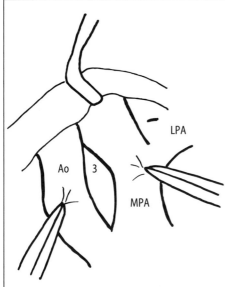

1.15 *(left)* The aorta is retracted laterally and the adventitia between the duct and the aortic arch is divided (3). When the intrapericardial length of the duct is short, it will be necessary to cut the pericardial reflection for safe passage of an instrument behind the duct. Care is taken to preserve the recurrent laryngeal nerve.

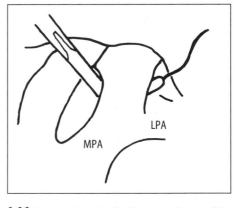

1.16 The duct is encircled with a strong ligature. If the tissues are delicate or the duct is at a very high pressure, ligation is performed immediately after going on cardiopulmonary bypass, when the duct is decompressed. When division is necessary (as in the arterial switch operation), this is done between two ligatures and each end is subsequently oversewn.

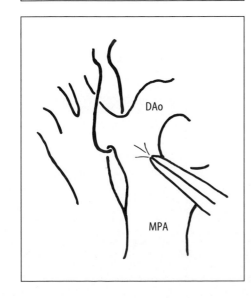

1.17 *(left)* Retraction of the duct itself rather than the main pulmonary artery, excessive traction on the main pulmonary artery, and confusion of the descending aorta with the left pulmonary artery, may lead to erroneous ligation of the aortic isthmus. The descending aorta is then perfused from the right ventricle and the patient may have blue feet.

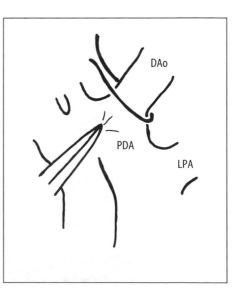

1.18 *(right)* Alternatively, excessive retraction of the duct towards the right may draw the descending aorta into the operative field. If it is mistakenly ligated, there is no distal perfusion of the lower body, while the pulmonary arteries remain at systemic pressure.

Suggested Reading

Connuck D, Sun JP, Super DM, Kirchner HL, Fradley LG, Harcar-Sevick RA, Salvator A, Singer L, Mehta SK. Incidence of patent ductus arteriosus and patent foramen ovale in normal infants. Am J Cardiol 2002;89:244.

Gross RE, Hubbard JP. The first successful case of surgical ligation of a patent ductus arteriosus. JAMA 1939;112:729.

Jones JC. Twenty-five years' experience with surgery of patent ductus arteriosus. J Thorac Cardiovasc Surg 1965;50:149.

Kelsey JR, Gilmore CE, Edwards JE. Bilateral ductus arteriosus representing persistence of each sixth aortic arch. Report of a case in which there was associated isolated dextrocardia and ventricular septal defects. Arch Pathol 1953;55:154.

Kirklin JW, Silver AW. Technique of exposing the ductus arteriosus prior to establishing extracorporeal circulation. Proc Staff Meet Mayo Clin 1958;33:423.

Kron IL, Mentzner RM Jr, Rheuban S, Nolan SP. A simple rapid technique for operative closure of patent ductus arteriosus in the premature infant. J Cardiovasc Surg 1984;37:422.

Laborde F, Noirhomme P, Karam J, Batisse A, Bourel P, Saint Maurice O. A new video-assisted thoracoscopic surgical technique for interruption of patent ductus arteriosus in infants and children. J Thorac Cardiovasc Surg 1993;105:278.

O'Donovan TG, Geck W. Closure of the complicated patent ductus arteriosus. Ann Thorac Surg 1978;25:463.

Pontius RG, Danielson GK, Noonan JA, Judson JP. Illusions leading to surgical closure of the distal left pulmonary artery instead of the ductus arteriosus. J Thorac Cardiovasc Surg 1981;82:107.

Rashkind WJ, Cuaso CC. Transcatheter closure of patent ductus arteriosus: successful use in a 3.5kg infant. Pediatr Cardiol 1979;1:3.

2 Anomalies of the Thoracic Aorta

2A Coarctation of the Aorta

Introduction

Coarctation of the aorta is a localized narrowing of the vessel which causes obstruction to blood-flow. Most commonly, it occurs in the thoracic aorta beyond the left subclavian artery, in proximity to the insertion of the arterial duct. More rarely, coarctation is found in the abdominal aorta, lower thoracic aorta or between the left subclavian and left common carotid arteries. The classical lesion of coarctation is a localized shelf of thickened tissue within the aortic lumen. This may represent ectopic ductal tissue or an infolding of the aortic wall consequent to abnormal flow patterns. Externally, in patients beyond the neonatal period, there is often a narrowing at the level of the coarctation shelf with post-stenotic dilatation of the distal vessel. Variable hypoplasia and/or elongation of the aortic segments proximal to the coarctation are not uncommon, particularly in the transverse aortic arch and isthmus. In older patients, collateral circulation around the coarcted segment may produce enlarged intercostal vessels which manifest as rib notching on the chest X-ray. The formation of aneurysms in either these intercostal vessels or the aorta, increases progressively after about five years of age.

Coarctation which occurs in association with only a persistently patent arterial duct or no other significant cardiac lesion is called "isolated" coarctation. This is in distinction to approximately 40% of cases in which there are additional intracardiac malformations. The most common of these is a ventricular septal defect. In general, patients with associated cardiac lesions tend to present at a younger age (generally, in the neonatal period) than do those with isolated coarctation. A two-leaflet aortic valve, which may or may not be hemodynamically significant, is also found in about 85% of patients with coarctation.

The surgical management of coarctation depends on the age of the patient, the type of associated malformations and the morphology of the coarctation itself. In the sick neonate, resuscitation is first carried out by administration of Prostaglandin E1, to reopen the arterial duct. This facilitates perfusion of the lower body either by dilating ductal tissue within the coarctation shelf or by allowing flow from the pulmonary artery into the descending aorta.

For isolated coarctation and patients whose associated lesions do not require intracardiac procedures, the standard surgical approach is through a left posterolateral thoracotomy. If there is significant hypoplasia of the transverse arch, this must be dealt with, as well as the obstruction at the coarctation site, either by extended aortoplasty or mobilization and anastomosis of the descending aorta to the intrapericardial ascending aorta.

For obstructions which are distal to the left subclavian artery, the choice of procedure broadly lies among subclavian flap angioplasty, resection with primary anastomosis (generally "end-to-end" or "side-by-side") or patch aortoplasty. Subclavian flap angioplasty enlarges both a hypoplastic isthmus and the coarcted segment with the patient's own tissue, thus conserving growth potential. However, the abnormal tissue of the coarctation shelf itself is generally incompletely removed and the arterial supply to the left arm is sacrificed, both of which constitute drawbacks associated with this procedure. Patch angioplasty is technically simpler than the other two options but carries a significant risk of late aneurysm formation opposite the prosthetic material. While resection with end-to-end anastomosis removes the coarctation segment with any abnormal tissue and permits tissue-to-tissue apposition, a circumferential suture line may predispose to recoarctation in small vessels. A modification of this technique in which the descending aorta is brought up to the lateral side of the isthmus and subclavian artery, the so-called "side-by-side" anastomosis, may avoid this complication. Extensive mobilization of all the vessels is necessary to make such an anastomosis without tension, which is of particular importance in cases with a hypoplastic aortic isthmus.

Repair of coarctation in association with intracardiac corrections has been done through a midline sternotomy, especially when a descending-to-ascending aortic anastomosis is necessary. While other types of repair are possible also from an anterior approach, most surgeons find that a thoracotomy is preferable for a reconstruction that is done within the left chest.

In older children or adults, isolated coarctation, which is the most common form among these age groups, can generally be managed by excision with end-to-end anastomosis. Exceptions to this are the long segment, isthmal hypoplasia (which usually requires patch angioplasty) and coarctation with aneurysm formation (where the affected aorta is replaced with an interposition graft). In these older patients, collateral development is important as a source of lower body perfusion during the period of aortic cross-clamping. When it is inadequate, provision for spinal-cord protection is mandatory, either with a temporary shunt or use of cardiopulmonary bypass for hypothermia and perfusion of the lower body.

Most recoarctations are now treated by the interventional cardiologist using balloon dilatation with or without stenting. When this is not successful or possible, a right-sided bypass graft may provide an alternative to repeat thoracotomy in selected cases. This procedure is particularly useful when there is associated hypoplasia of the transverse aortic arch.

2.1 Coarctation of the aorta.
Preductal coarctation. The lumen of the aorta is narrowed between the orifice of the left subclavian artery and that of the patent arterial duct, by both hypoplasia and infolding of the aortic wall (short arrow). The descending aorta is perfused from the persistently patent duct. This coarctation is the most common type found in association with ventricular septal defect. A preductal coarctation may be produced also by a shelf of ductal tissue extending around the aortic lumen. Not infrequently, these hearts also have lesions which potentially obstruct the left ventricular outflow tract.

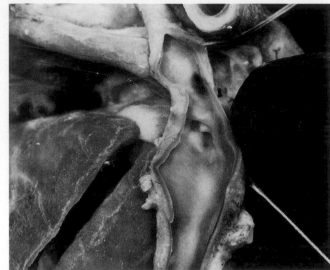

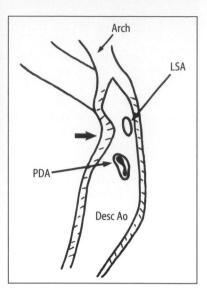

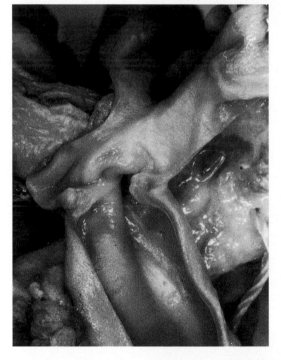

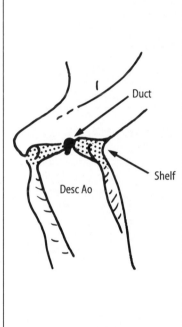

2.2 Paraductal (juxtaductal) coarctation. The aortic narrowing in this particular coarctation is due to excessive ductal tissue encroaching around the lumen directly opposite the aortic end of the arterial duct. The external appearance of such a coarctation may not suggest severe narrowing, even when the aortic lumen is nearly occluded by the shelf (stippled). Closure of the duct exacerbates the obstruction by further constriction of the aorta. This proliferation of ductal tissue constitutes the type of shelf often found in isolated coarctation and in hearts with intact ventricular septum.

2.3 *(right)* **Postductal coarctation.** The orifices of a small persistently patent arterial duct and the left subclavian artery both lie proximal to the coarctation shelf (stippled) in this case. This is an extremely rare type of coarctation. As the obstruction is beyond the duct, there is severe hemodynamic disturbance which is not influenced by ductal patency.

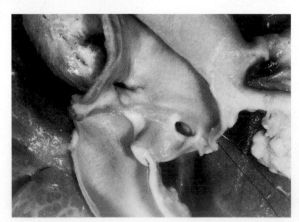

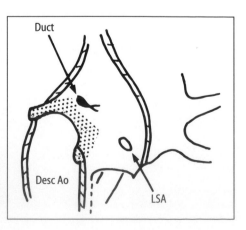

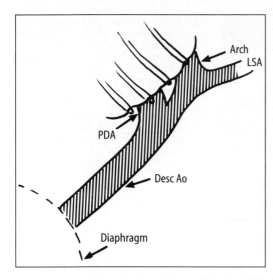

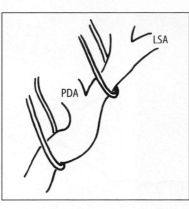

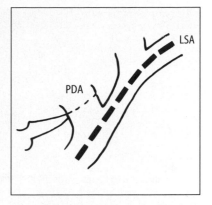

2.4 All of these types of coarctation are localized beyond the left subclavian artery and, accordingly, amenable to resection with "side-by-side" anastomosis. For this procedure, the aorta is exposed through a left posterolateral thoracotomy, and stay stitches on the incised posterior mediastinal pleura are used to retract the lung beneath a moist swab. The aorta is mobilized from the distal arch to the diaphragm, and the proximal left subclavian artery and arterial duct are also dissected (hatched area). When a narrow (paediatric) operating table is available, this dissection is facilitated by placing the patient at a 45° angle to the edge of the table.

2.5 Vessel loops passed around the aortic isthmus and descending aorta allow gentle traction on the vessels and facilitate the dissection. There are no intercostal or collateral vessels arising from the isthmus and rarely any immediately distal to the arterial duct.

2.6 The arterial duct is dissected circumferentially and encircled with a 5/0 monofilament suture, taking superficial bites in the adventitia. A line drawn with a skin marking-pencil on the front of the aorta, across the isthmus into the left subclavian artery (dashed line), will later help to maintain correct orientation of the vessels.

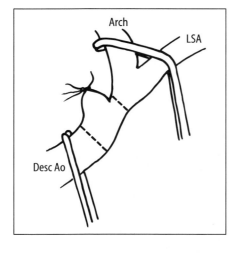

2.7 *(left)* A side-biting clamp is positioned across the left subclavian artery and distal aortic arch, the arterial duct is ligated and a second clamp is placed across the descending aorta. The aorta is then divided above and below the arterial duct (dashed lines), taking care to remove all duct tissue from both segments of the vessel.

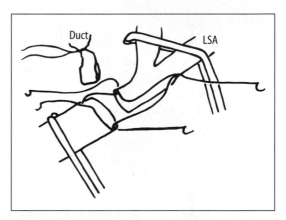

2.8 The lateral side of the proximal aortic segment is incised into the left subclavian artery. The diameter of the descending aorta is often equal to this distance, but, if necessary, the distal segment is opened slightly on its medial side to match the length of the proximal incision. The ligature on the arterial duct is gently retracted medially to remove it from the area of the anastomosis.

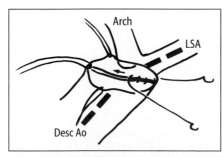

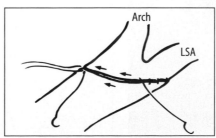

2.10 Continuous suturing with the second arm of the stitch completes the anterior layer of the anastomosis. The clamps are rotated slightly towards each other at this time to take any tension off the vessels.

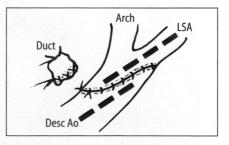

2.11 With the patient in steep Trendelenberg position, the distal and proximal clamps are slowly released. As confirmed by the position of the marking lines, the two segments of aorta lie "side-by-side" and have not been rotated. The remnant of aorta attached to the arterial duct is oversewn to ensure hemostasis. This technique achieves an anastomosis whose diameter is equal to the combined diameters of the isthmus and descending aorta, and does not risk narrowing the distal aortic arch.

2.9 The posterior wall of a continuous anastomosis is done forehand with a fine (7/0 in neonates; 6/0 in infants) double-ended monofilament suture, working inside the vessels. The orifice of the distal aortic arch must be differentiated from the cut edge of the vessel, particularly if the aortic isthmus is narrow. Rotation of the clamps slightly away from each other helps to expose the posterior walls of the vessels, as do additional stay-sutures on the free edges anteriorly, if needed. If the patient has been positioned at an angle on the operating table, the surgeon does the anastomosis from the opposite side of the table.

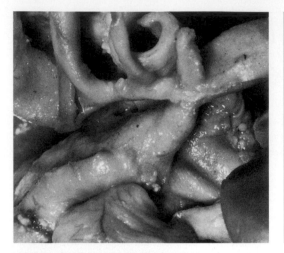

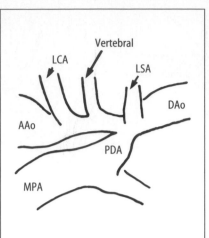

2.12 Coarctation of the aorta. Hypoplastic transverse aortic arch. The transverse aortic arch extends from the innominate or brachiocephalic artery to the origin of the left subclavian artery. The left carotid artery divides it into proximal and distal segments, either or both of which may be hypoplastic and/or elongated. In this example, the distal segment is severely narrowed with complete occlusion internally beyond a vertebral artery which originates directly from the arch (see Figure 2.13). The innominate (brachiocaphalic) branch is not seen.

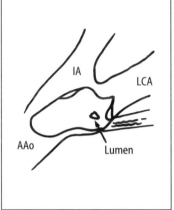

2.13 Internally, the lumen of the hypoplastic arch narrows, as in the previous case, to a diameter of about 1 mm after the origin of the left carotid artery, but without total occlusion distally. The proximal transverse aortic arch, between the innominate and left carotid arteries, is very short.

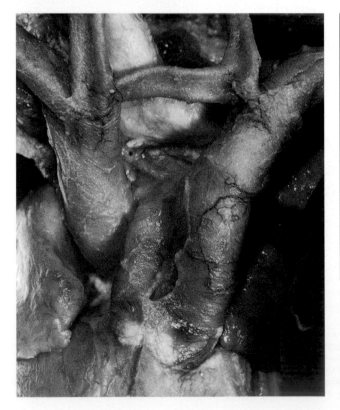

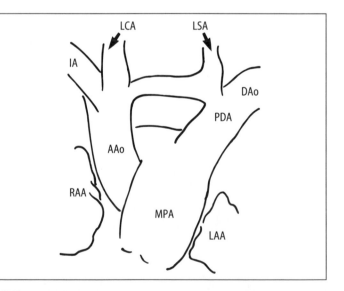

2.14 A segment of the aortic arch is considered to be hypoplastic when its external diameter is less than about 50% of the ascending aortic diameter or smaller than the descending aorta. The distal transverse arch in this heart is both hypoplastic and elongated, and internally the isthmus is completely occluded beyond the origin of the left subclavian artery. The arterial duct, which appears to give off the descending aorta, inserts opposite the subclavian artery, such that there is virtually no isthmus. The left carotid artery arises adjacent to the innominate artery, so that there is absence also of the proximal arch. This is the least common type of aortic arch hypoplasia. Such morphology is found more frequently when the mitral valve is abnormal or the left ventricle is small.

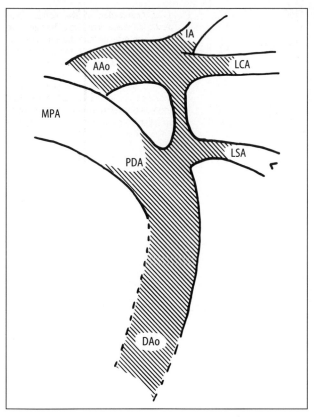

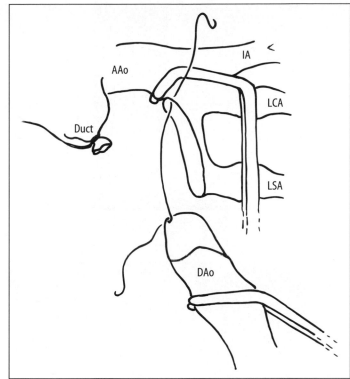

2.15 Repair of coarctation of the aorta with hypoplastic transverse aortic arch is carried out through a standard left posterolateral thoracotomy in the third intercostal space. Extensive dissection of the aorta (hatched area) is necessary to achieve adequate mobilization for a tension-free anastomosis. The descending aorta is dissected to the diaphragm, and the arterial duct, subclavian and left carotid arteries are dissected also. The pericardium is opened anterior to the phrenic nerve and the ascending aorta is freed from the main pulmonary artery. A vessel loop is passed around the intrapericardial ascending aorta, and the innominate artery and proximal transverse arch are mobilized. Exposure is then set up again in the posterior mediastinum and the vessel loop around the ascending aorta is passed posteriorly into the field, beneath the hypoplastic transverse arch.

2.16 For repair by extended arch reconstruction, the arterial duct is ligated and divided, using the ligature to retract the duct and pulmonary artery anteriorly and give access to the distal ascending aorta. Careful positioning of the proximal clamp is necessary to ensure cerebral blood-flow, as evidenced by pressure or oxygen saturation monitoring in the right radial or superficial temporal artery. The entire coarctation segment is resected with adjacent ductal tissue. The incision is carried along the concavity of the transverse aortic arch, proximal to the origin of the innominate artery and on to the ascending aorta. The descending aorta is opened on its lateral side if needed to match the length of the incision in the aortic arch, but this is rarely necessary. The descending aorta is then anastomosed to the distal ascending aorta and undersurface of the transverse arch with a running monofilament suture. The posterior wall is first constructed working inside the vessels, and the anterior, also suturing forehand, outside the vessels. The patient is placed in steep Trendelenberg position prior to the removal of the clamps, and the innominate and left carotid arteries are briefly occluded as the proximal clamp is released.

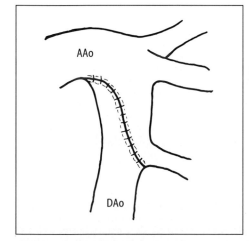

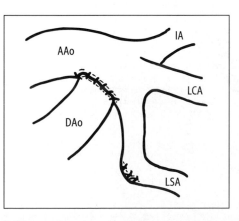

2.17 The completed anastomosis must extend far enough proximally to relieve the obstruction completely and all ductal tissue must be removed to prevent "recoarctation." In general, the suture line should start just proximal to the origin of the innominate artery, on the distal ascending aorta.

2.18 When there is extreme hypoplasia and elongation of the distal arch, an alternative technique is to bring the divided descending aorta to the distal ascending aorta, leaving the left subclavian artery as an end artery. In many instances, however, the diameter of the descending aorta is so wide in comparison to the length of the aortic arch that the anastomosis still extends distally beyond the origin of the innominate artery. On echocardiography postoperatively, as well as at the time of operation, the acute angle formed between the ascending and descending aorta gives a characteristic appearance which has been likened to the architectural structure of a Gothic arch. Hence, this procedure is also known as a "Gothic arch reconstruction." Full mobilization of the vessels is essential with this technique to prevent pressure on the left mainstem bronchus which passes through the arch.

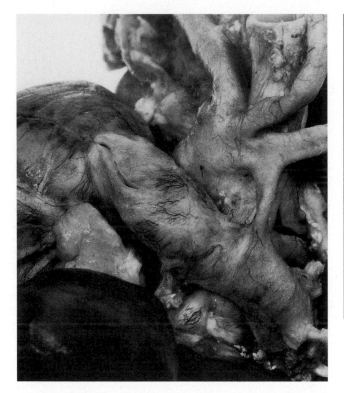

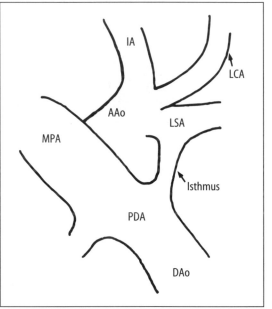

2.19 Coarctation of the aorta. Hypoplasia of the aortic isthmus. The great arteries are shown from the left side. Removal of the pericardium allows the right ventricle, the pulmonary trunk and the ascending aorta to be seen. The innominate and left carotid arteries arise close together with shortening of the distal aorta, a situation which has been called "bovine innominate trunk." The aortic isthmus is the segment of the aorta between the left subclavian artery and the insertion of the arterial duct. In this specimen it is long and narrow. Internally, there is also a discrete coarctation shelf at the distal end of the isthmus, just above the arterial duct. The persistently patent arterial duct, which clearly perfuses the descending aorta in this situation, is considerably larger than the diameter of the transverse aortic arch. When the lumen of the isthmus is completely occluded, there is said to be "atresia" of the aortic isthmus. In this situation, the ascending and descending aorta remain in continuity, in contrast to "interrupted aortic arch," where the segments of aorta are not connected to each other. A variety of surgical techniques, including subclavian flap angioplasty, patch angioplasty, and excision with end-to-end anastomosis, have been used to repair coarctation with hypoplasia of the aortic isthmus. Exposure for these procedures is also through a left posterolateral thoracotomy, but dissection of the aorta is more limited than that described for "side-by-side" anastomosis (see Figures 2.4–2.11) or extended aortoplasty (see Figures 2.15–2.18).

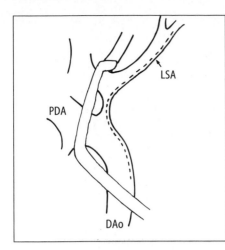

2.20 The incision for subclavian angioplasty extends from about 0.5 cm below the arterial duct, across the lateral side of the isthmus, and the full length of the subclavian artery whose first five or six branches are divided. A single side-biting clamp may be used to control the distal aortic arch, the arterial duct, and the descending aorta. The distal subclavian artery is carefully ligated prior to division.

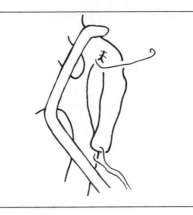

2.21 The "flap" of opened subclavian artery is turned down with continuous monofilament sutures after excision of any coarctation shelf within the lumen of the aorta (see Figures 2.2 and 2.3). Each half of the suture line is done forehand working towards the surgeon, from top to bottom. Rotation of the clamp rightward gives excellent exposure of the posterior portion. An additional stay-suture at the "toe" of the anastomosis helps to align the structures.

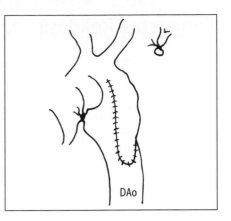

2.22 Suturing adjusts the flap to obtain maximal enlargement of the isthmus and to avoid narrowing the distal aortic arch. The arterial duct is routinely ligated after removal of the clamp.

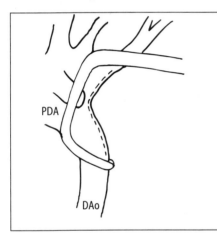

2.23 Patch angioplasty is conveniently done with a single, large side-biting clamp controlling all the vascular structures. This has been advocated as a very quick procedure for a sick neonate because minimal dissection is necessary, and is applicable also for long segment hypoplasia.

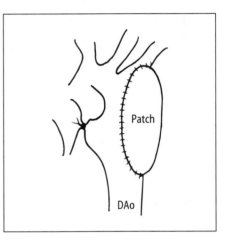

2.24 The aorta is opened on its lateral side from below the arterial duct onto the origin of the left subclavian branch.

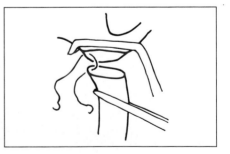

2.25 The patch provides generous enlargement of the coarctation segment but lacks growth potential.

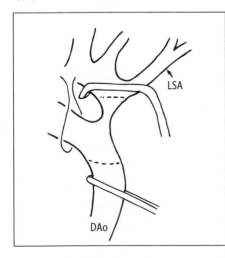

2.26 (left) For resection and end-to-end anastomosis, the proximal clamp may leave some perfusion through the enlarged left subclavian artery. This is particularly true in older patients for whom this is usually the procedure of choice. Collateral vessels proximal to the level of clamping on the descending aorta and the arterial duct are also dissected and controlled prior to opening the aorta.

2.27 (above right) The arterial duct is ligated and the coarctation is excised. Proximal and distal aortic segments are joined with continuous or interrupted sutures.

2.28 (below right) The completed anastomosis often extends into the left subclavian origin and on to undersurface of the arch to achieve a wide lumen. All ductal tissue is removed by this technique. After about seven years of age, the aorta has grown to approximately 70% its adult size and the risk of recoarctation is markedly less with this procedure than in younger patients.

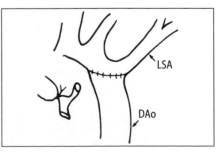

Suggested Reading

Becker AE, Becker MJ, Edwards JE. Anomalies associated with coarctation of the aorta. Particular reference to infancy. Circulation 1970;41:1067.

Ben-Shoshan M, Rossi NP, Korns ME. Coarctation of the abdominal aorta. Arch Pathol; 1973;95:221.

Bergdahl L, Ljungquist A. Long term results after repair of coarctation of the aorta by patch grafting. J Thorac Cardiovasc Surg 1980;80:177.

Bove EL, Minich LL, Pridjian AK, Lupinetti FM, Snider AR, Dick M, Beckman RH. The management of severe subaortic stenosis, ventricular septal defect and aortic arch obstruction in the neonate. J Thorac Cardiovasc Surg 1993;105:289.

Connolly HM, Schaff HV, Izhar U, Dearani JA, Warnes CA, Orszulak TA. Posterior pericardial ascending-to-descending aortic bypass: an alternative surgical approach for complex coarctation of the aorta. Circulation 2001;104 (12 Suppl 1) I133.

Elliott MJ. Coarctation of the aorta with arch hypoplasia: improvements on a new technique. Ann Thorac Surg 1987;44:321.

Hamilton DI, DiEusanio G, Sandrasagra FA, Donnelly RJ. Early and late results of aortoplasty with a left subclavian flap for coarctation of the aorta in infancy. J Thorac Cardiovasc Surg 1978;75:699.

Hart JC, Waldhausen JA. Reversed subclavian flap angioplasty for arch coarctation of the aorta. Ann Thorac Surg 1983;36:715.

Ho SY, Anderson RH. Coarctation, tubular hypoplasia, and the ductus arteriosus: a histological study of 35 specimens. Br Heart J 1979;41:268.

Karolczak MA, McKay R, Arnold R. Right-sided intrathoracic bypass graft for complex or recurrent coarctation of the aorta. European J Cardiothoracic Surg 1989;3:278.

Lacour-Gayet F, Bruniaux J, Serraf A, Chambran P, Blaysat G, Lasay J, Petit J, Kachaner J, Planche C. Hypoplastic transverse arch and coarctation in neonates, surgical reconstruction of the aortic arch: a study of sixty-six patients. J Thorac Cardiovasc Surg 1990; 100:808.

McKay R, Tyrrell MJ, Kakadekar AP. Aortic coarctation: surgical management simplified. In: Imai Y, Momma K (eds). Proceedings of the Second World Congress of Pediatric Cardiology and Cardiac Surgery. Futura Publishing Company, 1998, p 251.

Rahasinghe HA, Reddy VM, van Son JA, Black MD, McElhinney DB, Brook MM, Hanley FL. Coarctation repair using end-to-side anastomosis of descending aorta to proximal aortic arch. Ann Thorac Surg 1996;61:840.

Ungerleider RM, Ebert PA. Indications and techniques for midline approach to aortic coarctation in infants and children. Ann Thorac Surg 1987;44:517.

van Son JA, Asten WN, van Lier HJ, Daniels O, Vincent JG, Skotnicki SH, Lacquet LK. Detrimental sequelae on the hemodynamics of the upper limb after subclavian flap angioplasty in infancy. Circulation 1990;81:996.

von Kodolitsch Y, Aydin MA, Koschyk DH, Loose R, Schalwat I, Karck M, Cremer J, Haverich A, Berger J, Meinertz T. Predictors of aneurysmal formation after surgical correction of aortic coarctation. J Am Coll Cardiol 2002;39:617.

Vouhé PR, Trinquet F, Lecompte Y, Vernant F, Roux PM, Touati G, Pome G, Leca F, Neveux J-Y. Aortic coarctation with hypoplastic aortic arch: results of extended end-to-end aortic arch anastomosis. J Thorac Cardiovasc Surg 1988;96:557.

Waldhausen JA, Wahrwold PL. Repair of the coarctation of the aorta with a subclavian flap. J Thorac Cardiovasc Surg 1966;51:532.

Ziemen G, Jonas RA, Perry SB, Freed MP, Castaneda AR. Surgery for coarctation of the aorta in the neonate. Circulation 1986;74 (Pt 2):125.

2B   Interruption of the Aortic Arch

Introduction

The arch of the aorta is said to be "interrupted" when there is complete discontinuity between two of its parts. Although severe coarctation with obliteration of the aortic lumen ("aortic atresia") may produce a similar clinical and hemodynamic picture, there is no tissue connecting the vascular segments of an interrupted aortic arch. The most common site for interruption is between the left carotid and left subclavian arteries (Type B) which occurs in more than half of the cases. Type A (interruption beyond the left subclavian artery) constitutes about 40%, while the rare Type C (interruption between the innominate and left carotid arteries) is found in only about 5% of patients. The arch may be left- or right-sided, and the contralateral subclavian artery not uncommonly arises aberrantly as its last branch (see 2C, Vascular Rings). The descending aorta is invariably connected to the pulmonary artery by an arterial duct.

A ventricular septal defect is nearly always associated with interrupted aortic arch and its absence should suggest the alternative possibility of the more unusual aortopulmonary window. The defect may be either perimembranous or muscular and is commonly sub-arterial. In any of these, deviation of the outlet (infundibular) septum or anomalous muscle bundles may cause obstruction of the left ventricular outflow tract. Other anomalies which have been found in association with interrupted aortic arch include common arterial trunk, univentricular atrioventricular connection (double inlet ventricle) and, more rarely, transposition of the great arteries (discordant ventriculo-arterial connection).

The surgical management of interrupted aortic arch is directed towards reconstitution of the systemic great vessel and normalization of pulmonary blood-flow, each of which may be accomplished by several different methods. Direct anastamosis of the proximal and distal aortic segments is nearly always possible after mobilization of the vessels and conserves growth potential. Alternatively, a synthetic conduit may be interposed, but this invariably will be outgrown and thus commits the patient to reoperation. Arch reconstruction may be done through a lateral thoracotomy on the side of the descending aorta or through a midline sternal incision.

The technical options for the management of pulmonary blood-flow in interrupted aortic arch consist of pulmonary artery banding, complete separation of the systemic and pulmonary circulations by closure of the ventricular septal defect, or, in selected cases of so-called "single ventricle", an arterial switch procedure to interpose a hypoplastic or stenotic pulmonary artery between the ventricle and the pulmonary circulation. With the usual intracardiac morphology of an isolated ventricular septal defect, closure of the ventricular septal defect achieves single-stage, complete repair during the neonatal period and constitutes the procedure of choice when facilities for open-heart surgery in small babies are available. Some patients also require simultaneous relief of subaortic obstruction, usually by excision of the deviated infundibular septal muscle or anomalous subaortic muscle bundles. Pulmonary artery banding may be done as preliminary palliation when neonatal open-heart surgery is not feasible or when a "single ventricle" type of morphology ultimately necessitates the Fontan circulation. Alternatively, some of these patients are managed like hypoplastic left heart syndrome (see Chapter 19), using the main pulmonary artery for the systemic outflow from the heart and creating an alternative source of blood-flow to the lung.

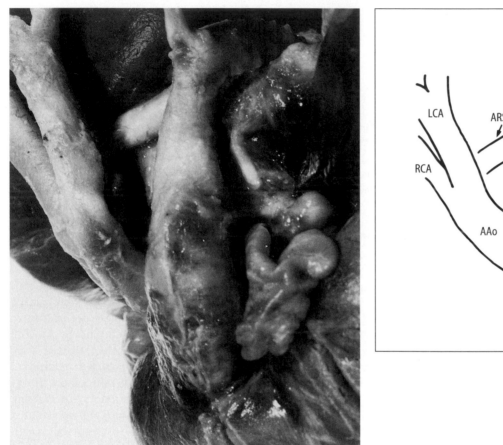

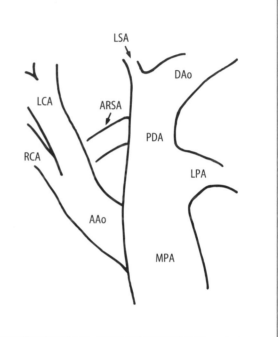

2.29 Interrupted aortic arch. Type B. The base of the heart and great arteries are seen partly from the left side, about midway between the appearances through a midline sternotomy and those through a left lateral thoracotomy. The ascending aorta gives off the right and left common carotid arteries. A large main pulmonary artery continues over the left bronchus as a patent arterial duct, perfusing the descending aorta. The actual distance between the upper and lower segments of the aorta during life is approximately as shown in this example. The left subclavian artery lies at the distal margin of the arterial duct. The right subclavian artery arises as the last branch of the left-sided descending aorta (the esophagus and trachea have been removed to show its position). The origin of the right pulmonary artery is just proximal to the left branch and obscured by the overlying main pulmonary artery. The relationships of the duct and descending aorta to the left bronchus are important, as insufficient mobilization of the descending aorta or anastomosis too far proximally on the ascending aorta may cause its external compression.

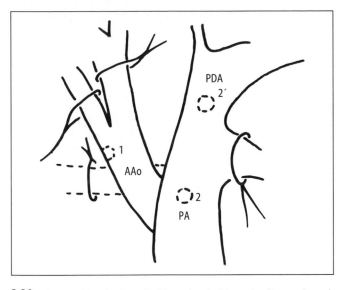

2.30 When complete primary repair of the aortic arch with associated intracardiac mal-formations is carried out through a midline sternotomy, branches of the pulmonary artery and ascending aorta are dissected for subsequent control, either with snares or temporary vascular clips. Surface cooling may accompany or precede these maneuvers, while hemodynamic instability may necessitate cardiopulmonary bypass prior to their completion. The ascending aortic purse-string is placed on the right lateral wall, precisely opposite the anticipated site of the aortic anastomosis (1). Alternatively, the innominate artery may be cannulated either directly or through a small vascular graft to continue cerebral perfusion during arch reconstruction. For perfusion of the descending aorta, a second purse-string generally is placed on the distal main pulmonary artery (2) or arterial duct (2'). Cannulation of the descending thoracic aorta through the posterior pericardium has been used also to maintain perfusion of the lower part of the body throughout the procedure.

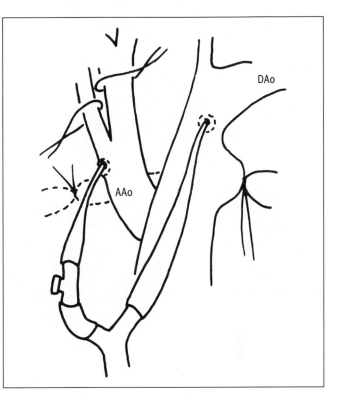

2.31 Cardiopulmonary bypass is instituted by cannulation of the small ascending aorta, followed by the duct or main pulmonary artery. The position of the ascending aortic cannula is critical to ensure flow to both the cerebral and coronary circulations. Immediately after commencement of perfusion, the right and left branch pulmonary arteries are occluded to prevent pulmonary congestion. If total circulatory arrest is employed, a single cannula is used in the right atrium for venous drainage. Otherwise, the superior and inferior caval veins are cannulated directly, taking care not to obstruct venous drainage from the lower half of the body. This can be ensured by leaving the inferior caval cannula rotated up into the right atrium until it is time to open the atrium itself. Cardioplegia is delivered through the ascending aortic cannula, after occlusion of the distal vessels.

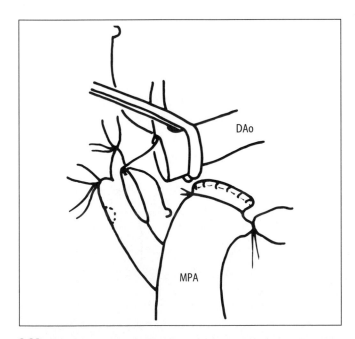

2.32 Under total circulatory arrest with the head vessels snared or reduced perfusion to the cerebral circulation distal to an aortic clamp, the arterial duct is ligated, divided, and oversewn. The descending aorta is mobilized extensively and drawn into the anterior mediastinum with a c-clamp. Division of the aberrant subclavian artery is often necessary to achieve this. After excision of all ductal tissue, the descending aorta is anastomosed end-to-side to the ascending aorta and origin of the left carotid artery with a continuous monofilament suture. The ascending aorta is the more delicate structure in this anastomosis, and it can be useful to support the posterior suture line with a strip of autogenous pericardium.

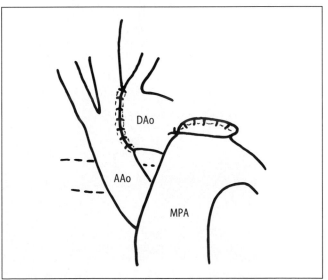

2.33 Completed arch repair achieves unobstructed pathways for blood-flow to the head and lower body, as well as to both pulmonary arteries. The associated ventricular septal defect is usually closed through the right atrium, although a doubly committed subarterial defect may require access through the pulmonary artery or right ventricle as well. Any interatrial communication is also closed.

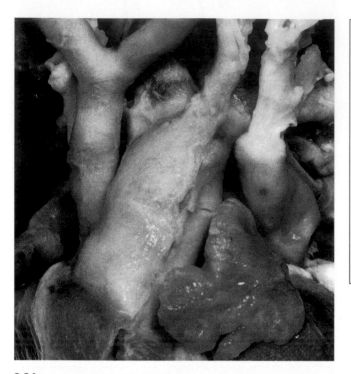

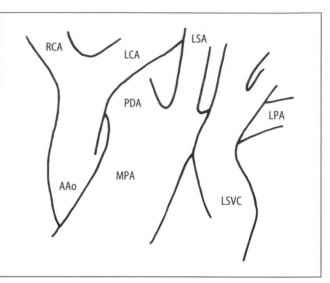

2.34 Interrupted right aortic arch. The descending aorta (which is not visible) in this patient lies to the right of the trachea and, even though the aortic arch is interrupted, it is designated a "right aortic arch". As the two carotid vessels arise from the ascending aorta, this is analogous to a Type B interruption of a left aortic arch. The left subclavian artery arises from the main pulmonary artery, proximally to the right-sided patent arterial duct. This situation is not uncommon with interrupted right aortic arch. When ductal tissue extends into the origin of the subclavian artery, there are said to be bilateral persistently patent arterial ducts, one giving rise to the descending aorta and the other to the left subclavian artery. In this specimen, a left superior caval vein drains to the coronary sinus. Interrupted right aortic arch is nearly always associated with Di George syndrome. A high proportion of cases also have a doubly committed subarterial ventricular septal defect.

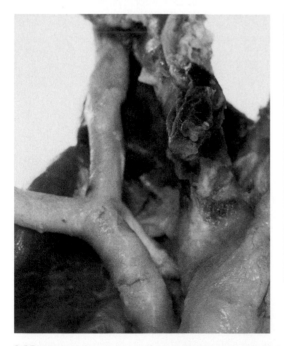

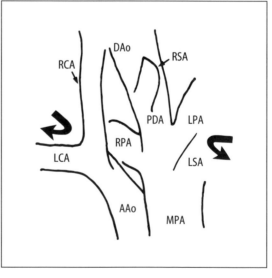

2.35 The above specimen is now viewed from the front but more distally downstream, with the carotid vessels rotated towards the right and the subclavian arteries towards the left. This exposes the descending aorta which is a continuation of the duct and gives off the right subclavian artery. All the structures shown in this illustration lie either to the front or the right side of the trachea.

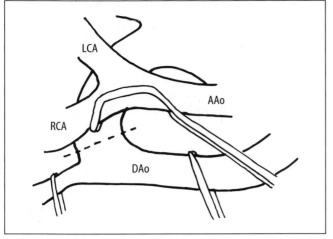

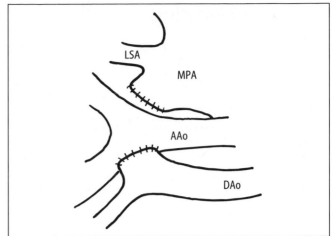

2.36 An alternative to primary complete repair as illustrated for the preceding heart (Figures 2.30–2.33) is reconstruction of the aortic arch through a thoracotomy. This must be done on the side of the descending aorta. The descending aorta and right subclavian artery are mobilized extensively and the arterial duct is dissected. A side-biting clamp is positioned on the ascending aorta and origin of the right carotid artery, leaving flow through at least the left and preferably both carotid vessels. In this case, the left subclavian artery will be perfused also from the main pulmonary artery.

2.37 An end-to-side anastamosis behind the superior caval vein restores continuity of the ascending and descending aorta. The arterial duct has been divided, taking care to avoid narrowing of the origin of the right pulmonary artery.

2.38 *(right)* In this case, the left subclavian artery, were it left attached to the left pulmonary artery, would "steal" blood into the pulmonary circulation and, accordingly, it is transferred to the left carotid artery. Trans-sternal extension of the thoracotomy will facilitate this anastomosis if it proves difficult to reach the vessel on the leftward side of the enlarged main pulmonary artery.

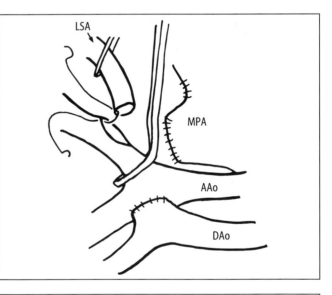

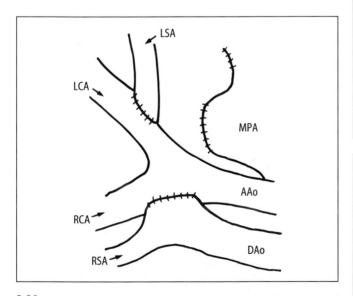

2.39 The completed reconstruction creates a right aortic arch with mirror-imaged branching. It may be desirable or necessary also to band the pulmonary artery for control of heart failure at this time.

2.40 *(right)* Interposition of a tube graft is an alternative technique for arch reconstruction, although it is rarely possible to implant a sufficiently large graft to obviate eventual reoperation. A conduit behind the superior caval vein may produce some displacement and obstruction of this vessel. Anastomosis to the more proximal ascending aorta is also possible and permits the graft to pass anteriorly to the superior caval vein. Cerebral perfusion during this anastomosis is maintained through the subclavian arteries prior to occlusion of the duct, and the left subclavian artery is subsequently transferred to the left carotid artery, as described above.

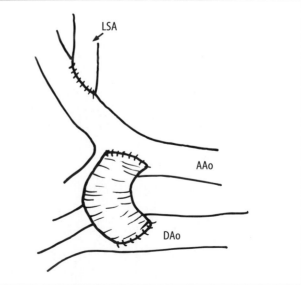

Suggested Reading

Celoria GC, Patton RB. Congenital absence of the aortic arch. Am Heart J 1959;58:407.

deLeon SY, Idriss FS, Ilbawi MN, Tin N, Berry T. Transmediastinal repair of complex coarctation and interrupted aortic arch. J Thorac Cardiovasc Surg 1981;82:98.

Freedom RM, Bain HH, Esplugas E, Dische R, Rowe RD. Ventricular septal defect in interruption of aortic arch. Am J Cardiol 1977;39:572.

Ho SY, Wilcox BR, Anderson RH, Lincoln JCH. Interrupted aortic arch – anatomical features of surgical significance. J Thorac Cardiovasc Surg 1983;31:199.

Jonas RA, Quaegebeur JM, Kirklin JW, Blackstone EH, Daicoff G. Outcomes in patients with interrupted aortic arch and ventricular septal defect, a multi-institutional study. J Thorac Cardiovasc Surg 1994;107:1099.

Karl TR, Sano S, Brawn W, Mee RB. Repair of hypoplastic or interrupted aortic arch via sternotomy. J Thorac Cardiovasc Surg 1992;104:688.

Kreutzer J, van Praagh R. Comparison of left ventricular outflow tract obstruction in interruption of the aortic arch and in coarctation of the aorta, with diagnostic, developmental, and surgical implications. Am J Cardiol 2000;86:856.

MacDonald MJ, Hanley FL, Reddy VM. Arch reconstruction without circulatory arrest: Current clinical applications and results of therapy. Semin Thorac Cardiovasc Surg Pediatr Card Surg Annu. 2002;5:95.

Moerman P, Dumoulin M, Lauweryns J, Vander Hauwaert LG. Interrupted right aortic arch in Di George syndrome. Br Heart J 1987;58:274.

Pierpoint MEM, Zollikofer CL, Moller JH, Edwards JE. Interruption of the aortic arch with right descending aorta. Ped Cardiol 1982;2:153.

Sell JE, Jonas RA, Mayer JE, Blackstone EH, Kirklin JW, Castaneda AR. The results of a surgical program for interrupted aortic arch. J Thorac Cardiovasc Surg 1988;96:864.

Yasui H, Kado H, Nakano E, Yonenaga K, Mitani A, Tomita Y, Iwao H, Yoshii K, Mizoguchi Y, Suhagawa H. Primary repair of interrupted aortic arch and severe aortic stenosis in neonates. J Thorac Cardiovasc Surg 1987;93(4):539.

2C Vascular Rings

Introduction

Vascular rings, by strict definition, are anomalies of the great vessels or their major branches which completely encircle the trachea and the esophagus in the superior mediastinum. In common usage, however, this definition is extended to include "slings" which do not completely surround the trachea and esophagus but may compress them. Some forms of the subclavian arterial steal syndrome are developmentally related and thus also are included in this category of vascular abnormalities.

The morphology of vascular rings can be understood most easily from developmental anatomy, although not all the variants which have been observed can be explained completely as derivatives of Edwards' hypothetical double aortic arch. At various times during

embryogenesis, six pairs of primitive branchial arches connect the ventral aortic sac with paired dorsal aortae. Retaining and combining the segments which may contribute ultimately to the definitive aortic arch produces a hypothetical situation – Edwards' double aortic arch with bilateral arterial ducts. Both the branching patterns of the usual left aortic arch and those of most arch malformations can then be described according to regression of one or more segments of this hypothetical double aortic arch (see Figs 2C(i), (ii), and (iii)).

The normal left aortic arch (which means that the aorta passes from the anterior to posterior mediastinum, to the left of the trachea and esophagus) results from disappearance of the right-sided dorsal aortic root between its points of fusion with the left-sided

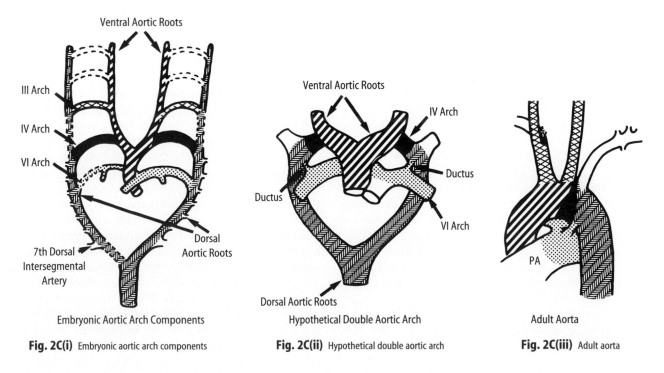

Fig. 2C(i) Embryonic aortic arch components

Fig. 2C(ii) Hypothetical double aortic arch

Fig. 2C(iii) Adult aorta

dorsal aorta and the seventh intersegmental artery. The seventh intersegmental arteries ultimately become the subclavian arteries, while the sixth aortic arches contribute to the pulmonary arteries. The fifth aortic arches have been identified only rarely and generally do not exist in the adult vascular system, although newer techniques of magnetic resonance imaging may redefine our understanding of this topic in the future. On the left side, however, the fourth arch becomes the transverse aorta between the carotid and subclavian arteries, while on the right side it persists at the origin of the right subclavian artery. The third aortic arches become the common carotid vessels. The first two become minor facial arteries. The left-sided aorta itself consists of ventral aortic root, persistent left fourth aortic arch and left dorsal aortic root.

A right aortic arch (i.e. one which passes to the right of the trachea and esophagus), conversely, results from regression of the left dorsal aortic root. Either a right or left definitive aortic arch may also be formed when the contralateral embryonic fourth arch disappears rather than the segment of dorsal aortic root beyond the seventh dorsal intersegmental artery. This produces subclavian arteries which arise as the last two branches of the aortic arch. The subclavian artery opposite to the side of the aortic arch then passes behind the esophagus and trachea as an "aberrant" left or right subclavian artery. Left aortic arch with aberrant right subclavian artery is the commonest aortic arch malformation. It occurs in 0.5–2.3% of autopsy and clinical series. Occasionally, the origin of the aberrant subclavian artery is from the more distal descending aorta and may have a broad base, called a "Kommerell's diverticulum."

Most vascular rings result from failure of the right dorsal aorta *and* fourth segmental arch to regress with variable persistence of the left-sided derivatives. There is thus a dominant right aortic arch. From a surgical perspective, this means that the vast majority of vascular rings (> 90%) are approached through a left thoracotomy, and it is usually the vascular segment passing to the right side of the trachea and esophagus which is conserved.

Double aortic arch results from persistence of both the left- and right-sided arches, each of which gives off its respective common carotid and subclavian artery. When the descending aorta is on the left (about 70% of cases), the right arch passes around the right tracheobronchial angle and behind the esophagus; conversely, when the aorta descends on the right side, the left arch continues posteriorly to the esophagus. Regardless of the side of the descending aorta, the right arch is larger than the left in 70–75% of cases, the two arches are of equal size in about 10% and the left is dominant in 15–20%. Atretic segments occur exclusively in the left arch, either between the left subclavian artery and the descending aorta or between the carotid and subclavian arteries. However, both arches are usually patent. Stenosis in the right arch has been seen only when there is also coarctation or atresia in the left arch. The arterial duct connects the underside of the left arch to the left pulmonary artery and is virtually never present on the right side. The right recurrent laryngeal nerve usually passes around the right arch (in contrast to its more common course around the subclavian artery), while the left is in its normal relation to the arterial duct. Double aortic arch is rarely associated with congenital cardiac malformations.

Both common types of right aortic arch – that with mirror-image branching and that with aberrant left subclavian artery – may produce vascular rings. In the case of the right arch with mirror-image branching, the first branch of the aorta is a left innominate artery (which divides into left carotid and left subclavian arteries), followed by the right common carotid and subclavian arteries. A complete vascular ring is produced only when the arterial duct or ligament arises distally to the right subclavian branch and passes behind the esophagus to the left pulmonary artery. In contrast to the other types of right aortic arch with mirror-image branching (where the arterial duct runs from the left innominate or subclavian artery to the left pulmonary artery or connects the undersurface of the aorta to the right pulmonary artery), this vascular ring is rarely associated with cardiac malformations. When there is *no* vascular structure crossing behind the esophagus in a right aortic arch with mirror-image branching (i.e. in the absence of a complete vascular ring), 98% of the patients *do* have associated congenital heart defects. The most common of these are tetralogy of Fallot and persistent arterial trunk (truncus arteriosus).

In right aortic arch with aberrant left subclavian artery, the aberrant subclavian artery arises from the dorsal aspect of the descending aorta as the fourth branch of the right aortic arch, being preceded by the left carotid, right carotid and right subclavian arteries. It then crosses the midline posteriorly to the esophagus and ascends to the left axilla. With few exceptions, an arterial duct connects this left subclavian artery to the left pulmonary artery, forming a complete, but loose, vascular ring. Congenital heart defects occur in less than 10% of patients with aberrant left subclavian artery. In tetralogy of Fallot with right aortic arch, however, the incidence of aberrant left subclavian artery is about 15%. The morphology in these patients is somewhat atypical in that the subclavian artery arises directly from the aorta without a diverticulum and the duct is nearly always absent. Hence there is no vascular ring in this subset of patients. Analogous to the aberrant left subclavian artery, the left innominate artery also may arise as the third branch of a right aortic arch and cross the midline posteriorly to the esophagus, forming a complete vascular ring with a duct between the base of the subclavian branch and the left pulmonary artery. This anomaly is extremely rare.

In a much less common variant of right aortic arch, the left subclavian or the innominate artery occupies a normal position but has no connection to the aortic arch. This occurs in 0.2–1.4% of cases with right aortic arch, most of whom have cyanotic congenital heart defects or other complex cardiac lesions. The left subclavian or the innominate artery in these cases is attached to the left pulmonary artery by an arterial duct and fills retrogradely from the left vertebral artery. Often, the distal aortic arch gives off a blind-ending diverticulum which is an angiographic clue to the presence of this anomaly. While not forming a vascular ring, this malformation is important to recognize when a systemic-pulmonary anastomosis is contemplated as there are no normal systemic vessels in the left chest.

Vascular rings are much less frequently found with a left aortic arch, if the controversial aberrant right subclavian artery is excluded. When the left aortic arch passes behind the esophagus to descend in the right chest, however, a complete vascular ring may result from an atretic right arch between the ascending and descending aortae or from a ligament or duct connecting the right pulmonary artery to a right subclavian artery which arises as the fourth branch of the aorta. These malformations must be approached surgically through a right thoracotomy.

The aberrant left pulmonary artery or pulmonary artery sling is the only vascular ring in which a vessel consistently passes between the trachea and the esophagus. In this malformation, the left pulmonary artery arises from the right pulmonary artery and courses behind the trachea to the hilum of the left lung. The aberrant left pulmonary artery compresses the right tracheobronchial angle and posterior trachea, while a ligament between the aorta and the normal site of origin of the left pulmonary artery completes a ring around the trachea. About half of these patients have complete tracheal rings and nearly all have some localized bronchial or tracheal compression by the vascular structures. The two surgical approaches to this anomaly are translocation of the left pulmonary artery and resection of the trachea with reanastomosis posterior to the left pulmonary artery.

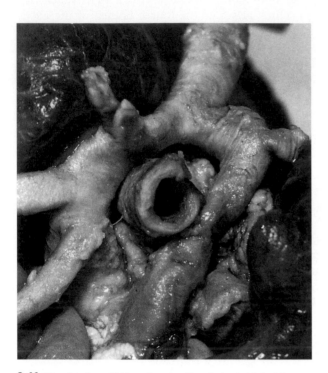

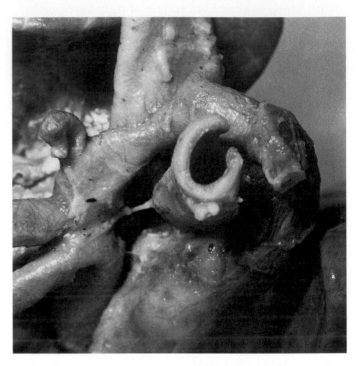

2.41 Vascular rings. Right aortic arch with patent arterial duct from an aberrant left subclavian artery.

2.42 Right aortic arch with aberrant left subclavian artery. The persistently patent arterial duct arises from the junction of the left subclavian artery and the aorta.

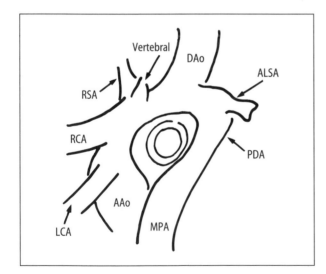

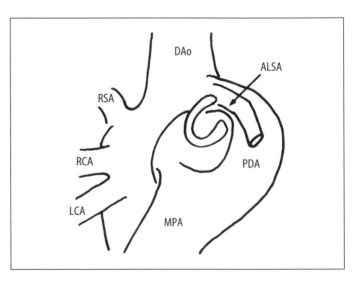

Both specimens are viewed from above, looking down on the divided trachea. They demonstrate a right aortic arch which, by definition, passes from the anterior to the posterior mediastinum on the right side of the trachea. The position of the descending aorta is determined independently from the arch and lies further to the left in the first specimen (Figure 2.41). With a right aortic arch, the left brachiocephalic vessels may arise either as a left innominate artery ("mirror-imaged branching"), or the left subclavian artery may be given off as the last branch ("aberrant left subclavian artery"). In both of the hearts seen here, the aortic arch gives off the left carotid artery as its first branch, followed by the right carotid and right subclavian arteries. A complete vascular ring, encircling the trachea and esophagus, is produced by the persistently patent arterial duct which connects the aberrant left subclavian artery or distal arch to the pulmonary artery. The arterial duct is nearly always a left-sided structure, even with a right aortic arch.

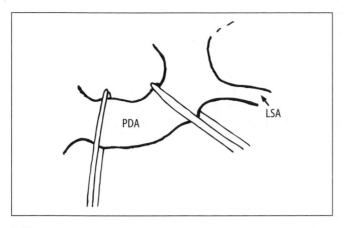

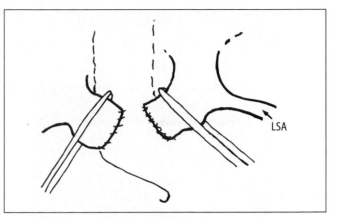

2.43 The vast majority of vascular rings, including the right aortic arch with the left arterial duct, are approached through a left thoracotomy. In this case, the left subclavian artery will probably be the only major systemic vessel found in the left chest, although the descending aorta may be visible after some dissection in the posterior mediastinum. The subclavian artery is identified and traced to the persistent arterial duct which is dissected circumferentially and occluded with two fine vascular clamps. The recurrent laryngeal nerve should pass around the arterial duct in the usual relationship.

2.44 After a trial of clamping to confirm the absence of pulmonary or systemic circulatory dependence on the arterial duct, it is divided and the two ends are oversewn. A smaller persistently patent arterial duct may be transfixed, ligated, and divided, while a ligamentum in this position is simply divided.

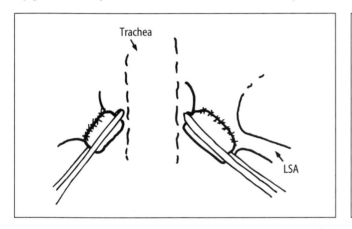

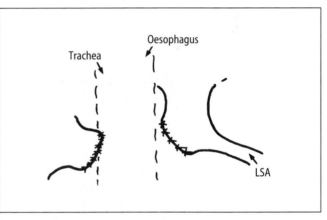

2.45 It is important to free completely the trachea and esophagus. Each end of the divided duct is retracted with its vascular clamp. Dissection is carried posteriorly along the descending aorta and origin of the left subclavian artery well behind the esophagus, and anteriorly to the pulmonary trunk in front of the trachea.

2.46 The ends of the divided vessels usually spring apart after removal of the clamps. When there has been long-standing tracheal compression, however, oedema or tracheomalacia may still contribute to airway obstruction for several weeks or months.

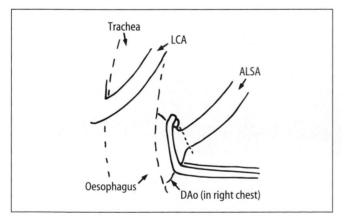

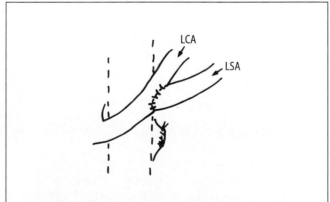

2.47 It is debatable whether the aberrant subclavian artery (left or right) by itself causes significant esophageal compression. This is probably more likely when the carotid vessels arise close together anteriorly, as seen on the second specimen (Figure 2.42). In such cases, dysphagia may be relieved by translocating the subclavian artery to the left carotid artery. The subclavian artery is followed to its origin from the descending aorta, which can be reached from the contralateral thorax through the posterior mediastinum.

2.48 It is then divided, and anastamosed to a vertical incision in the carotid artery, using temporary occlusion of the latter vessel with a side-biting clamp. While simple division of the aberrant subclavian artery with mobilization of its two ends will also relieve dysphagia, this compromises the blood supply to the arm and risks later development of a subclavian steal syndrome.

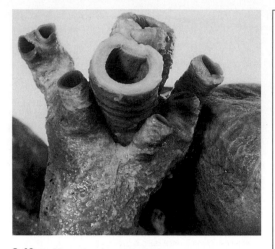

2.49 Double aortic arch: anterior view.

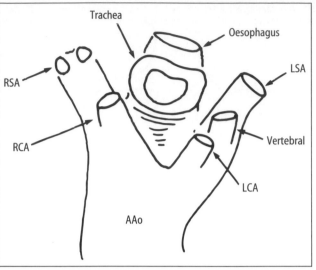

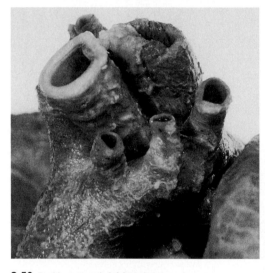

2.50 Double aortic arch: left lateral view.

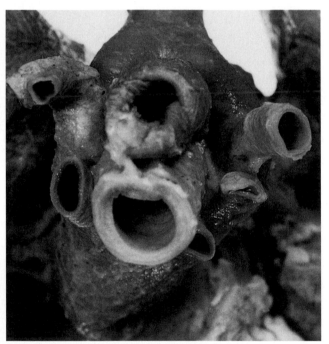

2.52 Double aortic arch: superior view.

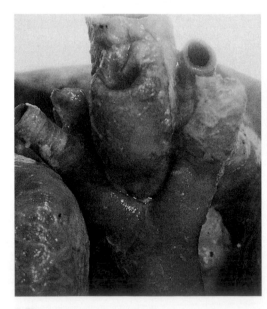

2.51 Double aortic arch: posterior view.

← **2.49–2.52 Vascular rings/double aortic arch.** This malformation represents a persistence of both right and left embryonic fourth branchial arches. Each arch gives off a sub-clavian and a carotid branch, which is the diagnostic hallmark of double aortic arch. The left or anterior arch lies in front of the trachea, while the right or posterior arch passes to the right of and posteriorly to the esophagus. The two arches then join behind the esophagus at the descending aorta, which is usually left-sided. Most commonly (about 75% of cases), the right posterior arch is the dominant or larger vessel, but occasionally the left is greater in size, or both may be equal (10%). Coarctation may occur in either arch but is more common in the left. Stenosis of the right arch has been observed only when there is coarctation or atresia in the left; a duct or ligament connecting the underside of the arch to the pulmonary artery has been found only on the left side. Constriction of the trachea and esophagus is produced by the vascular structures surrounding them. This specimen is slightly atypical in that the left vertebral artery arises directly from the arch, giving three branches rather than the usual two. Double aortic arch is not commonly associated with other congenital cardiac malformations.

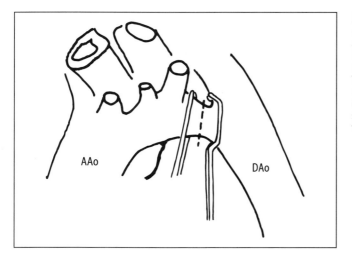

2.53 *(left)* The principles of the surgical management of vascular rings are to divide the encircling malformation at a point which does not compromise distal aortic perfusion, and to mobilize fully the constricted area of the trachea and esophagus. With a minor left arch, the usual point of division is between the left subclavian artery and descend-ing aorta. However, other areas of stenosis or hypoplasia may dictate an alternative site. The ligament or persistently patent arterial duct is divided also, allowing the left arch to rotate forwards and away from the trachea. This, in essence, converts the vascular ring into a right aortic arch with mirror-image branching, retroesophageal aorta and left-sided descending aorta. In cases of cyanotic heart disease, a minor left arch has been used for a palliative systemic-pulmonary anastamosis.

2.54 *(right)* When the posterior (right) arch is the smaller of the two, careful dissection into the posterior mediastinum, with rotation of the descending aorta forward, may be necessary to identify this structure. A minor arch is divided also at its junction with the descending aorta. The recurrent laryngeal nerve on the right side passes around the right arch and, on the left side, around the arterial duct. The segment of the arch thus divided should, accordingly, have no relation to this nerve.

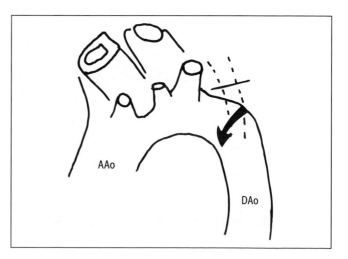

Suggested Reading

Antia AU, Otteson OE. Collateral circulation in subclavian stenosis or atresia; angiographic demonstration of retrograde vertebral-subclavian in two cases with right aortic arch. Am J Cardiol 1966;18:599.

Arciniegas E, Hakimi M, Hentzler JH, Farooki ZQ, Green EW. Surgical management of congenital vascular rings. J Thorac Cardiovasc Surg 1979;77:721.

Bayford D. An account of a singular case of obstructed deglutition. Mem Med Soc London 1794;2:275.

Berdon WE, Baker DH, Wung JT, Chrispin A, Kozlowski K, deSilva M, Bales P, Alford B. Complete cartilage-ring tracheal stenosis associated with anomalous left pulmonary artery: the ring-sling complex. Radiology 1984;152:57.

Berman W Jr, Yabek SM, Dillon T, Neal JF, Aki B, Burnstein J. Vascular ring due to left aortic arch and right descending aorta. Circulation 1981;63:458.

Dodge-Khatami A, Tulevski II, Hitchcock JF, de Mol BA, Bennink GB. Vascular rings and pulmonary arterial sling: from respiratory collapse to surgical cure, with emphasis on judicious imaging in the hi-tech era. Cardiol Young 2002;12:96.

Dunn JM, Gordon I, Chrispin AR, de Laval MR, Stark J. Early and late results of surgical correction of pulmonary artery sling. Ann Thorac Surg 1978;28:230.

Edwards JE. Anomalies of the derivatives of the aortic arch system. Med Clin North Am 1948;July:925.

Ergin MA, Jayaram N, LeConte M. Left aortic arch and right descending aorta: diagnostic and therapeutic implications of a rare type of vascular ring. Ann Thorac Surg 1981;31;82.

Izukawa T, Scott ME, Durrani F, Moes CAF. Persistent left fifth aortic arch in man. Report of two cases. Br Heart J 1973;35:1190.

Jonas RA, Spevak PJ, McGill T, Castaneda AR. Pulmonary artery sling: primary repair by by tracheal resection in infancy. J Thorac Cardiovasc Surg 1989;97:548.

Klinkhamer AC. Aberrant right subclavian artery, clinical and roentgenologic aspects. Am J Roentgenol Radium Ther Nucl Med 1966;97:438.

Klinkhamer AC. Esophagography in Anomalies of the Aortic Arch System. The Williams and Wilkins Company, Baltimore, 1969.

Knight L, Edwards JE. Right aortic arch, types and associated cardiac anomalies. Circulation 1974;50:1047.

Nikaidoh H, Riker WL, Idriss FS. Surgical management of "vascular rings". Arch Surg 1972;105:327.

Replogle RL. Left subclavian artery arising from obliterated ductus arteriosus, management during a Blalock shunt. Ann Thorac Surg 1968;5:153.

Stewart JR, Kincaid OW, Edwards JE. An atlas of vascular rings and related malformations of the aortic arch system. Springfield: Charles C. Thomas, Publisher, 1964.

3 Aortopulmonary Window

Introduction

Communications between the ascending aorta and pulmonary artery constitute a spectrum of malformations which is collectively designated "aortopulmonary window," "aortic septal defect," or "aorticopulmonary window." The communication is distal to the aortic and pulmonary valvar leaflets, but may be found in any position where the great vessels are contiguous, from the sinus of Valsalva to the origin of the brachiocephalic vessels.

Aortopulmonary windows have been subclassified into Type I (proximal defects between the left lateral wall of the ascending aorta and the pulmonary trunk), Type II (defects involving the right pulmonary artery and its origin – also called distal defects), and Type III (a large defect combining the other two types). It is probably more useful to view them as a continuum of pathology. The proximal communications tend to be very large and round or oval-shaped, while smaller, more rare and distal lesions may join the posterior aorta to the anterior right pulmonary artery, similar to a Waterston anastomosis. As suggested by the name

"window," there is usually no length to the communicating channel. The origin of the right pulmonary artery from the aorta is sometimes considered to be an example of the most extreme type of aortopulmonary window. Either the right or (less commonly) the left coronary artery may arise on the pulmonary side of the window. About half of the cases of aortopulmonary window occur as isolated lesions, while the other half has associated major or minor cardiac malformations. These include interrupted aortic arch, tetralogy of Fallot, persistently patent arterial duct, and ventricular septal defect.

Surgical repair of aortopulmonary window is done virtually always as an open heart procedure with cardiopulmonary bypass or, in small infants, with low flow or profound hypothermia and total circulatory arrest. A patch of Dacron or other material is used to close the defect, taking care to leave the orifices of the coronary arteries in continuity with the aorta. Associated malformations are generally repaired at the same time.

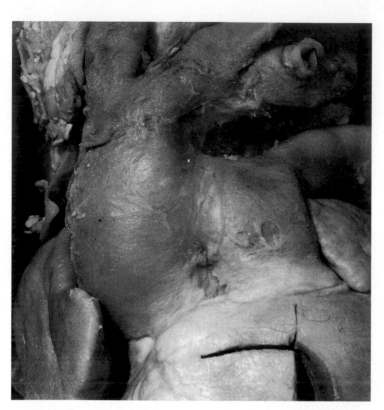

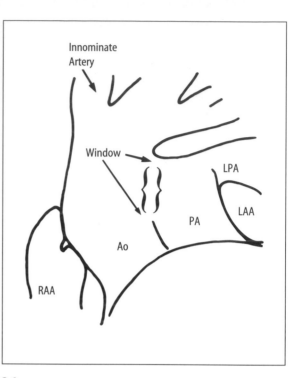

3.1 Aortopulmonary window. The external appearances of a large proximal defect are seen from the front.

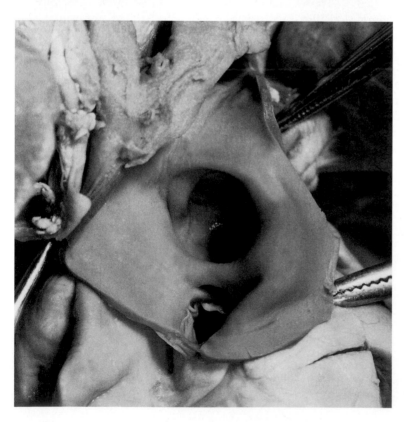

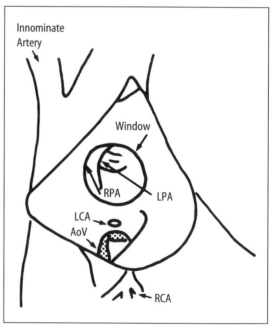

3.2 The aorta has been opened in the case above to show the large aortopulmonary window just above the orifice of the left coronary artery. The orifice of the right coronary artery lies close to the window, although this is not immediately apparent in the photograph. The origins of the right and left branch pulmonary arteries are seen through the window.

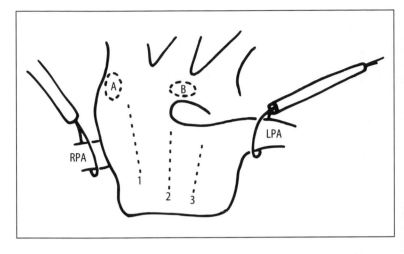

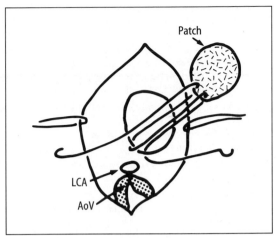

3.3 Repair of the aortopulmonary window may be done through an incision in the aorta (1), through the window itself (2) with a sandwich technique, or through an incision in the pulmonary artery (3). Cannulation must be sufficiently distal on the lateral side of the aorta (A) or transverse aortic arch (B) to permit safe application of a clamp above the window; the branch pulmonary arteries are temporarily occluded to maintain a perfusion pressure and prevent flooding of the lungs on bypass.

3.4 Exposure through an aortic incision allows visualization of the coronary arterial orifices, both of which must be identified with certainty. A patch of either prosthetic material or composite prosthetic material/pericardium is then inserted with a continuous monofilament suture. Sutures near the coronary orifice are placed accurately, with the patch at a distance for good visualization.

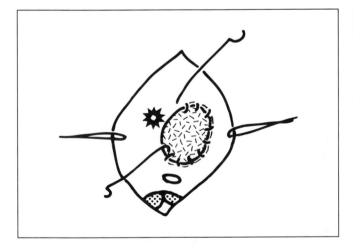

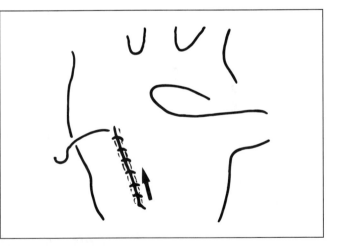

3.5 The patch is lowered down when the suture line has cleared the coronary arterial orifices. It may be carried into the pulmonary artery when a coronary artery lies on that side of the window. Alternatively, a flap of vessel wall may be used to tunnel the aorta to the coronary artery. As the suture line approaches the origin of the right pulmonary artery (star), it is deviated into the aorta to avoid any narrowing of that vessel.

3.6 The aortotomy is closed, working from proximal to distal end, so that the aortic leaflets and coronary arterial orifices may be visualized at the bottom of the suture line.

Suggested Reading

Burroughs JT, Schumutzer KJ, Linder F, Neuhans G. Anomalous origin of the right coronary artery with aortico-pulmonary window and ventricular septal defect. J Cardiovasc Surg 1968;3:142.

Casillas JA, Delcon JP, Villagra F, Checa SL, Sanchez PA, Gomez R, Fortuny R, MaBrito J. Aortopulmonary window with anomalous origin of the right coronary artery from the pulmonary trunk. Texas Heart Inst J 1986;13:323.

Castaneda AR, Kirklin JW. Tetralogy of Fallot with aorticopulmonary window. Report of two surgical cases. J Thorac Cardiovasc Surg 1977;74:467.

Doty DB, Richardson JV, Falkovsky GE, Gordonova MI, Burakovsky VI. Aortopulmonary septal defect; hemodynamics, angiography and operation. Ann Thorac Surg 1981;32:244.

Gula G, Chew C, Radley-Smith R, Yacoub M. Anomalous origin of the right pulmonary artery from the ascending aorta associated with aortopulmonary window. Thorax 1978;33:265.

Ho SY, Gerlis LM, Anderson C, Devine WA, Smith A. The morphology of aortopulmonary windows in regard to their classification and morphogenesis. Cardiol Young 1994;4:146.

Kirkpatrick SE, Girod DR, King H. Aortic origin of the right pulmonary artery; surgical repair without graft. Circulation 1967;36:777.

Kutsche LM, Van Mierop LHS. Anatomy and pathologenesis of aorticopulmonary septal defect. Am J Cardiol 1987;59:443.

Mori K, Ando M, Takao A, Ishikawa S, Imai Y. Distal type of aorto-pulmonary window; report of four cases. Br Heart J 1978;40:681.

Penkoske PA, Castaneda AR, Fyler DC, Van Praagh R. Origin of pulmonary artery branch from ascending aorta; primary surgical repair in infancy. J Thorac Cardiovasc Surg 1983;85:537.

Ravikumar E, Whight CM, Hawker RE, Celermajer JM, Nunn G, Cartmill TB. The surgical management of aortopulmonary window using the anterior sandwich patch closure technique. J Cardiovasc Surg 1988;29:629.

Richardson JV, Doty DB, Rossi WP, Ehrenhaft JL. The spectrum of anomalies of aortopulmonary septation. J Thorac Cardiovasc Surg 1979;78:21.

Van Praagh R, Van Praagh S. The anatomy of common aortico-pulmonary trunk (truncus arteriosus communis) and its embryologic implications. A study of 57 necropsy cases. Am J Cardiol 1965;16:406.

2 ·

Anomalies Related to the Atriums

4 Atrial Arrangement (Situs)/Isomerism/ Juxtaposition

Introduction

Within the human body, some structures occur in pairs and are mirror images of each other, while others show discrete characteristics which make them distinctly and identifiably different from their counterparts. The paired structures are arranged on either side of a midline, sagittal plane through the body and are said to be "symmetrical". Examples of symmetry are hands, feet, eyes, nerves, and muscles. In contrast, most of the non-parietal organs are "lateralized", such that their left and right sides are morphologically different. The right lung, for example, has three lobes and a short mainstem bronchus, whereas the left lung has two lobes and a long bronchus. The morphologically right atrium has a broad-based appendage which contains an extensive arrangement of pectinate muscles and is separated from the smooth, sinus portion of the atrium by a prominent muscular ridge, the terminal crest. In contrast, the left atrial appendage is long and narrow, also containing pectinate muscles, but with a narrow attachment to the body of the atrium and with multiple crenellations along its lower edges. There is no crest separating the pectinate muscles of this appendage from the smooth portion of atrium. It is the smooth portions of both atriums which usually receive the venous connections. It is thus possible to recognize a morphologically right atrium by the characteristics of its appendage or a morphologically right lung wherever it is found, even in an abnormal or unusual position, such as the left side of the body.

As one pattern of lateralization occurs in the vast majority of the population, this has been called "situs solitus", which is the Latin terminology meaning "usual arrangement" or "usual situs". With regard to the heart, situs solitus is a left-sided, morphologically left atrium and a right-sided morphologically right atrium. Very rarely, the morphologically left atrium is on the right side and vice versa, which is then designated "situs inversus" or just "inverted situs." This so-called mirror-image arrangement is not necessarily associated with any structural (as opposed to positional) abnormality of the heart.

Rather than having morphologically right and left appendages, however, some hearts have two appendages of the same type, which then makes them symmetrical or "isomeric." This is also rare but more common than is mirror image, and it is virtually always accompanied by complex cardiac malformations. Technically, it is only the atrial appendages which are isomeric, but if both appendages are of the morphologically right type, the condition is commonly called "right atrial isomerism," and with bilateral morphologically left appendages it is called "left atrial isomerism." In the majority of cases, all the thoracic organs (i.e. the heart and the lungs) follow the same pattern of symmetry or lateralization, so right atrial isomerism is usually found with bilateral right lungs and left atrial isomerism is usually found with bilateral left lungs. This is also called "bilateral right-sidedness" or "bilateral left-sidedness" respectively. The external appearances of the atriums and their appendages are readily observable in both the surgical operating theatre and the post-mortem laboratory. Their morphology thus conveys information about likely associated cardiac malformations, the conduction tissue in some instances, and abnormalities of other thoracic and/or abdominal viscera.

The abdominal organs also have a characteristic or "usual" arrangement which is a spleen on the left side and a liver on the right. Any deviation from this arrangement is called "heterotaxy," a definition of which is "anomalous placement or transposition of viscera or parts." Again, this may be an inverted arrangement, bilateral right-sidedness or bilateral left-sidedness. In bilateral right-sidedness, there is usually (but not invariably) absence of the spleen ("asplenia") and, in the latter, multiple spleens ("polysplenia"). Because certain groups of cardiac malformations tend to be associated with either polysplenia or aspenia, they have been called "heterotaxy syndromes," although within any such given syndrome, there are many varieties of malformed hearts. Usually, but again not invariably, the arrangement of the abdominal organs is the same as that of the atriums and lungs in the chest, such that there is concordance between thoracic and abdominal situs. Thus, left atrial isomerism is usually (70%) found with multiple spleens and right atrial isomerism with asplenia (82%). "Discordance" between the abdominal and thoracic organs, however, does occur and includes all the possible permutations and combinations of situs solitis, situs inversus, and isomerism.

From a morphological perspective, hearts with left isomerism tend to dominate clinical series, while those with right isomerism predominate in post-mortem collections, probably reflecting the poorer prognosis of the latter group. The most consistent anatomical associations with right isomerism are absent coronary sinus, total anomalous pulmonary venous connection, pulmonary obstruction, and univentricular atrioventricular connection. Left isomerism has a high incidence of azygos and hemiazygos continuation of the inferior caval vein and also biventricular heart. Both groups frequently have bilateral superior caval veins and deficiencies of the atrial septum. In right isomerism, the sinus node is generally duplicated bilaterally. In left isomerism it may not be found under the light microscope in serial sections or it may be abnormally small and situated in a bizarre position in the atrial myocardium. The location of the atrioventricular node depends on the ventricular topology (see Section 5). To a degree, the patterns of anomalies which are associated with bilateral left- or right-sidedness reflect a duplication or absence of the structures most characteristically found in either one or other of the atriums. Thus, the connection of the pulmonary veins and the coronary sinus, which are normally left atrial structures, tend to be more consistently abnormal or absent in right atrial isomerism, while interruption of the inferior caval vein and absence of the sinus node, as noted above, are more common in left atrial isomerism.

Juxtaposition, in contrast with atrial isomerism, refers to the position of the atrial appendages rather than their morphological characteristics. Normally, one atrial appendage is found on either side of the heart. Because both ends of the transverse sinus lie in open communication with the pericardial space, either atrial appendage may pass to the other side of the heart to be positioned behind the great vessels. The juxtaposed appendage thus lies above the normally situated one – that is, left above right with right juxtaposition and right above left with the more common left juxtaposition. In surgical practice, this is often obvious because desaturated blood gives the systemic right atrial appendage a blue colour, while the left atrial appendage is pinker. Left juxtaposition is always associated with complex cardiac malformations, frequently including transposition of the great arteries. The intracardiac anatomy may or may not be complex with right juxtaposition. Isomeric appendages may show either right or left juxtaposition.

Situs inversus, defective lateralization (isomerism), and juxtaposition do not, of themselves, ever indicate surgical intervention, but all may impact upon procedures for associated cardiac malformations. While operations on the surface or outside of the heart can be approached in the usual manner, when the inverted atrial arrangement is present, those within the atrium, the aorta, or the right ventricle usually require the surgeon to work from the opposite (left side) of the table. The anesthetic screen then needs to be placed more cephalad for a right-handed surgeon, and the cardiopulmonary perfusionist and scrub nurse will generally find themselves working in an unfamiliar arrangement.

The cardiac malformations found in isomeric hearts tend to be multiple and complex, such that careful planning is essential to accomplish successful repair within the constraints of cardiopulmonary bypass, myocardial ischemic and/or circulatory arrest times. Anomalies of systemic venous connection frequently require additional cannulations, and when the inferior caval vein is interrupted, the size of cannula placed in the superior caval vein which receives the azygos or hemiazygos continuation needs to be adequate to drain also the lower half of the body. Several hepatic veins may enter an atrium directly. Larger ones can often be cannulated directly outside the atrium with small, right-angled cannula to obtain a dry operating field. Alternatively, a pump-sucker is placed in the orifice, with or without periods of reduced flow or total circulatory arrest.

Because of their complexity, many patients with isomeric hearts undergo preliminary palliative procedures. In right atrial isomerism, for example, this is often a systemic-pulmonary shunt for pulmonary stenosis or atresia. It is helpful for planning subsequent investigation and cardiac repair to observe and note carefully the systemic and pulmonary venous connections in the operative findings at this time. Right atrial isomerism also has important clinical implications in that such patients are susceptible to bacterial infection with capsulated organisms (pneumococcus) and benefit from immunization and antibiotic prophylaxis.

In cases of left juxtaposition of the atrial appendages, the area of free right atrial wall and volume of the main atrial cavity may be markedly reduced. This can make insertion of an atrial baffle for a Mustard Procedure or creation of the systemic and venous pathways in the Senning operation, for example, technically difficult. A juxtaposed appendage in the transverse sinus may be a nuisance during pulmonary artery reconstruction for the repair of pulmonary atresia with ventricular septal defect and major aortopulmonary collateral vessels (see Chapter 18), but, alternatively, it constitutes a useful way of enlarging the right pulmonary artery when an atriopulmonary connection is used in the Fontan circulation. Usually, however, juxtaposition has little surgical import.

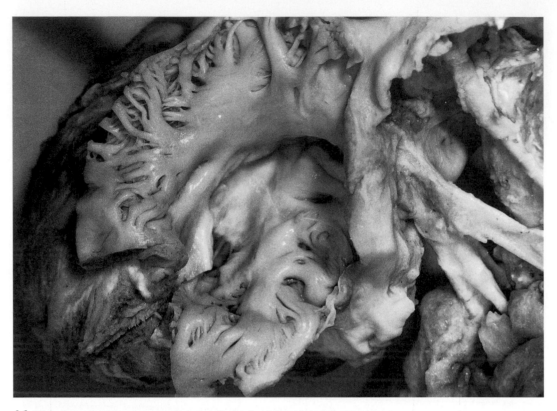

4.1 Mirror-imaged atrial arrangement (inverted situs). Left-sided morphologically right atrium.

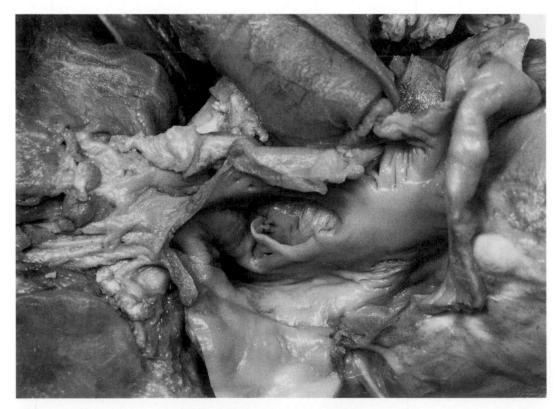

4.2 Mirror-imaged atrial arrangement (inverted situs). Right-sided morphologically left atrium.

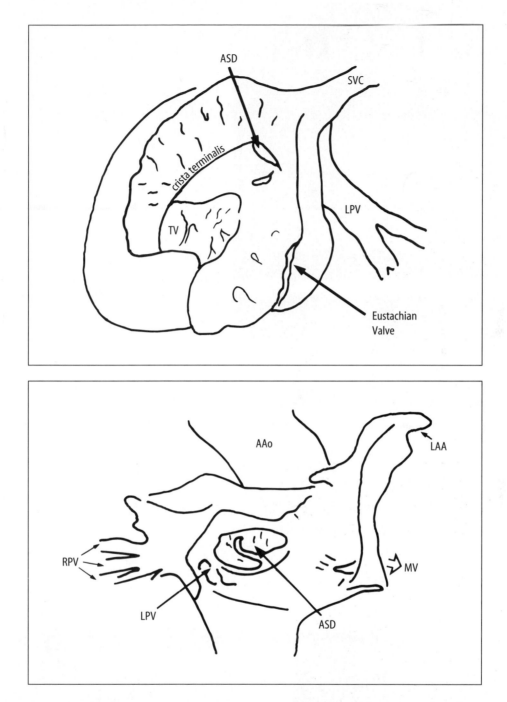

In the usual atrial arrangement (situs solitus), the morphologically left atrium lies on the left side of the heart and the morphologically right atrium on the right. Each can be identified by its typical characteristics – a blunt, wide-based appendage in the right atrium and a narrow, finger-like appendage in the left. The normal right atrium also receives the caval drainage into the smooth sinus portion. A terminal crest (crista terminalis) lies between this and the trabeculations of the appendage. The limbus of the oval fossa is a right atrial structure, while the left atrium contains the flap valve of the oval fossa. The atriums shown here have all these features. However, this heart also illustrates a mirror-imaged arrangement (situs inversus), with the morphologically left atrium on the right side of the heart and the morphologically right atrium on the left. There is an atrial septal defect of the oval fossa. The cardiac connections, valves and chambers are otherwise normal, although also mirror-imaged.

From a surgical point of view, operations within the atrium in a heart with a mirror-imaged arrangement usually have to be done with the surgeon standing on the left side of the operating table.

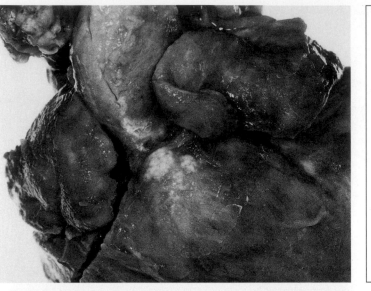

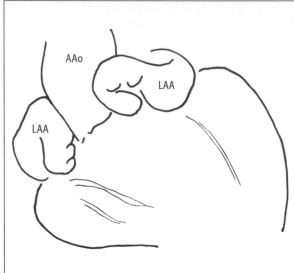

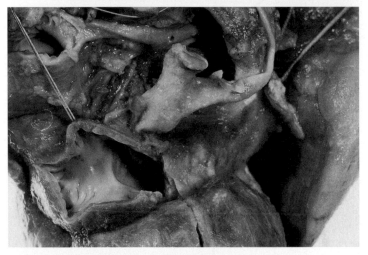

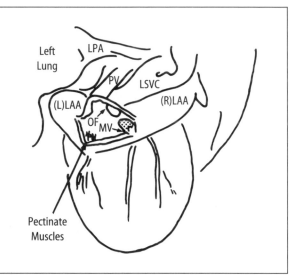

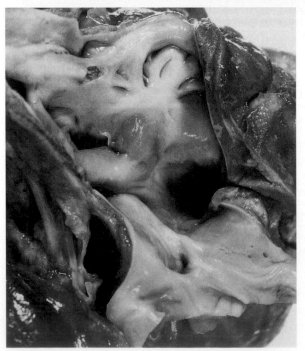

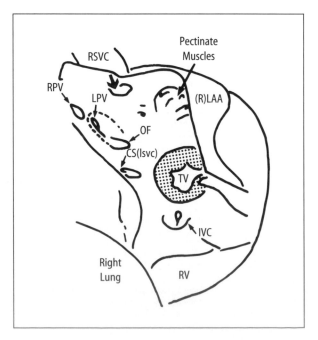

← **4.3** *(top)* **Left atrial isomerism.** Both appendages are long and narrow, with many constrictions along the lower edge. This feature, along with the absence of a terminal crest internally, is sufficient for identification of the morphologically left atrium and usually correlates with the bronchial morphology. In this heart, two ventricles are present in the usual spatial relationships. The ventriculo-arterial connection is a single outlet (aorta) with pulmonary atresia. The branch pulmonary arteries are connected to the right aortic arch and the left subclavian artery respectively. Although less consistent than in association with right atrial isomerism, obstruction to the pulmonary outflow is found in about half of hearts with left atrial isomerism.

4.4 *(centre)* Left-sided, morphologically left atrium in left isomerism, opened transversely across the posterior wall. Pectinate muscles of the appendage merge into the smooth sinus portion of the atrium without an intervening crest. The left-sided pulmonary veins connect to this atrium and there is a large defect of the oval fossa. Atypically, the left superior caval vein drains to a coronary sinus in this specimen. It is more common for a left superior caval vein to attach directly to the left-sided atrium between the appendage and the orifice of the pulmonary veins.

4.5 *(bottom)* Right-sided morphologically left atrium in left isomerism. Pectinate musculature is confined to the atrial appendage, but there is no crest separating it from the orifices of the superior and inferior caval veins. The right pulmonary veins also enter this atrium, while a slight distortion for the camera's lens shows the orifice of the left pulmonary veins in the left-sided atrium through a large atrial septal defect (dashed line). It is typical (63%) for the pulmonary veins to enter each side of a common atrium or two to each atrium ("two-plus-two") with left isomerism. More often (70–80%) in left isomerism, there is interruption of the inferior caval vein which drains to the left or right superior caval vein, and direct connection of the hepatic veins to one or both atriums. Because each ventricle is connected to a morphologically left atrium, the atrioventricular connection in this heart is ambiguous.

The surgical importance of isomerism relates to the conduction tissue, the management of venous drainage for cardiopulmonary bypass and the extremely complex cardiac malformations which accompany it. In left atrial isomerism, the sinus node, if found by light microscopy, is hypoplastic and abnormally positioned in the atrial musculature. The position of the atrioventricular node depends on the ventricular topology. For venous drainage, it is often necessary to use multiple cannulae (including a large one for the superior caval vein which receives an azygos or hemiazygos continuation of the inferior caval vein) or total circulatory arrest. A pump-sucker may be placed inside a small hepatic or caval vein directly from the opened atrium. The cardiac repair is generally individualized according to the ventricular mass (two ventricles or univentricular connection). Common atrium is frequently found with some variant of atrioventricular septal defect, pulmonary obstruction and both great arteries arising from the right ventricle in left atrial isomerism. Complete correction of such a heart would involve a complex atrial baffle to separate and lateralize the venous drainage, repair of the atrioventricular septal defect and relief of the pulmonary obstruction (often with a valved extracardiac conduit). In this particular heart, the correction of the venous drainage would be more straightforward than usual as enlargement of the atrial septal defect would permit channelling of the right pulmonary veins to the left-sided atrium. Systemic venous drainage is already lateralized to the right-sided atrium. It is often useful to conceptualize one type of venous drainage (pulmonary or systemic) as lying beneath the patch and the other superficial to it when planning such a baffle. When a Fontan-type of repair is elected, either for a less common univentricular connection or extremely complex morphology, it has often been constructed with cavopulmonary anatomosis, leaving any hepatic veins to drain directly into the atrium with the pulmonary veins. However, it is now appreciated that this leads to the formation of pulmonary arteriovenous fistulae by removing hepatic factors from the lung circulation. Accordingly, an intracardiac baffle or extracardiac conduit is now generally incorporated into the repair to also route the hepatic venous blood to the lungs.

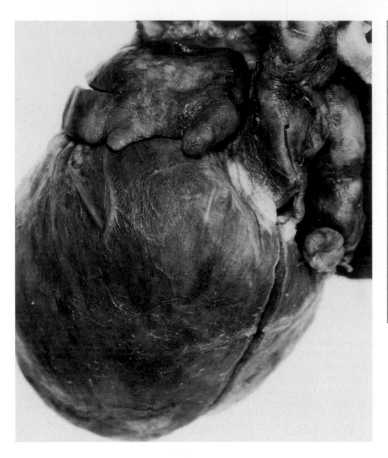

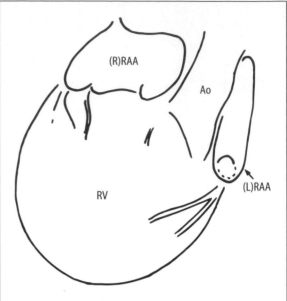

4.6 *(above)* **Right atrial isomerism.** The atrial appendages are shown in an anterior oblique view. Both the right- and left-sided appendages are blunt with a broad base. In this heart, the right lung has three lobes and the left has four, both with short, eparterial bronchi. All the pulmonary veins connect to the right superior caval vein (not seen). This heart also has an atrioventricular septal defect with two valvar rings (partial atrioventricular septal defect), extreme dominance of the right ventricle, and hypoplasia of the left ventricle. Both great arteries arise from the right ventricle. Internally there is a pulmonary stenosis. The right and left coronary arteries arise together from a single orifice.

The surgical implications of right atrial isomerism, in addition to frequent anomalies of the systemic venous connection, include a high incidence of univentricular atrioventricular connection and, almost without exception, total anomalous venous connection. Thus, most of these patients enter a program of staged management, firstly to regulate pulmonary blood-flow (often a systemic-pulmonary anastomosis for pulmonary atresia or stenosis) and relieve pulmonary venous obstruction, followed by cavopulmonary connections, and eventually completion of the Fontan circulation.

4.7 *(top)* Left-sided morphologically right atrium. The appendage is characteristically wedge-shaped with ➔ broad base. The pectinate muscles, which extend posteriorly, are separated from the superior caval orifice by a prominent muscle ridge (open arrows). Externally, this terminal crest is indicated epicardially as the terminal groove. No pulmonary veins connect to this chamber. There is also a defect of the oval fossa. The left-sided valve connects mainly to a dominant right ventricle. A small rudimentary left ventricle lies posteriorly (same heart as in Figures 4.6 and 4.8).

4.8 *(bottom)* Right-sided morphologically right atrium. The terminal crest separates the extensive ➔ pectinate muscles from the superior caval orifice (dashed line) and inferior caval orifice (which has been divided at the solid arrow). The terminal crest is indicated by a curved arrow. This heart also has a large atrial septal defect (asterisk) close to the slit-like orifice of the right superior caval vein. The smooth sinus portion of the atrium would be favorable for tunnelling inferior-to-superior caval veins in a lateral tunnel Fontan pathway. The coronary sinus is absent, which is typical of right atrial isomerism.

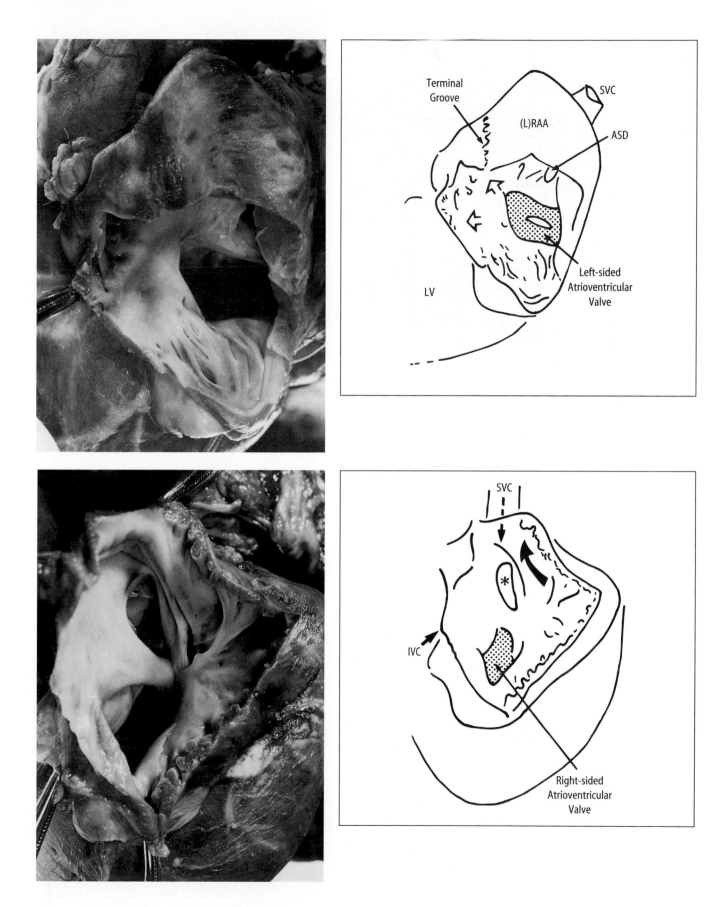

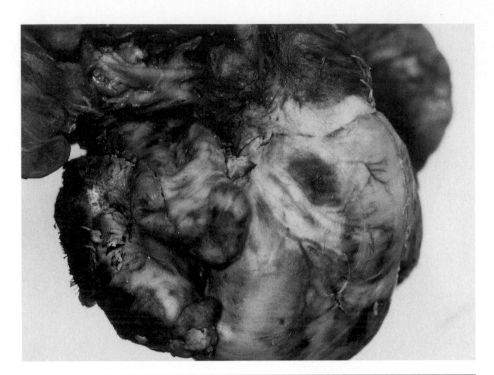

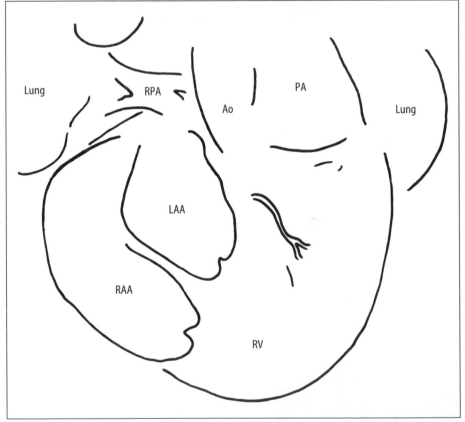

← **4.9 Right juxtaposition of the atrial appendages.** The heart is shown in an anterior view. The left atrial appendage has passed through the transverse sinus behind the aorta and lies above the right atrial appendage on the right side of the heart. Although not completely obvious in the photograph, the lower appendage is morphologically a right appendage, and the upper appendage is a morphologically left appendage (usual atrial arrangement). This heart also has generalized hypoplasia of the aortic arch and a small mitral valve, but the ventriculo-arterial connections are concordant. A pronounced bulge of the posterior part of the ventricular septum produces left ventricular outflow tract obstruction. There are also an atrial septal defect of the oval fossa and defects in the membranous and muscular ventricular septum. The pulmonary root is dilated. A persistent left superior caval vein drains to the coronary sinus (not shown).

Right-sided juxtaposition of the atrial appendages is rare by comparison with left-sided juxtaposition (see Figure 21.150). Whereas left juxtaposition is always associated with severe intracardiac malformations (usually cyanotic lesions with abnormal ventriculo-arterial connections), the remainder of the heart may or may not be malformed with right juxtaposition. The types of intracardiac morphology which have been described in association with right juxtaposition, however, may be more diverse, ranging from a simple atrial septal defect of the oval fossa to complex atrioventricular septal defects with isolated ventricular inversion and disturbances of the conduction tissue. The presence of juxtaposition of the atrial appendages does not exclude atrial isomerism, with both appendages having right or left morphology.

In addition to alerting the surgeon to the possibility of complex cardiac malformations, right juxtaposition may complicate access to the right pulmonary artery (for example, for a posterior atrio-pulmonary anastomosis) or to the back of the ascending aorta (for reimplantation of an anomalous left coronary artery). This is particularly true in reoperations where adhesions obscure the presence of an atrial appendage in the transverse sinus. Within the right atrium itself, distortion of the atrial anatomy and poor development of the limbus, causing an atrial septal defect to lie unusually high, have been encountered in a heart with right juxtaposition of the atrial appendages.

Suggested Reading

Allwork SP, Urban AE, Anderson RH. Left juxtaposition of the auricles with l-position of the aorta. Report of six cases. Br Heart J 1977;39:299.

Anderson RH, Macartney FJ, Shinebourne EA, Tynan M. Definitions of cardiac chambers. In: Anderson RH, Shinebourne EA (eds) Paediatric Cardiology 1977. Edinburgh and London: Churchill Livingstone 1978:16.

Anderson RH, Smith A, Wilkinson JL. Right juxtaposition of the auricular appendages. European J Cardiol 1976;4:495.

Anderson RH, Webb S, Brown NA. Defective lateralisation in children with congenitally malformed hearts. Cardiol Young 1998;8:512.

Azakie A, Merklinger SL, Williams WG, Van Arsdell GS, Coles JG, Adatia I. Improving outcomes of the Fontan operation in children with atrial isomerism and heterotaxy syndromes. Ann Thorac Surg 2001;72:1636.

Becker AE, Becker MJ. Juxtaposition of the atrial appendages associated with normally orientated ventricles and great arteries. Circulation 1970;41:685.

De Tommasi SM, Daliento L, Ho SY, Macartney FJ, Anderson RH. Analysis of atrioventricular junction, ventricular mass, and ventriculoarterial junction in 43 specimens with atrial isomerism. Br Heart J 1981;45:236.

Dickinson DF, Wilkinson JL, Anderson KR, Smith A, Ho SY, Anderson RH. The cardiac conduction system in situs ambiguus. Circulation 1979;59:879.

Freedom RM, Harrington DP. Anatomically corrected malposition of the great arteries. Report of 2 cases, one with congenital asplenia: frequent association with juxtaposition of the atrial appendages. Br Heart J 1974;36:207.

Hirooka K, Yagihara T, Kishimoto H, Isobe F, Yamamoto F, Mishigaki K, Matsuki O, Uemura H, Kawashima Y. Biventricular repair in cardiac isomerism. Report of seventeen cases. J Thorac Cardiovasc Surg 1995;109:530.

Ho SY, Munro JL, Anderson RH. Disposition of the sinus node in left-sided juxtaposition of the atrial appendages. Br Heart J 1979;4:129.

Kawahira Y, Kishimoto H, Kawata, Kiawa S, Ueda H, Nakajima T, Kayatani F, Inamura N, Nakada T. Morphologic analysis of common atrioventicular valves in patients with right atrial isomerism. Pediatr Cardiol 1997;18:107.

Kawashima Y, Kitamura S, Matsuda H, Shimazaki Y, Nakano S, Hirose H. Total cavopulmonary shunt operation in complex cardiac anomalies. J Thorac Cardiovasc Surg 1984;87:74.

Kirklin JW, Barratt-Boyes BG. Atrial isomerism. In: Cardiac Surgery, Morphology, Diagnostic Criteria, Natural History, Techniques, Results and Indications, 2nd edn. New York: Churchill Livingstone 1993;1585.

Macartney FJ, Partridge JB, Shinebourne EA, Tynan M, Anderson RH. Identification of atrial situs. In: Anderson RH, Shinebourne EA (eds) Paediatric Cardiology, Vol 5 1977. Edinburgh and London: Churchill Livingstone 1978:16.

Macartney FJ, Zuberbuhler JR, Anderson RH. Morphological considerations pertaining to recognition of atrial isomerism, consequence for sequential chamber localisation. Br Heart J 1980; 44:657.

Meluish BPP, Van Praagh R. Juxtaposition of the atrial appendages. A sign of severe cyanotic congenital heart disease. Br Heart J 1968;30:269.

Min JY, Kim CY, Oh MH, Chun YK, Suh YL, Kang IS, Lee HJ, Seo JW. Arrangement of the systemic and pulmonary venous components of the atrial chambers in hearts with isomeric atrial appendages. Cardiol Young 200;10:396.

Pacifico AD, Fox LS, Kirklin JW, Bargeron LM. Surgical treatment of atrial isomerism. In: Anderson RH, Macartney FJ, Shinebourne EA, Tynan M (eds) Paediatric Cardiology, Vol 5. London: Churchill Livingstone 1983:223.

Uemura H, Ho SY, Anderson RH, Yagihara T. The structure of the common atrioventricular valve in hearts having isomeric atrial appendages and double inlet ventricle. J Heart Valve Dis 1998;7:850.

Uemura H, Yagihara T, Kawahira Y, Yoshikawa Y. Anatomic biventricular repair by intraatrial and intraventricular re-routing in patients with left isomerism. Cardiol Young 2001;11:12.

Van Mierop LHS, Gessner IH, Schliebler GL. Asplenia and polysplenia syndromes. In: Birth Defects: Original Article series. Baltimore: Williams and Wilkins, 1972;5:36.

5 Atrial Septal Defect

Introduction

Communications which allow shunting of blood between left and right atriums are collectively called "atrial septal defects," although by strict definition only the defect of the oval fossa is actually within the interatrial septum. The oval fossa or "secundum" atrial septal defect thus lies in the middle of the floor of the right atrium. It may extend to the orifice of the inferior caval vein if there is a deficiency of limbic tissue, but does not reach the atrioventricular valves, coronary sinus or orifice of the superior caval vein. An atrial septal defect is distinguished from a patent oval fossa by the fact that there is sufficient tissue of the flap valve to close the latter, simply by pressing on the oval fossa from its left atrial side.

The "sinus venosus defects" include the superior caval defect, inferior caval defect, and posterior atrial septal defect, all of which lie within remnants of the right horn of the embryological sinus venosus and are separated from the oval fossa by the limbus. The superior caval defect, at the junction of the superior caval vein and right atrium frequently (90%) has associated anomalous connection of some of the right pulmonary veins. It is bounded inferiorly by the atrial septum, but has no superior border as the superior caval vein sits astride the defect. Similarly, the inferior caval vein overrides the inferior type of defect and may be connected more towards the left atrial side of the septal plane, while the right pulmonary veins form one margin of a posterior atrial septal defect. Any of these may coexist with an atrial septal defect of the oval fossa or patent oval fossa.

The "coronary sinus atrial septal defect" is one end of a spectrum of malformations constituting the unroofed coronary sinus syndrome. Because one wall of the coronary sinus is shared with the left atrium, a defect in this tissue produces an interatrial communication through the enlarged, but otherwise normal orifice of the coronary sinus. This is the only interatrial communication which has intimate relations with the atrioventricular node of the conduction system.

The "ostium primum" atrial septal defect is a type of atrioventricular septal malformation and accordingly is considered in Chapter 12.

Surgical closure of interatrial communications depends on the size and position of the defect as well as on an adequate ventricle and atrioventricular valve (usually to the left side) to accommodate the increased volume of blood formerly shunted through the defect. Where there is minimal tissue deficiency (patent oval fossa, some defects of the oval fossa), direct suture can be used to approximate the edges of the defect. This is often possible early after a conservative balloon atrial

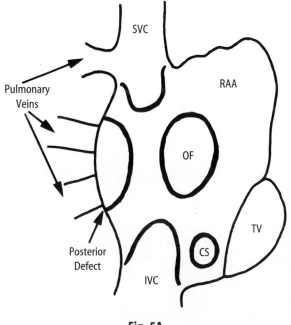

Fig. 5A

septostomy for transposition of the great arteries and when the oval fossa is stretched by a large interatrial shunt, as in total anomalous pulmonary venous connection.

In general, when the defect extends to a venous orifice (superior and inferior caval veins, pulmonary vein, coronary sinus), direct suture is inadvisable because inadequate tissue will result in narrowing of the venous pathway and/or tension on surrounding structures. This is true also of large oval defects in the oval fossa and those where absence of the limbus leaves a small margin of septum between the defect and the tricuspid valve. In these situations, a patch of autogenous pericardium usually suffices to close the defect, leaving the smooth side towards the left atrium. Alternatively, the sinus venosus defects can be repaired by turning in atrial flaps hinged on the caval orifice to direct the pulmonary veins across the defect to the left atrium. Because the right atrium is enlarged as a result of the left-to-right shunt, there is then ample free wall to reconstruct a caval pathway to the tricuspid valve, analogous with the Senning operation, or to connect the superior caval vein to the right atrial appendage. In these operations, the atrial incisions and suture lines are planned to avoid damage to the sinus node, its arteries, and the terminal crest, whenever possible. When the defect reaches the inferior caval vein, it is especially important to identify the Eustachian valve and to avoid suturing to its free margin as the mistaken edge of the defect. This erroneous maneuver directs the inferior caval vein to the left atrium and causes post-operative cyanosis.

Repair of coronary sinus defects depends also on the extent of unroofing within the left atrium and the presence or absence of a left superior caval vein and left innominate vein. In the absence of a left superior caval vein and the presence of a large communication in the left atrium, the orifice of the coronary sinus is closed with a patch, deviating the suture line within the wall of the coronary sinus to avoid trauma to the atrioventricular node. This leaves a right-to-left shunt of coronary venous blood to the left atrium, which is about 10% and clinically insignificant. A left superior caval vein which cannot be ligated must be redirected to the right atrium, either by patch-repair of the defect in the coronary sinus within the left atrium or by partitioning of the left atrium and closure of the orifice of the coronary sinus. Absent or small left innominate vein is the usual situation in left superior caval vein associated with unroofed coronary sinus. This rare type of atrial septal defect is often found in association with tricuspid atresia or tetralogy of Fallot, where failure to recognize it pre- or intraoperatively (by the presence of a large orifice of the coronary sinus) may lead to persistent cyanosis or heart failure after surgery.

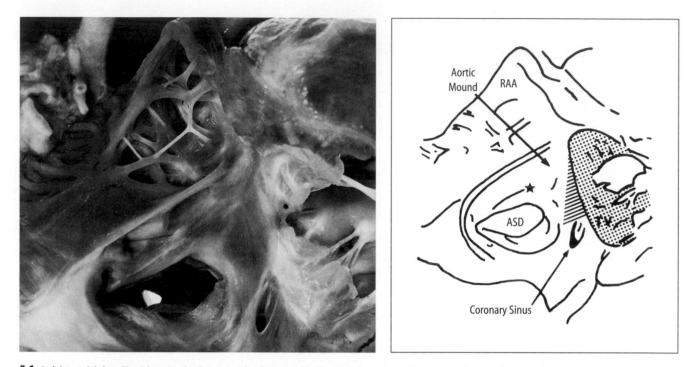

5.1 **Atrial septal defect.** The right atrium has been opened and orientated in the anatomic position to demonstrate a large atrial septal defect. The superior caval vein would lie towards the left upper portion of the illustration and the inferior caval vein at the bottom. The flap valve, or floor, of the oval fossa is almost completely absent, creating a large defect of which the margins are the intact limbus tissue (star). The atrioventricular node, at the apex of the triangle of Koch (striped area) is not closely related to such a defect. The coronary sinus is in the normal position and the tricuspid valve is normal. The anterior margin of the atrial septal defect lies near the aortic mound. In this area, the right coronary sinus of the aortic root bulges into the right atrium and can be damaged by a deep suture during closure of the atrial septal defect, particularly if the aorta is distended. This is also the area where an aneurysm of a sinus of Valsalva may rupture into the right atrium or endocarditis may produce an aorto-right atrial fistula. This type of atrial septal defect may be amenable to transcatheter device closure.

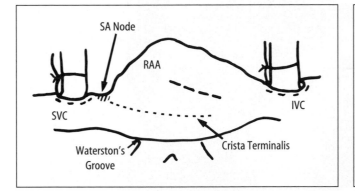

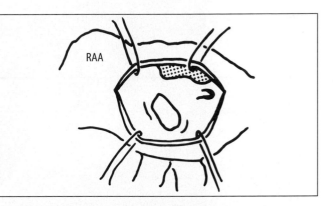

5.2 Cannulation of the superior caval vein above the sinus node, and the inferior caval vein at its junction with the right atrium gives excellent surgical access to most atrial septal defects. If pulmonary veins drain anomalously to the superior caval vein, this cannula is placed about 0.5 cm above their entrance. A short oblique atrial incision (long dashes) is made, starting in the lower part of the appendage and ending above the terminal groove.

5.3 After visualizing the atrial septal defect, the atrial incision is extended superiorly or inferiorly if needed, while looking inside the atrium for the position of the terminal crest. A short incision is usually adequate. The position of the coronary sinus, the pulmonary veins, the mitral and tricuspid valves, and the caval orifice should all be identified. This exposure is facilitated by four or five stay-sutures on the edge of the atriotomy.

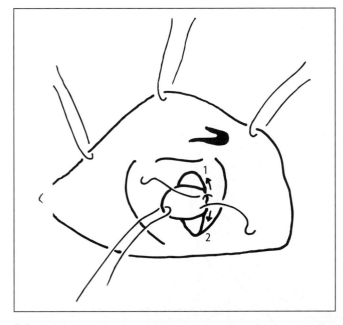

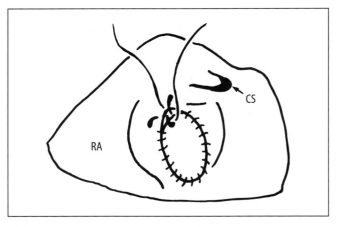

5.5 The suture line ends at the highest point in the atrium, which is usually just beneath the aortic mound. Prior to tying the suture, the lungs are inflated to evacuate air from the left atrium. This measure is then repeated to confirm secure closure and exclude additional defects. The atriotomy is closed, usually in two layers, allowing the right atrium to fill with blood and dispel air through the top of the suture line.

5.4 Where there is a large tissue deficiency or the defect extends to a venous orifice, closure with a patch is necessary to avoid distortion and tension of the septal remnant. Suturing begins on the right-hand margin of the defect, clearly visualizing its lower extent. By doing the side towards the coronary sinus (and hence conduction tissue) first, with the second arm of the suture held towards the surgeon's side and the scrub nurse following the suture, the more critical margins of the defect are clearly visualized.

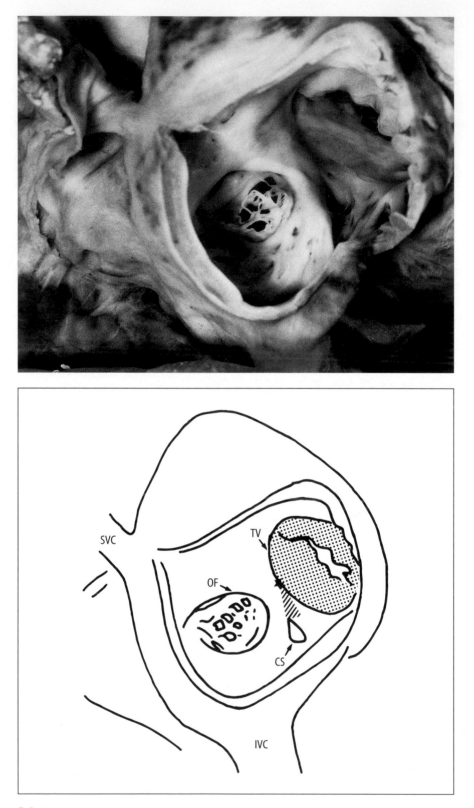

5.6 Atrial septal defect. The right atrium has been opened along the appendage from superior to inferior caval vein, such that the observer looks down on the tricuspid valve and atrial septum. The flap valve of the oval fossa is fenestrated, producing a large interatrial communication. The coronary sinus forms one side of the triangle of Koch (striped area), which has the atrioventricular node at its apex (star). Surgically, this defect would be managed by excision of the remnants of the flap valve and insertion of a patch (see Figs. 5.2–5.5).

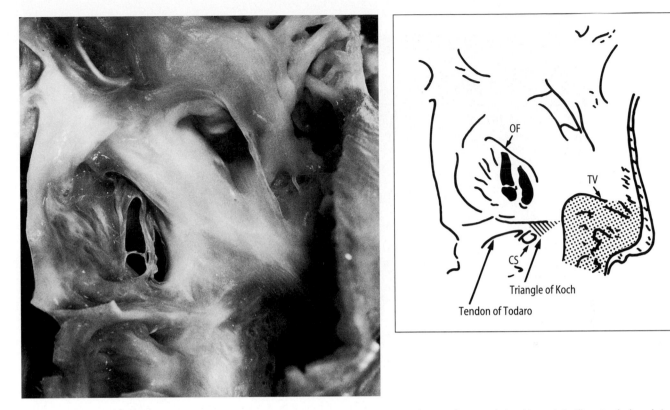

5.7 Atrial septal defect due to multiple fenestrations in the flap valve of the oval fossa. This specimen is shown in the anatomical position and also illustrates the boundaries of the triangle of Koch – namely, the tendon of Todaro, the tricuspid valvar annulus and the coronary sinus. The atrioventricular node lies within the triangle of Koch in hearts with concordant atrioventricular connections.

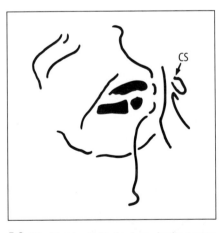

5.8 This defect is suitable for closure by direct suture because it does not extend to a venous orifice, there is ample well-formed tissue available in the limbus and the flap valve itself, and the oblong orientation of the defect allows side-to-side approximation without tension on either the remaining septum or conduction tissue. Closure is started at the bottom of the defect with a purse-string or three bites to be certain that a tunnel does not remain behind the suture line. This is tied with several knots and one end of the suture is held towards the patient's feet.

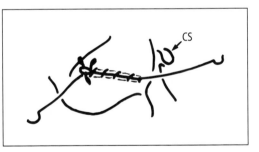

5.9 The lungs are inflated to evacuate air from the left atrium prior to pulling up the last bite at the top of the running suture. The second arm, which has provided gentle tension to align the defect for the first layer, is now used to complete closure with a second running stitch. It is important to keep these bites close to the first suture line, both to minimize tension on surrounding tissue and to avoid placement of sutures in the triangle of Koch. The lungs are reinflated to check the closure as there are often additional small fenestrations at the edges of the flap valve which often only become obvious after the major defect is closed.

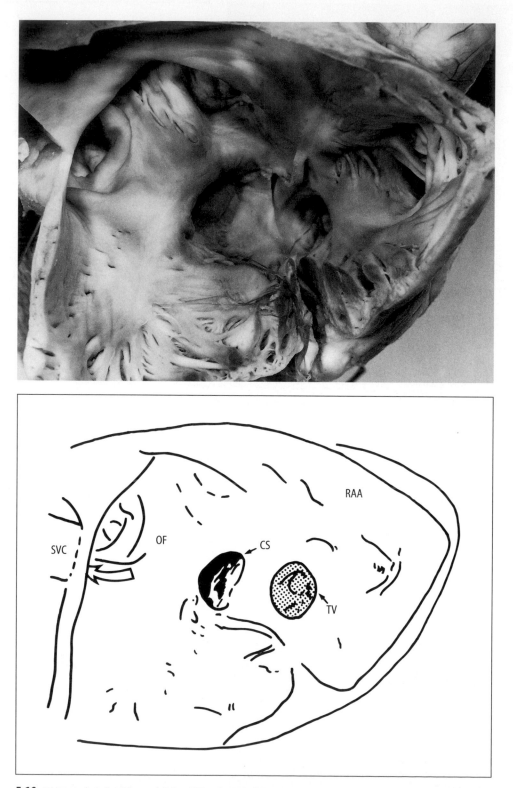

5.10 Coronary sinus "atrial septal defect." The tricuspid valve is hypoplastic and stenotic, and the oval fossa is displaced towards the superior caval vein (open arrow) by the enlarged orifice of the coronary sinus. This malformation is within the spectrum of unroofed coronary sinus (see Chapter 6). As such, it is outside the confines of the atrial septum per se, although it allows communication between the atriums.

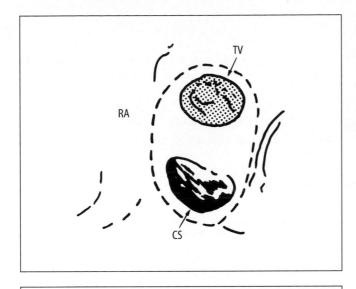

5.11 With any interatrial defect, it is necessary to confirm that both atrioventricular valves are present and adequate prior to closure of the communication. In this heart, the tricuspid valve is very small, so the surgical options lie between a "one-and-a-half" ventricle repair and a Fontan operation. Because of the very small and dysplastic tricuspid valve, the surgical repair is more likely to be a Fontan operation. In the case of an intra-cardiac tunnel procedure to accomplish this, both the coronary sinus and tricuspid valve may be left below a single patch, provided there is no valvar incompetence. The suture line is placed about 5 mm away from the tricuspid annulus (dashed line) to avoid injury to the conduction system which lies between the coronary sinus and the tricuspid annulus.

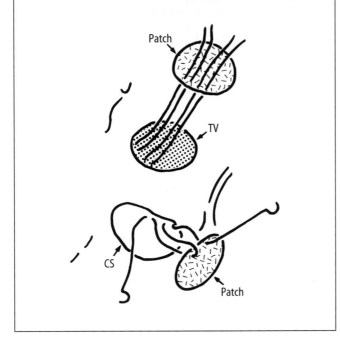

5.12 When there is incompetence of the tricuspid valve, it is isolated from the systemic circulation by separate closure of its orifice and that of the coronary sinus. This may be done with sutures placed from ventricle to atrium through the base of the leaflets, analogous to those for patch closure of a ventricular septal defect. The small amount of coronary venous blood returning directly to the right ventricle will still be ejected through the pulmonary artery if the ventricular septum is intact. In the area at risk for the conduction tissue, sutures in the patch of the coronary sinus are taken well inside the orifice. This is the same technique which would be used to close the orifice of the coronary sinus alone, were the tricuspid valve and right ventricle sufficiently large to permit the entire cardiac output to pass through them.

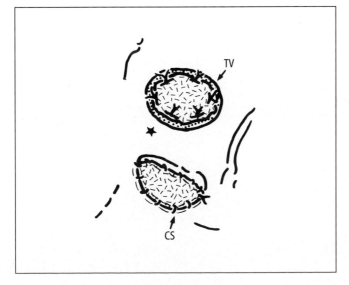

5.13 Both suture lines of the complete patches lie well away from the area of the atrioventricular node (star). Either may be done with continuous or interrupted technique, although placement around the tricuspid valve is facilitated by multiple interrupted sutures which can be supported by pledgets on their ventricular side in the presence of delicate leaflet tissue. When the tricuspid valve is adequate, the interatrial communication alone is closed with a patch in the orifice of the coronary sinus. An alternative procedure is to open the left atrium and repair the unroofed portion of the coronary sinus, if this can be patched, leaving its orifice to drain into the right atrium (see Figure 6.2).

Suggested Reading

Bedford DE. The anatomical types of atrial septal defect. Am J Cardiol 1960;6:568.

Cockerham JT, Martin TC, Gutierrez FR, Hartmann AFS, Goldring D, Strauss AW. Spontaneous closure of secundum atrial defect in infants and young children. Am J Cardiol 1983;52:1267.

Ferreira SM, Ho SY, Anderson RH. Morphological study of defects of the atrial septum within the oval fossa: implications for transcatheter closure of left-to-right shunt. Br Heart J 1992;67(4):316.

Hagen PT, Scholtz DG, Edwards WD. Incidence and size of the patent foramen ovale during the first 10 decades of life: an autopsy study of 965 normal hearts. Proc Staff meet Mayo Clin 1984;59:1489.

Hudson REB. The normal and abnormal interatrial septum. Br Heart J 1955;17:489.

Kirklin JW, Swan HJC, Wood EH, Burchall HB, Edwards JE. Anatomic, physiologic and surgical considerations in repair of interatrial communications in man. J Thorac Cardiovasc Surg 1955;29:37.

Lee ME, Sade RM. Coronary sinus septal defect. Surgical considerations. J Thorac Cardiovasc Surg 1979;78:563.

McKay R. Surgical management of the atrial septal defects. Heart Views 2002;3:68.

Quaegebeur J, Kirklin JW, Pacifico AD, Bargeron LM Jr. Surgical experience with unroofed coronary sinus. Ann Thorac Surg 1979;27:418.

Rose AG, Beckman CB, Edwards JE. Communication between coronary sinus and left atrium. Br Heart J 1974;36:182.

Ross DN. The sinus venosus type of atrial septal defect. Guy's Hosp Rep 1956;105:376.

Wilcox BR, Anderson RH. Surgical anatomy of the Heart. 2nd edn. London: Gower Medical Publishing 1992:p.76.

6 Unroofed Coronary Sinus

Introduction

The normal coronary sinus, which is a derivative of the left horn of the embryological venous sinus, runs in the posterior atrioventricular groove between the left atrium and the left ventricle. As it encircles the mural leaflet of the mitral valve, one wall of the coronary sinus is contiguous with the posterior wall of the left atrium. Having traversed the left atrium, it terminates in the right atrium between the oval fossa and tricuspid valve. Its orifice is guarded by the Thebesian valve.

Absence of part of the wall between the left atrium and coronary sinus produces an anatomical spectrum of anomalies that are referred to as the "unroofed coronary sinus syndrome." These range from a coronary sinus "atrial septal defect," in which there is free communication between the left and right atriums through the ostium of the coronary sinus (see Chapter 5), to complete "unroofing" or absence of the wall of the coronary sinus in the left atrium. In the latter case, the coronary veins drain directly into the atrial chambers. A persistent left superior caval vein is associated frequently with anomalies of the coronary sinus. When it is present, there is rarely (less than about one in five patients) a left innominate vein connecting it to the right superior caval vein. Moreover, the right superior caval vein may be small or absent.

Unroofed coronary sinus syndrome is found more frequently in association with tricuspid atresia and tetralogy of Fallot than with other congenital malformations. If unrecognized, the persistent atrial communication may result in profound hypoxia post-repair.

Surgical management depends on the extent of unroofing and the presence or absence of a left superior caval vein draining to the coronary sinus. Without a left caval vein, the unroofed coronary sinus may be directed to the left atrium by patch-closure of its ostium in the right atrium. The important anatomical landmark for this procedure is the triangle of Koch which contains the atrioventricular node at its apex, in close proximity to the coronary sinus (see Chapter 5). The resulting right-to-left shunt of coronary venous blood to the left atrium, about 10%, is clinically and hemodynamically insignificant.

When a left superior caval vein is present and must drain to the right atrium (i.e. the innominate vein is small or absent), the extent of unroofing guides management. A limited deficiency (partial unroofing) in the coronary sinus wall can be repaired with a pericardial patch or imbricated left atrial wall sutured to the edges of the coronary sinus in the left atrium. Alternatively, when there is extensive unroofing and the left superior caval vein drains to the roof of the left atrium, the choice lies between intracardiac and extracardiac repair. For the former, a pericardial baffle may be used to direct the pulmonary veins to the mitral valve, leaving all the systemic venous orifices above the patch and connected with the tricuspid valve through the orifice of the coronary sinus. An alternative procedure which achieves the same hemodynamic result is to tunnel the left caval vein across the roof of the left atrium with a pericardial patch and use flaps of atrial septum or a second patch of pericardium to close the orifice of the coronary sinus. This too results in geometrically satisfactory pathways for both systemic and pulmonary venous drainage, and also conserves good growth potential for both pathways. Extracardiac techniques include anastomosis of the divided left superior caval vein to the right atrial appendage, the right superior caval vein, or the left pulmonary artery. While the last mentioned tends to be done as a bidirectional cavopulmonary connection in the Fontan circulation, it has also been employed in biventricular repairs, such as that for tetralogy of Fallot.

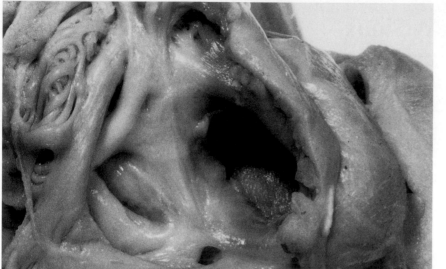

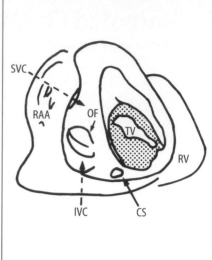

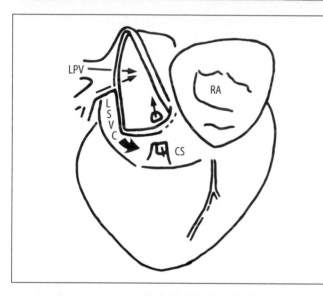

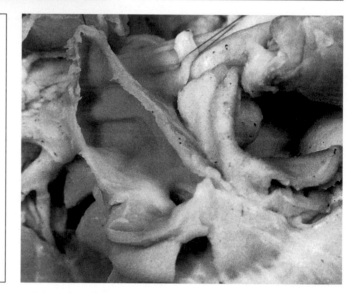

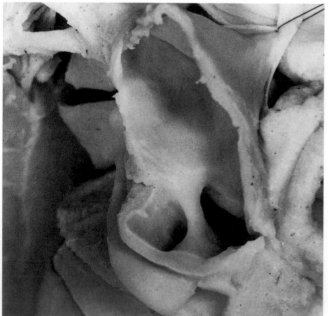

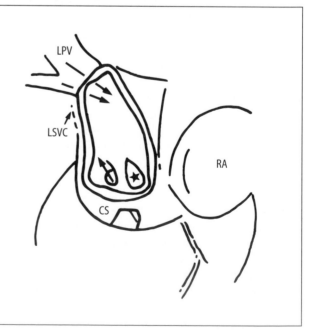

← **6.1** **Unroofed coronary sinus.** The right atrium has been opened from superior to inferior caval vein in a heart with imperforate mitral valve and unroofed coronary sinus. The superior and inferior caval veins drain into this chamber in the normal position, as does the coronary sinus. The right pulmonary veins, which are not seen, drain into the azygos system. The opening of the coronary sinus is unusually small, particularly considering that this is the only intracardiac route by which the left pulmonary venous return can leave the left atrium. The atrial septum is otherwise intact and the tricuspid valve is normal. In addition to the lesions shown below, this heart has double outlet right ventricle and coarctation of the aorta. The left ventricle is small and a perimembranous ventricular septal defect is present.

← **6.2** Posterior view of the left atrium in the heart shown in Figure 6.1. Most of the posterior wall and the left atrial appendage have been removed and a rectangular window has been cut into the enlarged coronary sinus which receives a persistent left superior caval vein. The left pulmonary veins are normally connected to the left atrium, but the right pulmonary veins (not seen) drain anomalously into an extracardiac descending vein. The coronary sinus is unroofed in its mid-portion (small arrow) into the left atrium and thus has "biatrial opening" into the right atrium through the ostium of the coronary sinus and into the left atrium through its unroofed portion.

← **6.3** This is a slightly different view of the specimen shown in Figure 6.2, rotated to demonstrate the position of imperforate mitral valve (star). The coronary sinus is unroofed near the mitral valve (arrow into left atrium). This is in contrast to a completely unroofed coronary sinus where the left superior caval vein would enter the left atrium between the left atrial appendage and the left pulmonary veins.

In the context of mitral valvar atresia, surgical management of this rare anomaly would include initial palliation by atrial septectomy to provide unobstructed drainage from the left atrium, repair of the associated coarctation and, if obstructed, right pulmonary veins and pulmonary arterial banding. Ultimately, it may be possible to create a Fontan circulation, at which time the left superior caval vein would be connected directly to the left pulmonary artery with a bidirectional cavopulmonary anastomosis.

Suggested Reading

Adatia I, Gittenberger-de Groot AC. Unroofed coronary sinus and coronary sinus orifice atresia. Implications for management of complex congenital heart disease. J Am Coll Cardiol 1995;25:948.

Chui I-S, Hegarty A, Anderson RH, de Leval M. The landmarks to the atrioventricular conduction system in hearts with absence or unroofing of the coronary sinus. J Thorac Cardiovasc Surg 1985;90:297.

de Leval MR, Ritter DG, McGoon DC, Danielson GK. Anomalous systemic venous connection. Surgical considerations. Mayo Clinic Proc 1975;50:599.

Mantini E, Grondim CM, Lillehei EW, Edwards JE. Congenital anomalies involving the coronary sinus. Circulation 1966;33:317.

Quaegebeur J, Kirklin JW, Pacifico AD, Bargeron LM Jr. Surgical experience with unroofed coronary sinus. Ann Thorac Surg 1979;27:418.

Reddy VM, McElhinney DB, Hanley FL. Correction of left superior vena cava draining to the left atrium using extracardiac techniques. Ann Thorac Surg 1997;63:1800.

Rumisek JD, Piggot JD, Weinberg PM, Norwood WI. Coronary sinus septal defect associated with tricuspid atresia. J Thorac Cardiovasc Surg 1986;92:142.

Sand ME, McGrath LB, Pacifico AD, Mandeke NV. Repair of left superior vena cava entering the left atrium. Ann Thorac Surg 1986;42:560.

van Son JA, Black MD, Haas GS, Falk V, Hambsch J, Onnasch JF, Mohr FW. Extracardiac repair versus intracardiac baffle repair of complex unroofed coronary sinus. Thorac Cardiovasc Surg 1998;46:371.

Winter FS. Persistent left superior vena cava. Survey of world literature and report of 30 additional cases. Angiology 1954;5:90.

7 Division of the Left Atrium (Cor Triatriatum)

Introduction

The normal left atrium has a characteristic, hooked appendage which is separated from a smooth-walled portion by a narrow junction. No terminal crest is present. There are no remnants of venous valves but the flap valve of the oval fossa is present on the septal surface. During normal development, the pulmonary veins join together in a common venous chamber which becomes incorporated into the left atrium producing the smooth sinus portion, thus transporting blood directly to the left-sided atrioventricular valve and ventricle. That part of the left atrium which contains its appendage and the vestibule to the mitral valve, develops from the cardiac mass itself.

Partitioning of the left atrium is a rare but important malformation. Many variants have been reported which involve more complex anomalies such as persistent left superior caval vein, unroofed coronary sinus and pulmonary venous connection to the coronary sinus. Other important associated anomalies encompass variations of anomalous pulmonary venous connection, which are the result of degrees of failure of the common venous chamber to meet the left atrium (see Chapter 8). Division of the left atrium also has been explained historically in this context, as a result of either malincorporation of the common pulmonary vein or entrapment of the common pulmonary vein by the developing left sinus horn. However, the co-existence of divided left atrium with total anomalous pulmonary venous connection is then rendered difficult to explain. Be that as it may, it is accepted currently that there is no structure in normal development of the left atrium which represents a substrate for the fibromuscular partition in classic cor triatriatum. This contrasts with partitioning of the right atrium in which the anatomical substrates for division are present in foetal life. Associated ventricular septal defects, abnormal ventriculo-arterial connections, isomerism of the atrial appendages and mirror image atrial arrangement are some of the other anomalies which have also been described with divided left atrium.

The fibromuscular partition in the classic division of the left atrium, is always attached to the atrial septum, separating the left atrium into proximal and distal chambers. The proximal chamber receives the pulmonary veins and sometimes part of the flap valve of the oval fossa. The left atrial appendage, the mitral valve and part of, or sometimes the entire flap valve of the oval fossa, are found in the distal chamber, which is immediately above the mitral valve. In this uncommon anomaly, the left proximal or upper (common pulmonary venous) chamber has a direct communication with the distal chamber in about 90% of cases. This is usually a small orifice and may lie anywhere in the fibromuscular partition. Occasionally, there are multiple orifices. Alternatively, without an orifice in the partition, the proximal chamber drains to the right atrium directly through an atrial septal defect. In these hearts, a separate defect in the oval fossa is necessary to bring pulmonary venous return back to the lower (distal) chamber in the left side of the heart. Even with normal pulmonary venous drainage to the left atrium in association with partitioning, there is frequently a stretched oval fossa or an atrial septal defect (secundum type). Classical division of the left atrium should not be confused with the supravalvar mitral ridge (or "membrane"), which lies immediately adjacent to the mitral valve and thus below the orifice of the left atrial appendage and the flap valve of the oval fossa (see Chapter 10).

From the surgical point of view, the classic cor triatriatum may be considered an intermediate situation where the common venous chamber is connected as is usual to the left atrium, but internally a partition remains between the entrance of the pulmonary veins and the left atrium proper. The principle of surgical management in partitioning of the left atrium is to achieve unobstructed drainage of all the pulmonary veins to the distal chamber and hence across the mitral valve. Depending upon the complexity of the anomaly and the size of the patient, this is done either on cardiopulmonary bypass with periods of reduced flow or under total circulatory arrest. For the usual classic anatomy of this lesion, the atrial chamber with the greatest enlargement on the right (surgeon's) side of the heart is selected for access. When there is absence of a septal defect between the right atrium and the proximal chamber, the chamber with the greatest enlargement usually will be the proximal or upper common pulmonary venous chamber itself. This places the obstructing diaphragm ahead and towards the surgeon's right.

When the right atrium is enlarged by a left to right shunt, it is opened for access to either the proximal or distal chambers through atrial septal defects. In the latter case, the diaphragm lies towards the surgeon's left. Because endocardium flows smoothly from atrium to both sides of the fibromuscular partition, it is not possible to recognise its junction with the atrial wall. Therefore, the orifice is first identified and incised outward, noting the thickness of the fibromuscular diaphragm, which increases as the atrial wall is approached. Having reached the junction of the diaphragm and atrium, the partition is excised circumferentially with scissors. Excessive tension on the diaphragm during this manoeuvre may button-hole the atrial wall, resulting in a communication with the pericardial space, particularly in small infants. Unlike the atrioventricular groove, however, there are no important structures in this region and the defect is simply repaired by direct suture. When some of the pulmonary veins connect to structures other than the left atrium or proximal chamber, additional procedures may be necessary to direct them across the mitral valve.

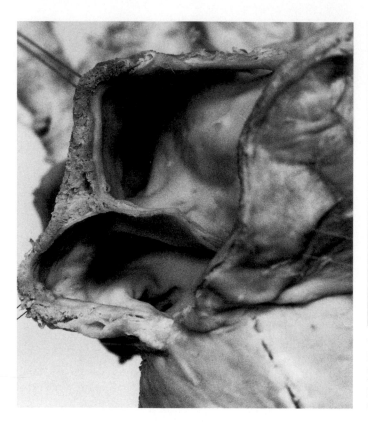

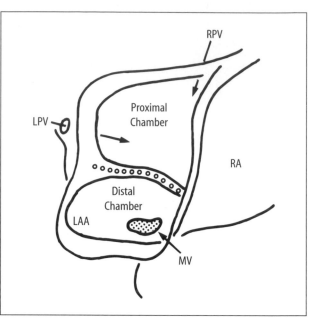

7.1 Division of the left atrium (cor triatriatum). The heart is viewed from behind, after excision of most of the posterior wall of the distal and proximal left atrial chambers. Blood-flows into the proximal (upper) chamber from the pulmonary veins (solid arrows). The distal (lower) chamber contains the mitral valve and a small left atrial appendage. The two chambers are separated by a thick fibromuscular diaphragm (open circles).

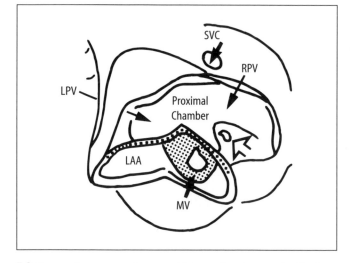

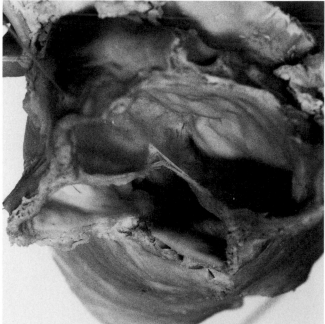

7.2 The same heart now seen from a cranial view to show the eccentric orifice (open arrow) between proximal and distal chambers. No communication is present between either chamber and the right atrium. The fibromuscular diaphragm (dotted line) extends from the top of the left atrial appendage to the opposite wall of the atrium. Solid arrows indicate the openings of the pulmonary veins into the proximal chamber, as well as the position of the superior caval vein entering the right atrium.

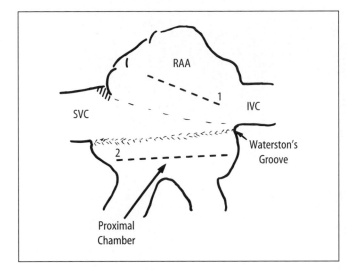

7.3 The diaphragm may be approached through the right atrium (1) if an atrial septal defect is present or through the proximal chamber of the left atrium (2). In the absence of an interatrial communication, the latter will be large and easily accessible on the right side of the heart. The pulmonary veins, by definition, connect to the proximal chamber, unless they drain anomalously. Waterston's groove indicates the position of the intratrial septum.

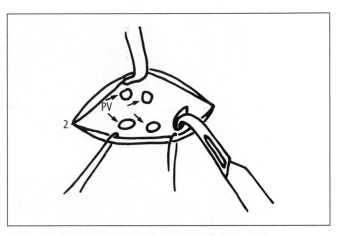

7.4 The pulmonary veins are identified by passing a right-angled instrument into their orifices and palpating it behind the heart. The orifice in the diaphragm may be central or lateral, but lies in a different plane, to the surgeon's right. After positive identification, a hook knife (12 blade) is used to extend the opening to the atrial wall. In this area, the diaphragm becomes thicker and more muscular (see Figure 7.1).

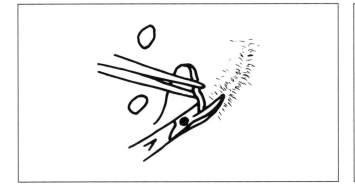

7.5 Having found the atrial wall, curved scissors are used to excise completely the diaphragm which is held under slight tension with forceps or a retraction suture. The blades of the scissors slide along the wall of the distal and proximal chambers. There is no obvious demarcation between the diaphragm and atrial wall, but the slight increase in thickness can be appreciated when the excision is carried deeper into the wall of the atrium. If this area is "buttonholed," it is simply repaired with fine monofilament sutures as (unlike the interatrial septum) there are no important structures related to the diaphragm externally.

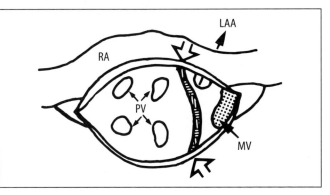

7.6 Complete excision of the diaphragm leaves a raw area of exposed muscle (open arrows) between the endocardium of the proximal chamber, which is often thickened, and that of the distal chamber. The mitral valve and orifice of the left atrial appendage are inspected in the distal chamber. The atrium is irrigated with saline to remove any fragments of muscle or fibrous tissue. The atriotomy (which need not extend into the distal chamber) is then closed with continuous running sutures from either end of the incision.

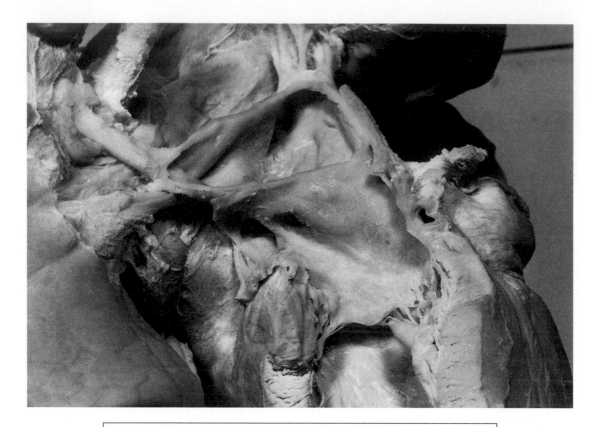

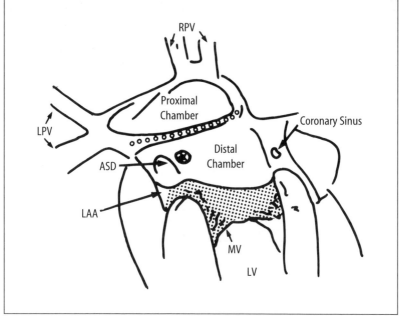

7.7 Division of the left atrium. The specimen has been opened vertically from the top of the proximal chamber (which receives the pulmonary veins), across the distal chamber (containing the mitral valve and a hypoplastic left atrial appendage) and left ventricle. It is seen from the back. The proximal and distal chambers are separated by a thick fibromuscular partition (open circles) and communicate through a small orifice (star). A patent oval fossa connects the left atrium with the right atrium through a small atrial septal defect. The coronary sinus is in the usual position above the mitral valve and thus not related to the membrane within the left atrium.

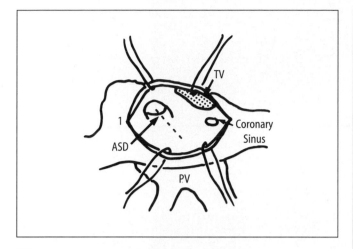

7.8 The oval fossa usually lies within the distal chamber in partitioning of the left atrium and, when patent, enlargement of the right atrium makes this an attractive approach for removal of the partition (see Figure 7.3, incision 1). The atrial septum is incised (dotted line) for access to the distal left atrial chamber.

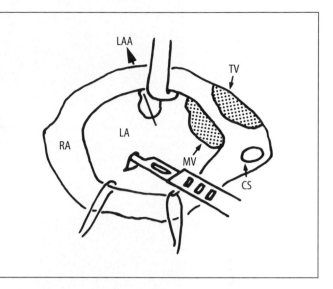

7.9 From this approach, the orifice in the diaphragm lies ahead and to the surgeon's left. It is incised in a convenient direction, looking for the increase in muscle thickness which indicates that the free atrial wall is approaching. If the upper proximal chamber also connects to the right atrium through a second interatrial defect without any orifice in the partition, a right-angle instrument is passed into the proximal chamber and used to press down the partition, such that a stab-incision can be made safely.

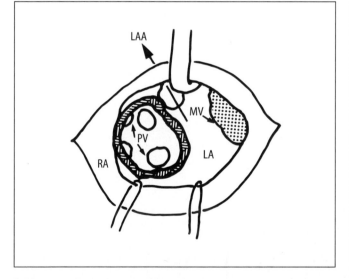

7.10 Having identified the edge of the partition, curved scissors are used to excise the entire diaphragm (see Figure 7.5). This produces free communication between the pulmonary veins in the proximal chamber and the mitral valve in the distal chamber.

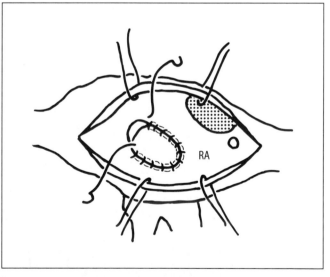

7.11 The enlarged atrial septal defect usually requires a patch for secure closure. If the operation has been done under total circulatory arrest, the left heart is filled with saline to evacuate air prior to completion of the suture line. The right atrium is closed with a continuous monofilament suture in two layers.

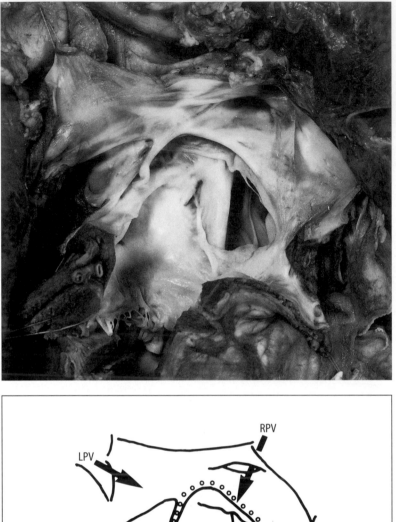

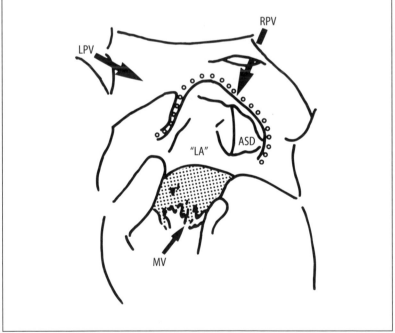

7.12 "Forme fruste" partitioning of the left atrium. The front of the left atrium and the ventricle have been removed so that the left side of the atrial septum, the posterior wall of the left atrium and the aortic (anterior) leaflet of the mitral valve are seen "en face." The morphology has been somewhat distorted for the camera by removal of some of the anterior wall of the atrium in order to better demonstrate the arch of the membrane. The left atrium is partially divided by fibrous tissue (open circles) which separates the openings of the pulmonary veins from the rest of the atrial chamber. A large atrial septal defect in the oval fossa connects the left to the right atrium. The remaining anatomy of this specimen is complex.

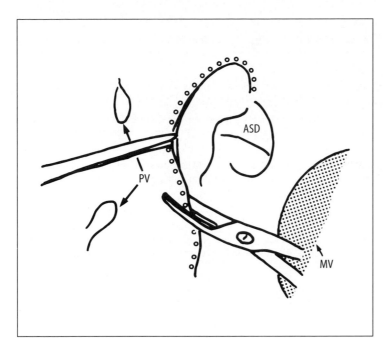

7.13 Partial division of the left atrium or "forme fruste" partitioning is a finding which is not altogether rare at the time of operation. It is seen in hearts with other complex malformations, such as atrioventricular septal defect or uni-ventricular atrioventricular connection. The partition may be a small unobstructive ridge of tissue or, as illustrated in this specimen, a well-developed membrane extending several centimetres into the atrium. As the surgical procedure in such hearts often involves a complex atrial baffle or closure of an interatrial communication, it is important to recognize that the fibrous tissue is not the atrial septum. It is then excised completely.

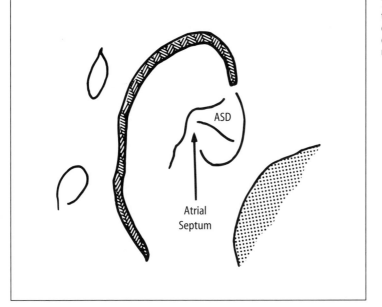

7.14 Having removed the arch of fibrous tissue, it is possible to identify clearly the morphology of the atrium and to plan the surgical repair, which is not otherwise influenced by the position of the membrane attachment. Failure to excise the tissue, or following its free edge or base with an intra-atrial baffle, may result in post operative pulmonary venous obstruction.

Suggested Reading

Anderson RH. Understanding the nature of congenital division of the atrial chambers. Br Heart J 1992;68:1.

Al-Fadley F, Galal O, Wilson N, Aloufi S. Cor triatriatum associated with total anomalous pulmonary venous drainage in the setting of mitral atresia and a restrictive interatrial communication. Pediatr Cardiol 2002;13:125.

Arciniegas E, Farooki ZA, Hakimi M, Perry BL, Green EW. Surgical treatment of cor triatriatum. Ann Thorac Surg 1981;32:571.

Jegeir W, Gibbons JE, Wiglesworth FW. Cor triatriatum: clinical, hemodynamic, and pathologic studies: surgical correction early in life. Pediatrics 1963;31:255.

Jorgensen CR, Ferlie RM, Varco RI, Lillehei CW, Eliot RS. Cor triatriatum: review of the surgical aspects with a follow-up report on the first patient successfully treated with surgery. Circulation 1967;36:101.

Kirk RJB, Pollock JCS. Concommitant cor triatriatum and coronary sinus total anomalous pulmonary venous connection. Ann Thorac Surg 1987;44:203.

Marin-Garcia J, Tandon R, Lucas RV Jr, Edwards JE. Cor triatriatum: study of 20 cases. Am J Cardiol 1975;35:59.

Richardson JV, Doty DB, Siewers RD, Zuberbuhler JR. Cor triatriatum (subdivided left atrium). J Thorac Cardiovasc Surg 1981;81:232.

Thilenius OG, Bharati S, Lev M. Subdivided left atrium: an expanded concept of cor triatriatum sinistrum. Am J Cardiol 1976;37:743.

Van Praagh R, Consini I. Cor triatriatum: pathologic anatomy and a consideration of morphogenesis based on 13 postmortem cases and a study of normal development of the pulmonary vein and atrial septum in 83 human embryos. Am Heart J 1969;78:379.

8 Anomalous Pulmonary Venous Connection

Introduction

The pulmonary veins normally attach to the morphological left atrium. Any deviation from this gives rise to an anomalous pulmonary venous connection. The anomalous connection usually, but not invariably (see Chapter 7), brings about anomalous drainage of the pulmonary veins to the systemic venous side of the circulation and, hence, physiologically, a left-to-right shunt. The malformation is said to be "total" anomalous pulmonary venous connection when none of the pulmonary veins connect to the left atrium and "partial" when some are connected normally and some anomalously.

The common sites of anomalous connections are to either a left ascending vein, the coronary sinus, the right atrium, or to abdominal veins. In total anomalous connection, these types are further described according to the site of drainage in relation to the heart. "Supracardiac" designates a connection which drains above the heart. This is usually to a left ascending vertical vein (the equivalent of a left superior caval vein), an azygos vein, or the right superior caval vein. "Cardiac" types enter the heart directly, either by connections to the right atrium or through the coronary sinus. The latter may be immediately into the coronary sinus or via a left-sided caval vein. "Infracardiac" drainage is to channels which pass below the diaphragm, including the portal vein, ductus venosus, hepatic veins, and inferior caval vein. As these sites all return blood to the heart, there is the potential for streaming of pulmonary venous blood across the oval fossa, which may reduce the degree of cyanosis. Usually, all four pulmonary veins join a confluence which then drains to a single site. However, individual veins connect to different channels in about 10% of post-mortem specimens, producing a "mixed" type of total anomalous pulmonary venous connection. A final rare group are the so-called "double connections" in which the pulmonary venous confluence drains through two patent channels, usually to

the coronary sinus and the left ascending vein (see Fig. 8A).

From a clinical standpoint, the presence or absence of obstruction to pulmonary venous drainage is also important. Supracardiac connections to the left ascending vein or to the right superior caval vein may or may not be obstructed by compression of the ascending channel between the left or right main bronchus and the pulmonary artery. Infracardiac channels are nearly always obstructed by virtue of their small size or blood having to pass through the liver, while drainage to the coronary sinus is occasionally restricted at the junction of the common venous channel with the coronary sinus. Obstruction may also occur within the channel itself or at the level of a restrictive atrial septal defect, which is obligatory for return of blood to the left side of the heart. These types of obstruction must be differentiated from pulmonary venous obstruction which is due to lesions within the veins themselves and of grave prognosis.

The principles of surgical management of anomalous pulmonary venous connections are to achieve unrestricted drainage of the pulmonary veins to the left atrium without compromise of important systemic venous pathways, to close all communications between the systemic and pulmonary circulations and to conserve growth potential in both the systemic and pulmonary venous channels. When a common pulmonary venous channel is present, this is usually anastomosed directly to the left atrium. The exception to this generalization is coronary sinus connections that are not obstructed, in which drainage to the left atrium is generally achieved by excision of the roof of the coronary sinus and part of the atrial septum (see Chapter 6). Other variants are managed by direct anastomosis of the anomalous veins to the left atrium or its appendage, or by various tunnelling procedures. In all these operations, growth potential for the connections

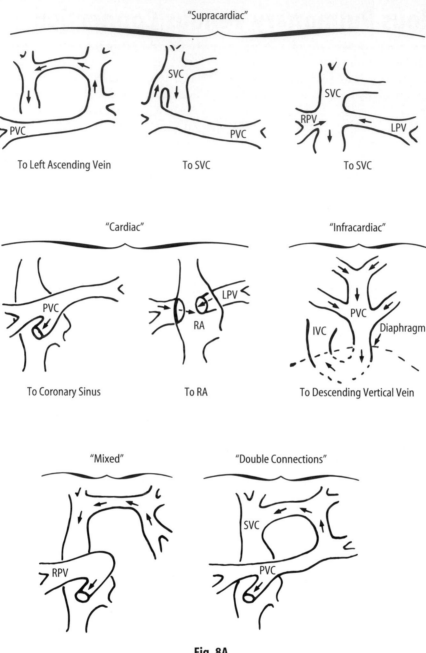

Fig. 8A

and pathways is maximized by incorporating as much native cardiac tissue as possible and, when practicable, using absorbable suture material. It is also important to avoid injury to the conduction tissue within the right atrium (of particular concern in repair of coronary sinus connections) and damage to the phrenic and recurrent laryngeal nerves, which are closely related to the left ascending channel or right superior caval vein and the frequently associated persistently patent arterial duct, respectively. These complications are rarely fatal but can result in both short- and long-term disability following an otherwise anatomically and hemodynamically satisfactory repair.

Controversy remains regarding the optimal approach for anastomosis of the pulmonary venous confluence to the left atrium. Using the posterior or external approaches, the heart is elevated upwards towards the right or displaced to the left. The atrial septal defect is closed from the left side and the anastomosis is done outside the heart, necessitating a three-dimensional spatial conceptualization of how it will lie when the heart is replaced in the pericardium. This technique gives good visualisation of the pulmonary veins and permits a very wide anastomosis. Alternatively, the heart is left in situ and the venous confluence is approached across the atrial septum and through the posterior left atrial wall. This anastomosis is constructed exactly where it will lie and readily allows insertion of a pericardial patch for closure of the interatrial communication, but access in small infants requires incisions across three parts of the heart (extending horizontally across the terminal crest of the right atrium, the interatrial septum and the posterior wall of the left atrium), which could have long-term implications for atrial function and cardiac rhythm. A superior approach between the ascending aorta and a superior caval vein, with or without division of the ascending aorta, is a third option which is said to be useful in patients with supracardiac or some types of mixed connections. The interatrial communication is closed either by direct suture or with a patch of pericardium, as dictated by its size and position. It is possible at this time to enlarge the size of the left atrium by translocating the septum or patch towards the right. The connection between the pulmonary venous confluence and an ascending or descending vein is either ligated or divided, the latter increasing the amount of tissue which is available also to enlarge the left atrium. Although in the past, leaving the ascending or descending channel patent was advocated to decompress the left side of the heart or to take oxygenated blood to the liver respectively, such maneuvers are now rarely employed in the modern era of improved cardiopulmonary bypass and myocardial management.

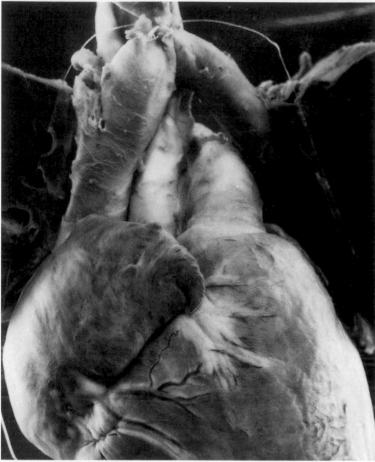

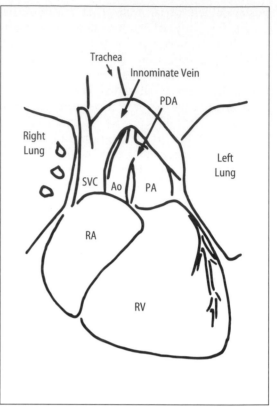

8.1 Partial anomalous pulmonary venous connection. A mounted heart is seen from the front with both lungs and the trachea attached. The left upper lobe pulmonary vein, seen at the top of the left lung, is connected to the innominate vein.

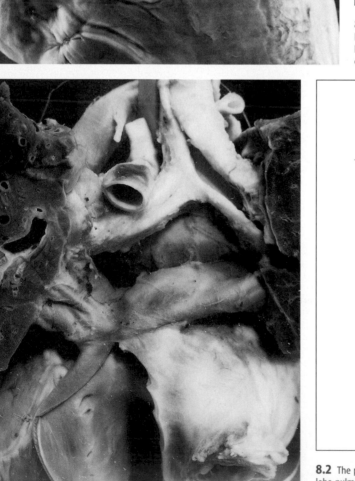

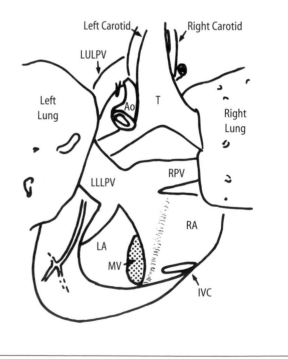

8.2 The posterior view of the heart illustrated in Figure 8.1 shows the left upper lobe pulmonary vein passing forwards to the innominate vein. The right and left lower pulmonary veins enter the left atrium which has been opened vertically.

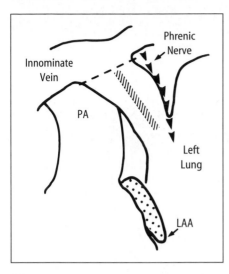

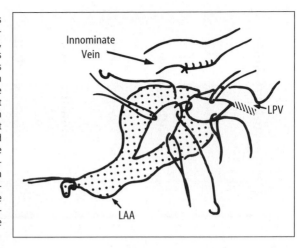

8.4 *(right)* The innominate vein is closed by direct suture and the pulmonary vein is mobilized to the lung, using the marked line to maintain its orientation. The left atrial appendage is retracted forward with a stay-suture on its tip. The limiting diameter of the appendage is its neck, so it is important to carry the incision across this junction on to the posterior wall of the left atrium. The pulmonary vein is incised anteriorly, just enough to match the atrial opening. An end-to-side anastomosis is constructed between the vein and the left atrium/left atrial appendage, taking care not to purse-string the running monofilament suture and letting the appendage come down to the vein.

8.3 *(above)* A single anomalous vein from one pulmonary lobe can be left uncorrected with little hemodynamic consequence, but intrapulmonary collateral channels may allow other segments to drain anomalously through this route, as suggested in this case by the large size of the vein. In the most commonly employed technique, successful translocation of the vein depends on an accurate anastomosis to the atrial appendage, with conservation of the three-dimensional geometric relationships of the anomalous vein to the lung. The operation can be done through a left thoracotomy using temporary occlusion of the left pulmonary artery, without cardiopulmonary bypass. However, a more controlled anastomosis is possible in the arrested heart. The pericardial reflection is divided and reflected laterally, noting that the phrenic nerve lies on the side of the ascending channel. A side-biting clamp is placed on the innominate vein and the left pulmonary vein is resected with as much length as possible. Rotation of the table towards the surgeon improves exposure for these maneuvers. A sterile pen is used to mark the anterior surface of the distended vein from its innominate connection to the lung hilum.

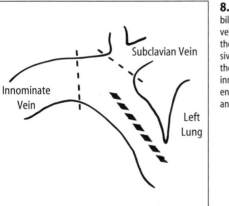

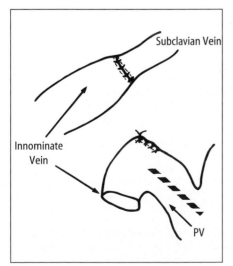

8.6 *(left)* A different technique which reduces the possibility of kinking, and hence obstructing the pulmonary vein, is to resect a segment of the innominate vein with the anomalous channel. It is necessary to mobilize extensively the innominate and left subclavian veins, as well as the proximal left internal jugular vein to do this. The innominate vein is then divided just proximal to the entrance of its internal jugular and subclavian tributaries and as far medially as possible (dashed lines).

8.5 *(above)* On completion, the left atrial appendage is extended outwards to the left as the front wall of the pulmonary venous channel and the back wall (pulmonary vein) reaches on to the posterior wall of the left atrium. Leaving as much pulmonary vein as possible between the anastomosis and lung hilum allows the vein to resume its upward curve and drain without kinking or obstruction, despite the changing of its direction of flow by more than 90°.

8.7 *(left)* The two ends of the innominate vein are joined with an end-to-end anastomosis, using a continuous monofilament suture. The upper incision in the segment of innominate vein which remains attached to the pulmonary vein is oversewn. This segment and the pulmonary vein are mobilized to the lung hilum, again taking care to preserve the phrenic nerve.

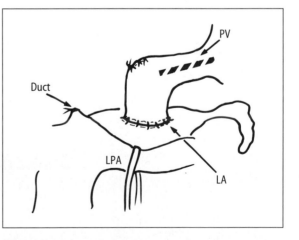

8.8 *(above)* The arterial duct or ligament is divided, and the proximal left pulmonary artery is mobilized and retracted forwards to expose the roof of the left atrium. Using the marked line on the front of the venous channel to maintain the correct orientation, the segment of innominate vein is anastomosed to a transverse incision on the roof of the atrium. This brings the pulmonary vein to drain to the left atrium through a large connection with less than 90° of rotation and does not use the more delicate tissues of the atrial appendage for the anastomosis. Its excellent patency rate justifies the more extensive operative procedure, which also conserves growth potential by tissue-to-tissue apposition.

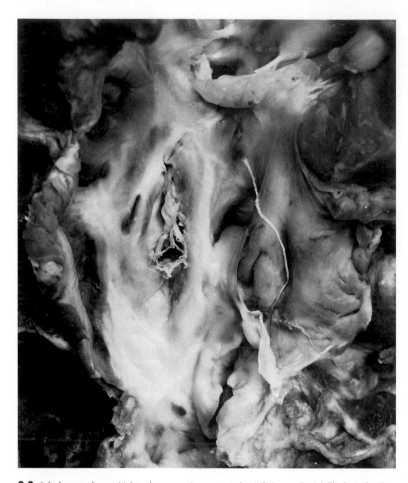

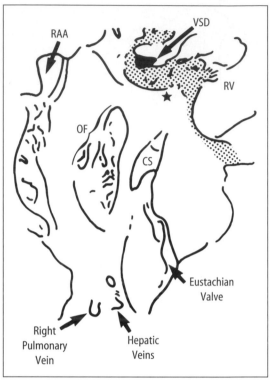

8.9 Scimitar syndrome (right pulmonary veins connected to inferior caval vein). The heart has been opened along the right atrial appendage and down the inferior caval vein below the diaphragm. There is a fenestrated atrial septal defect of the oval fossa and a perimembranous ventricular septal defect under the septal leaflet of the tricuspid valve. The coronary sinus is enlarged as a result of the drainage into it of a persistent left superior caval vein, which is not seen. The entrance of the right pulmonary veins, at the level of the hepatic veins, is unusually low in this specimen. A well-developed Eustachian valve (valve of the inferior caval vein) is present. The approximate position of the atrioventricular node is marked by a star. Hypoplasia of the right lung, which may or may not receive a pulmonary artery, often causes the heart to be rotated towards the right chest (dextrocardia) with anomalous connection of the right pulmonary veins to the inferior caval vein. Part of the right lung may be sequestrated and there are frequently anomalous systemic arteries from the coeliac axis to the sequestration. The term 'Scimitar' derives from the X-ray appearance of the anomalous vein which produces a comma- or sickle-shaped shadow in the right chest.

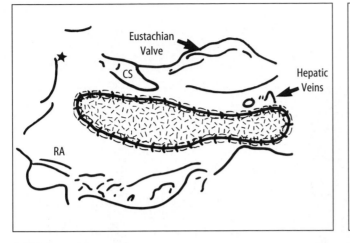

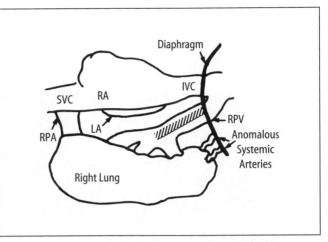

8.10 The conventional repair of Scimitar syndrome consists of enlargement of the interatrial communication by complete resection of the septum and tunnelling the anomalous vein through the atrial septal defect to the left atrium with a long pericardial patch. A period of circulatory arrest or femoral venous cannulation is necessary to place the patch between hepatic and pulmonary veins, and the tunnel must spiral at least 90° from the venous orifice on the side of the inferior caval vein to the atrial septal defect. There is thus a risk of obstruction to either the pulmonary or the hepatic/inferior caval veins. Moreover, this procedure is difficult in young patients.

8.11 A more satisfactory approach is via a right thoracotomy in the fifth intercostal space, with cannulation of the aorta, and the superior and inferior caval veins directly. Because it receives less than half of the pulmonary venous drainage, the left atrium tends to be small and confined behind the heart. The right pulmonary vein is traced to the diaphragm and its anterior surface marked with a line. Any anomalous systemic arteries are easily identified through this approach and divided prior to bypass. If indicated, a pulmonary sequestration can be resected before cardiopulmonary bypass or at the end of the procedure, after the administration of protamine.

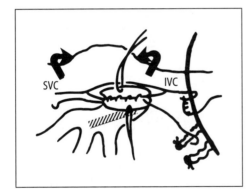

8.12 The clearly marked pulmonary vein is divided at the diaphragm or its junction with the inferior caval vein. The left atrium is small and to the left of the spine, but leftward rotation of the right atrium brings it into good view on the right side of the chest. After aortic cross-clamping, a longitudinal incision is made on the left atrium, which is then anastomosed to the opened-out pulmonary vein, using the marked line to avoid rotation.

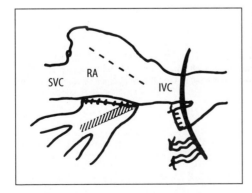

8.13 Upon completion, the anastomosis rotates to the back of the chest, producing a direct pathway for pulmonary venous drainage in the anatomical position. The usual oblique right atrial incision (dashed line) is then used to repair an atrial septal defect (present in about 30% of cases) or other associated anomalies. This approach is suitable for patients of all ages, although total circulatory arrest or periods of reduced flow may be preferable to cardiopulmonary bypass for visualization of the heart in small infants.

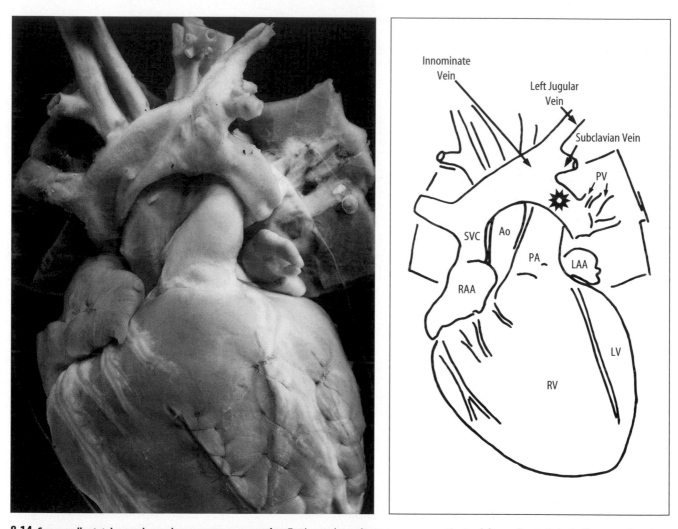

8.14 Supracardiac total anomalous pulmonary venous connection. Total anomalous pulmonary venous connection to a left ascending vertical vein. The mounted specimen is viewed anteriorly. The ascending vein (star) has been opened above its junction with the posterior common venous sinus to show segmental veins from the left upper lobe entering the left vertical vein by separate orifices. In this heart, the ascending channel passes in front of the pulmonary artery and thus is not obstructed. Alternatively, it may run between the left pulmonary artery and the left bronchus, in which case a vice-like mechanism compresses the vein. The left phrenic nerve (not seen) is closely applied to the lateral side of the ascending vein outside the pericardium. The innominate vein, right atrium and right ventricle are all enlarged as a result of the pulmonary venous return to the right side of the heart, while the left ventricle is small and does not reach the cardiac apex.

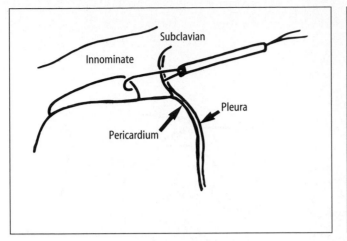

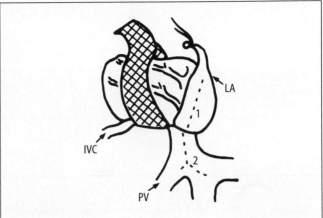

8.15 Using a vertical midline sternotomy, the left ascending vein is dissected extrapericardially, after removal of the thymus gland. The phrenic nerve on its lateral side is identified and preserved. Isolation of the vein at its junction with the innominate vein ensures that isolated pulmonary veins entering high up on the ascending channel will not be left draining anomalously. A snugger is placed around the ligature so that the channel may be closed during circulatory arrest and reopened to vent the left side of the heart during rewarming.

8.16 When a posterior approach is used, the surgeon moves to the left side of the operating table. Under total circulatory arrest, the venous cannula is removed and the heart is elevated towards the right in a gauze sling which has been passed into the oblique sinus behind the inferior caval vein. A ligature on the tip of the left atrial appendage helps to expose its posterior atrial wall, which is opened transversely (1). Unless there is obstruction of the pulmonary veins, the confluence (2) is left intact to keep the operative field dry at this time.

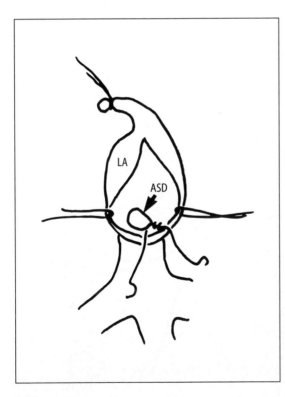

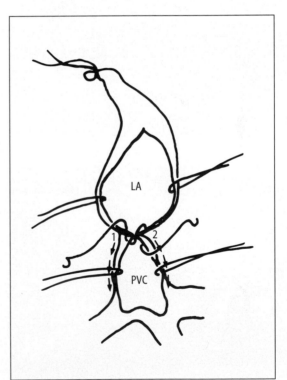

8.17 The atrial septal defect is closed, taking care not to incorporate the Eustachian valve at the lower margin and thus direct inferior caval return to the left atrium. Usually, direct suture is possible, but a large defect may require a pericardial patch. A central venous line can be retrieved across the atrial septal defect at this time for post-operative left atrial pressure monitoring.

8.18 The pulmonary venous confluence is opened (dashed line 2 in Figure 8.16) directly through the posterior pericardium which serves to buttress the suture line. Starting at the most distal point, a running 7/0 monofilament suture is used to approximate the left atrium to the confluence, allowing the left atrial appendage and heart to come down as the suture line progresses. It is neither necessary nor desirable to extend the incision in the confluence to the right pulmonary veins, as the channel will be adequate for their drainage towards the left. If additional length is needed, the atrial incision may be extended into the appendage and the pulmonary confluence into the ascending vertical vein. However, this is rarely necessary and the appendage, being thinner than the pulmonary venous confluence or left atrium, tends to bleed easily.

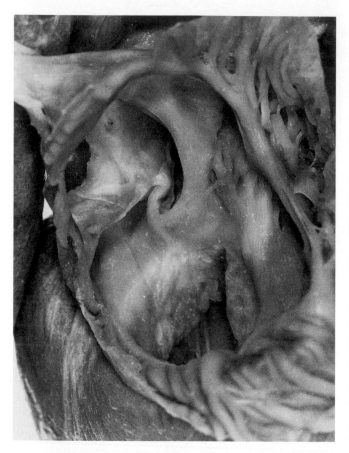

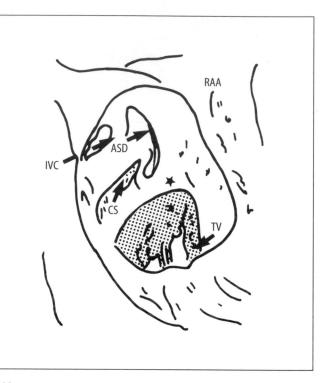

8.19 Total anomalous pulmonary venous connection to the coronary sinus. The right atrium has been opened along its appendage, showing an enlarged orifice of the coronary sinus and a defect of the valve of the oval fossa (atrial septal defect). A star indicates the position of the atrioventricular node at the apex of the triangle of Koch, above the tricuspid valve.

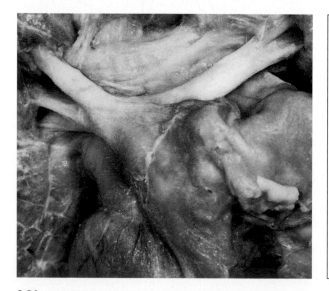

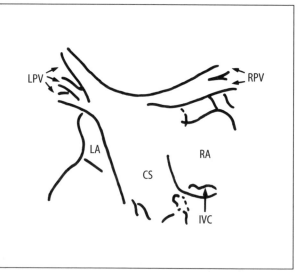

8.20 Posterior aspect of the heart shown above. All the pulmonary veins are connected to the enlarged coronary sinus which is in the normal position. In this case, the pulmonary venous confluence is attenuated and the veins all virtually enter the coronary sinus directly.

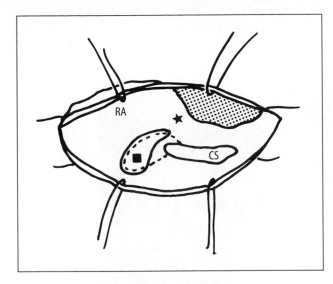

8.21 Surgical repair of total anomalous pulmonary venous connection to the coronary sinus is done through a right atriotomy, either on cardiopulmonary bypass with intermittent low flow or, in small infants, with profound hypothermia and total circulatory arrest. The posterior limbus and flap valve of the oval fossa (square) are excised, connecting the atrial septal defect with the orifice of the coronary sinus. These incisions are planned away from the area of the conduction tissue (star).

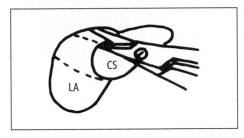

8.22 The common wall between the coronary sinus and left atrium is excised (as opposed to merely unroofing the coronary sinus by incision). The side towards the mitral valve is incised first, working from the orifice back towards the left pulmonary veins. The direction of this incision may be first explored by placing a pair of forceps into the coronary sinus through its orifice.

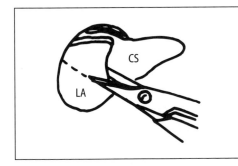

8.23 The upper margin of the coronary sinus is divided, taking care not to button-hole the posterior atrial wall. If an external communication is made, it is carefully repaired outside the heart to avoid narrowing the circumflex coronary artery.

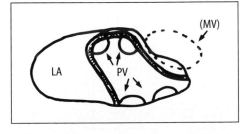

8.24 Leaving a small margin of coronary sinus tissue ensures an intact atrium without any risk of pulmonary venous obstruction. The right pulmonary veins frequently join the coronary sinus to the right of its orifice (actually in the pulmonary venous confluence) and, paradoxically, have greater risk of post-repair obstruction than the left veins. This is especially true if there is a well-developed pulmonary venous confluence which is narrowed at its junction with the coronary sinus. A clue to this situation, if it has not been demonstrated pre-operatively, is difficulty in visualizing the orifices of the right pulmonary veins after excision of the wall of the coronary sinus.

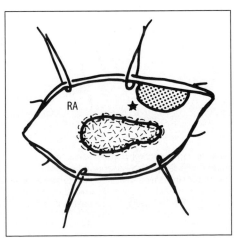

8.25 The atrial septal defect and the orifice of the coronary sinus are closed with a single peri-cardial patch, leaving the pulmonary veins and coronary sinus to drain within the left atrium. The suture line may be deviated inside the mouth of the coronary sinus to avoid the atri-oventricular node (star), but should come back on to the right atrial wall in front of the right pulmonary veins. While the combination of these two commonly used techniques (coronary sinus unroofing and tunnelling of its orifice across the atrial septum) usually achieves free drainage of both the right and left pulmonary veins, in cases where there is obstruction between the pulmonary venous confluence and the coronary sinus, it is necessary to anastomose the venous confluence directly to the posterior wall of the left atrium.

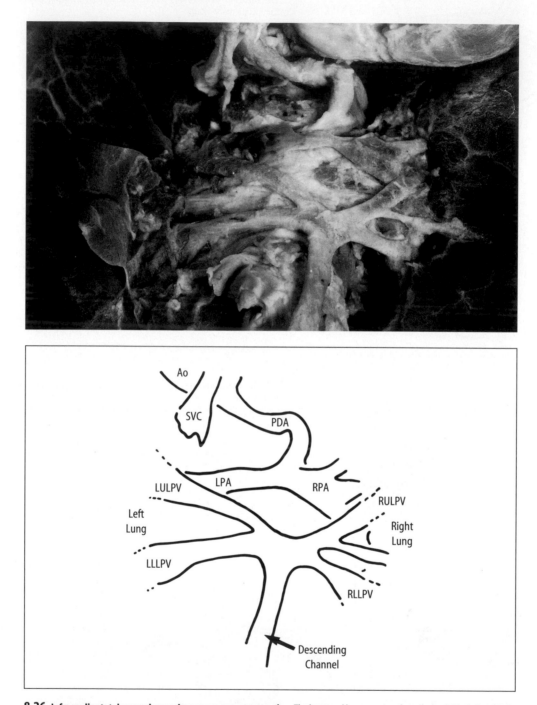

8.26 Infracardiac total anomalous pulmonary venous connection. The heart and lungs are seen from the back. The left and right pulmonary veins join a confluence which drains below the diaphragm by means of a descending channel. While all the veins in this case join the confluence at approximately the same level, it is not uncommon to have one or the other lower pulmonary vein connected near the diaphragm, the so-called "Christmas tree" arrangement. The remainder of the anatomy in this heart is complex, with pulmonary atresia and confluent branch pulmonary arteries supplied by a persistently patent arterial duct.

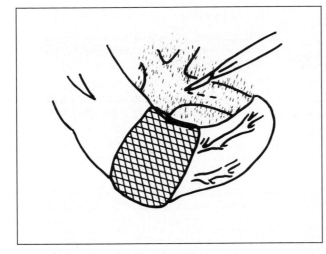

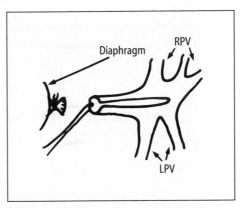

8.27 Repair of infracardiac total anomalous pulmonary venous connection is generally done with profound hypothermia and total circulatory arrest. The arterial duct is ligated immediately after going on bypass and a small incision is made through the posterior pericardium into the descending channel to decompress the obstructed pulmonary veins.

8.28 Under total circulatory arrest, with the heart elevated (see Figure 8.16) and the surgeon working from the left side, the descending channel is dissected to the diaphragm. When the pulmonary veins enter in a Christmas-tree fashion, it is important to identify the lowest vein. The descending channel is then ligated, divided and oversewn. A traction suture is placed on the cardiac end of the descending vein to maintain its orientation and it is incised upwards, taking care to stay in the midportion and not enter the orifice of a pulmonary vein.

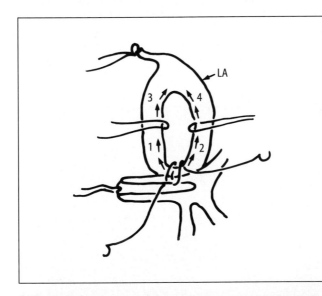

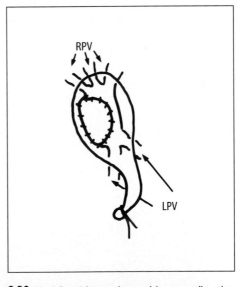

8.29 The pulmonary venous confluence tends to lie towards the diaphragm rather than directly behind the left atrium with infracardiac drainage. Division of the descending vein allows it to be brought up to the atrium without any tension. After closure of the atrial septal defect (see Figure 8.17), the confluence and descending channel are connected to the left atrium with a running monofilament suture. Dividing the suture line into four quadrants helps to avoid twisting the veins.

8.30 The left atrial appendage and heart are allowed to come down into the pericardium as the anastomosis progresses. On completion, the descending channel and pulmonary venous confluence effectively enlarge the volume of the left atrium, leaving the pulmonary veins themselves supported by the posterior pericardium and undistorted.

Suggested Reading

Arciprete P, McKay R, Watson GH, Hamilton DI, Wilkinson JL, Arnold R. Double connections in total anomalous pulmonary venous connection. J Thorac Cardiovasc Surg 1986;92:146.

Blake HA, Hall RJ, Manion WC. Anomalous pulmonary venous return. Circulation 1965;32:406.

DeLeon MM, DeLeon SY, Roughneen PT, Vitullo DA, Cetta F, Lagamayo L, Fisher EA. Recognition and management of obstructed pulmonary veins draining to the coronary sinus. Ann Thorac Surg 1997;63:741.

DeLisle G, Ando M, Calder AL, Zuberbuhler JR, Rochenmacher S, Alday LE, Mangino O, Van Praagh S, Van Praagh R. Total anomalous pulmonary venous connection:a report of 93 autopsied cases with emphasis on diagnostic and surgical considerations. Am Heart J 1976;91:99.

Giamberti A, Deanfield JE, Anderson RH, de Leval MR. Totally anomalous pulmonary venous connection directly to the superior caval vein. Eur J Cardiothorac Surg 2002;21:474.

Jonas RA, Smolinsky A, Mayer JE, Castenada AR. Obstructed pulmonary venous drainage with total anomalous pulmonary venous connection to the coronary sinus. Am J Cardiol 1987;59:431.

Kakadekar A, McKay R, Tyrrell M. Experience with total anomalous pulmonary venous connection (TAPVC) in a provincial pediatric cardiac program. Heart Views 2001;2:174.

Kawashima Y, Matsuda H, Nakano S, Miyamoto IC, Pugino M, Kozaka T, Manabe H. Tree-shaped pulmonary veins in infracardiac total anomalous pulmonary venous drainage. Ann Thorac Surg 1977;23:436.

Nakib A, Moller JH, Kanjuh VI, Edwards JE. Anomalies of the pulmonary veins. Am J Cardiol 1967;20:77.

Neill CA. Development of the pulmonary veins with reference to the embryology of anomalies of pulmonary venous return. Pediatrics 1956;18:880.

Neill CA, Ferencz C, Sabiston DC, Sheldon H. The familial occurrence of hypoplastic right lung with systemic arterial supply and venous drainage "scimitar syndrome". The Johns Hopkins Medical Journal 1960;107:1.

Roe BR. Posterior approach to correction of total anomalous pulmonary venous return. Further experience. J Thorac Cardiovasc Surg 1970;59:748.

Serraf A, Belli E, Roux D, Sousa-Uva M, Lacour-Gayet F, Planche C. Modified superior approach for repair of supracardiac and mixed total anomalous pulmonary venous drainage. Ann Thorac Surg 1998;65:1391.

Tucker BL, Lindesmith GG, Stiles QR, Meyer BW. Superior approach for correction of the supracardiac type of total anomalous pulmonary venous return. Ann Thorac Surg 1976;22:374.

Van Praagh R, Harken AH, DeLisle G, Ando M, Gross RE. Total anomalous pulmonary venous drainage to the coronary sinus: A revised procedure for its correction. J Thorac Cardiovasc Surg 1972;64:132.

Van Praagh S, Carrera ME, Sanders S, Mayer JE Jr, Van Praagh R. Partial or total direct pulmonary venous drainage to right atrium due to malposition of septum primum. Anatomic and echocardiographic findings and surgical treatment: a study based on 36 cases. Chest 1995;107:1488.

Vargas FJ, Kreutzer GO. A surgical technique for correction of total anomalous pulmonary venous drainage. J Thorac Cardiovasc Surg 1985;90:410.

Ward KE, Mullins CE, Huhta JC, Nihill MR, McNamara DG, Cooley DA. Restrictive interatrial communication in total anomalous pulmonary venous connection. Am J Cardiol 1986;57:1131.

Wukasch DC, Deutsch M, Reul GJ, Hallman GL, Cooley DA. Total anomalous pulmonary venous return: review of 125 patients treated surgically. Ann Thorac Surg 1975;19:622.

9 Anomalous Systemic Venous Connection

Introduction

The most common pattern of systemic venous connection to the heart is that of right-sided superior and inferior caval veins joining the morphologically right atrium. Variations from this "normal" arrangement probably occur in more than 0.5% of the population but rarely produce outward manifestations because the anomalous pathway still returns deoxygenated systemic blood to the right side of the circulation. Their interest from the morphologist's perspective lies in their reflection of developmental anatomy, although the frequency of abnormal connections negates the use of systemic venous connections as a guide to identification of cardiac chambers in complex malformations. In addition to correction of the anomalous venous connection itself, their importance in clinical work relates to venous access to the heart (for example, in cardiac catheterization or placement of transvenous pacemaker leads), management of cardiopulmonary bypass and technical modifications to the repair of the cardiac malformations with which they are associated.

The anomaly encountered most frequently is a left superior caval vein, manifesting a persistence of the left anterior cardinal vein. It occurs in 3–5% of congenitally malformed hearts and one of every 350 post-mortem examinations. The left superior caval vein is formed at the junction of the left internal jugular and subclavian veins. It passes vertically downwards in front of the left pulmonary artery, in the fold of Marshall, and terminates near the base of the left atrial appendage, usually in the coronary sinus. The left phrenic nerve lies along its lateral aspect. In about 40% of cases, a left innominate vein also connects the left superior caval vein to a right superior caval vein. In about 40% of patients with a left superior caval vein, there are associated cardiac defects (atrial septal defect being the most common). A deficiency in the wall of the coronary sinus will cause a left superior caval vein to drain anomalously into the left atrium – the so-called "unroofed coronary sinus"

syndrome." Unroofing may occur anywhere along the shared wall between the left atrium and coronary sinus, but most defects are found near the orifice of the coronary sinus or in its midportion. When the coronary sinus is completely absent, the left superior caval vein terminates directly in the roof of the left atrium, which then communicates with the right atrium through a defect at the anticipated site of the orifice of the coronary sinus.

Much less commonly, the inferior caval vein or hepatic veins connect directly to the left atrium. An extremely rare malformation is drainage of the right superior caval vein to the left atrium. The infrahepatic segment of the inferior caval vein may be absent, in which case systemic venous return passes either to the azygos (right) or hemiazygos (left) vein. These two veins terminate in the right and left superior caval veins respectively. In such patients, the hepatic veins usually join the right atrium directly by single or multiple orifices. A further anomaly, generally seen in patients with obstructed outflow of the left atrium (mitral valvar atresia), is a venous channel which lies between the roof of the left atrium and a systemic vein other than the left superior caval vein, passing *behind* the pulmonary artery and left bronchus. This has been called the "levoatrial cardinal vein" and probably serves to decompress the left atrium by blood-flowing from the cardiac chamber into the systemic vein, as opposed to the usual drainage of the vein into the heart.

With the advent of surgical interventions based upon non-invasive cardiac investigations, precise and complete definition of systemic venous anomalies is not invariably available to the surgeon pre-operatively. An enlarged coronary sinus on echocardiography usually can be traced to the persistent left superior caval vein but, in the absence of a contrast (bubble) study, the presence of a connecting innominate vein and the possibility of unroofed coronary sinus often remain uncertain. Completely unroofed coronary sinus with a left caval vein terminating in the left atrium may be missed altogether, because the patients rarely have clinical cyanosis and the coronary sinus is not enlarged on echocardiography. A clue to this diagnosis at the time of surgery is an unexpectedly small orifice at the mouth of the coronary sinus in the presence of a large left caval vein. Similarly, an unusually large azygos or hemiazygos vein which is discovered during thoracotomy for a systemic-pulmonary shunt or repair of aortic coarctation, should suggest the possibility of interruption of the inferior caval vein with azygos continuation. In this situation, it cannot be divided for access to the pulmonary artery or other vascular structures.

Beyond their obvious importance in the management of cardiopulmonary bypass, anomalies of systemic venous connection may also complicate otherwise standard surgical procedures. A large left superior caval vein limits exposure of the left branch pulmonary artery, making the reconstruction of a stenotic segment – for example, in tetralogy of Fallot – technically challenging. High direct cannulation and extensive mobilization of the vein are necessary in this situation to gain access to the left pulmonary artery. Even a small persistent left superior caval vein in continuity with the innominate vein may steal a significant proportion of the pulmonary blood-flow after bidirectional cavopulmonary anastomosis on the right side or flood the operative field (washing out cardioplegia) during

cardiopulmonary bypass. These small channels should, therefore, be sought routinely and ligated securely. They may be divided with impunity when necessary for access to the left pulmonary artery or veins. If a hemodynamically important caval vein drains to the coronary sinus, the ostium of the coronary sinus must be left in the systemic venous atrium after intra-atrial repairs. In atrioventricular septal defect, this means that the atrial patch is brought posteriorly around the annulus of the left atrioventricular valve. In the Senning operation, it requires the coronary sinus to be cut back to drain into the caval pathway. One final dilemma is the discovery of a pressure monitoring line from the femoral vein entering the right atrium directly in a patient for bidirectional cavopulmonary anastomosis when pre-operative cardiac catheterization has demonstrated an azygos continuation of the inferior caval vein. This indicates a dual system of venous channels from the lower half of the body. Occlusion of the azygos vein may leave inadequate lower body venous drainage, while failure to occlude it will certainly allow run-off from the pulmonary artery to the right atrium (venovenous shunt) and produce profound hypoxia after cavopulmonary anastomosis. Options here include construction of a complete Fontan circulation (if possible) or intraoperative femoral venography to determine the relative importance of the two systems. If this shows that sacrifice of the azygos vein is not possible, a Fontan circulation with an adjustable atrial septal defect or generous fenestration is probably the best approach.

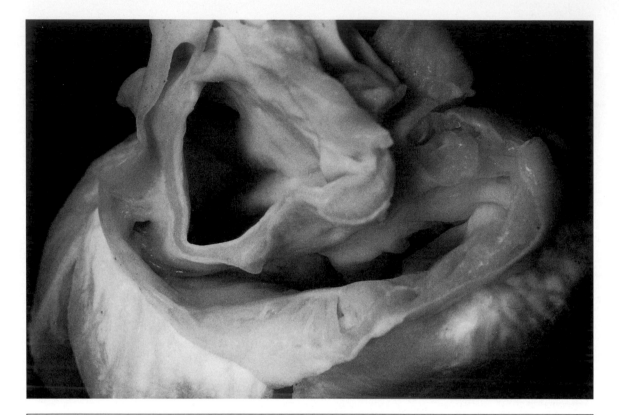

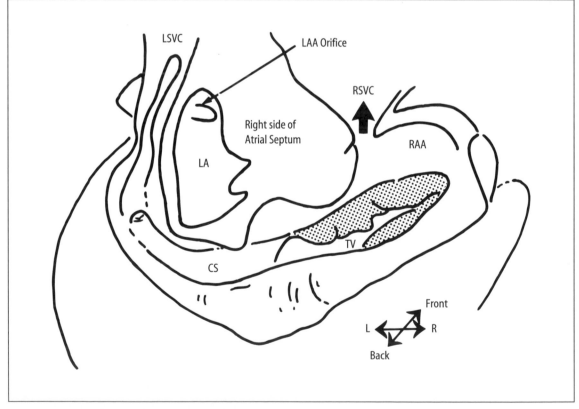

9.1 Left superior caval vein draining to the coronary sinus. The heart is viewed from the back with the top of the atriums and coronary sinus removed. A persistent left superior caval vein enters the enlarged coronary sinus which terminates normally in the right atrium. The atrial septum has been rotated leftward to show the normal entrance of the right superior caval vein into the right atrium.

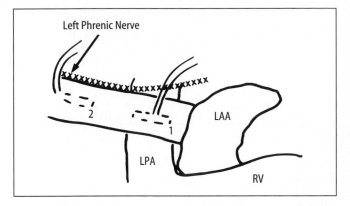

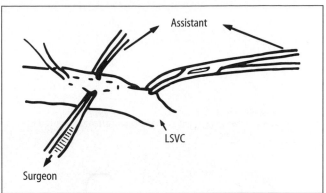

9.2 When the left superior caval vein is very small (1–2 mm), it should be ligated to prevent washout of the cardioplegia and myocardial reperfusion during aortic cross-clamping. However, while a larger vein may be snared during bypass if an innominate vein is present and left internal jugular pressure does not exceed about 18–20 mm Hg., drainage is preferable whenever its size approaches that of the right superior caval vein. Direct cannulation has the advantage of leaving the right atrium free for surgical access. The left atrial appendage is depressed downward, taking care not to compress branches of the left coronary artery. Depending on the level of cannulation (1- routinely; 2- for a cavopulmonary connection or access to a left pulmonary artery), a tape is passed around the vein in front of the left pulmonary artery or higher. Extreme care should be exercised to avoid injury to the phrenic nerve which lies on the lateral side of the vein extra-pericardially. The purse-string for cannulation is a narrow rectangle to avoid subsequent narrowing of the vessel.

9.3 After cardiopulmonary bypass has been established, the superior caval vein is retracted downward by the assistant using a curved clamp which has caught the anterior vessel wall. A second fine curved clamp is used by the assistant's other hand to place slight tension opposite the surgeon's forceps in the middle of the purse-string. Using a pointed knife (no. 11 blade), an incision is made from below upwards with the knife blade facing upwards. The incision is gently dilated with a curved mosquito which is also passed up the vein to be certain of the angle for cannulation and to exclude any obstruction (for example, by a central venous cannula).

9.4 *(left)* A right-angle, thin-walled metal or plastic cannula with side holes, is inserted, using the tip of the bevel to gently enter the vein.

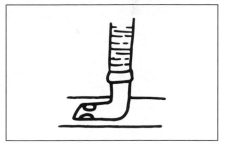

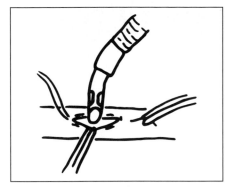

9.5 Once the entire tip of the cannula is within the lumen of the vessel, the cannula is rotated 90° clockwise and advanced to the right-angled bend. If any resistance is encountered, the cannula is completely withdrawn and the pathway explored again to avoid dissection of the vein. The cannula is secured with the snugger ("keeper"), carefully avoiding any rotation or twisting which would bring the side or end holes against the wall of the vein.

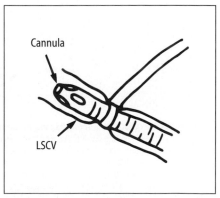

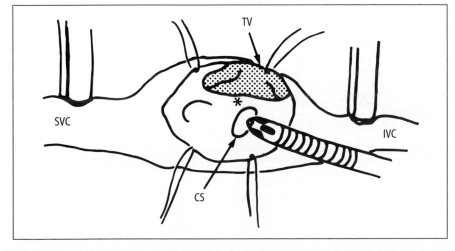

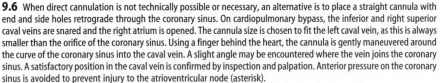

9.6 When direct cannulation is not technically possible or necessary, an alternative is to place a straight cannula with end and side holes retrograde through the coronary sinus. On cardiopulmonary bypass, the inferior and right superior caval veins are snared and the right atrium is opened. The cannula size is chosen to fit the left caval vein, as this is always smaller than the orifice of the coronary sinus. Using a finger behind the heart, the cannula is gently maneuvered around the curve of the coronary sinus into the caval vein. A slight angle may be encountered where the vein joins the coronary sinus. A satisfactory position in the caval vein is confirmed by inspection and palpation. Anterior pressure on the coronary sinus is avoided to prevent injury to the atrioventricular node (asterisk).

9.7 The cannula is held in the left superior caval vein by the snugger which is positioned just below the side-holes. If excessive venous return obscures landmarks in the right atrium during cannulation, pump flow is decreased briefly to visualize the coronary sinus and insert the cannula. The cannula may be left in place until the right atrium is nearly closed and the inferior caval vein unsnared to accommodate return from the coronary sinus, or it may be removed with a sucker in the right atrium during closure.

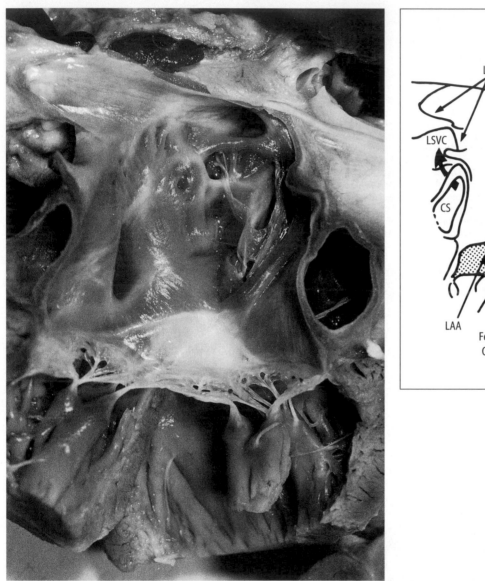

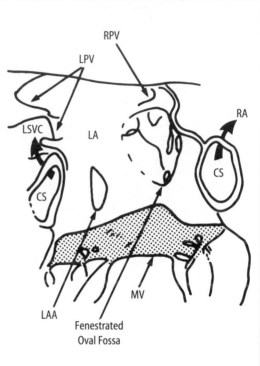

9.8 **Left superior caval vein draining to coronary sinus.** Left atrial view. The heart has been cut vertically across the atrioventricular junction and opened out like a book hinged on the aortic leaflet of the mitral valve. The posterior wall of the left atrium has also been rotated upwards to show the entrance of the pulmonary veins. A left superior caval vein joins the greatly enlarged coronary sinus beside the orifice of the left atrial appendage. Although the coronary sinus was intact prior to dissection of this heart, its divided end towards the right atrium now demonstrates the location where a coronary sinus interatrial communication would be found and its relation to the oval fossa defect (fenestrated). The mitral valve is supported by two papillary muscles, but the intercordal spaces are partially filled by leaflet tissue, resulting in short tendinous cords and the potential for an obstructive "funnel-type" valve. Unroofing of the coronary sinus may occur at any point either side of the two cut ends shown in this photograph, causing a left superior caval vein to drain into the left atrium

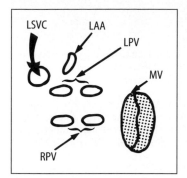

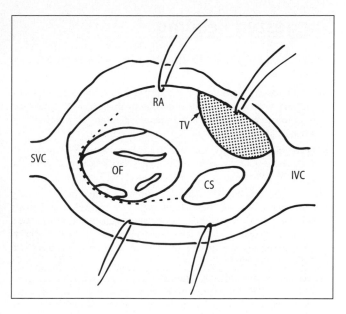

9.10 *(right)* One method of repair of unroofed coronary sinus syndrome is to baffle the left superior caval vein across the roof of the left atrium. Exposure is set up through an oblique incision in the right atrium. The septum is incised towards the limbus and the coronary sinus atrial septal defect (dashed line).

9.9 *(above)* As shown schematically in a surgeon's view of the left atrium, when the coronary sinus is completely unroofed, a persistent left superior caval vein always enters the roof of the left atrium in between the orifices of the left atrial appendage and the left upper pulmonary vein. If the vein has been cannulated directly, it will be possible to feel the cannula in the lumen with an instrument passed upwards from the left atrium, which aids positive identification of the systemic venous orifice. Alternatively, under circulatory arrest, gentle inflation of the lungs will return pink blood from the pulmonary veins, also helping to demonstrate the entrance of the left pulmonary veins and hence that of the left superior caval vein by exclusion.

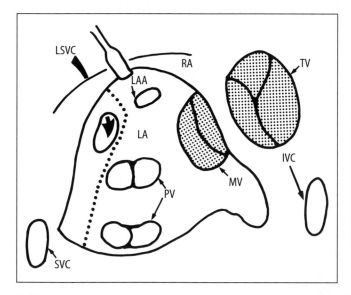

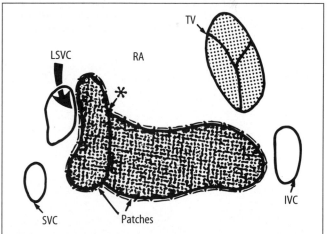

9.11 Retraction of the atrial septum leftward displays the orifice of the left superior caval vein in the left atrium. A patch is sutured across the back of the left atrium between the orifice of the left superior caval vein and pulmonary veins/left atrial appendage (dotted line). Anteriorly, the patch is brought to the remnant of atrial septum, partitioning the left atrium into upper and lower chambers.

9.12 Even a small remnant of atrial septum (such as that left after excision of the fenestrated oval fossa) is useful to distance the suture lines from the conduction tissue. The atrial septal defects (in the oval fossa and coronary sinus) are closed in continuity with a patch which lies at right angles to the upper one coming across the top of the left atrium. It is useful in this situation to use two separate patches which simplifies the geometry of the complex pathways. They are then joined together (asterisk). Everything behind the baffle (pulmonary veins) will drain to the mitral valve and everything in front (caval veins) will drain to the tricuspid valve.

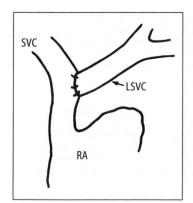

9.13 *(left)* An alternative technique consists of anastomosing the divided left superior caval vein to the side of the right superior caval vein or the right atrial appendage, with closure of the coronary sinus interatrial communication. This requires the presence of a reasonably good-size right caval vein and extensive mobilization of both vessels. As the left superior caval vein comes to lie in front of the aorta, it may be at risk of damage during any subsequent resternotomy.

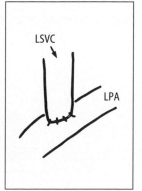

9.14 When the right ventricle or tricuspid valve is hypoplastic, another option is to place the divided left caval vein on the left pulmonary artery as a bidirectional cavopulmonary anastomosis – a so-called "one and three-quarter ventricle" repair. Unlike the right pulmonary artery which lies at a right angle to the superior caval vein, the left pulmonary artery passes obliquely backwards. Marking the anterior surface of the caval vein prior to its division helps to maintain the proper orientation for the anastomosis. If an innominate or hemiazygos vein is present, this is occluded to prevent retrograde flow of blood from the higher-pressure pulmonary artery into the systemic venous circulation.

Suggested Reading

Campbell M, Deuchar DC. The left-sided superior vena cava. Br Heart J 1954;16:423.

Chiu I-S, Hegerty A, Anderson RH, de Leval MR. The landmarks to the atrioventricular conduction system in hearts with absence or unroofing of the coronary sinus. J Thorac Cardiovasc Surg 1985;90:297.

de Leval MR, Ritter DG, McGoon DC, Danielson GK. Anomalous systemic venous connection. Surgical considerations. Mayo Clin Proc 1975;50:599.

Edwards JE, DuShane JW. Thoracic venous anomalies I. Vascular connection between the left atrium and the left innominate vein (levoatriocardinal vein) associated with mitral atresia and premature closure of the foramen ovale (case 1). II. Pulmonary veins draining wholly into the ductus venosus (case 2). Arch Pathol 1950;49:517.

Fischer DR, Zuberbuhler JR. Anomalous systemic venous return. In: Anderson RH, Macartney FJ, Shinebourne EA, Tynan M (eds) Paediatric Cardiology, Vol 1. Edinburgh: Churchill Livingstone, 1987;497.

Freedom RM, Culham JAG, Rowe RD. Left atrial to coronary sinus fenestration (partially unroofed coronary sinus): Morphological and angiocardiographic observations. Br Heart J 1981;46:63.

Gueron M, Hirsh M, Borman J. Total anomalous systemic venous drainage into the left atrium. Report of a case of successful surgical correction. J Thorac Cardiovasc Surg 1969;58:570.

Kadletz M, Black MD, Smallhorn J, Freedom RM, Van Praagh S. Total anomalous systemic venous drainage to the coronary sinus in association with hypoplastic left heart disease: more than a mere coincidence. J Thorac Cardiovasc Surg 1997;144:282.

Kakadekar A, McKay, R, Tyrrell MJ. Isolated right superior caval vein to left atrium connection: Non-invasive neonatal diagnosis. Cardiol Young 1999;9:310.

Lee ME, Sade RM. Coronary sinus septal defect. Surgical considerations. J Thorac Cardiovasc Surg 1979;78:563.

McElhinney DB, Reddy VN, Moore P, Hanley FL. Bidirectional cavopulmonary shunt in patients with anomalies of systemic and pulmonary venous drainage. Ann Thorac Surg 1997;63:1676.

Sand ME, McGrath LB, Pacifico AD, Mandke NV. Repair of left superior vena cava entering the left atrium. Ann Thorac Surg 1986;42:560.

Winter FS. Persistent left superior vena cava. Angiology 1954;5:90.

10 Supravalvar Mitral Ring

Introduction

Supravalvar mitral ring is a rare anomaly. Thick fibrous tissue extends from the left atrial endocardium to form a diaphragm, which is often circumferential, between the left atrium and the leaflets of the mitral valve. The membrane is usually attached directly to the aortic (anterior) mitral leaflet, several millimetres inside the valvar annulus. It spirals back up to the atrial wall above the mural (posterior) mitral leaflet. The left atrial appendage and the pulmonary veins thus lie together on one side of the membrane, while the leaflets of the mitral valve are on the other. The degree of obstruction caused by the diaphragm is variable but tends to be more severe when the ring is an isolated anomaly. This occurs in about half of the cases and the mitral valve then tends to be normal. In the other half, there are associated lesions, usually involving either the mitral valve itself, the left ventricular outflow tract or the aorta. Surgical removal of the ring can be done by blunt dissection, analogous to enucleation of the fibrous tissue in subaortic stenosis. This technique offers the advantage of removing some of the thickened surrounding endocardium so that both the leaflets and the annulus of the mitral valve are fully mobilized. Following complete removal of the ring in this manner, the mitral annulus appears to spring open by several millimetres.

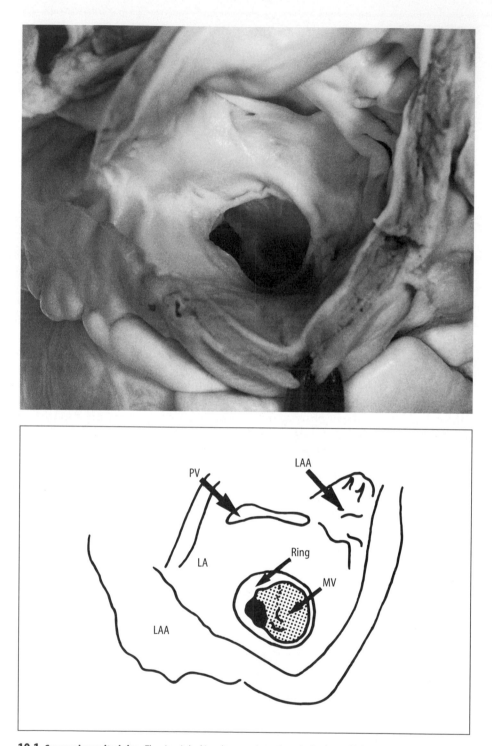

10.1 Supravalvar mitral ring. The view is looking downwards on the mitral valve and left atrium. The ring consists of tough fibrous tissue which encroaches on to the aortic (anterior) mitral leaflet (head of arrow) and is otherwise contiguous with the thickened left atrial endocardium. In contrast with partitioning of the left atrium, both the pulmonary veins and left atrial appendage lie above the membrane and the mitral valve below.

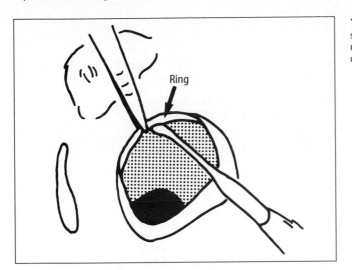

10.2 The ring is approached either through the left atrium or across the interatrial septum. Blunt dissection with a Watson-Cheyne is begun between the ring and the aortic mitral leaflet, elevating the ring with slight traction. Because the valve leaflet is more delicate than the ring, it is gently peeled away from the fibrous tissue.

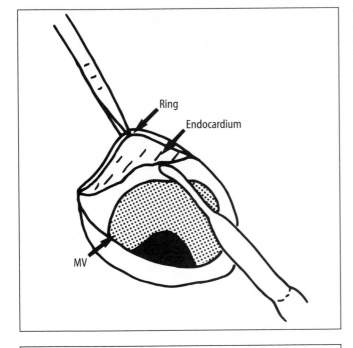

10.3 Having found the plane between the ring and anterior mitral leaflet, dissection is carried outwards into the endocardium and also posteriorly, where the ring is usually attached at the junction of the mural leaflet and the annulus. Carrying the dissection several millimetres outside the mitral annulus removes the thickened surrounding endocardium and allows the mitral valve to open up fully.

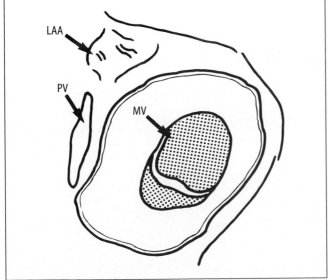

10.4 After removal of the ring, the valve is inspected carefully for damage as well as possible associated lesions involving the leaflets, tendinous chords or papillary muscles. These are dealt with as necessary to achieve a competent and unrestricted orifice (see Chapter 14).

Suggested Reading

Anabtawi IW, Ellison RG. Congenital stenosing ring of the atrioventricular canal (supravalvar mitral stenosis). J Thorac Cardiovasc Surg 1965;49:994.

Carpentier A, Branchini B, Cour JC, Asfaow E, Villani M, Deloche A, Relland J, D'Allaines C, Blondeau P, Piwmica A, Parenzan L, Brom G. Congenital malformations of the mitral valve in children. J Thorac Cardiovasc Surg 1976;72:854.

Chung KJ, Manning JA, Lipchik EO. Isolated supravalvar stenosing ring of the left atrium: diagnosis before operation and successful surgical treatment. Chest 1974;65:25.

Collins-Nakai RL, Rosenthal A, Castaneda AR, Bernhard WF, Nadas AS. Congenital mitral stenosis: a review of 20 years' experience. Circulation 1977;56:1039.

Coto EO, Judez VM, Juffe A, Rufilanchas JJ, Tellez G, Maronas J, Aymerich DF. Supravalvar stenotic mitral ring. J Thorac Cardiovasc Surg 1976;71:537.

Davichi F, Moller JH, Edwards JE. Diseases of the mitral valve in infancy. Circulation 1971;43:565.

McKay R, Ross DW. Technique for relief of discrete subaortic stenosis. J Thorac Cardiovasc Surg 1982;84:917.

Neirotti R, Kreutzer G, Galindez E, Becu L, Ross D. Supravalvar mitral stenosis associated with ventricular septal defect. Am J Dis Child 1977;131:862.

Rogers HM, Waldron BR, Murphy DFH, Edwards JE. Supravalvar stenosing ring of the left atrium in association with endocardial sclerosis (endocardial fibroelastosis) and mitral insufficiency. Am Heart J 1955;50:777.

Shone JD, Sellers RD, Anderson RC, Adams P Jr, Lillehei CW, Edwards JE. The developmental complex of 'parachute mitral valve', supravalvar ring of the left atrium, subaortic stenosis and coarctation of the aorta. Am J Cardiol 1963;11:714.

3

Four-chambered Hearts with Concordant Atrioventricular and Ventriculo-arterial Connections

11 Ventricular Septal Defect (Interventricular Communication)

Introduction

A ventricular septal defect is a communication – less elegantly called a "hole" – through which the cavities of the left and right ventricles are connected with each other. It is the most common congenital cardiac malformation. Ventricular septal defects occur as "isolated" or "primary" malformations, which are discussed in this chapter, or as intrinsic components of more complex cardiac lesions. The latter include such malformations as tetralogy of Fallot, common arterial trunk and atrioventricular septal defect, and will be considered in the subsequent relevant sections.

The term "isolated" ventricular septal defect implies the presence of concordant atrioventricular and ventriculo-arterial connections. Such defects, however, not infrequently have major or minor associated lesions of the heart and/or great arteries, the most common being a persistently patent arterial duct, coarctation of the aorta, subvalvar aortic obstruction and mitral valvar anomalies. Truly isolated ventricular septal defects make up about half of those in surgical series and a much smaller proportion of hearts seen at post-mortem examination.

Isolated ventricular septal defects may occur in any part of the septum. The position of the defect has distinct implications for its relations to the specialized conducting tissue and leaflets of the atrioventricular or semilunar valves, its margins for closure and the potential for either spontaneous closure or development of valvar complications.

Efforts to categorize ventricular septal defects anatomically, however, have resulted in conflicting and confusing classifications (see Suggest Reading), none of which is entirely faultless for both morphological and clinical application. In part, this situation derives from the fact that the left and right sides of the ventricular septum do not match each other precisely (i.e. a defect opening into the inlet portion of the right ventricle, for example, may communicate with the outlet portion of the left ventricle). Apart from these circumstances, there are differences in the septal components of the normal heart, upon which some classifications have been based, and those with ventricular septal defects, to which the classification is then applied. An example of this latter situation is that part of the septum which lies in the outlet of the heart, but in the normal heart is so small that it cannot be distinguished without careful dissection. It lies at the ventricular end of the discrete sleeve of outlet myocardium which is the subpulmonary infundibulum. However, in many congenitally malformed hearts, the septal portion between the ventricular outlets is a well-developed, easily identifiable structure and there is no difficulty in relating it to a ventricular septal defect. Under extreme conditions, such as double outlet right ventricle, the outlet part of the septum may be totally a right ventricular structure. Other pitfalls include nomenclature derived from developmental biology and classifications which depend on cardiac structures that are themselves either inconsistent or difficult to identify (such as the "supraventricular crest"). Some classifications have proved too simple to convey the relevant anatomical information, while others are too complex for practical application.

For the purposes of this chapter, ventricular septal defects are described arbitrarily according to where they open within the right ventricle. The rationale for this is that virtually all isolated ventricular septal defects are approached surgically on the right ventricular side of the septum. The left ventricular opening of the defect, however, is illustrated also in each case and, wherever useful, reference is made to other systems of commonly used terminology.

In a four-chambered heart with usual atrioventricular and ventriculo-arterial connections, the right and left ventricle can each be separated into three components – namely, the inlet, the apical (trabecular) and outlet portions. Each of these is separated from its counterpart on the other side of the heart by a portion of the interventricular septum, but the boundaries of the inlet, apical and outlet parts of the ventricles are mismatched from one side to the other. Despite this arrangement, it is helpful for the surgeon to be able to identify landmarks within the right ventricle which indicate its inlet, outlet and trabecular regions, each encompassing its own area of septum. These three portions abut on and radiate outwards from the smaller membranous intraventricular septum that borders the inner curvature of the heart. Most defects are situated around this area. Accordingly, the "inlet" septum of the right ventricle is the part which is bounded on the right ventricular side by the tricuspid valvar leaflets and the point of attachment of its subvalvar apparatus to the septal surface. The "outlet" septum is that part which lies above (distally to) the body of the septomarginal trabeculation. In the presence of a septal defect at the outlet of the heart, if a bar of muscle can be seen below the arterial valves and separating them, this structure is the "outlet" septum. The remaining part of the septum reaches to the apex of the heart and is the "trabecular" or "apical" portion. The medial papillary muscle complex is taken as the border between the inlet and outlet of the right ventricle and thus lies anteriorly (to the surgeon's left hand) to inlet defects and posteriorly (to the surgeon's right hand) to outlet defects, as viewed through the tricuspid valve.

Small defects which are exclusive to the membranous septum are extremely rare. When a ventricular septal defect extends to the membranous septum from a part of the muscular septum, there is fibrous continuity between the aortic, tricuspid and usually the mitral valves. This area of fibrous continuity forms one border of the defect. Such ventricular septal defects are called "perimembranous" or "paramembranous" and invariably extend well beyond the membranous septum, although they are sometimes confined to either the inlet, trabecular or outlet portions of the right ventricle. They are then classified as either "perimembranous inlet," "perimembranous trabecular" or "perimembranous outlet" defects, which means that the defect opens into that portion of the septum which is designated as such in the right ventricle. "Malalignment" defects may also be perimembranous or may have completely muscular margins. In the case of large perimembranous defects which extend into more than one component of the right ventricle, the terms "conjoined" or "confluent" have been used to emphasize their extent.

The conduction system consistently lies along the posterior margin of perimembranous defects (to the surgeon's right hand, as viewed from the right atrium). Perimembranous outlet defects tend to be related more to the anterosuperior leaflet than to the septal leaflet of the tricuspid valve, and their excavation towards the outlet septum may cause the aortic valve to override the

defect. While the basic position of the conduction tissue remains posterior to the perimembranous outlet defect, it is less likely to be on the immediate crest of the septum than it would be with the perimembranous inlet defect.

Defects which reach to the pulmonary valve frequently have as their superior margin an area of fibrous continuity between the aortic and pulmonary valves, the so-called "absence of the outlet septum." Because they lie immediately beneath both arterial outlets, these defects have been called "doubly committed," "subarterial," or "juxta-arterial" ventricular septal defects. Commonly, the doubly committed subarterial defect has a muscular lower rim formed by fusion between the ventriculo-infundibular fold and the septomarginal trabeculation which separates the defect from the tricuspid valve and the conduction tissue. Alternatively, however, such ventricular septal defects may extend to the membranous septum, in which case there is fibrous continuity between all four cardiac valves and the posterior margin is closely related to the conduction tissue.

Those defects which do not involve the membranous area have completely muscular borders and may occur in any part of the septum. Moreover, they may be multiple or coexist with a perimembranous defect. A posterior (inferior), muscular defect, for example, opening into the inlet of the right ventricle is separated from the tricuspid valve by a rim of muscle. The axis of the conduction system then passes anteriorly to this type of defect, generally following the shortest pathway from atrioventricular node to ventricular septum, and will be found related to the margin towards the surgeons' left hand, again working through the tricuspid valve. Other muscular defects (mid-trabecular, apical and multiple defects along the septomarginal trabeculation) may be close to fascicles of the conduction tissue, but are not usually related to the more important, proximal non-branching bundle. When muscular and perimembranous defects coexist, the conduction axis may run between them, in the position predicted from the perimembranous defect.

The presence of a defect opening into the inlet and/or trabecular component of the right ventricle, and less commonly into the infundibular region, gives rise to the potential for straddling and overriding of the atrioventricular valves. A valve is said to override the ventricular septum when its annulus moves over the inappropriate ventricle. It is said to straddle when some of its subvalvar components, either papillary muscles or cords, pass through the defect and are attached in the inappropriate ventricle. Straddling and overriding may coexist or each can be found in isolation. By convention, the atrioventricular valve is assigned to the ventricle which lies below half or more of its diameter. Thus, extreme straddling and overriding – i.e. by more than

50% of either the tricuspid or mitral valve, will convert a biventricular atrioventricular connection into double inlet left or double inlet right atrioventricular connection, respectively. Both straddling tricuspid and mitral valves are usually associated with malalignment between the atrial and ventricular septums. This may have an influence on the course of the conduction tissues. Similarly, more than 50% overriding of the aortic or pulmonary valve into its complementary ventricular outlet, which already carries its own appropriate arterial trunk, will result in a double outlet right or double outlet left ventriculo-arterial connection.

The principles of surgical management of ventricular septal defects are to achieve secure and unobstructed separation of the systemic and pulmonary circulations without damage to the conduction system or cardiac valves. This may be a technically straightforward exercise or one of the most demanding undertakings in congenital heart surgery, depending on the location of the defect and the presence of associated lesions. In general, most ventricular septal defects are approached through the right atrium and tricuspid valve which can be detached to facilitate exposure of a defect under its septal or anterosuperior leaflet. The muscular doubly committed subarterial ventricular septal defect, however, is often closed using a combined transatrial/transpulmonary approach or through a right ventriculotomy, while the large apical muscular defect (where there is usually an absence of the distal left anterior descending coronary artery) is exposed through a limited fishmouth ventriculotomy. In older patients with ventricular septal defect and aortic regurgitation, both lesions may be approached through the aortic valve.

Small muscular defects are generally closed with mattress sutures supported by pericardial or Dacron pledgets. Perimembranous and large muscular defects should be patched to avoid tension on the closure and distortion of cardiac valves. The surgeon must conceptualize also, in three dimensions, the position which the patch will assume in the filled, beating heart, to prevent subsequent obstruction of the left or right ventricular outflow tract. In this regard, intraoperative or postoperative echocardiography is an invaluable tool for both education and quality assurance. Straddling valves and intrinsic outflow tract obstruction are treated on their own merits (see also Chapters 13, 14, 15, and 16).

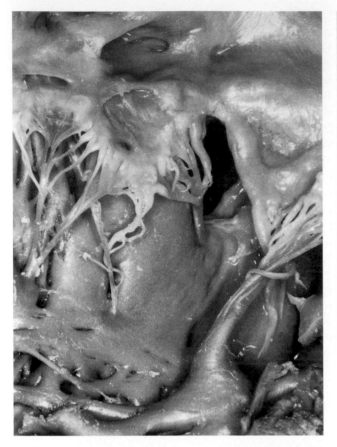

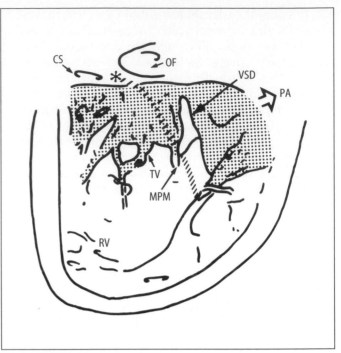

11.1 Perimembranous, confluent inlet/trabecular ventricular septal defect. Right ventricular side. The long axis of the defect extends into the trabecular septum, while its posterior margin lies behind the medial papillary muscle, just in the inlet septum. The medial side of the anterosuperior leaflet of the tricuspid valve is thickened and devoid of tension apparatus. The open arrow indicates the direction of the right ventricular outflow, and the asterisk indicates the approximate position of the atrioventricular node.

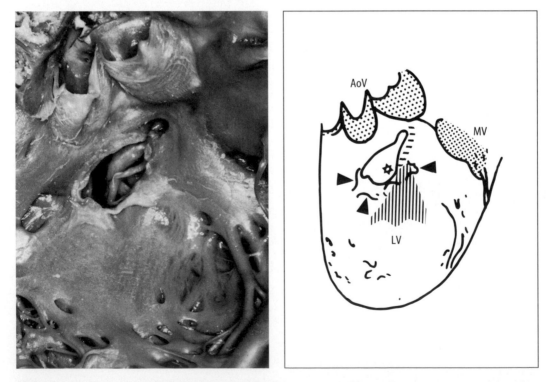

11.2 Left ventricular side. The perimembranous ventricular septal defect has accretions of fibrous tissue around its margins (arrows) and the tricuspid valve is visible through it (star). There is a small area of fibrous continuity between the aortic valve and the tricuspid valve through the ventricular septal defect. The conduction tissue runs from the remnant of membranous septum, usually away from the crest of the muscular septum, to branch out as the left bundle.

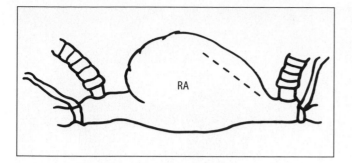

11.3 Using bicaval cannulation, a right atrial approach and closure on cardiopulmonary bypass is possible for nearly all perimembranous ventricular septal defects. The atrium is opened about 5 mm from the atrioventricular groove (dashed line).

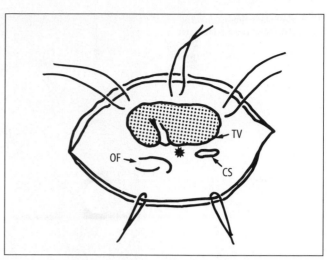

11.4 Exposure of the ventricular septal defect is facilitated by stay-sutures at 10 o'clock 12 o'clock, and 2 o'clock on the tricuspid annulus. A gap or "cleft" in the septal tricuspid leaflet is often present and extends to the central fibrous body. The atrioventricular node (star) lies between this and the coronary sinus.

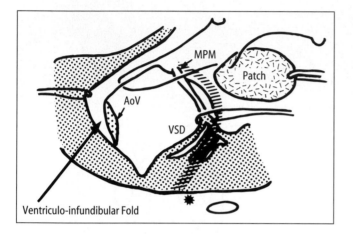

11.5 For a continuous suture technique, the patch is held towards the patient's foot and the first bite in the heart is taken near the junction of the infundibular septum and the ventriculo-infundibular fold. Gentle tension on this suture helps to expose the upper margin of the defect, as does retraction of the tricuspid valve with additional fine stay-sutures.

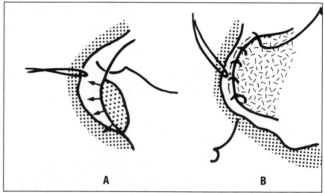

11.6 Sutures are placed radially around the aortic valve to avoid distortion of the leaflets (A). After the patch has been lowered down and the transition stitch has been placed from the ventriculo-infundibular fold through the tricuspid valve leaflet (B), the lower edge of the patch is elevated to permit inspection on its left ventricular side to ensure that the aortic valve is undamaged and the suture line is secure.

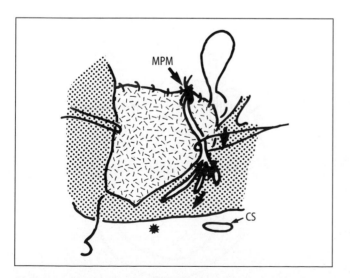

11.7 The second arm of the suture is taken clockwise, with forehand bites from the ventricular septum to the patch. The patch is split around the medial papillary muscle and repaired in this area. Along the lower margin, bites are taken parallel to (arrows) and about 5 mm from the edge of the ventricular septal defect to avoid the conduction tissue (see Figure 11.5).

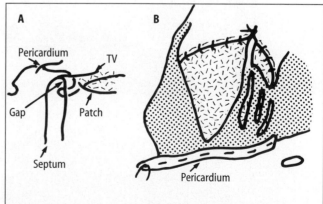

11.8 At the posterior junction of septum and tricuspid valve, a transition suture leaves a small gap (A) where the penetrating bundle may pass. Sutures on the septal tricuspid leaflet itself are placed 2–3 mm from its base. A strip of pericardium (B) is used to support the running mattress suture on the tricuspid septal leaflet.

11.9 Perimembranous, confluent trabecular/outlet ventricular septal defect. Right ventricular side. The medial papillary muscle complex lies posteriorly to the defect and one major cord inserts on its margin.

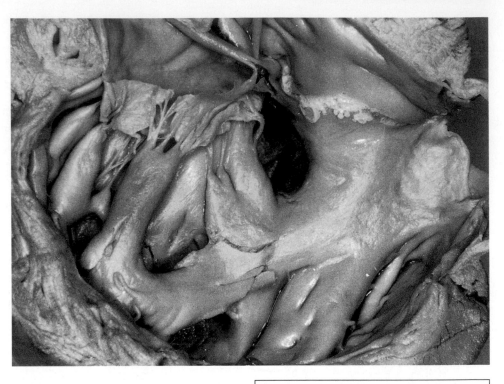

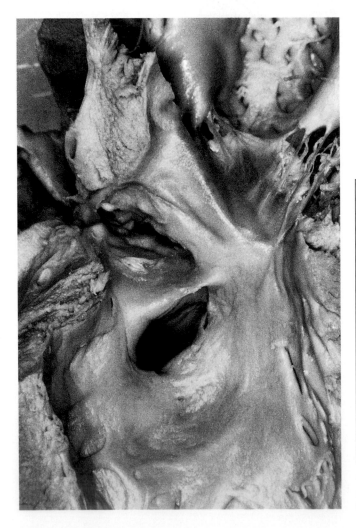

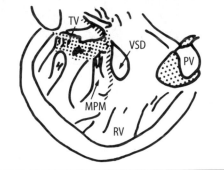

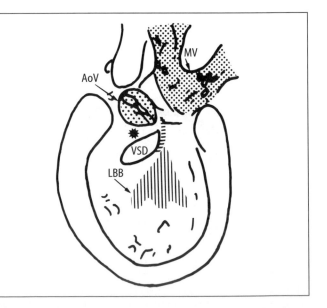

11.10 On the left ventricular side, a muscle bar (star) between the defect and aortic valve provides the potential for subaortic obstruction. The aortic valve has three leaflets of disparate sizes. This patient also has coarctation of the aorta.

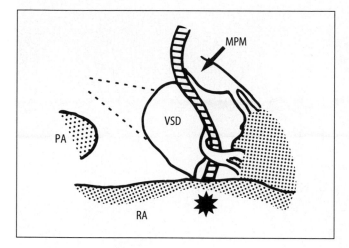

11.11 Surgical exposure of the defect is obtained through the right atrium and tricuspid valve. The atrioventricular node (star) lies at the apex of the triangle of Koch and the axis of the conduction tissue passes along the posterior margin of the defect towards the medial papillary muscle – the surgeon's right-hand side. The left ventricular outflow tract may be enlarged safely by excision of a wedge of outlet septum (dotted lines).

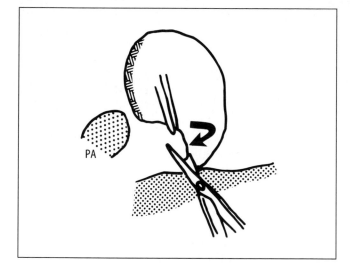

11.12 In this heart, the muscle bar on the left ventricular side of the septum, between the upper margin of the defect and the aortic valve, could still potentially obstruct the subaortic area after closure of the ventricular septal defect. It is removed by sharp excision, lifting the lower edge into the right ventricle and taking care to avoid injury to the valve. The aortic valvar leaflets themselves must be clearly visualized. As exposure of the valve is limited to its ventricular surface, however, a separate aortotomy would be required to carry out a valvotomy or repair of the valve, if needed.

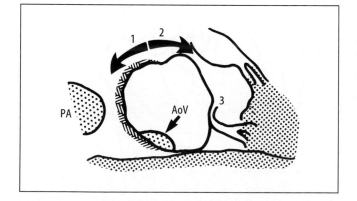

11.13 The enlarged ventricular septal defect is closed, as described for the preceding specimen, carrying a continuous suture line first counterclockwise around the upper margin of the defect (1), and then clockwise along the posterior margin (2). In the areas of muscle resection, multiple mattress sutures pledgeted with Teflon or pericardium will facilitate a secure closure. A rim of muscle is left between the aortic and pulmonary valves for suture placement. The patch is split to accommodate the major cords on the crest of the ventricular septal defect (3) and to avoid the conduction tissue.

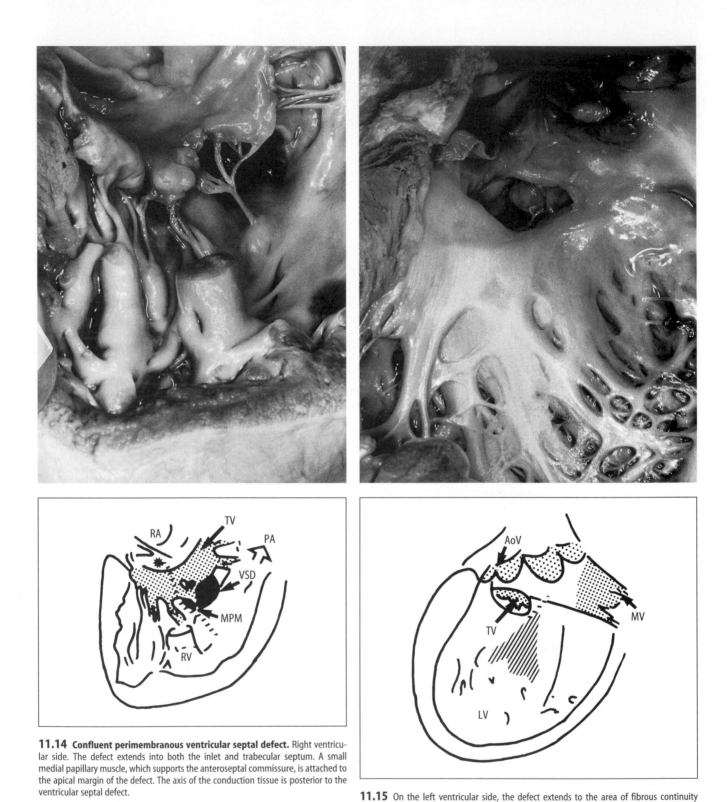

11.14 Confluent perimembranous ventricular septal defect. Right ventricular side. The defect extends into both the inlet and trabecular septum. A small medial papillary muscle, which supports the anteroseptal commissure, is attached to the apical margin of the defect. The axis of the conduction tissue is posterior to the ventricular septal defect.

11.15 On the left ventricular side, the defect extends to the area of fibrous continuity among the aortic, mitral, and tricuspid valves. Tricuspid valvar leaflet is seen through the ventricular septal defect.

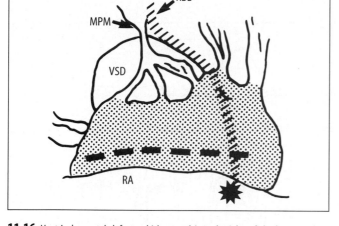

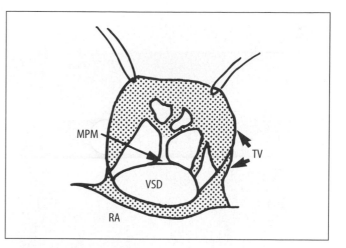

11.16 Ventricular septal defects which extend into the inlet of the heart are best approached through the right atrium. Because the defect is perimembranous (it reaches the tricuspid valve), the penetrating bundle (slashed line) passes from the atrioventricular node (star) to the ventricular septum on the surgeon's right-hand side of the defect. When tricuspid subvalvar apparatus complicates exposure of the margins, the septal leaflet is detached about 4 mm from and parallel to its base (dashed line).

11.17 Rotation of the septal tricuspid valvar leaflet away from the surgeon, towards the cavity of the right ventricle, gives excellent access to the ventricular septal defect. The base of the leaflet which remains attached to the annulus may also be placed under tension, if needed, with fine stay-sutures.

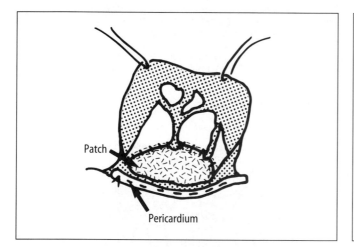

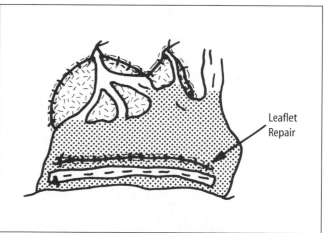

11.18 The defect is closed with a patch, either as described in Figures 11.3–11.8, or starting in the mid-portion of the attached base of tricuspid septal leaflet and working forward both clockwise and counter clockwise around the defect. Sutures in the area of the septal leaflet are placed 2–3 mm from the base of the leaflet and supported with pericardium, leaving the cut edge for subsequent valve repair. The patch is split and repaired around major papillary muscles and cords as needed.

11.19 The septal leaflet is repaired by direct suture, separately from closure of the ventricular septal defect. If the tissue is extremely delicate, as in a small infant, this suture line is pledgeted also with pericardium. The valve is then tested by an injection of saline into the right ventricle to confirm that there is no major incompetence.

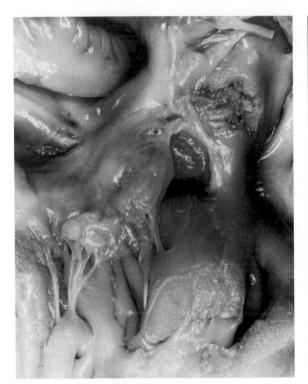

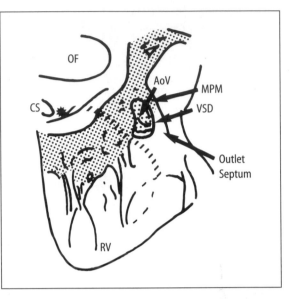

11.20 Perimembranous inlet/outlet ventricular septal defect. Right ventricular view. The medial papillary muscle complex lies on the anterior margin of the defect and the conduction tissue along the posterior margin. The outlet septum is hypoplastic and deviated, such that the aortic valve overrides the defect and the trabecular septum, but the right ventricular outflow is not obstructed. The aortic leaflet prolapses into the defect.

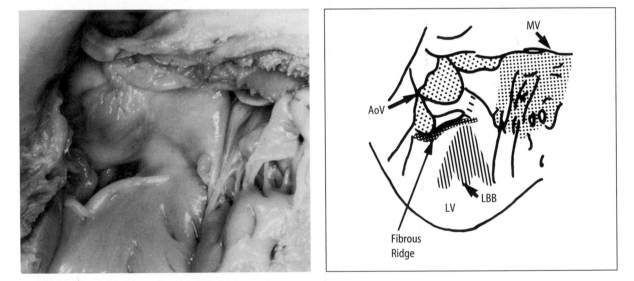

11.21 Left ventricular aspect. The defect runs posteriorly towards the area of aortic-mitral fibrous continuity. An accretion of fibrous tissue on the apical margin potentially leads to subaortic obstruction following closure of the defect. Prolapse of the aortic valvar leaflet into the ventricular septal defect is better appreciated from this view.

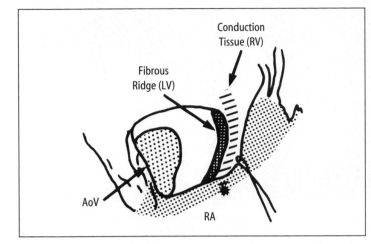

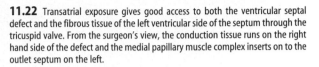

11.22 Transatrial exposure gives good access to both the ventricular septal defect and the fibrous tissue of the left ventricular side of the septum through the tricuspid valve. From the surgeon's view, the conduction tissue runs on the right hand side of the defect and the medial papillary muscle complex inserts on to the outlet septum on the left.

11.23 The free edge of the fibrous ridge is grasped with forceps through the ventricular septal defect and put under tension away from the septum. It is then peeled off the endocardium by blunt dissection, lifting the fibrous tissue away from the septum. Pressure on the margin of the ventricular septal defect or the crest of the septum in this area may produce heart block.

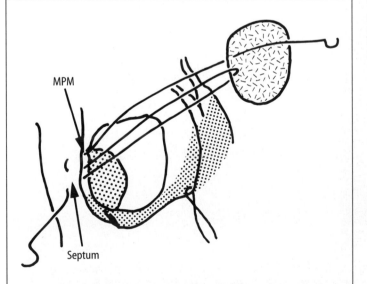

11.24 The anterior rim of the defect contains some tricuspid leaflet tissue and the medial papillary muscle complex, neither of which is composed of strong material. Accordingly, sutures are brought through the margin radially to the aortic valve (taking care not to damage the leaflet) and then mattressed in the thickened muscle of the outlet septum.

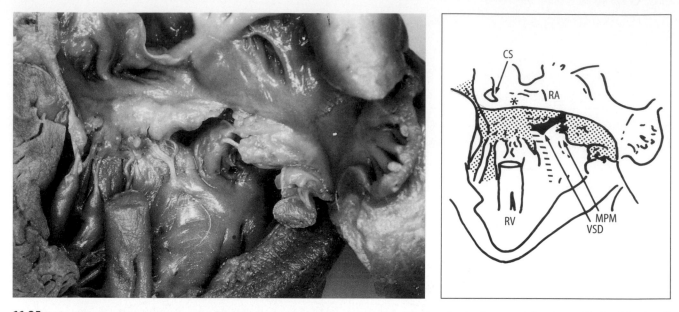

11.25 Perimembranous inlet ventricular septal defect. Right ventricular side. The opening of the defect is confined to the septum below the septal leaflet of the tricuspid valve. The conduction tissue runs posteriorly to the ventricular septal defect, usually with the penetrating bundle at the corner and non-branching bundle on the left ventricular side of the septum. An asterisk in the right atrium indicates the approximate position of the atrioventricular node. The tricuspid valve straddles the defect into the left ventricle. The anteroseptal commissure and medial papillary muscle complex are anterior to the defect. There is no gross evidence of malalignment between the atrial and ventricular septums in this heart.

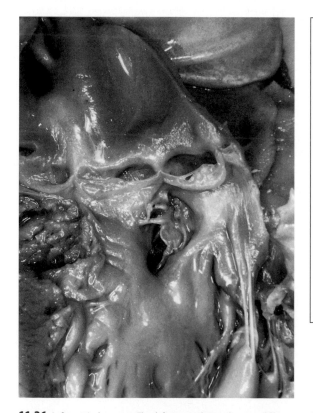

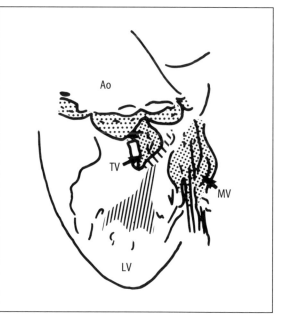

11.26 Left ventricular aspect. The defect extends into the area of fibrous continuity between the mitral, tricuspid, and aortic valves. The tricuspid valvar leaflet is seen through the defect and has cords attached to both the anterior margin of the ventricular septal defect on the left ventricular side of the septum and to the base of the aortic valve leaflet. This is "minor" straddling of the tricuspid valve.

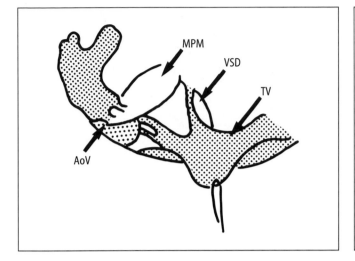

11.27 Seen in surgical orientation through the right atrium, the medial papillary muscle forms the leftward margin of the ventricular septal defect and the penetrating bundle lies to the right-hand side. Retraction of the septal leaflet pulls the straddling cords and aortic valve into view.

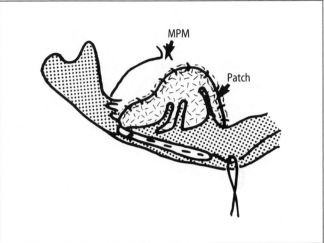

11.28 The cords are detached from the aortic leaflet and the defect is closed with a patch. Sutures along the anterior (left-hand) margin are passed through the medial papillary muscle complex, while those on the posterior (right-hand) margin are deviated about 3–5 mm rightward from the margin of the defect to avoid the conduction tissue.

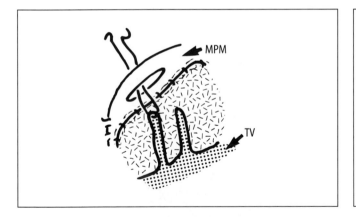

11.29 As these are major cords supporting the anteroseptal commissure, reattachment is important to achieve a competent tricuspid valve. A slit is incised into the medial papillary muscle and each cord is drawn into it with a fine monofilament mattress suture.

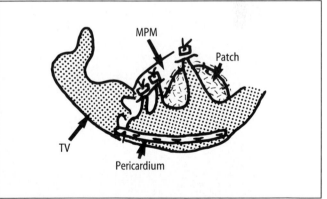

11.30 The papillary muscle is closed over the cords with several mattress sutures supported by pledgets of autogenous pericardium. Partial approximation of the anteroseptal commissure at its apex is done also to improve competency of the valve, incorporating the pericardial strip which has been placed to support the suture-line for the patch along the septal leaflet of the tricuspid valve.

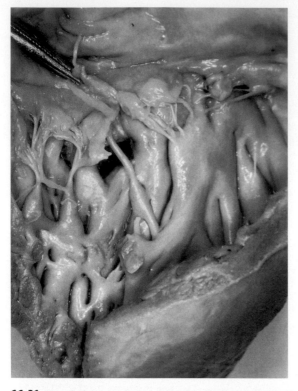
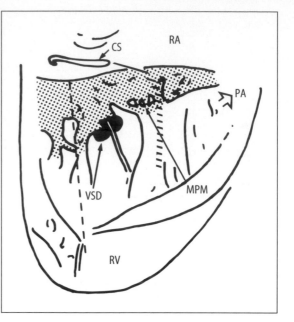

11.31 **Muscular inlet ventricular septal defect.** Right ventricular side. The defect is surrounded completely by muscle and lies beneath the septal leaflet of the tricuspid valve, proximal to papillary muscle attachments. It extends almost to the posterior wall of the heart (dashed line). The conduction tissue passes anteriorly to the defect, towards the medial papillary muscle complex.

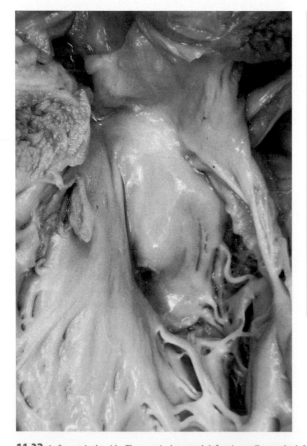
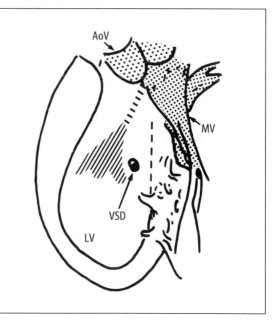

11.32 Left ventricular side. The ventricular septal defect is smaller on the left side of the septum and lies close to the posterior wall of the heart (dashed line). It is remote from the penetrating and non-branching bundle of the conduction tissue, and from the aortic and mitral valves.

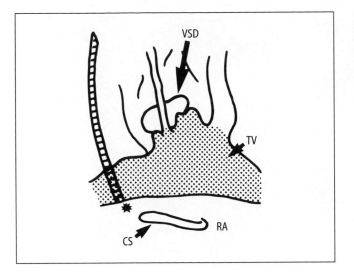

11.33 Muscular ventricular septal defects opening to the inlet of the right ventricle are approached from the right atrium through the tricuspid valve, of which the septal leaflet is retracted if necessary. The atrioventricular node (star) lies at the apex of the triangle of Koch, and the conduction system is to the left-hand side of the defect, as seen by the surgeon in this exposure.

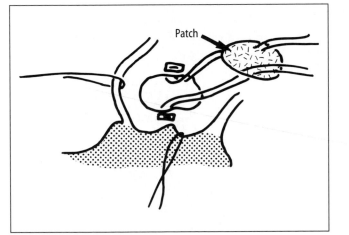

11.34 The placement of pledgeted mattress sutures from the right to the left ventricular side of the defect on two (or four) sides, everts the margin and defines the edges of the defect. These sutures are then passed through the patch which is lowered down on to the septum.

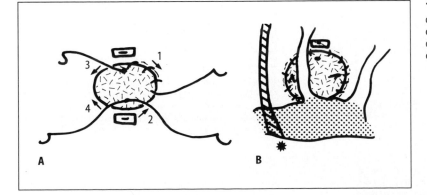

11.35 The patch is set down firmly into the ventricular septal defect and septal muscle and sutured continuously with bold bites to obliterate any space behind trabeculations (A). This is conveniently done in four quadrants. The completed patch is close to neither the conduction tissue nor the tricuspid subvalvar apparatus (B).

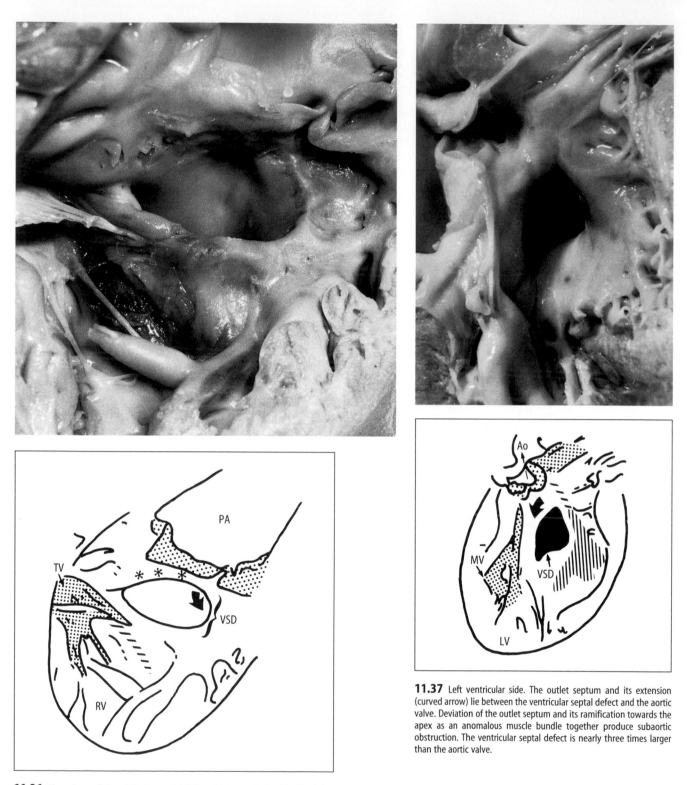

11.36 Muscular outlet ventricular septal defect. Right ventricular side. The defect opens to the outlet of the right ventricle and the pulmonary valve overrides the defect and the trabecular septum. The outlet septum (asterisks) is rather flattened and hypoplastic. It is deviated into the left ventricular outflow tract, where it spirals down (curved arrow) to become a prominent muscular bundle. This arrangement produces subaortic obstruction. Conduction tissue lies normally in relation to the tricuspid valve and medial papillary muscle. It is judged to be not too close to the margins of the ventricular septal defect in this heart. This patient has associated coarctation of the aorta.

11.37 Left ventricular side. The outlet septum and its extension (curved arrow) lie between the ventricular septal defect and the aortic valve. Deviation of the outlet septum and its ramification towards the apex as an anomalous muscle bundle together produce subaortic obstruction. The ventricular septal defect is nearly three times larger than the aortic valve.

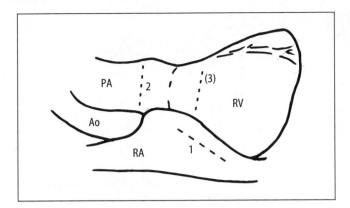

11.38 A muscular outlet ventricular septal defect is usually approached through the right atrium (1), although a pulmonary arteriotomy (2) may also facilitate closure. A right ventriculotomy (3) gives good access but is rarely necessary.

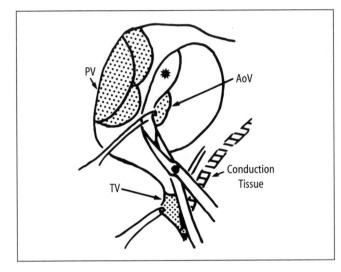

11.39 Working through the tricuspid valve and ventricular septal defect, a retraction suture is used to pull the outlet septum (star) down into the right ventricle and visualize the aortic valve leaflets. The outlet septum, which is obstructing the left ventricular outflow, is excised.

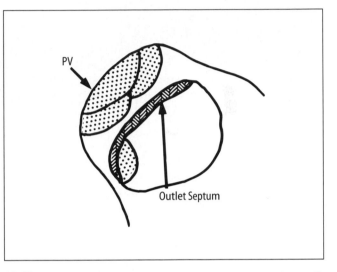

11.40 Removal of the muscular bar relieves the subaortic obstruction and essentially converts the ventricular septal defect to a "doubly committed subarterial" defect, with only a thin remnant of outlet septum remaining between the aortic and pulmonary valvar leaflets.

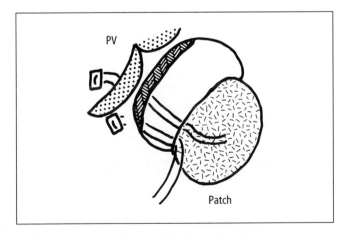

11.41 The upper left-hand margin of the defect may support sutures below the pulmonary valve or, alternatively, interrupted mattress sutures are passed through the ventriculo-arterial junction from the pulmonary arterial side.

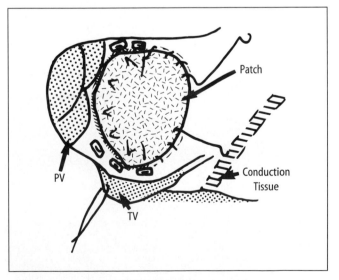

11.42 The lower right-hand portion of the suture line is carried continuously along the margin of the defect, which is not very close to the conduction tissue. The defect has a completely muscular rim and does not extend to the tricuspid valve. Accordingly, sutures need not be placed through the septal tricuspid leaflet.

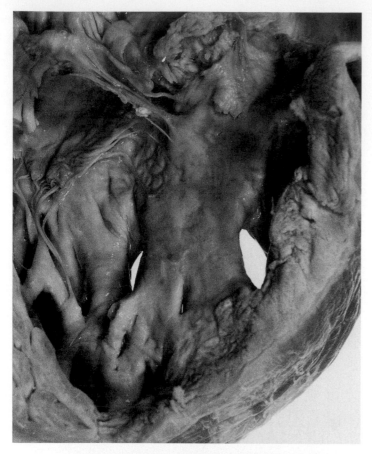

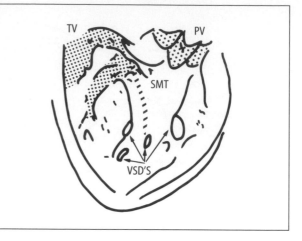

11.43 Multiple muscular ventricular septal defects. Right ventricular view. This shows several defects opening into the trabecular septum, related to either side of the large septomarginal trabeculation. The distal right bundle branch may run close to one of the smaller defects. This anomaly is also called "Swiss cheese septum" because of its resemblance to the multiple holes found in a slice of Swiss cheese.

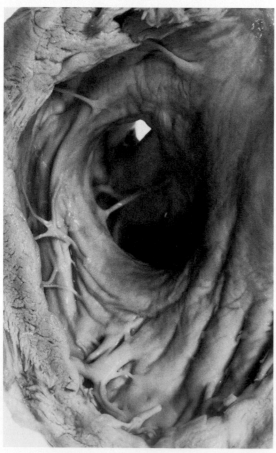

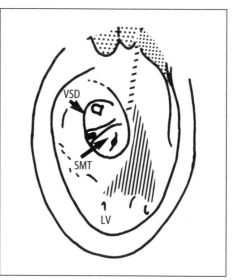

11.44 The left ventricular view shows that there is one large defect, which would be almost closed by the septomarginal trabeculation of the right ventricle, were it attached to the remainder of the muscular septum. Two small defects are seen through the septomarginal trabeculation. This case also has coarctation of the aorta.

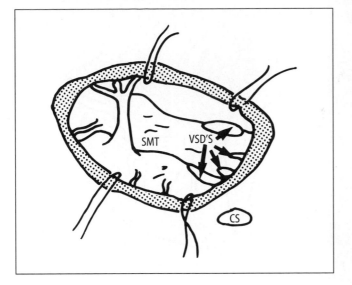

11.45 Multiple muscular ventricular septal defects in the right ventricle are, in essence, produced by failure of the septomarginal trabeculation to close a single large left-sided defect. Exposed through the tricuspid valve, the defects lie anywhere within, or adjacent to, the margins of the septomarginal muscle mass. The perimembranous and outlet regions should be inspected also for possible additional defects. The main axis of the conduction tissue is not related to the muscular trabecular defects.

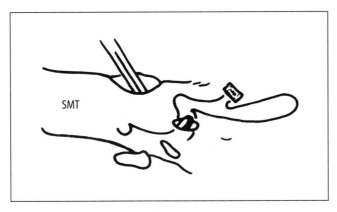

11.46 Defects within the septomarginal trabeculation are closed by interrupted, pledgeted mattress sutures. Their identification is facilitated by passing a right-angled instrument through the defect from the left ventricle, which is entered either through one of the larger ventricular septal defects or via the atrial septum and the mitral valve. The tip of the instrument elevates the defect towards the surgeon and differentiates its margins from muscular trabeculations.

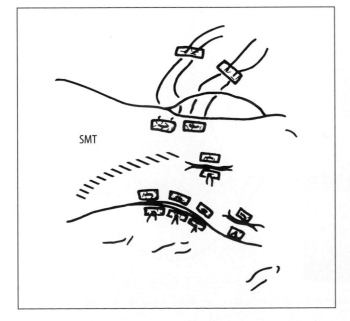

11.47 At the edge of the septomarginal trabeculation, defects are closed by approximation of this muscle bundle to the remainder of the septum. The mattress sutures at either end therefore include an area where the muscles overlap. If a large defect reaches the anterior wall of the heart, sutures may be passed through the right ventricular free wall. In this instance, however, in distinction to the situation of an apical muscular defect, the anterior descending (interventricular) coronary artery does extend to the apex of the heart and must be protected from injury. The largest and most superior ventricular septal defect is used to locate smaller defects and then is closed last, filling the left ventricle to displace air before the final suture is tied. As muscular trabeculations may easily be confused with ventricular septal defects, particularly in a hypertrophied right ventricle, it is useful for the surgeon to set a time limit for closure of the defects, such that myocardial ischemic time does not become excessively prolonged. Intraoperative transesophageal echocardiography should be done routinely in such cases to exclude major residual shunts.

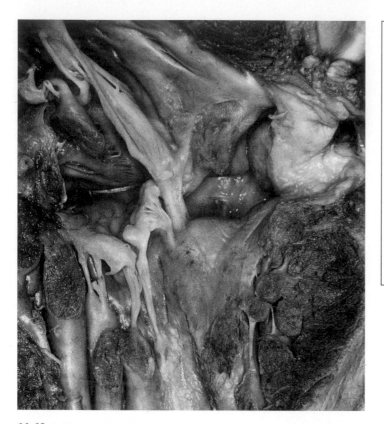
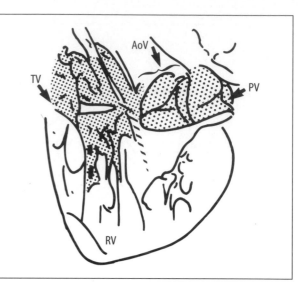

11.48 Perimembranous, doubly committed subarterial ventricular septal defect. Seen from the right ventricle, the aortic and pulmonary valves are in fibrous continuity in the roof of the defect, which is thus committed to both great arteries. The muscular outlet septum is completely absent. In contrast with most subarterial ventricular septal defects, this one is also perimembranous because it extends to the tricuspid valve. The conduction system is close to its posterior margin because the posterior limb of the septomarginal trabeculation does not extend to the ventriculo-infundibular fold as a muscular border between the defect and the conduction tissue. The pulmonary valve is thickened and stenotic. The tricuspid valvar leaflets are also thickened.

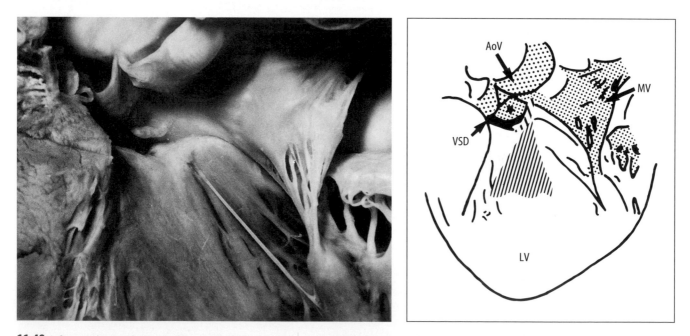

11.49 Left ventricular view showing the fibrous continuity between the aortic and mitral valves. Tricuspid valvar tissue (star) is visible through the ventricular septal defect. All four cardiac valves are thus in fibrous continuity in this heart.

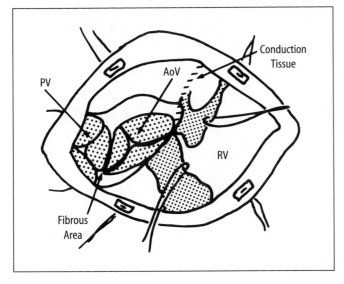

11.50 A doubly committed subarterial ventricular septal defect which extends to the membranous septum usually requires a combined approach through the pulmonary artery and the tricuspid valve for exposure , but a right ventriculotomy, as illustrated here, will also give good access to both the perimembranous and subarterial margins. Traction sutures on the anterosuperior and septal tricuspid leaflets elevate the lower part of the defect towards the surgeon. The conduction tissue lies on the right-hand margin of the defect, unprotected by muscle in this example.

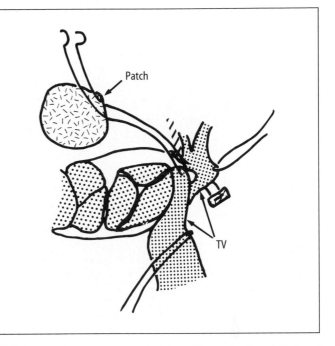

11.51 The first suture is passed through the base of the septal and anterior leaflets of the tricuspid valve from the atrial to the ventricular side and then through the patch. The small "frap" of leaflet tissue which is commonly present may be safely incorporated in the suture. This will close any gap between the valvar leaflets, when present, and avoid a small residual shunt without endangering the conduction tissue.

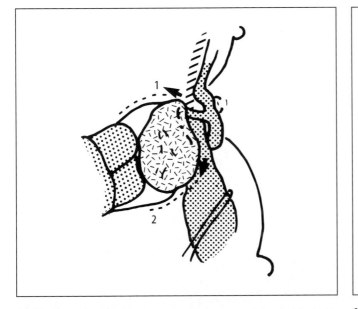

11.52 The first suture is tied down and the patch is displaced into the left ventricle through the ventricular septal defect. Using the first arm (1), sutures are placed parallel to the ventricular septal defect and about 3–4 mm from its crest, weaving through tricuspid valvar tissue as necessary to avoid the conduction axis. The second arm (2) runs as a mattress suture along the septal tricuspid leaflet and on to the ventriculo-infundibular fold. A V-shaped depression is often present in this region, where it is important to place sutures at the bottom of the muscular mound, rather than approximating its edges, which leaves a shunt behind the patch.

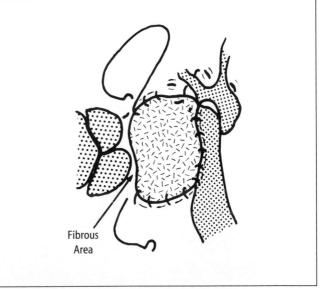

11.53 There may be sufficient fibrous tissue in the area of aortic-pulmonary valvar continuity to support horizontally placed sutures between the valvar leaflets. If not, interrupted mattress sutures should be passed from the pulmonary artery between the valves to complete attachment of the patch around the upper part of the defect (see Figure 11.41). In this particular heart, the hypoplastic tricuspid valve probably would require a simultaneous cavopulmonary connection, and the stenotic pulmonary and tricuspid valves would make exposure of the ventricular septal defect through either valvar orifice extremely difficult. More commonly, the pulmonary valve is considerably enlarged in the presence of a doubly committed subarterial ventricular septal defect and gives good access to the upper portion, if not the entire suture line. A final consideration is to avoid subpulmonary obstruction by the patch. In some cases, resection of subpulmonary muscle bundles or placement of a small patch on the infundibulum of the right ventricle is necessary to do this.

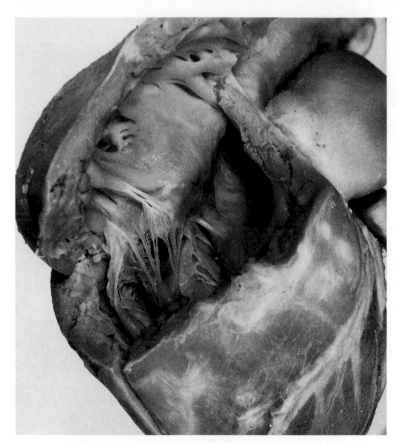

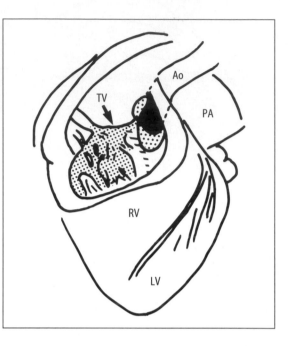

11.54 Perimembranous doubly-committed subarterial ventricular septal defect. The right ventricle is small, as is the aortic root. Both arterial valves override the defect and, from this view, appear to arise mainly from the left ventricle. However, from the left ventricle (Figure 11.56), at least the aorta seems to be connected to the right ventricle. This case illustrates the difficulty of establishing ventriculo-arterial connections in hearts with extensive absence of the outlet septum.

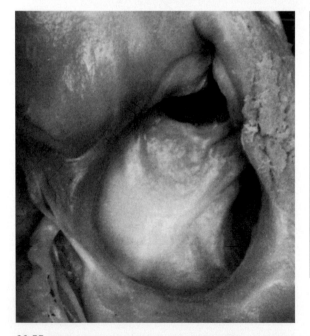

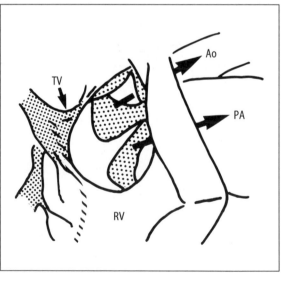

11.55 A close-up view of the defect shows that there is fibrous continuity among the aortic, pulmonary, and tricuspid valves, as seen from the right ventricle. The area of conduction tissue runs along the posterior margin of the ventricular septal defect.

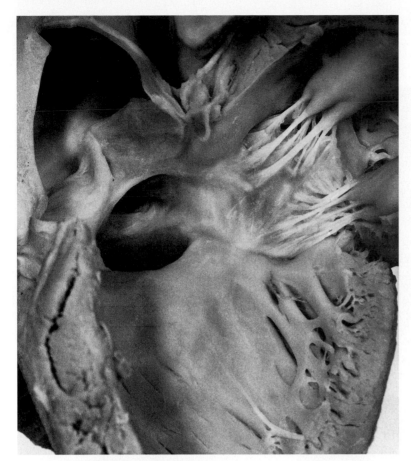

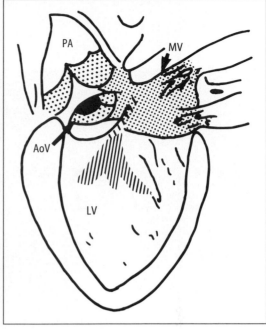

11.56 The left ventricular view shows that there is also fibrous continuity among the aortic, pulmonary, and mitral valves. The aortic valve is seen through the ventricular septal defect and appears to arise from the right ventricle, while the pulmonary valve and pulmonary artery appear committed to the left ventricle.

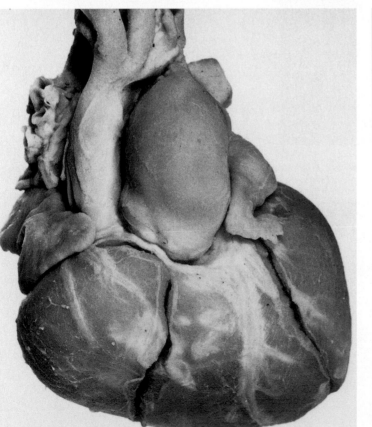

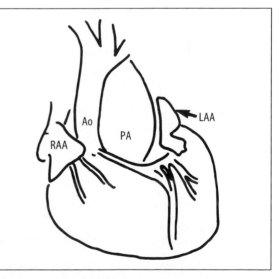

11.57 Anterior view of the heart shown in Figures 11.54–11.56. The dilated pulmonary root lies to the left of and slightly anteriorly to the aortic root, but the external appearances of the heart do not immediately suggest a diagnosis of transposed great arteries or double outlet left ventricle. The left main coronary artery, however, passes anteriorly to the pulmonary root, and this pattern is seen most frequently in complete transposition of the great arteries. In that situation, the aorta most often lies more anteriorly than is seen in this heart. Surgical correction of this heart probably would require an arterial switch, closure of the ventricular septal defect, leaving the left ventricle connected to the pulmonary artery (neo-aorta), and possibly bidirectional cavopulmonary anastomosis to partially bypass the small right ventricle. Given these considerations, the ventricular septal defect would probably no longer be considered "isolated" in this case.

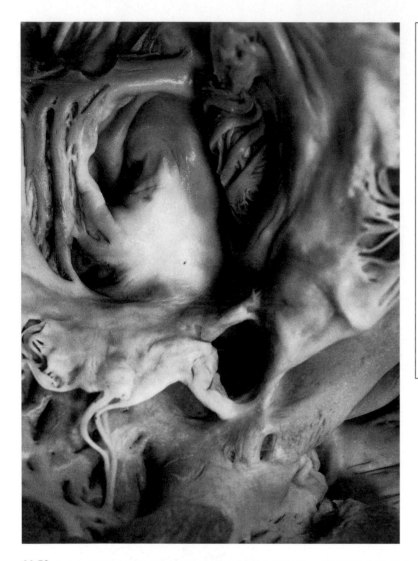

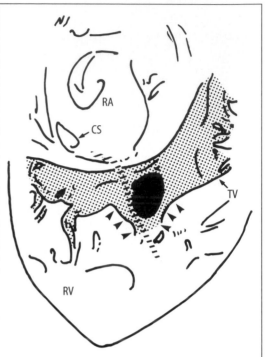

11.58 Perimembranous trabecular ventricular septal defect with left ventricular to right atrial communication (infra-annular Gerbode defect). Seen from the right side, fibrosis around the perimembranous trabecular defect has caused the surrounding tricuspid valvar leaflets to become firmly adherent to the muscular septum (arrow heads). The tension apparatus of the valve has been obliterated in this area. As a result of the failure of the thickened tricuspid valve leaflets to coapt, the left ventricle is in direct communication with the right atrium through the ventricular septal defect. The annulus of the tricuspid valve and the atrioventricular septum, however, are intact. The defect is surrounded entirely by tricuspid leaflet tissue. Progressive fibrosis in such a ventricular septal defect may compromise the conduction tissue which lies posteriorly to the defect. This anomaly should not be confused with the more rare supra-annular Gerbode ventricular septal defect, which is a communication between the left ventricle and right atrium above the annulus of the tricuspid valve, through a defect in the atrioventricular membranous septum.

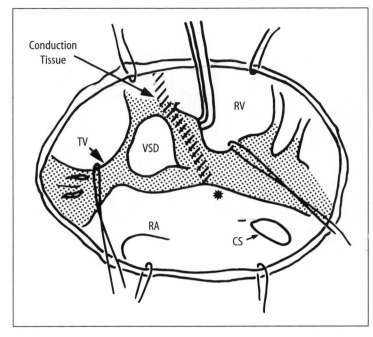

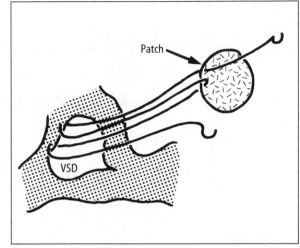

11.60 Patch closure with a continuous suture technique is begun along the apex of the defect, taking generous bites of thickened tricuspid valvar tissue. This area is remote from the specialized conduction tissue.

11.59 This defect is exposed through the right atrium. Traction sutures on the tricuspid valve help to define its margins. The conduction tissue passes from the apex of the triangle of Koch (star) to the right of the defect and may be protected by fibrous tissue. A right-angled instrument is used to explore beneath the tricuspid valve for additional communications.

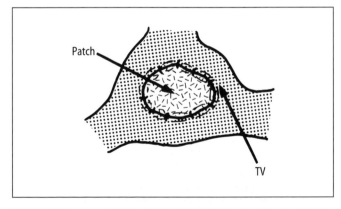

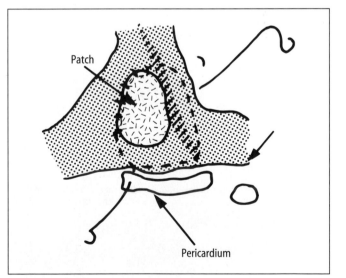

11.61 If all the communication with the left ventricle lies above the tricuspid leaflet, the patch may be sutured entirely to the fibrous tissue of the valve. The conduction tissue should not be at risk in this situation.

11.62 If there are additional communications between the left and right ventricle through gaps in the fibrous tissue, the ventricular septal defect is closed like a perimembranous defect (see Figures 11.3–11.8, and 11.13). The patch is then attached to the muscular septum, taking bites away from, and parallel to, the lower margins of the defect. A pericardial strip may not be essential to reinforce sutures in the tricuspid valve leaflet when it is thickened to this degree. It may be necessary to detach the septal tricuspid valvar leaflet to gain access for insertion of such a patch (see Figures 11.16–11.19).

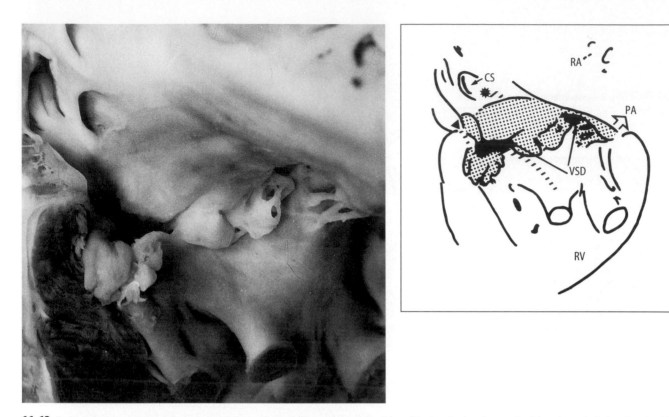

11.63 Perimembranous inlet ventricular septal defect with straddling and overriding tricuspid valve. As viewed across the right atrioventricular junction, the defect extends to the posterior wall of the heart and there is gross malalignment of the atrial and ventricular septums. The cavity of the right ventricle is small. The atrial septum is intact.

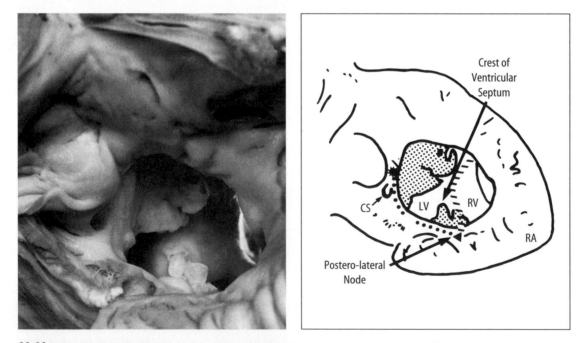

11.64 Right atrial view looking down upon the tricuspid valve. The septal malalignment produces both overriding and straddling of the tricuspid valve into the left ventricle. A hypoplastic node may be present at the apex of the triangle of Koch (star), but the atrioventricular connection is through an anomalous posterolateral node (triangle) where the ventricular septum reaches the atrioventricular junction. There may also be islets of conduction tissue between the two nodes (dotted lines).

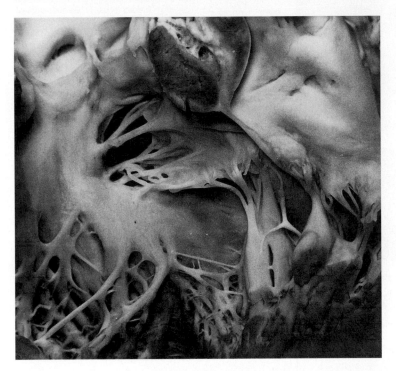

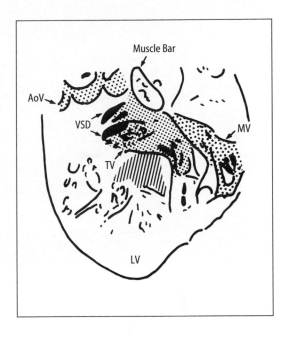

11.65 Left ventricular view, showing the tricuspid valvar leaflet attached anteriorly to the margin of the ventricular septal defect and posteriorly to a well-developed papillary muscle in the left ventricle. The mitral valvar annulus is displaced posteriorly by a large muscle bar which separates it from the aortic valve. This muscle, along with a small rim of the posterior limb of the septomarginal trabeculation which passes through the ventricular septal defect, forms a complete muscular subaortic conus within the left ventricle. The axis of the conduction system lies posteriorly to the defect. Rhythm disturbances are associated frequently with this type of malformation.

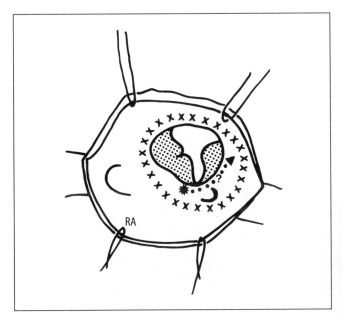

11.66 The hypoplastic right ventricle and extreme straddling of the tricuspid valve favour a Fontan-type of repair in this heart. If the tricuspid valve is competent, this could be accomplished by anastomosis of both ends of the divided superior caval vein to the right pulmonary artery, closure of the main pulmonary artery (or division and anastomosis of the cardiac end to the aorta to bypass left ventricular outflow obstruction) and closure of the right atrioventricular junction. The latter is done by suturing a patch about 5 mm above the valve annulus (crosses), with deviations around the coronary sinus and posterolateral node (triangle) to avoid damage to the conduction tissue. If valve closure were needed for regurgitation, suture placement in the tricuspid valvar leaflet itself would be necessary to conserve atrioventricular conduction.

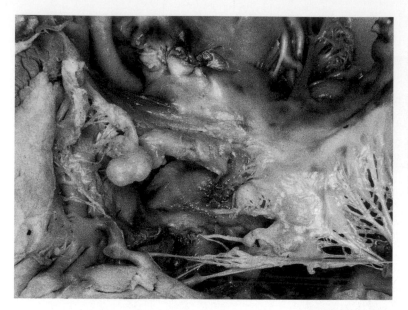

11.67 Perimembranous inlet ventricular septal defect with straddling and overriding tricuspid valve. Right atrioventricular junction. Like the preceding heart (Figures 11.63–11.66), malalignment of the atrial and ventricular septums brings the tricuspid valve to override the left ventricle but to a lesser degree than that which is seen in Figure 11.63. A portion of the septal leaflet (asterisk) also straddles across the defect into the left ventricle. The defect does not quite extend to the posterior wall of the heart, but there is fibrous continuity between the mitral and tricuspid valves, such that this could be regarded as a "ventricular septal defect of the atrioventricular canal type." However, in this particular heart, the ventricular conduction tissue does not contact the atrial conduction tissue and heart block is present. The atrial conduction tissue is likely to be represented by clusters of node-like cells on the atrial side of the tricuspid annulus. A defect in the atrial septum has been sutured.

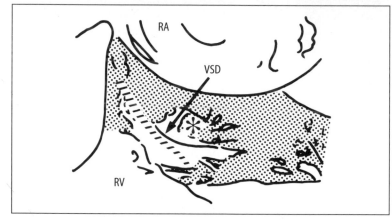

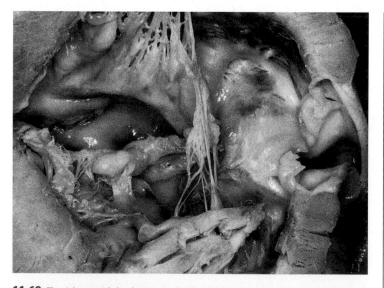

11.68 The right ventricle has been opened with a fish-mouth incision from apex to inlet/base and is viewed looking upwards towards the inlet and the outlet. The tricuspid valve is thickened in several areas. The anterior portion of the septal leaflet (asterisk) passes through the ventricular septal defect and the anterosuperior leaflet is enlarged and dysplastic. The pulmonary valve is also thickened and the right ventricle is hypertrophied.

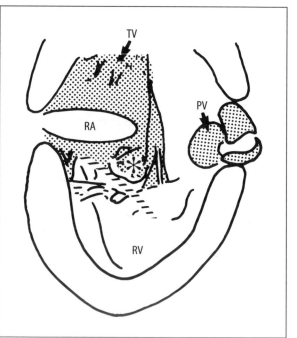

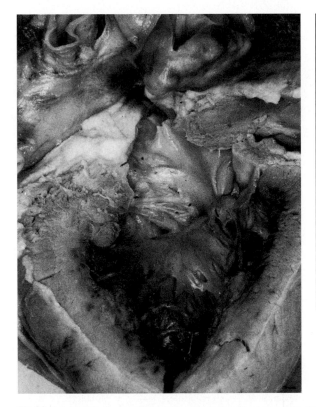

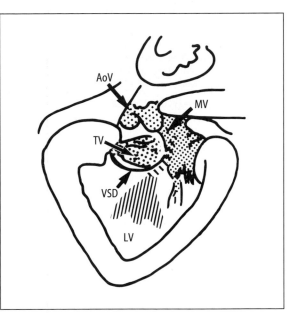

11.69 Left ventricle. The straddling portion of the tricuspid valve is attached to a papillary muscle on the anterior wall of the left ventricle, in the subaortic area. This is major or severe straddling of the tricuspid valve and has resulted in severe left ventricular outflow tract obstruction with a small cavity and hypertrophied left ventricle. Conservative, biventricular surgical repair of this heart by repositioning of the tricuspid papillary muscle or tricuspid valve replacement and closure of the ventricular septal defect would be extremely high risk due to the combination of left ventricular outflow obstruction, an abnormal pulmonary valve, pulmonary hypertension and complete congenital heart block. A theoretical alternative possibility would be to create a pulmonary-to-aorta connection (Damus-Kaye-Stansel) with a systemic-to-pulmonary artery shunt, using the right ventricle for systemic outflow during the neonatal period. Staged management would then proceed through a bidirectional cavopulmonary connection, when the pulmonary resistance had fallen, to a Fontan circulation. However, the severe biventricular hypertrophy again mitigates against a successful outcome and cardiac transplantation probably would be a better option for such a patient.

Suggested Reading

al-Marsafawy HMF, Ho SY, Redington AN, Anderson RH. The relationship of the outlet septum to the aortic ouflow in hearts with interruption of the aortic arch. J Thorac Cardiovasc Surg 1995; 109:1225.

Anderson RH, Becker AE, Tynan M. Description of ventricular septal defects – or how long is a piece of string/ Editorial review. Int J Cardiol 1986;13:267.

Anderson RH, Wilcox BR. The surgical anatomy of ventricular septal defect. J Cardiac Surg 1992;7:17.

Becu LM, Fontana RS, Du Shane JW, Kirklin JW, Burchell HB, Edwards JE. Anatomic and pathologic studies in ventricular septal defect. Circulation 1956;24:349.

Bove EL, Minich LL, Pridjian AK, Lupinelti FM, Snider AR, Dick M 2nd, Beekman RH 3rd. The management of severe subaortic stenosis, ventricular septal defect and aortic arch obstruction in the neonate. J Thorac Cardiovasc Surg 1993;105:289.

Capelli H, Andrade JL, Somerville J. Classification of the site of ventricular septal defect by 2-dimensional echocardiography. Am J Cardiol 1983;51:1474.

Gerbode F, Hultgren H, Melrose D, Osborn J. Syndrome of left ventricular – right atrial shunt: successful surgical repair of defect in 5 cases with observation of bradycardia on closure. Ann Surg 1958;148:433.

Goor DA, Lillehei CW. Septal defects in congenital malformations of the heart; embryology, anatomy. Operative considerations. New York, Grune and Stratton 1978.113.

Kawashima Y, Fujita T, Mori T, Ihara K, Manabe H. Transpulmonary arterial closure of ventricular septal defect. J Thorac Cardiovasc Surg 1977;74:191.

Kirklin JW, Harshbarger HG, Donald DE, Edwards JE. Surgical correction of ventricular septal defect; anatomic and technical considerations. J Thorac Cardiovasc Surg 1957;33:45.

Latham RA, Anderson RH. Anatomical variations in the atrioventricular conduction system with reference to ventricular septal defects. Br Heart J 1972;34:185.

Lev M. The architecture of the conduction system in congenital heart disease III. Ventricular septal defect. Archives of Pathology 1960; 70:529.

McGoon DC, Danielson GK, Wallace RB, Puga FJ. Surgical implications of straddling atrioventricular valves. In: Becker AE, Losekoot G, Marcelletti C, Anderson RH (eds) Paediatric Cardiology, Vol 3. Edinburgh, Churchill Livingstone, 1981:431.

McKay R, Battistessa SA, Wilkinson JL, Wright JP. A communication from the left ventricle to the right atrium: a defect in the central fibrous body. Int J Cardiol 1989;23:117.

McNicholas K, de Laval M, Stark J. Taylor JFN, Macartney FJ. Surgical treatment of ventricular septal defect in infancy. Primary repair versus banding of the pulmonary artery and later repair. Br Heart J 1979;41:133.

Milo S, Ho SY, Macartney FJ, Wilkinson JL, Becker AE, Wenink AC, Gittenberger de Groot AC, Anderson RH. Straddling and overriding atrioventricular valves. Morphology and classification. Am J Cardiol 1979;44:1122.

Pacifico AD, Soto B, Bargeron LM Jr. Surgical treatment of straddling tricuspid valves. Circulation 1979;60:655.

Riemenschneider TA, Moss AJ. Left ventricular – right atrial communication. Am J Cardiol 1967;19:710.

Serraf A, Lacour-Gayet F, Brumiaux J. Surgical management of isolated multiple ventricular septal defects. J Thorac Cardiovasc Surg 1992;103:437.

Soto B, Becker AE, Moulaert AJ, Lie JT, Anderson RH. Classification of ventricular septal defects. Br Heart J 1980;43:332.

Truex RC, Bishof JK. Conduction system in human hearts with interventricular septal defects. J Thorac Cardiovasc Surg 1958;35:421.

Turner SE, Hornung T, Hunter S. Closure of ventricular septal defects: a study of factors influencing spontaneous and surgical closure. Cardiol Young 2002;12:357.

Ueda M, Becker AE. Morphological characteristics of perimembranous ventricular septal defects and their surgical significance. Int J Cardiol 1985;8:149.

Van Praagh R, McNamara JJ. Anatomic types of ventricular septal defects with aortic insufficiency. Diagnostic and surgical considerations. Am Heart J 1968;73:604.

Wenink ACG, Oppenheimer-Dekker A, Moulaert AJ. Muscular ventricular septal defects: a reappraisal of the anatomy. Am J Cardiol 1979;43:259.

12 Atrioventricular Septal Defect

Introduction

The atrioventricular septal defects comprise a diverse group of malformed hearts which are defined by a common atrioventricular junction guarding the inflow to the ventricular mass. This common junction arises by virtue of a deficiency in the "sandwich" of membranous, muscular and other layers of fibrous tissue that normally separates the mitral and tricuspid valves. This "sandwich" has been called the "atrioventricular septum." The deficiency manifests itself as a constellation of abnormalities involving the interatrial septum immediately above the valves, the interventricular septum immediately below the valves, and the valvar leaflets themselves. In addition, other major cardiac defects may be found in association with an atrioventricular septal defect, including tetralogy of Fallot, double outlet right ventricle, persistent arterial trunk (truncus arteriosus), transposition of the great arteries (discordant ventriculo-arterial connections), and congenitally corrected transposition (the combination of discordant ventriculo-arterial and discordant atrioventricular connections). When atrioventricular septal defects occur with atrial isomerism, they are often accompanied by anomalies of systemic and/or pulmonary venous connections.

Central to the description of atrioventricular septal defects is the morphology of the atrioventricular valve. In contrast to the normal three-leaflet tricuspid valve and the two-leaflet mitral valve, each of which is hinged on a complete annulus separated and supported by fibrous or muscular tissues (Figure 12A), the valve guarding a common atrioventricular junction has a total of five or six leaflets within a single annulus. Two of these leaflets, the most superior and inferior, may span the septum to lie above both ventricles and are thus designated the superior and inferior bridging leaflets, respectively. When the superior and inferior bridging leaflets are joined together, the valve tissue is partitioned into right and left segments, producing separate valvar orifices. Most commonly this area of fusion is attached to the ventricular septum and may completely obliterate the interventricular communication. This results in the so-called "partial atrioventricular septal defect", "partitioned orifice," or "primum atrial septal defect" (see Fig. 12B).

In the absence of such fusion, the bridging leaflets lie freely between the right and left atriums and ventricles. This is generally called a "complete defect" or "atrioventricular septal defect with common orifice." While the term "intermediate" has been used for defects which have separate valvar orifices and both interatrial and interventricular communications, there is no general consensus regarding other morphological features which should define such an intermediate group. Anatomically, it is more appropriate to describe any atrioventricular septal defect as having a common atrioventricular junction with either one or two valvar

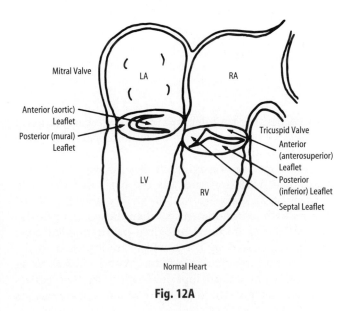

Fig. 12A

Mitral Valve

LA   RA

Anterior (aortic) Leaflet

Posterior (mural) Leaflet

LV   RV

Tricuspid Valve

Anterior (anterosuperior) Leaflet

Posterior (inferior) Leaflet

Septal Leaflet

Normal Heart

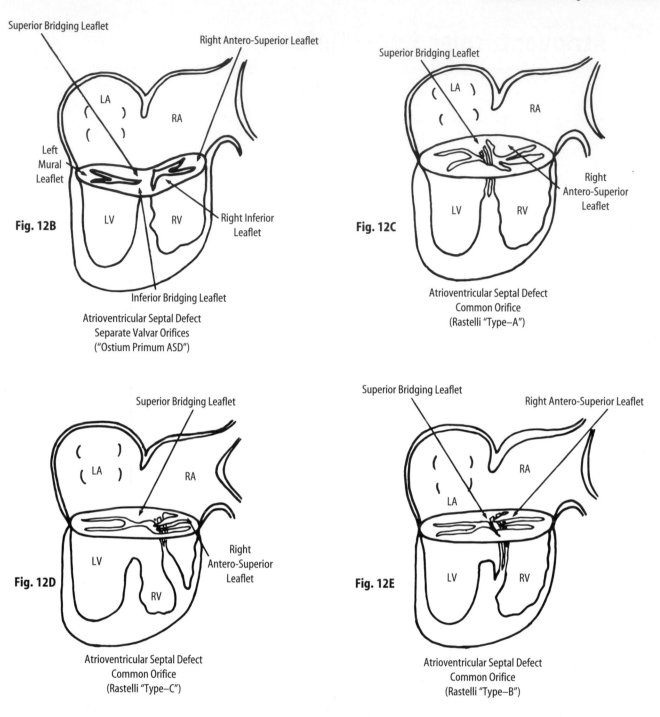

Fig. 12B
Atrioventricular Septal Defect
Separate Valvar Orifices
("Ostium Primum ASD")

Fig. 12C
Atrioventricular Septal Defect
Common Orifice
(Rastelli "Type–A")

Fig. 12D
Atrioventricular Septal Defect
Common Orifice
(Rastelli "Type–C")

Fig. 12E
Atrioventricular Septal Defect
Common Orifice
(Rastelli "Type–B")

orifices, making no reference to the degree of shunting through the defect (which is a physiological rather than an anatomical attribute).

The superior bridging leaflet shows the most anatomical variation and was the basis of the widely used Rastelli classification of atrioventricular septal defects with common orifice. When the superior bridging leaflet has minimal bridging, its right-sided edge will be supported by cords which are attached to the crest of the ventricular septum. When viewed along with the right antero-superior leaflet, the two leaflets together may give the appearance of one leaflet which is

divided into left and right sides, both of which are attached to the crest of the ventricular septum. This is the Rastelli Type A defect (see Fig. 12C).

At the other extreme, the superior bridging leaflet spans further along the right-sided valvar orifice. It is undivided and usually unattached to the septum. There is a corresponding rightward displacement of its sub-valvar apparatus and a proportionate shortening of the right antero-superior leaflet, giving the Rastelli Type C defect (see Fig. 12D).

In a Rastelli Type B defect, the superior bridging leaflet has an intermediate degree of spanning and is supported by a papillary muscle attached more apically to the right side of the ventricular septum (see Fig. 12E).

It is now recognized that these three "types" are only discrete points (perhaps seen more often than others) along a continuous spectrum of the bridging of the superior leaflet.

The morphology of the inferior bridging leaflet is more constant and this leaflet is nearly always attached to the posterior part of the septum with a variable amount of bridging. Rarely, however, it is divided and each side is attached to the crest of the ventricular septum, resulting in a six-leaflet valve. Two other leaflets – namely, the right inferior (also called the "right lateral") and right antero-superior (also called "right superior") – are committed completely to the right ventricle, while one other, the left mural (or "left lateral") leaflet, lies completely above the left ventricle. In some hearts, it may be difficult to differentiate the inferior bridging leaflet from the right inferior leaflet, this giving the appearance of a four-leaflet common valve rather than one which has five or six leaflets. Moreover, the area occupied by any one leaflet is highly variable.

It is apparent from this description that the left atrioventricular orifice, whether defined naturally by septal attachments or surgically by suturing to patch material, will be guarded by a three-leaflet valve which is distinctly different from the normal mitral valve. The leftward components of the superior and inferior bridging leaflets coapt with the mural leaflet and with each other. This latter area of contact has been called a "cleft" to emphasize its potential for regurgitation and a "commissure" to underscore its functional significance as a component of the valvar orifice. However, neither is anatomically accurate because suture of the atrioventricular septal defect "cleft" (in contrast to an isolated cleft) does not achieve a normal mitral valve, nor are the edges of the leaflets supported by the subvalvar cords and papillary muscles which define the angles between the zones of apposition of a normal atrioventricular valvar "commissure." Designation of this area as the "zone of apposition" between superior and inferior bridging leaflets serves to clarify these concepts. The annulus of a normal mitral valve is apportioned roughly 65% to the posterior (mural or lateral) leaflet and 35% to the anterior (aortic) leaflet. In contrast, in atrioventricular septal defect, the extent of the mural leaflet is variable, but usually occupies only about 25% of the circumference of a left atrioventricular orifice.

Subvalvar support of the leaflet tissue is also highly variable. The two commissures between the bridging and mural leaflets of the left-sided valve are usually attached through tendinous cords to separate papillary muscles on the lateral wall of the left ventricle. Displacement of a papillary muscle towards the septum may cause it to lie across the ventricular inflow or outflow, while approximation of the two papillary muscles may result in a type of "parachute valve." When the superior bridging leaflet lacks well-defined tendinous cords, its attachment to the ventricular septum also may narrow the left ventricular outflow. Other variations in the leaflet tissue itself include tethering of the right-sided portion of the superior bridging leaflet to the ventricular septum (analogous to Ebstein malformation) and also the accessory orifice. This latter variant consists of a miniature valvar orifice with its own cords and papillary muscle within a leaflet – usually the left mural, but occasionally the left or right side of the inferior bridging leaflet.

The angiographic hallmark of atrioventricular septal defect – the "goose-neck" appearance of the left ventricle – results from a disproportion between the inlet and outlet dimensions of the ventricular cavity. In the normal heart these are about equal, but unwedging of the aorta from between the mitral and tricuspid valves by the common orifice elongates the ventricular outlet. There is thus a longer area of continuity between the aortic valve and the left atrioventricular valve, such that the left ventricular outflow tract is defined by the ventricular free wall, the superior bridging leaflet and (depending on the interventricular communication), a variable amount of interventricular septum. While obstruction to this elongated outflow is not common, it may result from either attachments of the superior bridging leaflet in the subaortic area or any of the other mechanisms which produce a subaortic stenosis in hearts with a normal atrioventricular junction (see Chapter 16).

A deficiency of the inlet septum is an invariable finding in atrioventricular septal defect. When the valvar tissue is displaced downward and attached to the crest of the septum (resulting in a "partial" defect), the potential interventricular communication is closed and there is no channel for interventricular shunting. In the "complete" form, there is a defect in the inlet septum which may extend beneath the entire length of the common valve and further excavate the outlet septum anteriorly, or may be confined to small intercordal areas beneath either the superior or inferior bridging leaflet. Usually, the interventricular communication is deeper under the superior bridging leaflet and becomes more shallow at the back of the heart.

Similarly, defects in the interatrial septum immediately above the valve range from small, slit-like openings over one leaflet, to very large deficiencies spanning the entire length (superior to inferior) of the atrioventricular junction. In combination with defects of the oval fossa, this may produce a functional common atrium. A rare but surgically important variant consists of the complete attachment of both bridging leaflets to the entire length of the *atrial* septum, which produces an

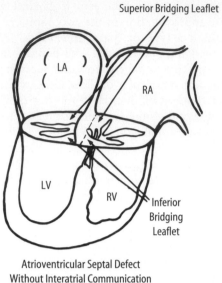

Superior Bridging Leaflet

LA

RA

LV

RV

Inferior
Bridging
Leaflet

Atrioventricular Septal Defect
Without Interatrial Communication
Separate Valvar Orifices

Fig. 12F

atrioventricular septal defect without interatrial communication – the converse of a "primum atrial septal defect" (see Fig. 12F). This malformation differs from an inlet ventricular septal defect or perimembranous ventricular septal defect of the "atrioventricular canal type" by virtue of the bridging leaflets. These may give the appearance of a straddling mitral or tricuspid valve. There is also malalignment of the atrial septum relative to the ventricular septum, which leaves a potential communication from the left ventricle to the right atrium, through the right zone of apposition, following closure of the interventricular communication. But unlike ventricular septal defect with straddling tricuspid valve, the conduction tissue remains in the expected position. Extremely rarely, both the interatrial and interventricular communications are absent, which produces an "atrioventricular septal defect with neither atrial septal defect nor ventricular septal defect."

The specialized conduction tissue in atrioventricular septal defects is displaced posteriorly, such that the atrioventricular node lies between the orifice of the coronary sinus and the crest of the ventricular septum in the so-called "nodal triangle." The non-branching bundle then runs anteriorly from its junction with the atrioventricular valve ring along the crest of the ventricular septum, approximately to its mid-point. By this time, it has given off the left bundle branches and continues towards the medial papillary muscle complex as the right bundle branch. These relationships are constant whether or not there is an interventricular communication. Thus, the conduction tissue lies immediately below the inferior bridging leaflet also in a "primum atrioventricular septal defect."

Ventricular size is the final morphological variable among hearts with atrioventricular septal defects. Either the left or right ventricle may be pathologically small, with corresponding enlargement of the opposite chamber. Usually, but not invariably, hypoplasia of a ventricle is associated with off-setting of the atrial septum towards that side of the heart. In its extreme form, this displacement results in one atrium connecting to both ventricles, the so-called double-outlet right or left atrium.

Surgical management of patients with atrioventricular septal defect has evolved rapidly as a result of the improved understanding of morphology, experience with open heart surgery in small infants, and better techniques for atrioventricular valve repair. As palliative pulmonary artery banding in most situations now carries a risk equal to or greater than complete correction, primary repair is nearly always the procedure of choice. In patients with a large interventricular communication (90% of whom have Down's syndrome), this is done electively by about three months of age to avoid pulmonary damage or earlier if needed for uncontrolled heart failure. When shunting is predominantly or exclusively at atrial level and atrioventricular valve regurgitation is mild or absent, the patients (90% of whom are chromosomally normal) experience few symptoms and usually come to elective operation after about two years of age. Experimental work, however, suggests that earlier correction might also benefit this group of patients. The presence of valvar incompetence exacerbates heart failure in either group, as does associated coarctation of the aorta, a large persistently patent arterial duct, or unbalanced ventricles. During early infancy, it is usually possible to undertake surgical intervention guided by non-invasive investigations, and cardiac catheterization adds little information to high-quality echo-Doppler studies. Following this protocol, however, patients are assumed to have reversible pulmonary hypertension (until about six months of age) and a persistently patent arterial duct (which is closed routinely at the time of open heart surgery).

The goal of surgical repair is to abolish all shunting (at atrial, ventricular and/or ductal levels) and atrioventricular valve regurgitation, while ensuring adequate outflow tracts for both ventricles and an intact conduction system. This has been reliably accomplished by a variety of techniques, none of which has been clearly demonstrated, as yet, to achieve superior results in either short-term or long-term follow-up.

Operation is done through the right atrium on cardiopulmonary bypass with very low cannulation of the inferior caval vein to ensure access to the posterior part of the defect. Alternatively, in very small infants and those with a large left superior caval vein, profound hypothermia and circulatory arrest may be preferred. When there are associated conotruncal anomalies such as tetralogy of Fallot, persistent arterial trunk (truncus arteriosus), or double outlet right ventricle, a right ventriculotomy is usually required for access to the anterior extension of the interventricular communication. Intraoperative transesophageal echocardiography is particularly useful in this malformation, both before repair to elucidate functional morphologic details and afterwards to confirm a complete and accurate correction.

For patients with a common orifice ("complete" atrioventricular septal defect), options are to carry out the repair with either separate patches for the interventricular and interatrial communications (the "two-patch technique") or division of the valvar leaflets and closure of both defects with a single patch. Both techniques rely on accurate placement of an initial marking suture at the point of coaptation of the bridging leaflets over the crest of the ventricular septum to define the subsequent right and left atrioventricular valvar orifices. The two-patch technique, in theory, may avert distortion or dehiscence of the valvar leaflets because their existing position is unchanged by sandwiching them between the patches. The most serious residual defect should then be a small interatrial or interventricular septal communication. However, placement of a patch beneath the bridging leaflets may be technically challenging, particularly at the back of the heart. While division of the inferior and superior bridging leaflets for repair with a single patch affords clear exposure of the ventricular septum, proper reattachment of the leaflets to the patch is critical for valvar function and may be more difficult with the limited, delicate tissues of young infants. In both procedures, minor tendinous cords on the right side of the septum are divided as needed for patch placement, while major ones are conserved by splitting the patch to go around them. Various materials have proved satisfactory for closure of the interventricular communication – Dacron (in a two-patch procedure), bovine pericardium, and gluteraldehyde-preserved autogenous pericardium being among the more commonly used. Pericardium is always preferred in the atrium, however, to avoid hemolysis from any residual jet of left atrioventricular valvar regurgitation against the patch. The right-hand side of the patch for the ventricular septal defect, as viewed by the surgeon working through the right atrium, is intimately related to the conduction tissue. Either of two suturing methods may reliably avoid heart block. In the two-patch technique, an extension of the patch is taken posteriorly around the right atrioventricular valvar annulus, down the free wall of the right ventricle and back on to the septal surface, well below the area of the penetrating bundle. Alternatively, sutures are placed superficially just on the right side of the crest of the ventricular septum, ending at the atrioventricular valvar annulus, and thus superficial to the conduction tissue.

With regard to closure of the interatrial communication, the patch may be extended from the valvar leaflet posteriorly on to the right atrial wall and around the back of the coronary sinus (leaving this structure to drain into the left atrium below the patch), or it may come around the annulus of the left atrioventricular valve to reach the free margin of the atrial septum (leaving the orifice of the coronary sinus in the right atrium). In the first technique, the suture line crosses above the penetrating bundle in leaflet tissue, while in the second (which must be used when a large left superior caval vein drains to the coronary sinus), it stays completely to the left side of the conduction tissue. The latter method also gives the possibility of performing a limited annuloplasty on the left atrioventricular valve where the suture line passes around its annulus.

One final surgical controversy relates to the optimal management of the left-sided zone of apposition ("cleft") between the superior and inferior bridging leaflets. While there is general agreement that regurgitation through this area should be repaired, usually by "cleft closure," optimal treatment of a non-regurgitant valve is less clear. Those who regard this area as a functional commissure advocate its patency in a three-leaflet valve which conserves the maximal functional orifice, possibly at an increased risk of subsequent late incompetence. Closure of the zone of apposition produces a two-leaflet valve which may improve late function and possibly overall patient survival, but at a cost of valvar stenosis in some cases. Intraoperative transesophageal echocardiography may help to resolve this controversy in the future.

Major or minor variations in morphology and associated malformations, which occur frequently in this group of cardiac defects, impact directly on the surgical outcome and are treated on their own merits. Additional muscular ventricular septal defects may be difficult to identify under papillary muscles within the trabeculated right ventricle, but the scooped-out inlet septum often allows them to be exposed and closed on the left side of the septum. Resection of fibrous or muscular narrowing of the left ventricular outflow tract can be done, working through the atrioventricular valve without risking damage to the conduction tissue, which is not related to the subaortic area in these patients. However, outflow obstruction resulting from the attachments of the left atrioventricular valve may not be amenable to resection and it then becomes necessary either to replace the valve or to manage the lesion as a "single ventricle." When the left atrioventricular valve is replaced, either primarily or at reoperation, prosthetic obstruction of the elongated left ventricular outflow must be avoided by use of a low-profile device and/or positioning it within the left atrium. A right thoracotomy approach gives excellent exposure for such procedures when they are done as reoperations.

Malfunction of the left atrioventricular valve following correction of atrioventricular septal defects is a major cause of both reoperation and non-survival. It may be caused by any of the mechanisms that affect the mitral valve in a normal heart and similar techniques of repair are applicable in most situations. An accessory orifice, however, tends to be associated with valvar stenosis and is therefore not closed routinely. Similarly, the so-called "intermediate" forms of atrioventricular septal defect, with a tongue of tissue connecting the superior and inferior bridging leaflets, are prone to left atrioventricular valve obstruction when the "cleft" is approximated. A previously competent valve may be rendered regurgitant by prolapse of the leaflet, when its height is altered by the ventricular septal patch or by loss of subvalvar attachments. Intraoperative comparison with published values for normal valve sizes and transesophageal echocardiography are particularly useful to quantitate valvar function, identify the causes of malfunction and guide surgical repair.

When there is severe dominance of one ventricle, either before or after correction, mortality following two-ventricle repair becomes prohibitive. This probably occurs at a cavity ratio of about 3:1–4:1, although the methods of estimating ventricular dominance remain imprecise and other, as yet poorly defined factors, also may be contributory. In the case of left ventricular dominance, partial bypass of the inadequate right heart with a bidirectional cavopulmonary anastomosis (the so-called "one-and-a-half-ventricle repair") is a reasonable alternative. Right ventricular dominance is more difficult to manage. While in theory such patients should be candidates for a Fontan-type circulation, the overall outcome in this group remains suboptimal.

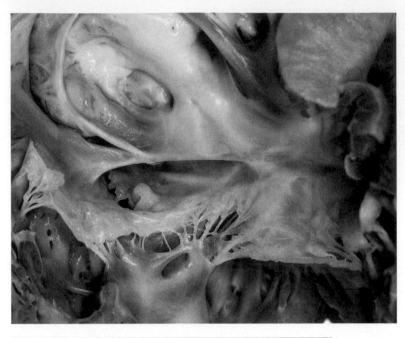

12.1 Atrioventricular septal defect with partitioned valvar orifice. The heart has been opened across the atrioventricular junction to display the septal surface of the right atrium and right ventricle. The oval fossa contains a small "secundum" atrial septal defect (defect of the oval fossa), which is separated from the "ostium primum" defect by a well-developed interatrial septum. The right atrioventricular valve is supported by a large septomarginal trabeculation and the left atrioventricular valve is partly seen through the defect. The coronary sinus is minimally displaced in this heart. The conduction tissue passes immediately beneath the posterior half of the atrioventricular valve and then towards the medial papillary muscle complex.

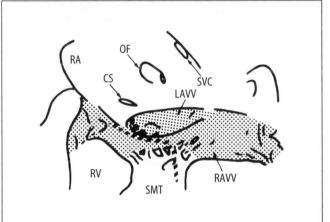

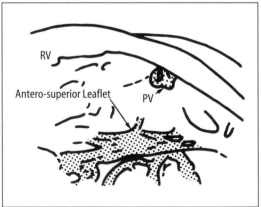

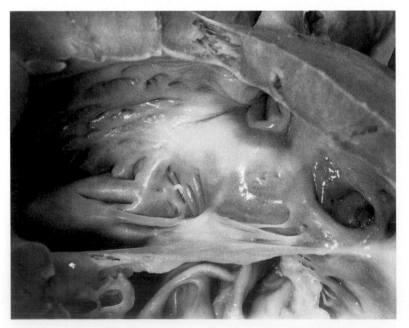

12.2 The outlet portion of the right ventricle is shown to illustrate the attachments of the anterosuperior leaflet of the right atrioventricular valve to the ventricular septum.

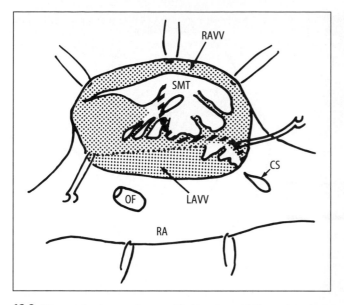

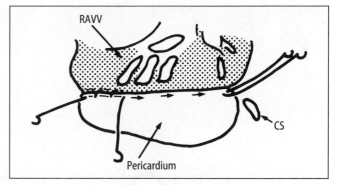

12.4 The distance between the two sutures is measured and a patch of pericardium is cut to the approximate size and shape of the interatrial defect. Anchoring the two ends of the patch with slight tension and the smooth side down (towards the left atrium) helps to expose the suture line. The patch is attached to the right atrioventricular valve leaflet using a monofilament suture, usually with a simple running stitch.

12.3 Using cardiopulmonary bypass with bicaval cannulation and moderate hypothermia, a "partial" atrioventricular septal defect is exposed by a long oblique incision in the right atrium. If a vent is not placed directly into the left atrium, the defect in the oval fossa may be used conveniently for this purpose. The right and left atrioventricular valves are inspected through the interatrial communication, as are the right and left ventricular outflow tracts. Double-ended sutures are then placed anteriorly and posteriorly, through the right atrioventricular valve at its junctions with the atrial septum. The conduction tissue will lie under the surgeon's right hand for about half the length of the value.

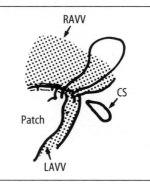

12.7 *(left)* At the right-hand (posterior) marking suture, stitches are deviated onto the left atrioventricular valvar annulus to avoid injury to the conduction tissue. These bites are superficial in and parallel to the valve annulus. If needed, they can also effect a limited annuloplasty of the left atrioventricular valve.

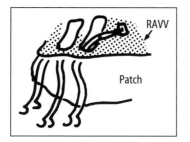

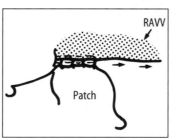

12.5 When the valve tissue is very delicate, interrupted mattress sutures supported by small pledgets of pericardium are passed from the ventricular side of the valve, immediately adjacent to its septal attachment, into the atrium and then through the pericardial patch. Occasionally, an Ebstein-like attachment of the right side of the superior bridging leaflet to the ventricular septum makes it necessary to place these sutures through the left atrioventricular valve anteriorly (on the surgeon's left-hand side).

12.6 Still another alternative suture technique is a continuous locking stitch ("blanket stitch"), which prevents purse-stringing of the suture line and brings the patch into firm apposition with the valve leaflet.

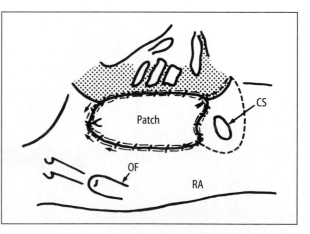

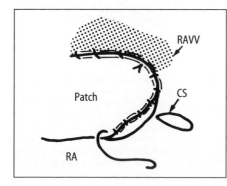

12.8 When the suture line has progressed beyond the coronary sinus, it is anchored with a locking stitch and brought back onto the atrial septum. Competence of the left atrioventricular valve is tested by injection of saline at this point. A few sutures placed within the left atrium are usually necessary to bring the patch back to the free edge of the atrial septum.

12.9 *(above)* The suture line is completed at the highest point of the right atrium, such that filling the left side of the heart evacuates air. Usually, this requires bringing the second arm of the suture counter-clockwise for a short distance to the edge of the septum. The small secundum atrial defect is closed separately by direct suture. An alternative technique, which also avoids the conduction tissue, is extension of the patch along the base of the right atrioventricular valve to its posterior (inferior) leaflet and then onto the atrial septum behind the coronary sinus (dashed line), leaving the coronary sinus to drain into the left atrium.

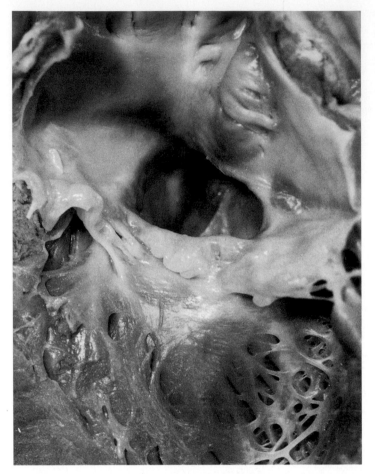

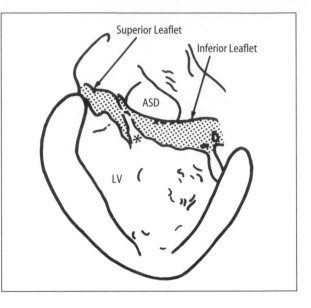

12.10 Atrioventricular septal defect with partitioned valvar orifice. The left atrioventricular junction of the specimen illustrated in Figures 12.1 and 12.2. The superior and inferior leaflets of the left atrioventricular valve are separated by the zone of apposition (a "cleft" or "commissure") (asterisk) which extends to the septum and is thus complete. The interatrial communication is large. The outflow of the left ventricle lies beneath the superior leaflet of the left atrioventricular valve. The conduction tissue runs posteriorly beneath the inferior leaflet.

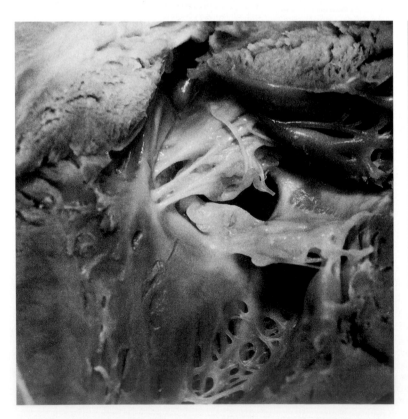

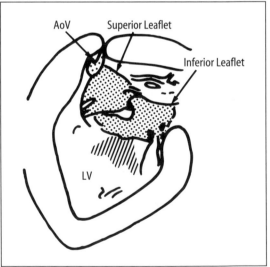

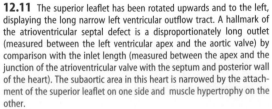

12.11 The superior leaflet has been rotated upwards and to the left, displaying the long narrow left ventricular outflow tract. A hallmark of the atrioventricular septal defect is a disproportionately long outlet (measured between the left ventricular apex and the aortic valve) by comparison with the inlet length (measured between the apex and the junction of the atrioventricular valve with the septum and posterior wall of the heart). The subaortic area in this heart is narrowed by the attachment of the superior leaflet on one side and muscle hypertrophy on the other.

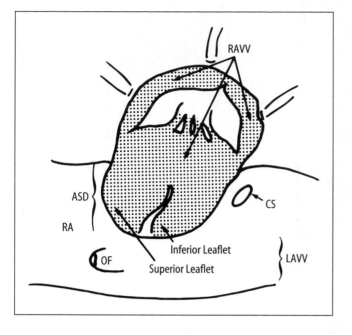

12.12 Narrowing of the left ventricular outflow in atrioventricular septal defects with either common atrioventricular orifice or separate valvar orifices can be approached through the right atrium in the completely relaxed heart. The large atrial septal defect provides access to the left atrioventricular valve, while the "cleft" permits retraction of the superior leaflet to expose the subaortic area.

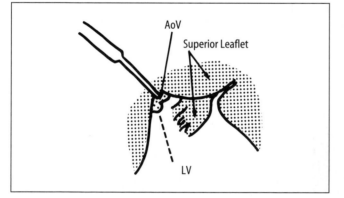

12.13 A small nerve root or nerve hook retractor (depending on the size of the patient) is used to elevate the superior leaflet until the aortic valve is seen. Since the conduction tissue lies more posteriorly than in the normal heart, there is no risk of injury to the penetrating bundle. An incision is made below the aortic valve into the muscular subaortic outflow (dashed line).

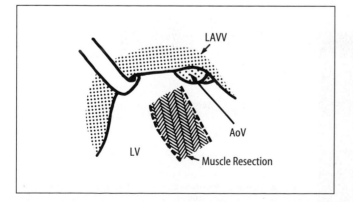

12.14 Rotating the retractor rightward exposes muscle on the lateral side of the outflow tract, where a second vertical incision is made. Muscle between the two incisions is then resected and cardioplegia is infused into the aortic root to exclude damage to the aortic valve. After sufficient muscle has been removed, the left ventricle is irrigated vigorously to remove any fragments of tissue which constitute potential systemic emboli. The operation is completed by repair of the left atrioventricular valvar regurgitation (if needed) and closure of the interatrial communication (see Figures 12.4–12.9).

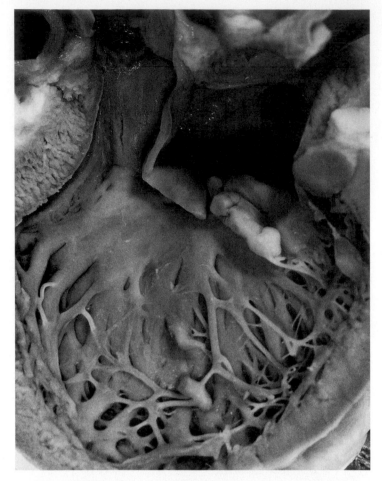

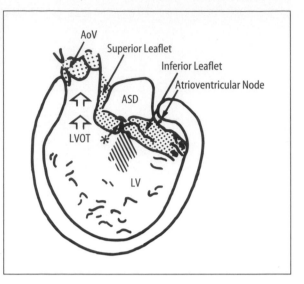

12.15 Atrioventricular septal defect with partitioned valvar orifice. Septal surface of the left ventricle. The zone of apposition ("cleft") (asterisk) in the left atrioventricular valve lies between the superior and inferior leaflets and is directed towards the atrial septum. The superior leaflet has no intercordal spaces at its attachment to the ventricular septum. The left ventricular outflow (open arrows) is long and narrow but, in contrast to the specimen illustrated in Figure 12.11, there is no obstruction because the attachment of cords from the left atrioventricular valve are confined beneath the leaflet.

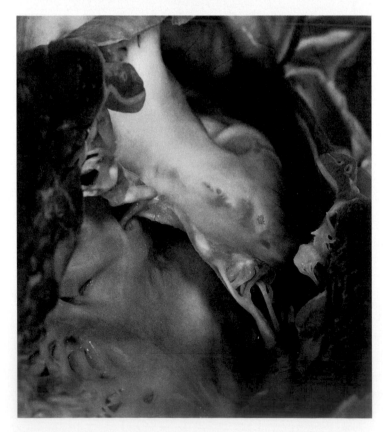

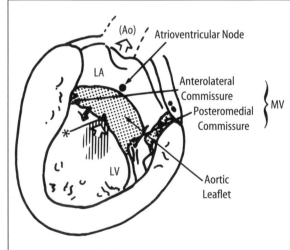

12.16 Isolated "cleft" in the aortic leaflet of the mitral valve in a heart which, apart from anomalous pulmonary venous connection, is normal. The septal surface of the left ventricle is shown for comparison with Figure 12.15. Attachments from the two normal commissures on either side of the left ventricular outflow (open arrow) anchor the leaflet across the subaortic area and produce obstruction. The "cleft "(asterisk) in the aortic (anterior) mitral valvar leaflet is directed towards the left ventricular outflow tract rather than the atrial septum.

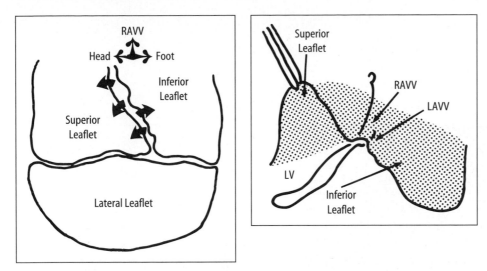

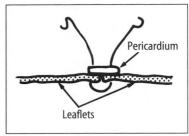

12.18 *(left)* A suture is placed at the apex of the zone of apposition, which usually extends to the ventricular septum, passing each end of a double-armed needle from the ventricular to atrial side of the superior and inferior leaflets. Often there is a small gap in the valve tissue where the leaflets attach to the ventricular septum.

12.17 *(above)* While routine closure of the zone of apposition remains controversial, thickening of the leaflets here indicate significant regurgitation which may be eliminated by approximation of the superior and inferior leaflets. Exposure is set up through the right atrium via the atrial septal defect (which can be enlarged if needed). Injection of cold saline into the left ventricle confirms the regurgitation and demonstrates the leaflet morphology.

12.20 *(above)* The pericardial buttress is wide enough to cover the valvar "cleft" and slightly longer than the opposing surfaces of the superior and inferior leaflets.

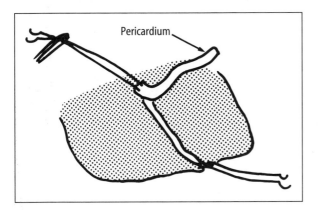

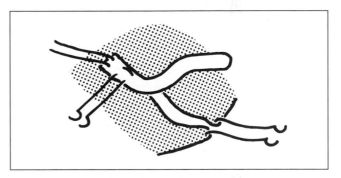

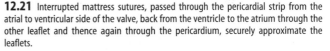

12.19 *(above)* Orientation of the zone of apposition is nearly always oblique rather than exactly perpendicular to the septum. A second suture is placed at the point where the free edges of the leaflets meet, as determined again by the injection of saline into the ventricle. This suture should line up the two sides of the "cleft." The first suture is then passed through a pericardial buttress and held under slight tension.

12.21 Interrupted mattress sutures, passed through the pericardial strip from the atrial to ventricular side of the valve, back from the ventricle to the atrium through the other leaflet and thence again through the pericardium, securely approximate the leaflets.

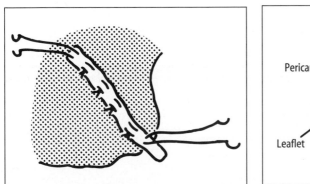

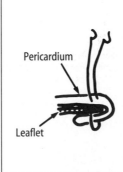

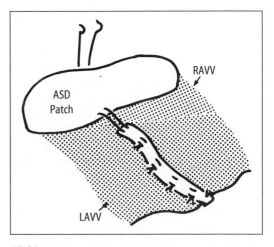

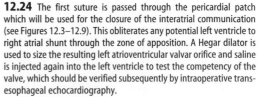

12.22 At the free edge of the leaflet, both ends of the simple suture are passed through the pericardial buttress.

12.23 The end of the pericardial strip is turned under the free edges of the valvar leaflets and secured within the loop of the single suture.

12.24 The first suture is passed through the pericardial patch which will be used for the closure of the interatrial communication (see Figures 12.3–12.9). This obliterates any potential left ventricle to right atrial shunt through the zone of apposition. A Hegar dilator is used to size the resulting left atrioventricular valvar orifice and saline is injected again into the left ventricle to test the competency of the valve, which should be verified subsequently by intraoperative transesophageal echocardiography.

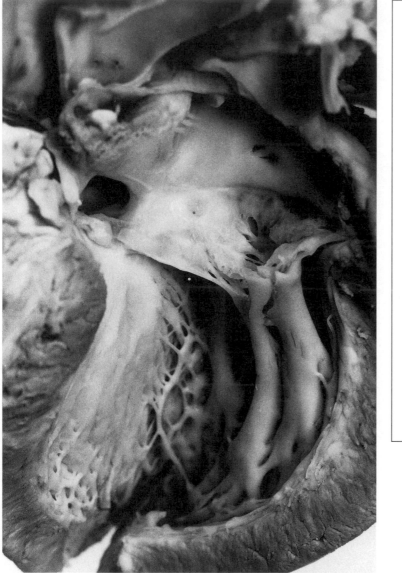

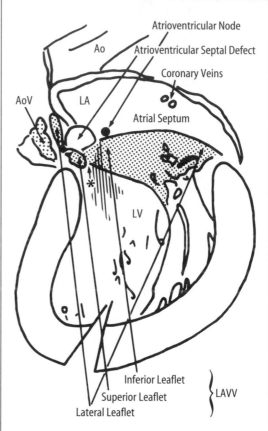

12.25 Atrioventricular septal defect with partitioned valvar orifice. The heart has been opened through the lateral leaflet of the left-sided atrioventricular valve to show the left atrioventricular junction and outflow tract. The atrial septum is fused for most of its length with the large inferior leaflet, leaving a small interatrial communication above the tiny superior leaflet and zone of apposition (asterisk). The single papillary muscle has two columns which are fused and placed eccentrically to produce a "parachute" type of support for the lateral and inferior valvar leaflets. The cords are short and poorly liberated from the leaflet tissue. This anatomy differs from the classical "parachute" mitral valve where the two leaflets and commissures are normally formed but supported by a single, central, papillary muscle. The zone of apposition between the superior and inferior leaflets has no subvalvar supporting apparatus (cords or papillary muscles) but functions as a commissure. The subaortic outflow region is extremely narrow as a result of muscular hypertrophy and attachment of the leaflets to the ventricular septum which is covered by endocardial fibrosis.

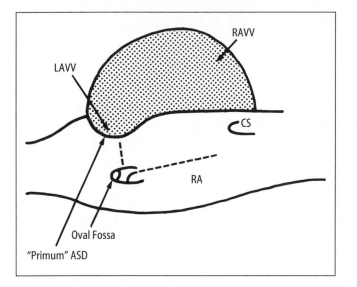

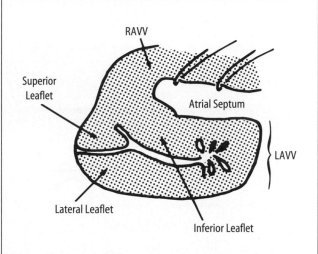

12.26 This heart illustrates very unfavorable morphology. The first decision (ideally made preoperatively) is whether obstruction of the left-sided atrioventricular valve and subaortic region can be relieved sufficiently to perform a two-ventricle repair or whether the malformation should be managed as a single ventricle, taking into consideration the patient's age, pulmonary vascular resistance, atrioventricular valvar regurgitation, myocardial function, and prospects for heart transplantation. Should a two-ventricle repair be attempted, the approach to the left atrioventricular valve is through the right atrium. The "primum" defect and oval fossa are connected and the septum is incised near the free wall of the right atrium (dashed lines). This leaves its attachment to the leaflet tissue intact (which may be important for valve function) and avoids working near the conduction system. When a Fontan circulation is planned, this flap of septum is completely removed, conserving a small rim of tissue above the valve leaflet.

12.27 Rotation of the atrial septal flap towards the left exposes the left atrium and left atrioventricular valve. In the area of the "primum" defect, the attachment of the ventricular septum defines the left-sided and right-sided valves, but this may not be obvious from the atrium until a right-angled instrument is passed under the valve to explore the septum. Usually, there is off-setting of the atrial septum and ventricular septum when both are attached to the leaflets. The valve is tested by injection of saline into the ventricle and its morphology (which can be difficult to understand) is carefully studied.

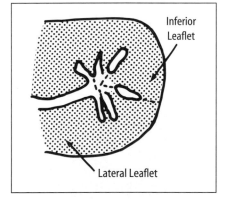

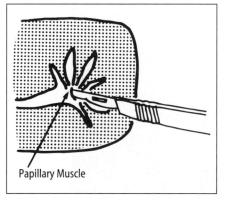

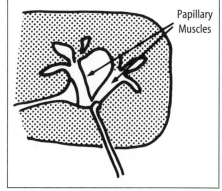

12.28 The "parachute" portion of the left atrioventricular valve is treated in a manner similar to a classical "parachute valve." The cords are liberated by division of any tissue in the intercordal spaces (dashed line). If a portion of the leaflet, supported on both sides by cords, is fused together, this can be opened to the annulus as a commissure (dashed line).

12.29 The fused papillary muscle is divided perpendicularly to the line of valve closure. This incision is carried towards the base of the papillary muscle, being careful to conserve cordal attachments and adequate muscle to support both sides of the valve.

12.30 Following valvotomy, the separate papillary muscles should permit the valve to open, while the mobilized cords retain leaflet coaptation.

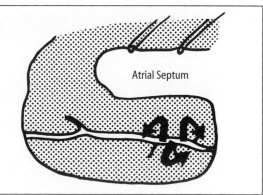

12.31 The valvar orifice is sized and its competence tested by injection of cold saline into the ventricle. There is nearly always some (mild-to-moderate) regurgitation. Intraoperative transesophageal echocardiography is essential to estimate if this will be acceptable post-operatively. A two-ventricle repair is completed by relief of the subaortic obstruction (see Figures 12.13–12.14), closure of the zone of apposition (if needed) and closure of the atrial septal defects. The patch can be safely sutured to the margins of the "primum" atrial septal defect in this heart because the atrial septum is already attached to the valve over the area of conduction tissue.

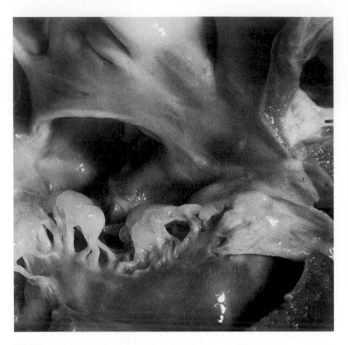
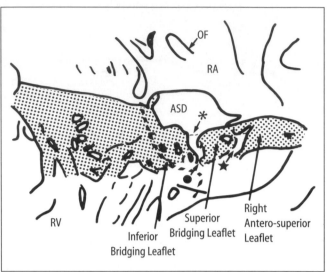

12.32 Atrioventricular septal defect with common orifice. Right atrioventricular junction. There is minimal bridging of the superior leaflet, making this a Rastelli "Type-A" defect. The superior bridging leaflet of the left atrioventricular valve is attached to the right side of the crest of the ventricular septum, leaving a bare area (star) on the crest, between its attachment and that of the right anterosuperior leaflet. The zone of apposition (asterisk) separates the inferior bridging leaflet from the superior bridging leaflet, leaving a second, exposed area on the crest of the septum between them (dot). The conduction tissue will lie posteriorly from this area on the crest of the ventricular septum. The interatrial communication is large, extending the full length of both superior and inferior bridging leaflets, while the interventricular communication consists of multiple, small areas between cordal attachments of the atrioventricular valve.

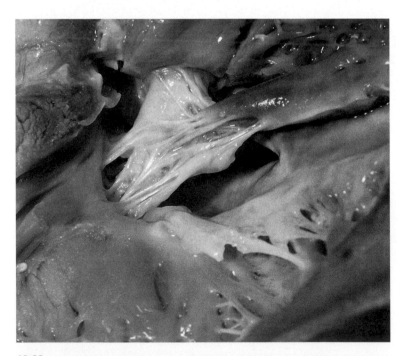
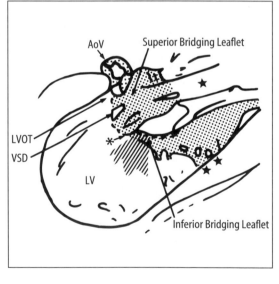

12.33 Left ventricular outflow. The mural leaflet and free wall of the left ventricle have been rotated upward to show the attachment of the superior bridging leaflet to the crest of the septum. Three papillary muscles (stars) support the leftward components of the atrioventricular valve. The "cleft" or zone of apposition (asterisk) between the superior and inferior bridging leaflets is not supported by a papillary muscle. This feature differentiates it from a true commissure. The left ventricular outflow is elongated and slightly narrow.

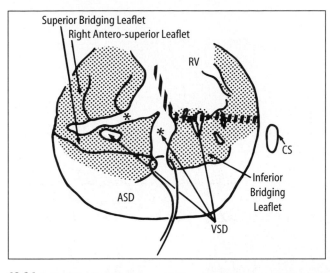

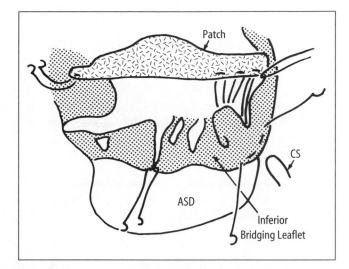

12.34 A standard right atrial exposure with bicaval cannulation is used for the repair of atrioventricular septal defects with a common valvar orifice ("complete atrioventricular septal defect"). In the surgeon's view, the conduction system passes from the nodal triangle in front of the posteriorly displaced coronary sinus, along the crest of the septum, approximately to the junction of the superior and inferior bridging leaflets. The valve is tested and a suture is placed at the point where the superior and inferior bridging leaflets meet above the septum. The asterisks correspond to the bare area of the septum, as shown in Figure 12.32.

12.35 A patch is cut to fit the highly variable shape of the interventricular communication, leaving an extension of about 1 cm posteriorly, to avoid stitching in the area of the conduction tissue. This part of the patch is sutured to the base of the right-sided atrioventricular valvar leaflet, from its attachment at the atrial septum to the right ventricular free wall, with a continuous mattress stitch. In young patients with delicate leaflets, the suture line is usefully supported with a strip of pericardium on the atrial aspect of the valve.

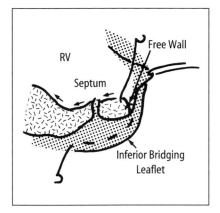

12.36 *(left)* At the right ventricular posterior wall, the suture line leaves the atrioventricular valve, passes down the free wall of the ventricle and back on to the septum below the position of the conduction tissue.

12.37 *(right)* When the suture line has passed beyond the junction of the superior and inferior bridging leaflets (the "zone of apposition"), it comes up on to the crest of the ventricular septal defect between the attachments of the superior bridging and the right anterosuperior leaflets.

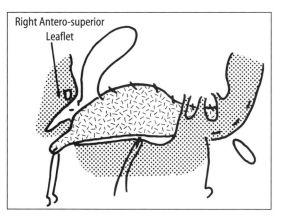

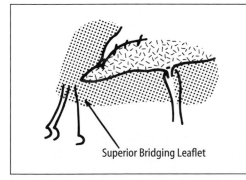

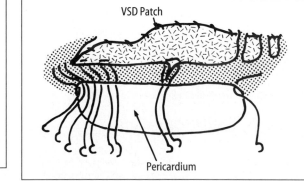

12.38 Anteriorly, there is a small extension of the interventricular communication beneath the undivided portion of the superior bridging leaflet. This is closed with the small tongue of patch material. At the junction of the atrioventricular leaflet with the atrial septum, both the mattress suture on the upper edge of the patch and the running suture are passed through the valvar leaflet into the right atrium. Maintaining the height of the leaflet in this area is important to avoid narrowing of the left ventricular outflow tract or, alternatively, causing leaflet prolapse with resulting atrioventricular valvar regurgitation.

12.39 The interatrial defect is closed with a second patch of pericardium, sandwiching the superior and inferior bridging leaflets between the two patches, with interrupted mattress sutures. Pericardium minimizes hemolysis, if there should be a residual jet of atrioventricular valvar regurgitation against the patch postoperatively. Left atrioventricular valvar regurgitation is repaired as needed (see Figures 12.8–12.24), and the remainder of the patch is inserted as for closure of a partial defect (see Figures 12.5–12.9). Alternatively, in older patients with thicker valvar tissue, a continuous running technique may be used for the suture line. Depending on the specific morphology, the ventricular patch may be more conveniently placed, starting anteriorly and working towards the area of junction between the valvar leaflet and the atrial septum, and then posteriorly towards the region of the conduction tissue.

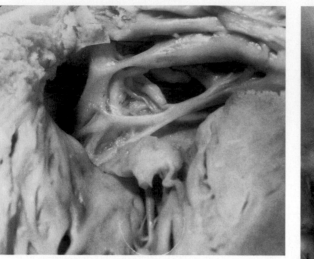

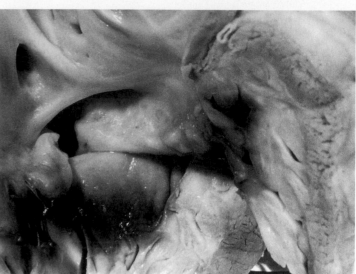

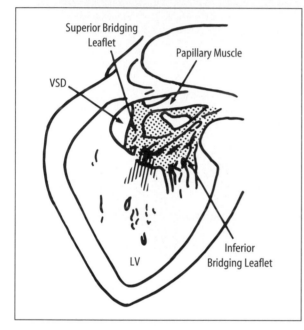

12.40 **Atrioventricular septal defect with common valvar orifice.** Left ventricular outflow. There is extreme bridging of the left superior leaflet (Rastelli "Type C") and right ventricular outflow tract obstruction (tetralogy of Fallot). The superior bridging leaflet does not attach to the ventricular septum and is supported by a papillary muscle which has been rotated upwards and counter-clockwise. The aortic valve is dextroposed over the right ventricle and hence is not seen.

12.41 Right atrioventricular junction. The interatrial communication is moderately large. A papillary muscle in the right ventricle supports the superior bridging leaflet which has no septal attachment. Anteriorly, it blends with the atrial septum (small open triangle). The axis of the conduction tissue passes anteriorly from the posterior nodal triangle, along the crest of the ventricular septal defect to the junction of the superior and inferior bridging leaflets.

Fig 12.42➔

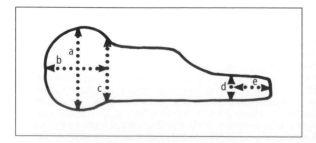

12.44 Repair of atrioventricular septal defect with tetralogy of Fallot differs from that of uncomplicated atrioventricular septal defect in 1) cannulation of the superior caval vein, which needs to be sufficiently high to permit the option of a bidirectional cavopulmonary anastomosis; 2) relief of the right ventricular outflow obstruction, and 3) the shape of the patch for the ventricular septal defect. The "comma" or "tear-drop" shaped patch is extended for the distance of aortic overriding (a) and the length by which the defect excavates into the infundibular (outlet) septum (b). Other measurements include the depth of the interventricular communication beneath the superior (c) and inferior (d) bridging leaflets, as well as a posterior extension (e) to pass around the right atrioventricular valve away from the conduction tissue. The superior bridging leaflet is nearly always unattached and undivided (Rastelli "Type C") in association with tetralogy of Fallot or with persistent arterial trunk (truncus arteriosus).

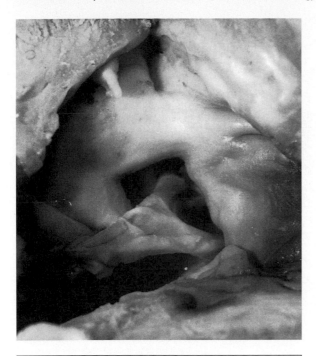

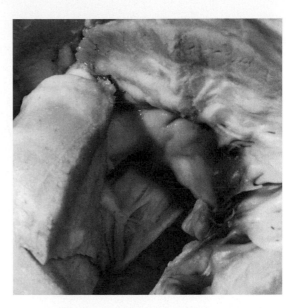

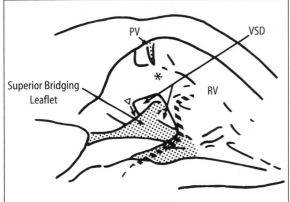

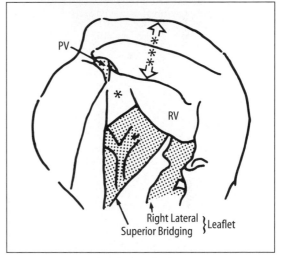

12.42 Right ventricular outflow. The portion of right ventricular free wall supporting the papillary muscle in the previous view has been rotated towards the right and downwards, demonstrating anterior displacement of the outlet septum (asterisk) and severe subpulmonary obstruction. The ventricular septal defect is large and excavates into the outlet septum beyond the superior bridging leaflet, the *ventricular* surface of the rightward portion of which is seen in this exposure. The only attachment (now unseen) of this leaflet is to the interatrial septum (open triangle). Conduction tissue lies on the crest of the posterior half of the defect. The aortic valve, although overriding the ventricular septal defect, is not seen.

12.43 The right ventricular outflow is rotated slightly more counter-clockwise than in the preceding view to show the small pulmonary valve above the hypertrophied and displaced outlet septum (single asterisk). There is severe hypertrophy of the right ventricle (triple asterisk), of which virtually all the cavity is seen in these two last views. A clearly defined right antero-superior leaflet is not seen in this heart.

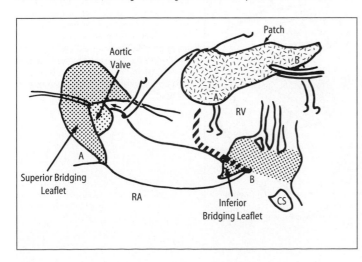

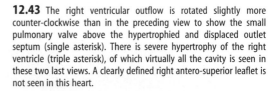

12.45 The patch (see Figure 12.44 – opposite page) for the ventricular septal defect in complete atrioventricular septal defect with tetralogy of Fallot can usually be inserted working through the atrium, although extreme overriding around the aorta may make the upper margin more easily accessible through a ventriculotomy. Sutures are placed radially around the aortic valve until they reach the junction of the valve or the outlet septum with the superior bridging leaflet (A). At this point, both the continuous suture and a second, double-armed mattress suture are brought from the patch, through the valvar leaflet, into the right atrium. The remainder of the repair is similar to other complete atrioventricular septal defects (Figures 12.34–12.39 and 12.4–12.9). A second mattress suture at the junction of the inferior bridging leaflet with the atrial septum (B) is useful to prevent distortion of the atrioventricular valves. Obstruction to the right ventricular outflow is managed as in tetralogy of Fallot. The extremely hypertrophied and small right ventricle in this heart, which will be further compromised by the ventricular septal patch, would require a bidirectional cavopulmonary anastomosis (see Figures 27.27–27.30) to partially bypass the right ventricle. This "one-and-a-half ventricle repair" usually also incorporates an orthotopic pulmonary homograft valve.

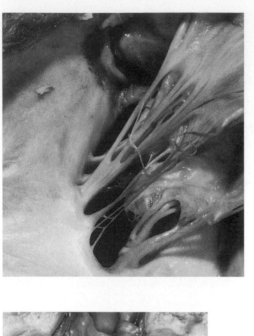

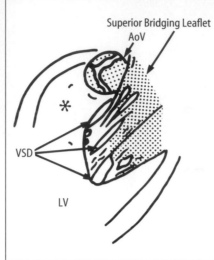

12.46 Atrioventricular septal defect with common valvar orifice. Left ventricular outflow tract. This series of hearts demonstrates the variability of the left ventricular outflow which results from differences in the attachment of the superior bridging leaflet, the size and position of the interventricular communication, and the leaflet tissue itself. In this heart, a relatively normal leaflet attaches to the crest of a deep ventricular septal defect (Rastelli "Type A") with multiple intercordal spaces extending over the full length of the attachment. Even though the aortic valve slightly overrides the defect, insertion of the patch to close the interventricular communication on the right side of the septum should not in any way compromise the widely patent left ventricular outflow tract (asterisk).

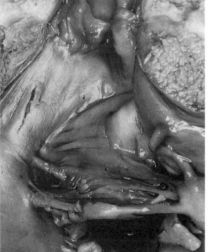

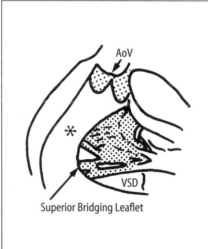

12.47 In contrast to the previous specimen, a long narrow left ventricular outflow (asterisk) has been defined by the extensive attachment of a thickened, dysplastic superior bridging leaflet to the greater part of the septum. Some intercordal spaces exist more apically, but the diameter of the outflow is less than that of the aortic valve. If the left atrioventricular valve is replaced, excision of the leaflet attachment, with careful positioning of the ventricular septal patch and possibly septal myectomy (see Figures 12.12–12.14), may achieve sufficient relief of the obstruction for a successful two-ventricle repair.

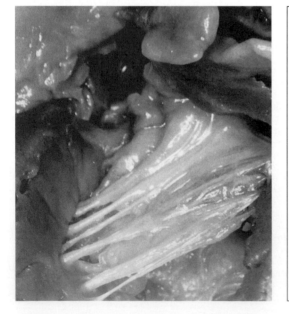

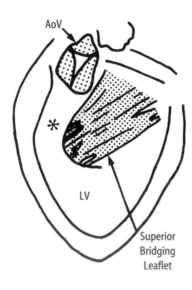

12.48 Extensive attachment of the superior bridging leaflet to the crest of the ventricular septal defect with obliteration of the intercordal spaces again causes subaortic narrowing of the left ventricular outflow tract (asterisk). In this heart, the entire subaortic length of the leaflet is bound down. Relief of the obstruction may not be possible, even with excision of the atrioventricular valve. Such cases become candidates for management as a "single" ventricle, using the pulmonary valve as a systemic outflow for the heart.

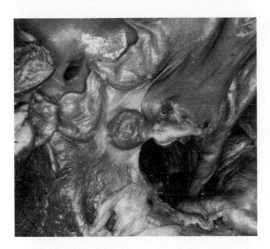

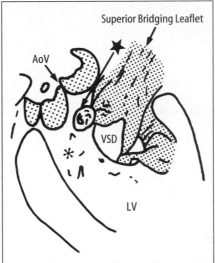

12.49 The superior bridging leaflet in this specimen is completely attached to the inter-ventricular septum for only a short distance below the aortic valve (essentially Rastelli "Type C") and the left ventricular outflow (asterisk) is wide. However, partial obstruction results from a button of fibrous tissue (star) extending from the atrioventricular valve into the subaortic area.

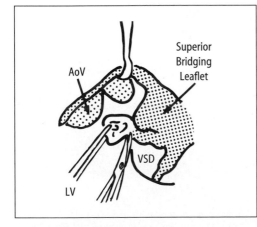

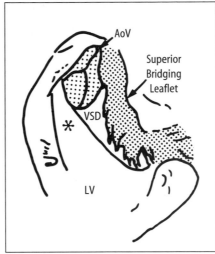

12.50 The superior bridging leaflet in this heart is completely unattached and free floating above the defect in the interventricular septum (Rastelli "Type C"). The aortic valve is displaced to the right ventricular side of the septum, such that the outflow of the left ventricle (asterisk) is through the ventricular septal defect.

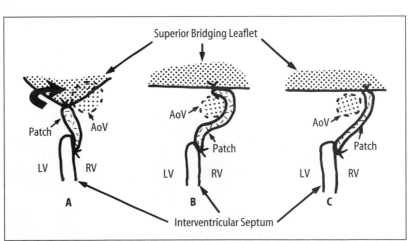

12.51 Most of the left ventricular outflow obstruction shown in Figure 12.49 can be relieved by resection of the fibrous nodule. Exposure in the relaxed heart is obtained through the right atrium and atrial septal defect by retraction of the superior bridging leaflet towards the patient's head. Sharp dissection detaches the tissue from the valvar leaflet, which is then inspected for damage. Infusion of cardioplegia into the aortic root will confirm that the aortic valve remains competent and the diameter of the outflow tract is calibrated with a Hegar dilator.

12.52 When the superior bridging leaflet is free floating, placement of the patch over the ventricular septal defect critically impacts on the left ventricular outflow tract, particularly if the aorta is dextroposed towards the right ventricle. A shallow patch (A) pulls the superior bridging leaflet down towards the ventricular septum, both narrowing the outflow of the left ventricle and producing atrioventricular valvar regurgitation. A patch inserted at the correct level (B) can still restrict the subaortic area if the extension around the aortic valve ("comma-shape" – see Figure 12.44) is inadequate. Correct placement of the patch (C) leaves the level of the superior bridging leaflet unaltered, with an open outflow to the aortic valve. If this compromises the *right* ventricular cavity or outflow, a bidirectional cavopulmonary anastomosis can be incorporated into the repair.

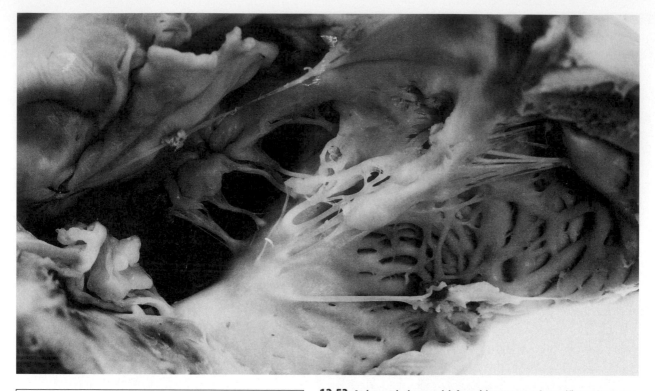

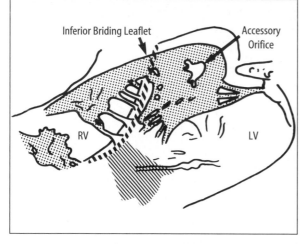

12.53 Atrioventricular septal defect with common valvar orifice and accessory orifice. The posterior part of the heart is viewed from the atrial side, showing a long discrete raphé between the right and left components of the inferior bridging leaflet, both of which are supported by multiple cords attached to the ventricular septum. A long non-branching and bifurcating bundle of atrioventricular conduction axis is vulnerable on the exposed crest of the ventricular septal defect. In the leftward portion of the leaflet, an accessory orifice is supported circumferentially by tendinous cords. The right inferior leaflet is not seen in this view.

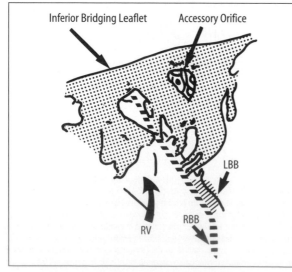

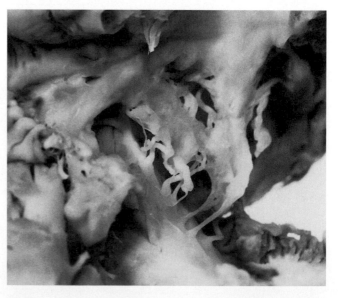

12.54 An oblique view of the inferior bridging leaflet, as seen from the atrium, looking down towards the left ventricle. The conduction tissue lies subendocardially on the exposed crest of the ventricular septum and there is an accessory orifice in the inferior bridging leaflet on its leftward portion. This is an unusual position for an accessory orifice.

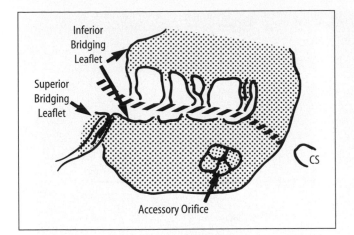

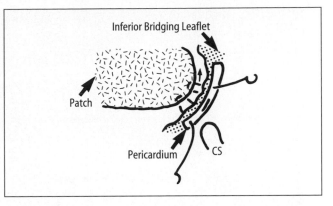

12.55 Repair is performed through a standard right atrial exposure with bicaval cannulation. An accessory orifice predisposes to obstruction of the left atrioventricular valve, so the superior and inferior bridging leaflets are approximated *only* where they meet over the crest of the ventricular septum. The valve (and accessory orifice, which is essentially a tiny valve within the leaflet) is tested by injection of saline into the ventricle. The conduction tissue, which usually lies beneath the inferior bridging leaflet, is exposed in this heart by virtue of the deep split in the inferior bridging leaflet.

12.56 In order to avoid placement of stitches in the area of the conduction tissue, an extension of the patch for the ventricular septal defect is sutured to the base of the rightward portion of the inferior bridging leaflet, from its junction with the atrial or ventricular septum for about 1 cm above the free right ventricular wall. This suture line is supported with a small strip of pericardium.

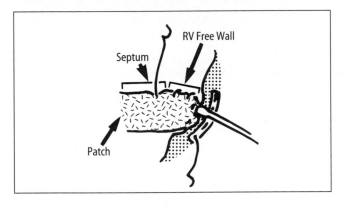

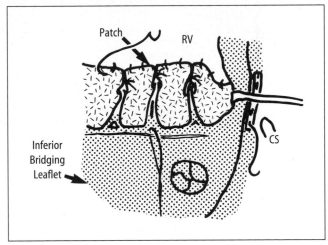

12.57 The patch is then lowered into the ventricle, and the suture line proceeds down the free wall of the right ventricle and back to the right ventricular side of the septum, well below the conduction tissue on the crest of the septum. Attachments of the leaflet tissue often make exposure of this area difficult and it may be necessary to divide some secondary cords.

12.58 Even though the rightward components of the inferior bridging leaflet will be attached to the patch for the ventricular septal defect, the preservation of major cords helps to position the leaflet at the correct level and may improve its function. This can be done by splitting the patch up to the level of cordal insertions and reapproximating the Dacron to itself with interrupted sutures.

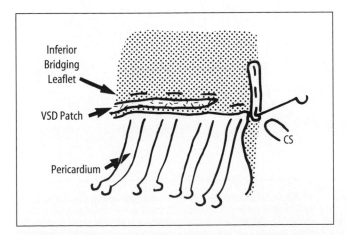

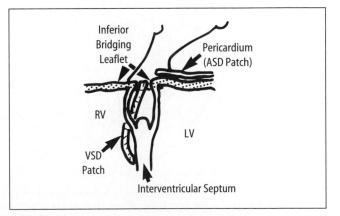

12.59 Both the right and leftward components of the inferior bridging leaflet are attached to the Dacron (ventricular) and pericardial (atrial) patches with multiple interrupted mattress sutures (or, in older patients, a continuous suture). When the leaflet tissue is very delicate, a second strip of pericardium may be used to support the sutures on the rightward side of the valve. The accessory orifice is not distorted in any way.

12.60 Using this technique, there are no sutures that could damage the conduction tissue close to the crest of the ventricular septum. The patch over the ventricular septal defect leaves a small recess of the right ventricle in continuity with the left ventricle posteriorly, which may produce interesting post-operative angiographic appearances, but is of no functional significance. The remainder of the pericardial patch is used to close the interatrial communication (see Figures 12.7–12.9).

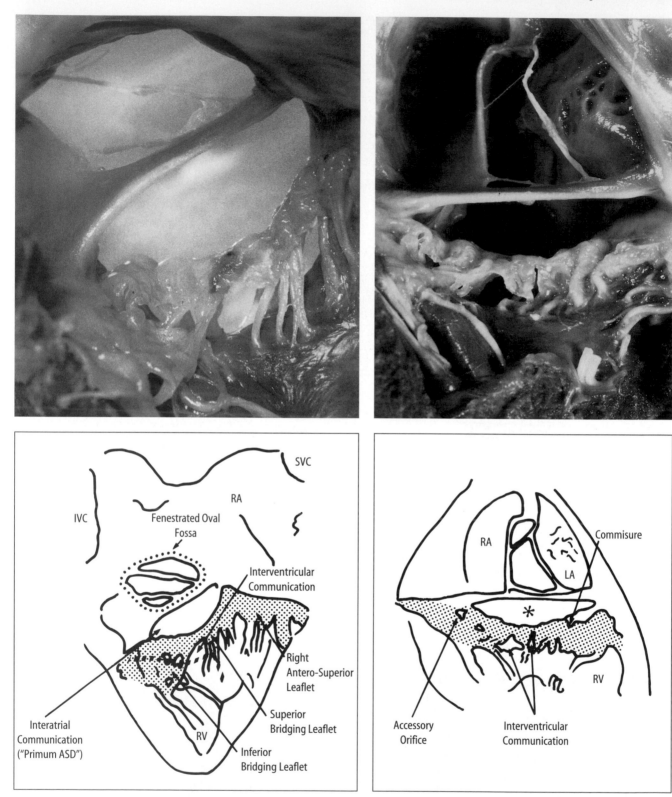

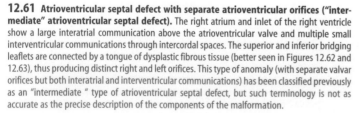

12.61 Atrioventricular septal defect with separate atrioventricular orifices ("intermediate" atrioventricular septal defect). The right atrium and inlet of the right ventricle show a large interatrial communication above the atrioventricular valve and multiple small interventricular communications through intercordal spaces. The superior and inferior bridging leaflets are connected by a tongue of dysplastic fibrous tissue (better seen in Figures 12.62 and 12.63), thus producing distinct right and left orifices. This type of anomaly (with separate valvar orifices but both interatrial and interventricular communications) has been classified previously as an "intermediate" type of atrioventricular septal defect, but such terminology is not as accurate as the precise description of the components of the malformation.

12.62 Septal aspect of the right atrium and right ventricle showing the fenestrated oval fossa (through which the left atrium is seen), the interatrial communication (asterisk) and multiple interventricular communications. An accessory orifice is present in the right-sided component of the inferior bridging leaflet. The coronary sinus is absent. The commissure which is seen lies between the superior bridging leaflet and the right anterosuperior leaflet.

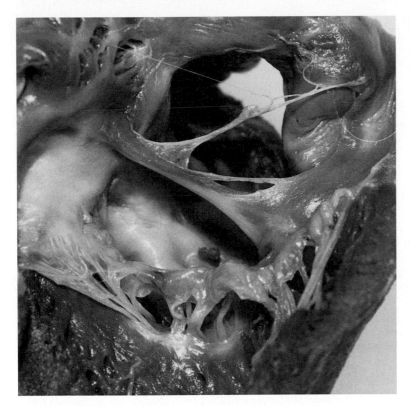

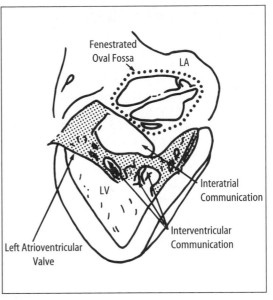

12.63 Left side of the septum. There is a large fenestrated defect of the oval fossa, as well as a large "primum" atrial septal defect. Shunting at the ventricular level occurs through multiple intercordal spaces beneath the superior and inferior bridging leaflets which are joined by a tongue of connecting tissue.

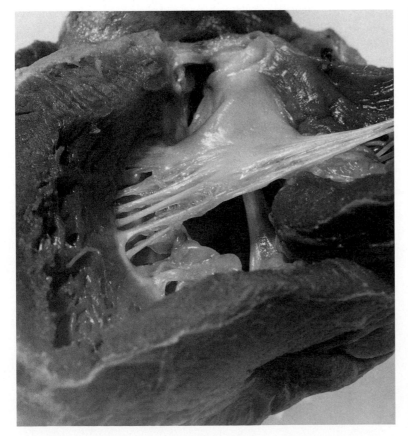

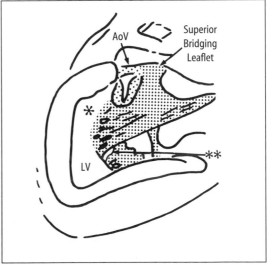

12.64 Left ventricular outflow. The leftward component of the superior bridging leaflet is attached directly to the ventricular septum in the subaortic area (single asterisk), thus narrowing the outflow tract. A tongue of dysplastic tissue (double asterisk) connects the two bridging leaflets above the interventricular communication. The left ventricular cavity, virtually all of which is seen in this illustration, is very small. Even though this heart has separate left and right atrioventricular orifices of approximately equal size, the presence of subaortic obstruction, which is not amenable to surgical relief, and a small left ventricular cavity mitigate against two-ventricle repair. Depending on the pulmonary vasculature and atrioventricular valvar function, a Fontan circulation (see Section 5) could be a surgical option.

Suggested Reading

Anderson RH, Ho SY, Falcao S, Daliento L, Rigby ML. The diagnostic features of atrioventricular septal defect with common atrioventricular junction. Cardiol Young 1998;8:33.

Atik E, Soares AM, Aiello VD. Common arterial trunk associated with atrioventricular septal defect. Cardiol Young 1999;9:617.

Bano-Rodrigo A, Van Praagh S, Trowitzsch E, Van Praagh R. Double-orifice mitral valve: a study of 27 post mortem cases with developmental, diagnostic and surgical considerations. Am J Cardiol 1988;61:152.

Becker AE, Anderson RH. Atrioventricular septal defects. What's in a name? J Thorac Cardiovasc Surg 1982;83:461.

Bharati S, Lev M, McAllister HA Jr, Kirklin JW. Surgical anatomy of the atrioventricular valve in the intermediate type of common atrioventricular orifice. J Thorac Cardiovasc Surg 1980;79:884.

David I, Castenada AR, Van Praagh R. Potentially parachute mitral valve in common atrioventricular canal: Pathologic anatomy and surgical importance. J Thorac Cardiovasc Surg 1982;84:178.

Ebels T, Anderson RH, Devine WA, Debich DE, Penkoske PA, Zuberbuhler JR. Anomalies of the left atrioventricular valve and related ventricular septal morphology in atrioventricular septal defects. J Thorac Cardiovasc Surg 1990;99:299.

Hanley FL, Fenton KN, Jonas RA, Mayer JE, Cook NR, Wernovsky G, Castenada AR. Surgical repair of complete atrioventricular canal defects in infancy. Twenty-year trends. J Thorac Cardiovasc Surg 1993;106:387.

Kadoba K, Jonas RA. Replacement of the left atrioventricular valve after repair of atrioventricular septal defect. Cardiol Young 1991;1:383.

Lee CN, Danielson GK, Schaff HV, Puga FJ, Mair DD. Surgical treatment of double orifice mitral valve in atrioventricular canal defects. J Thorac Cardiovasc Surg 1985;90:700.

Lev M. The architecture of the conduction system in congenital heart disease. I. Common atrioventricular orifice. AMA Arch Pathol 1958;65:174.

McGrath LB, Kirklin JW, Soto B, Bargeron LM Jr. Secondary left atrioventricular valve replacement in atrioventricular septal (AV canal) defect: A method to avoid left ventricular outflow tract obstruction. J Thorac Cardiovasc Surg 1985;89:632.

Piccoli GP, Gerlis LM, Wilkinson JL, Lozsadi K, Macartney FJ, Anderson RH. Morphology and classification of atrioventricular defects. Br Heart J 1979;42:621.

Piccoli GP, Wilkinson JL, Macartney FJ, Gerlis LM, Anderson RH. Morphology and classification of complete atrioventricular defects. Br Heart J 1979;42:633.

Rastelli G; Kirklin JW, Titus JL. Anatomic observations on complete form of persistent common atrioventricular canal with special reference to atrioventricular valves. Mayo Clin Proc 1966;41:296.

Rowlatt UF, Rimoldi HJ, Lev M. The quantitative anatomy of the normal child's heart. Pediatr Clin North Am 1963;10:499.

Sigfusson G, Ettedgui JA, Silverman NH, Anderson RH. Is a cleft in the anterior leaflet of an otherwise normal mitral valve an atrioventricular canal malformation? J Am Coll Cardiol 1995;26:508.

Silverman NH, Ho SY, Anderson RH, Smith A, Wilkinson JL. Atrioventricular septal defect with intact atrial and ventricular septal structures. Int J Cardiol 1984;5:567.

Stark J, McKay R, Anderson RH, Pacifico A et al. Atrioventricular septal defect with common valve orifice but without atrial component: In Jimines MO, Martinez MA (eds), "Paediatric Cardiology," pp 260–4. Ediciones Norma SA, Madrid 1988.

Studer M, Blackstone EH, Kirklin JW, Pacifico AD, Soto B, Chung GKT, Kirklin JK, Bargeron LM, Jr. Determinants of early and late results of repair of atrioventricular septal (canal) defects. J Thorac Cardiovasc Surg 1982;84:523.

Tlaskal T, Hucin B, Kostelka M, Chaloupecky V, Marek J, Tax P, Janouaek J, Kueera V, Hruda J, Reich O, Skovranek J. Repair of tetralogy of Fallot associated with atrioventricular septal defect. Cardiol Young 1998;8:105.

Wetter J, Sinzobahamvya N, Blaschczok C, Brecher A-M, Grävinghoff LM, Schmaltz AA, Urban AE. Closure of the zone of apposition at correction of complete atrioventricular septal defect improves outcome. Eur J Cardiothorac Surg 2000;17:146.

Weintraub RG, Brawn WJ, Venables AW, Mee RB. Two patch repair of complete atrioventricular septal defect in the first year of life. J Thorac Cardiovasc Surg 1990;99:320.

13 Tricuspid Valvar Anomalies

Introduction

In the assessment of congenital malformations, the tricuspid valve is evaluated in relation to its junction with the appropriate atrium, the valvar leaflets and its tension apparatus. The normal morphologically tricuspid valve has three leaflets. They are situated in septal, antero-superior and inferior positions. The inferior leaflet is sometimes referred to as the mural leaflet. The leaflets are separated from each other by three commissures. These commissures are the anteroseptal, the supero-inferior and the inferoseptal respectively. The anteroseptal commissure is supported by a complex of cords, the most prominent of which arises from the medial papillary muscle (of Lancisi). This muscle itself may be either a single structure or part of a group of small muscles and cords from the posterior limb of the septomarginal trabeculation. It is usually complemented by a further arrangement of cords arising directly from the septum. The largest muscle which supports the tricuspid valve is the anterior papillary muscle. This is invariably a single structure and supports the supero-inferior commissure. The inferior papillary muscle, supporting the inferoseptal commissure, may be single or represented by several muscles. The methods of attachment of the tricuspid valve are extremely variable, but an important and consistent feature that distinguishes the tricuspid valve from the mitral valve is that the septal leaflet is attached by cords directly to the ventricular septum.

Congenital malformations can implicate either the whole or part of the valve. Some of these are lesions which may similarly affect mitral or common valves, but others, such as Ebstein's malformation, have a predilection for the tricuspid valve and only rarely involve morphologically mitral valves or common valves. In Ebstein's malformation, the atrioventricular junction is in its appropriate position, but the proximal attachment of the valve is downwardly displaced so that the leaflets are delaminated more apically than usual and directly from the myocardium. The degree of displacement is extremely variable. In the area that is displaced, the leaflet tissue appears to be absent. It is generally the septal and inferior leaflets that are affected, but occasionally the antero-superior leaflet may also be minimally displaced along the ventriculo-infundibular fold. The leaflets can be thin or extremely thick and dysplastic. Cauliflower-like excrescences of valvar tissue, which are variable in size, are sometimes present along the valve. The severity of Ebstein's malformation is marked by the extent of the displacement, but this is never beyond the junction between the inlet and the trabecular portions of the right ventricle. However, the distal attachments of the valvar leaflets, in particular those of the antero-superior leaflet, may be grossly abnormal and dysplastic to the extent of producing an imperforate variant of Ebstein's malformation. This is one type of tricuspid atresia. Between the extremes, there are many intermediate patterns, some of which, in addition to causing valvar regurgitation, restrict the passage of blood to the pulmonary valve. For example, the anterior leaflet may have linear attachments to the junction between the septum and the anterior wall of the right ventricle.

Myocardial changes in Ebstein's malformation are well described. Thinning and dilatation of the inlet portion of the right ventricle, which has become part of the functional right atrium because of the valvar displacement, produces a so-called "atrialized ventricle." The outlet portion of the right ventricle may also be thin-walled. The abnormalities underlying development of the tricuspid valve in Ebstein's malformation also produce the substrate for accessory atrioventricular conduction pathways and ventricular pre-excitation. The lesion is often associated with Wolff-Parkinson-White syndrome. Calcification of the mitral valve and annulus has been described in association with these lesions and there have been reports of increased fibrosis of the ventricular septum and the left ventricular wall.

Atrial and ventricular septal defects are frequently associated with Ebstein's malformation and, conversely, Ebstein-like valves are found in pulmonary atresia with intact septum, discordant atrioventricular connections and with atrioventricular septal defects.

Other lesions of the tricuspid valve, as isolated malformations, are comparatively rare. While imperforate tricuspid valves may be found with a normal atrioventricular junction and concordant atrioventricular connections, they are more common with atrioventricular septal defect or as the right-sided atrioventricular valve in double inlet left ventricle. A degree of dysplasia of the leaflets in a normally attached valve not infrequently accompanies a ventricular septal defect, but this rarely produces hemodynamically important obstruction or regurgitation. Double orifices are occasionally present with more complex cardiac lesions and are often supported by their own dedicated tension apparatus. These valves have a tendency to be obstructive, as do valves with poor commissural development and a small orifice. "Parachute" tricuspid valves which are supported by only a single papillary muscle, and also complete failure of the leaflets of the tricuspid valve to form (unguarded orifice), are usually associated with pulmonary valvar atresia with intact ventricular septum. Annular distension may occur as an isolated lesion, but more frequently reflects other cardiac pathology, such as pulmonary hypertension with right ventricular dilatation or with cardiomyopathies, such as arrhythmogenic right ventricular dysplasia or mitochondrial myopathy.

Overriding of the tricuspid annulus forms the basis for the classification of anomalies in atrioventricular connection which range between the extremes of usual atrial arrangement with concordant atrioventricular connections and double inlet left ventricle. Frequently, overriding is associated with straddling of the tricuspid valve in which the tendinous cords of the valve are attached in both ventricles, thus "straddling" the ventricular septum. For this to occur, there must be a ventricular septal defect, and the occurrence of straddling indicates malalignment between the atrial and ventricular septal structures. In this way, the axis of the conduction tissue is affected. The atrioventricular connection is displaced to a posterolateral location where the ventricular septum meets the valvar annulus. Occasionally, the tricuspid valve straddles through a more anteriorly situated ventricular septal defect and then produces subaortic obstruction.

Because most of the anomalies of the tricuspid valve occur in association with other cardiac malformations, their recognition and management is usually in the context of surgery for complex congenital defects. Here, their implications may range from trivial to profound, from the inconvenience of closing a ventricular septal

defect through a slightly small tricuspid valvar orifice to the necessity of incorporating a partial or complete right heart bypass during the repair of complex transposition of the great arteries. Fortunately, high quality echocardiography usually alerts the surgeon to structural abnormalities of the valve preoperatively.

Obstruction at the level of the right atrioventricular orifice may be due to a small but anatomically normal valve, or to a valve which has dysplastic, fused leaflets attached to short, thick tendinous cords and papillary muscles. An interatrial communication is usually present and permits right-to-left shunting which "masks" the hemodynamic importance of the lesion preoperatively. Fused leaflets are opened as widely as possible by sharp division in the normal position of the commissures, with mobilization of the cords or attachments to the ventricular myocardium as needed. In the case of a valve supported by a single papillary muscle ("parachute valve"), the head of the papillary muscle is also incised vertically to its base. The resulting incompetence from valvotomy can often be improved, if not abolished, with some type of annuloplasty. The potential for enlargement of the orifice is much less in small but normally formed tricuspid valves because the annulus is limited by the right coronary artery and the conduction tissue. In these cases, it may be necessary to incorporate a bidirectional cavopulmonary anastomosis for a "one-and-a-half" ventricle repair, or consider extracardiac interposition of a homograft valve between the right atrium and the right ventricle, if the latter is of exceptionally good size. Extrapolating from clinical studies of the tricuspid valve in pulmonary atresia with intact ventricular septum, it is probably safe to accept a final orifice which is within about two or three standard deviations of the mean normal for the patient's body surface area.

Repair of tricuspid regurgitation is often possible both in Ebstein's malformation and other congenital malformations beyond early infancy. For Ebstein's malformation, intervention is indicated for cyanosis, heart failure or arrhythmias. The feasibility of repair depends on the size and mobility of the antero-superior leaflet, which can be assessed by echocardiography. By one of a number of techniques, the antero-superior leaflet is brought into apposition with the septal surface and then functions as a monocusp valve. Plication of the atrialized portion of the right ventricle may or may not be of hemodynamic importance, but is usually carried out at the time of valve repair. Associated defects, the most common being atrial and ventricular septal defects, are repaired at the same time, and ablation of accessory conduction tissue pathways is sometimes also incorporated into the procedure. The principles of mitral valve repair – namely, the provision of good leaflet mobility and coaptation – are equally applicable to the tricuspid valve and accomplished by the same technical maneuvers of leaflet retraction, cordal shortening and annuloplasty (see Chapter 14).

The neonate with severe tricuspid valve regurgitation due to Ebstein's malformation is a particularly difficult problem because pulmonary hypertension exaggerates the importance of the valve, resulting in "functional" pulmonary atresia and absence of forward right ventricular flow. Initially, these patients are managed with prostaglandin to provide blood-flow through the arterial duct. However, if their condition does not improve (which may take several days), conversion to "tricuspid atresia" by surgical closure of the valve and creation of a systemic-pulmonary shunt may be life-saving. At all ages, abnormalities which involve both right and left ventricular myocardium in Ebstein's malformation may influence surgical outcome.

When satisfactory repair cannot be achieved, tricuspid valve replacement is done, usually with a tissue prosthesis to avoid the potentially greater incidence of thrombosis with a mechanical valve and anti-coagulation. A stent-mounted valve is placed at the level of the anatomical tricuspid valvar annulus, leaving the coronary sinus below the prosthesis to avoid stitches in proximity to the conduction system. It is important also to orientate the struts of the valve away from the area of the conduction tissue on the ventricular septum. When a homograft semilunar valve is used, the coronary sinus is cut back to drain in the left atrium, and the conduction tissue passes between the upper and lower suture lines. In both cases, the native tricuspid valve tissue is not resected, but rather incorporated into the suture line for additional support wherever possible. More recently, homograft tricuspid valves themselves have been implanted in the anatomical position with encouraging early results.

Other lesions of the tricuspid valve include classical tricuspid atresia, in which the right atrioventricular connection is completely absent. As this is a major component of congenital heart disease, it will be considered separately in Chapter 24.

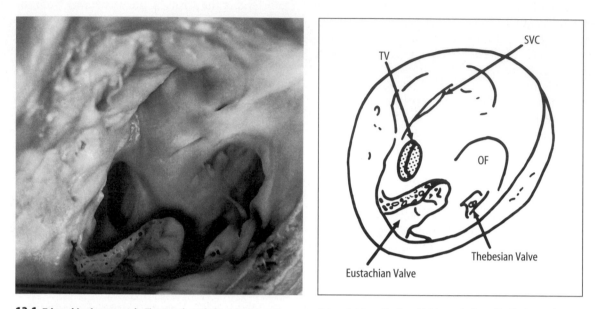

13.1 Tricuspid valvar stenosis. The view through the right atrium shows a small stenotic tricuspid valve which has a single small orifice in an otherwise normal heart. There is a large (aneurysmal) persistent valve of the coronary sinus (Thebesian valve). The persistent venous valve (Eustachian valve) has a filigree, "windsock" appearance and the flap valve of the oval fossa (unseen) is patent. It is extremely rare to find valvar tricuspid stenosis without other associated cardiac defects.

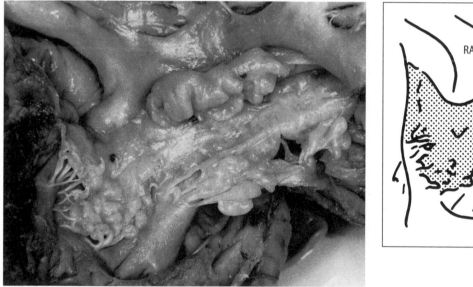

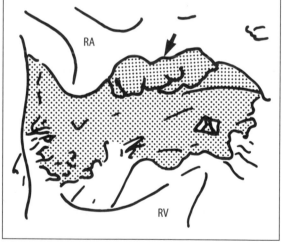

13.2 For comparison with the above heart, a grossly dysplastic and stenotic tricuspid valve is shown in the right atrial view of a heart which also has discordant ventriculo-arterial connections (transposed great arteries) and ventricular septal defect (see Figure 21.82). Duplication of fibrous material produces a mass of accessory tissue at the annular attachment of the antero-superior leaflet (arrow), and the body of the leaflet is thickened and knobbly. Shortened cords tether the leaflets to a hypertophied papillary muscle.

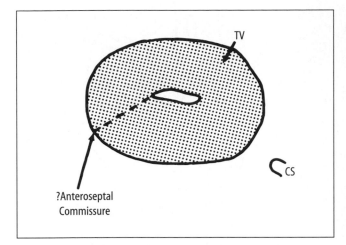

13.3 Preoperative transesophogeal echocardiography provides invaluable information regarding the size of the tricuspid valvar annulus, the mobility of the leaflets, and morphology of the subvalvar supporting apparatus. Operation is done through the right atrium with moderately hypothermic cardiopulmonary bypass (28° C) and bicaval venous cannulation, taking care to site the superior caval cannula high up in case the valvar orifice proves to be inadequate, necessitating a bidirectional cavopulmonary anastomosis. The valve may initially appear to be a thick diaphragm with complete lack of commissures. There is sometimes a slight depression in the leaflet where subvalvar cords attach on its undersurface.

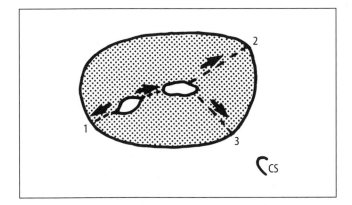

13.4 A small incision is made in the "dimple" area using a sharp knife (no. 12 blade or opthomology microblade, depending on the size of the patient) in order to view the subvalvar region. This is kept away from the orifice, such that it can be closed without prejudicing valvar function if the site proves to be inappropriate.

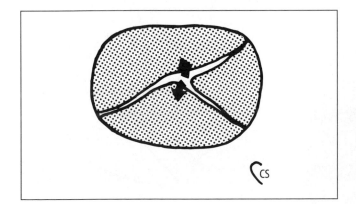

13.5 The leaflet is opened to form commissures between cordal attachments and to obtain the maximal orifice. Any fused cords are also mobilized and incisions into thickened papillary muscles may improve leaflet mobility. There is usually some incompetence of the valve, but a ring to support the annulus is not generally implanted before the patient is fully grown. The size of the orifice is calibrated and compared with normal values for the patient's body surface area. If the valve orifice and/or right ventricle remain inadequate, the right heart may be partially bypassed with a superior caval vein to right pulmonary artery anastomosis ("one-and-a-half" ventricle repair – see Figures 27.27–27.32).

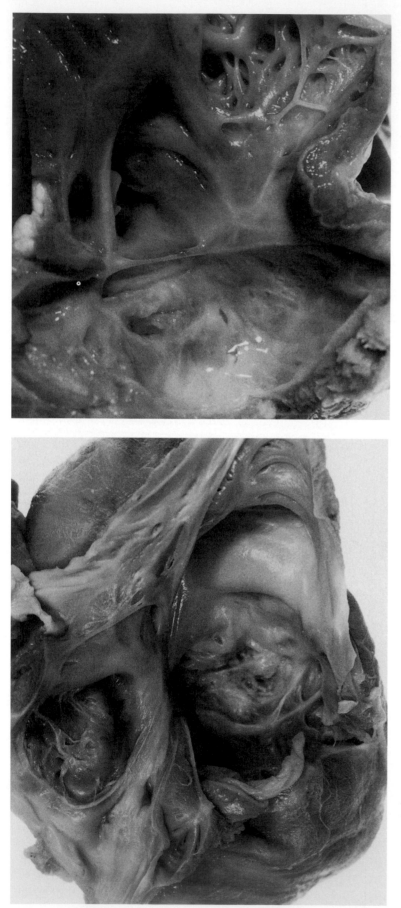

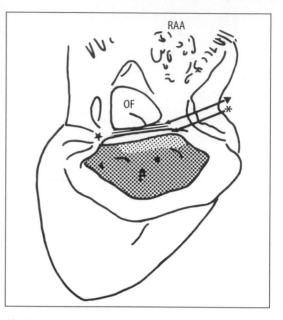

13.6 Imperforate right-sided atrioventricular valve. Atrioventricular septal defect. The right atrium has been opened above the atrioventricular groove and rotated upwards. There is an atrioventricular septal defect with partitioned orifice (ostium primum atrial septal defect), the right side of which is extensively adherent to the right ventricular wall (dense stippling) and has no orifice. Immediately above the valvar tissue, there is a small interatrial communication (asterisk). The valve of the oval fossa is absent and the atrial septum is represented by only a muscular strand (triangle). The cavity of the right ventricle is small. Pulmonary atresia is also present. Dysplastic tension apparatus (not seen) from the imperforate portion of the valve (light stippling) straddles into the left ventricle below the aortic valve. The position of the atrioventricular node is indicated by the star.

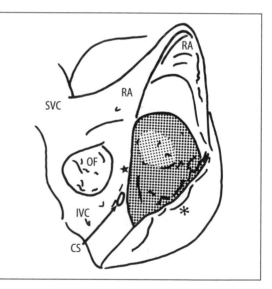

13.7 Imperforate tricuspid valve in Ebstein's malformation. The dilated right atrium has been opened and retracted to the atrioventricular junction which is guarded by an imperforate tricuspid valve (stippling). The valve is extensively adherent to the right ventricular wall (dense stippling) and the atrialized portion of the right ventricle is thin-walled (asterisk). The atrial septum is intact but the valve of the oval fossa is ragged. The atrioventricular node (star) occupies its usual position at the apex of the triangle of Koch, but other accessory conduction pathways are likely to be present around the annulus of the tricuspid valve. A massive subaortic muscular bulge of the ventricular septum (unseen) produces anatomical subaortic stenosis.

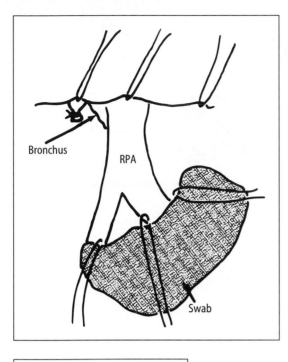

Bronchus

RPA

Swab

13.8 Patients with an imperforate tricuspid valve, in the absence of a ventricular septal defect, have no pulmonary blood-flow from the heart and are "duct dependent" from birth. A systemic pulmonary shunt is therefore needed, usually in the first few days of life. Having ensured the presence of an adequate atrial septal defect, this can be done through a right thoracotomy. The lung is retracted behind a moist swab, using fine stay-sutures between adventitia in the hilum and the edges of the incision. The pulmonary artery is dissected outside the pericardium, which is retracted medially with superficial stay-sutures to the chest wall after division of the azygos vein. This maneuver tends to elevate the superior caval vein and the patient should be observed for any reduction in systemic blood pressure. If the pulmonary artery is difficult to identify, it is helpful to recall that it is the vessel which lies immediately in front of the right bronchus. It is important to expose the pulmonary artery medially as far as possible, and the lower branch should be positively identified to avoid placing the anastomosis on the upper lobe branch. There are usually some dense fibrous bands which need division behind the pericardium to expose fully the upper surface of the vessel.

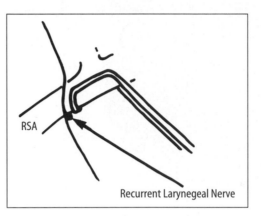

RSA

Recurrent Larynegeal Nerve

13.9 The dissection is continued upwards in the paratracheal tissues to expose the subclavian artery at its origin and to make a "bed" in which the shunt will lie. Usually, this involves division of the azygos vein. Alternatively, the artery is identified in the apex of the chest and dissected back towards the mediastinum. It is encircled with a vessel loop and the position of the vagus nerve with its recurrent laryngeal branch is observed. The nerve is displaced slightly laterally, such that a side-biting clamp can be placed comfortably on the origin of the subclavian artery.

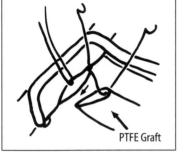

PTFE Graft

13.10 A polytetrafluoroethylene graft (usually 4 mm in diameter for a neonate) is trimmed slightly obliquely and joined to a longitudinal incision in the subclavian artery with a continuous 7/0 monofilament suture. The posterior wall of the anastomosis is done first, working inside the vessel and towards the surgeon.

13.11 The front layer of the anastomosis is also done forehand, working towards the surgeon, outside the vessel.

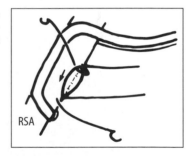

RSA

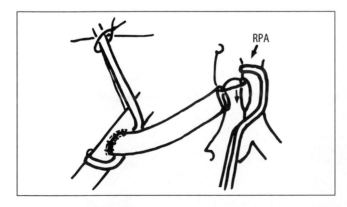

RPA

13.12 The clamp on the subclavian artery is not released but rather rotated upwards and held at the top of the field by a suture to the skin incision. With a second fine side-biting clamp on the main pulmonary artery, the distal end of the graft is trimmed transversely and anastomosed to a longitudinal incision on the upper surface of the pulmonary artery, in the same manner. A stay-stitch on the anterior side of the pulmonary artery incision is often helpful to expose the initial posterior suture line. Just before the suture is tied down, the proximal clamp is released momentarily to flush air from the graft. The suture is then tied, and distal and proximal clamps are removed in quick succession to avoid clot formation in the graft. There is always some bleeding through stitch holes in the prosthetic graft, but this generally abates after a few minutes of packing with dry swab.

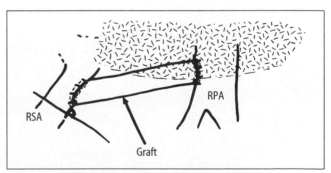

RSA

RPA

Graft

13.13 With release of the stay-sutures, the lower part of the shunt is largely behind the superior caval vein and the graft takes a straight course. This is a good position because the shunt will be readily accessible between the aorta and superior caval vein at median sternotomy. The pulmonary artery is palpated to confirm that a thrill from the shunt is present, the systolic and diastolic blood pressures are observed for any evidence of an excessively large shunt, and the graft is inspected for signs of serous leak from its surface prior to closure of the chest. Using this technique, it is possible to do the operation with minimal assistance.

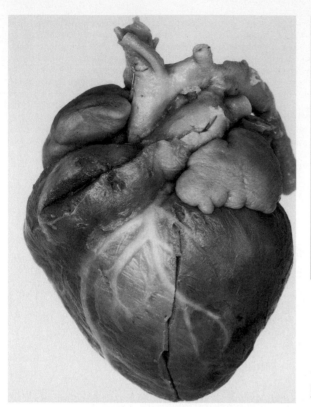

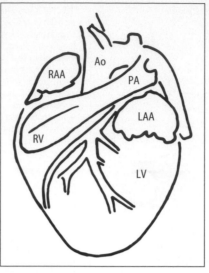

13.14 Imperforate tricuspid valve with Ebstein's malformation. An anterior view of the heart shows an enlarged left ventricle and a small right ventricle giving off the pulmonary artery. The atriums are in the usual (solitus) arrangement, but their walls are thickened.

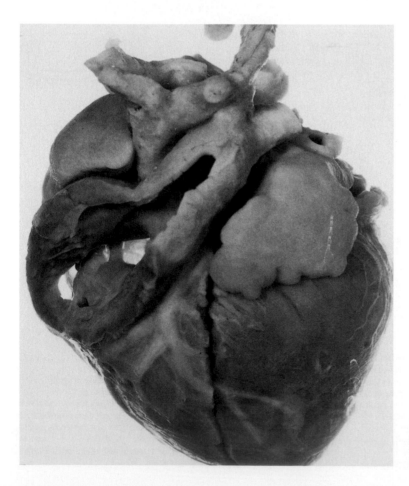

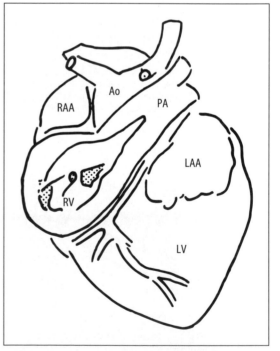

13.15 The anterior wall of the small right ventricle has been opened to demonstrate the anterosuperior leaflet of the tricuspid valve which is transilluminated from its atrial side. A well-developed subpulmonary outlet septum is present.

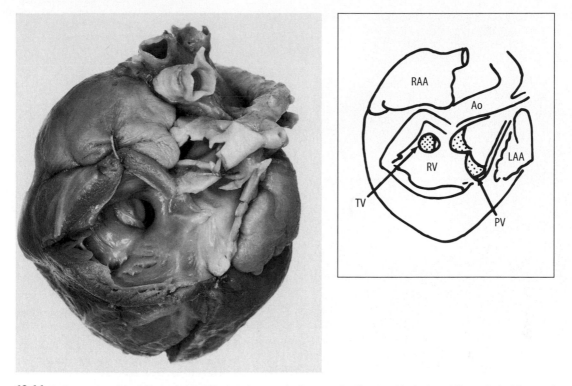

13.16 Further opening of the right ventricular outflow reveals a normal pulmonary valve. The tricuspid valve is partially seen in the inlet part of the ventricle.

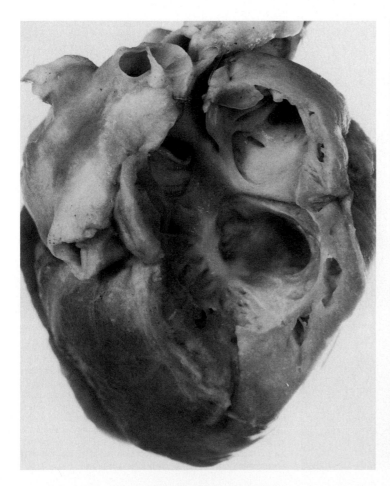

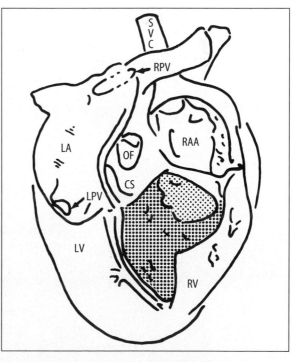

13.17 A posterior view of the heart with the right atrium opened into the atrioventricular junction shows the atrialized right ventricular sinus (dark stippling). The septal, inferior, and antero-superior leaflets of the tricuspid valve are all adherent to the myocardium of the right ventricle. In addition to an imperforate tricuspid valve (light stippling), the antero-superior leaflet also contributes to the obstruction of the right ventricular outlet. This is a very extreme and rare form of Ebstein's malformation which would present and need to be treated as pulmonary and right atrioventricular valvar atresia.

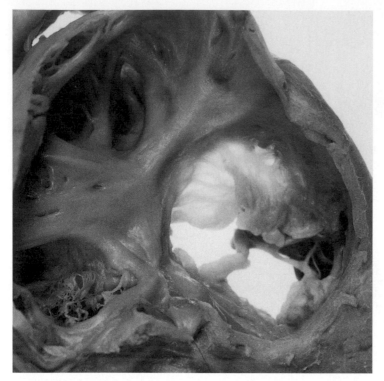

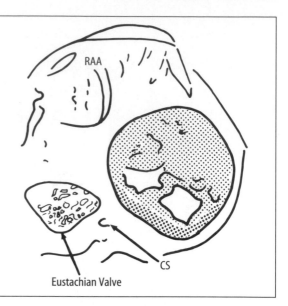

13.18 Ebstein's malformation of the tricuspid valve. Shown from above, the tricuspid valve has a mild Ebstein-like malformation with septal and inferior leaflets being adherent to the ventricular septum and posterior wall of the right ventricle (dense stippling). The anterior leaflet is large and mobile. The valve of the inferior caval vein (Eustachian valve) is prominent and has a filigree appearance. The atrial septum is intact.

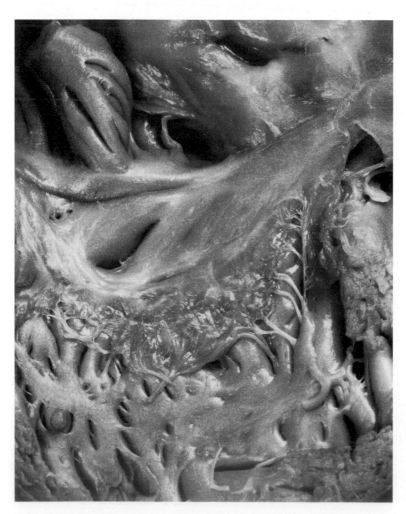

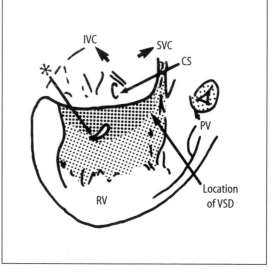

13.19 Another heart with Ebstein's malformation of the tricuspid valve has been opened across the junction of the right atrium and right ventricle to show the proximal portion of the septal and inferior leaflets attached to the septum and posterior wall of the right ventricle (dense stippling). The atrialized posterior wall is very thin and shows a crevice (asterisk). The orifice of the coronary sinus lies just above the annulus of the definitive tricuspid valve. The atrial septum is intact. Microscopic examination of serial sections through a paraffin block containing the atrioventricular conduction tissue shows minor peculiarities of the conduction tissue. The pulmonary valve (not seen) is normal. The position of a perimembranous ventricular septal defect is indicated.

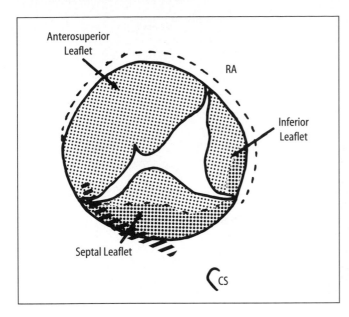

13.20 The large mobile antero-superior leaflet makes this type of Ebstein's morphology suitable for valve repair. After studying the function of the leaflets, the inferior leaflet and about two-thirds of the antero-superior leaflet are detached with a supporting cuff of endocardium (dashed line). The incision does not extend to the area of the atrioventricular node or the penetrating bundle of the conduction tissue.

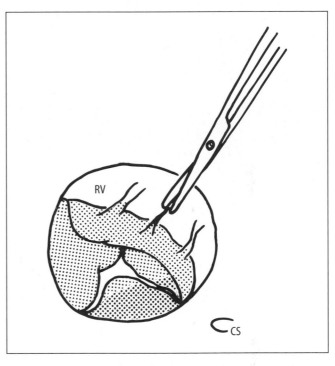

13.21 The detached leaflets are mobilized by the division of muscular and fibrous tissue which attach them to the ventricular endocardium. If the cords are fused, they too are mobilized by the fenestration of intercordal tissue.

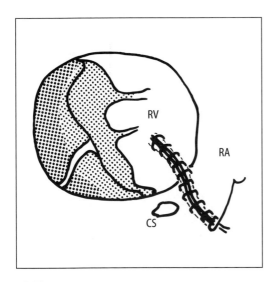

13.22 Both the ventricle and the atrium are plicated at about 5 o'clock, staying posterior to the coronary sinus. The ventricular plication is in its thin, atrialized portion and serves to narrow the ring of the tricuspid valve. The atrial portion reduces the size of the enlarged right atrium. This is done with an unpledgeted continuous suture, taking care not to injure important coronary arterial branches externally.

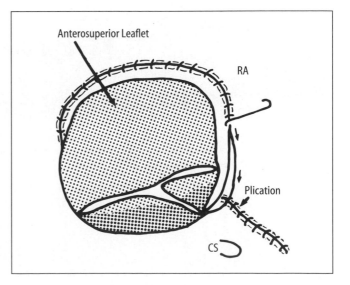

13.23 The repair is completed by rotation of the leaflets clockwise and reattachment of their muscular cuff at the level of the "true" tricuspid valve annulus. This brings the large anterior leaflet across most of the valvar orifice, such that it functions as a "monocusp" valve. In some cases the anterior papillary muscle requires repositioning to achieve a competent valve. In older patients, a supporting ring may be added to prevent the redevelopment of incompetence. Any atrial septal defect is routinely closed with a patch and associated lesions (ventricular septal defect, pulmonary stenosis or accessory conduction pathways) are dealt with on their own merits.

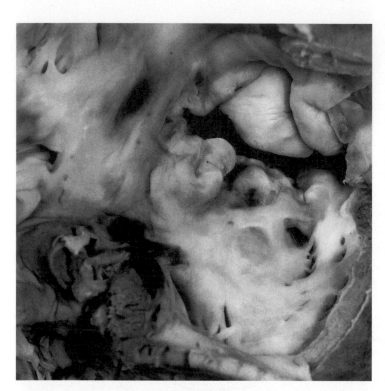

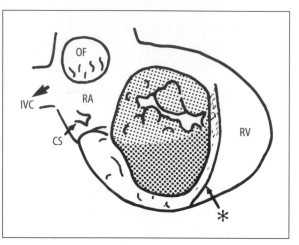

13.24 **Ebstein's malformation.** Looking down from above, the tricuspid valve can be seen to have extensive adherence of the inferior leaflet to the posterior wall of the right ventricle (dense stippling), while the "atrialized" portion of the ventricle is thin-walled (asterisk). All three leaflets are thickened and dysplastic (compare with Figure 13.18). The atrial septum is intact.

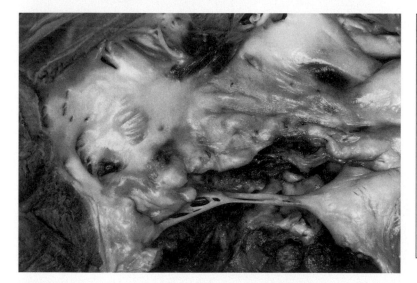

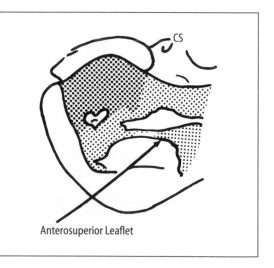

13.25 In another view, the tricuspid valve has been opened to demonstrate its thickened leaflets (light stippling) and the paucity of tendinous cords and intercordal spaces. A cord from the inferior leaflet crosses the right ventricular cavity and attaches to the antero-superior leaflet. A large portion of the right ventricle is "atrialized" (dense stippling) by the adherent leaflets.

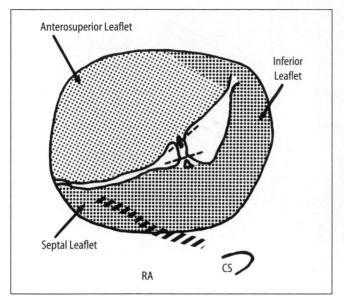

13.26 The likelihood of successful repair is much less certain in this patient due to the thickening of the antero-superior leaflet upon which valvar function is critically dependent, as the other two leaflets are completely adherent to the ventricle. However, the antero-superior leaflet is of good size and reasonably mobile and, with echocardiographic guidance, conservation of the valve could be attempted. The bridge of tissue between the inferior and antero-superior leaflets is first divided.

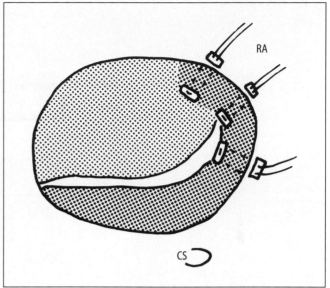

13.27 To approximate the anatomical tricuspid valvar annulus with the functional atrioventricular junction, pledgeted mattress sutures are placed at the lowest point of the "atrialized" ventricle and woven vertically through the leaflet and myocardium. Externally, the heart is inspected to place the stitches between major coronary arterial branches.

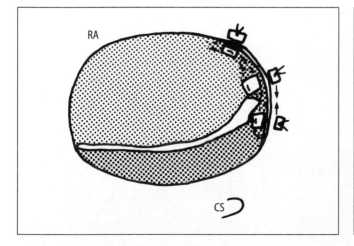

13.28 The sutures are tied down, which brings the antero-superior leaflet to the level of the anatomical tricuspid valvar annulus. A "double-size" pledget placed where the annulus will be plicated is useful.

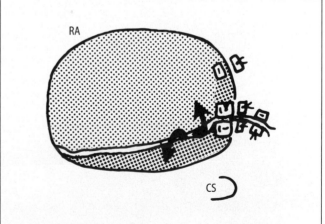

13.29 The annulus of the valve is reduced with a horizontal pledgeted mattress suture, which brings the antero-superior leaflet into apposition with valvar tissue on the ventricular septum. Mobility and competence of the valve are tested by injection of saline into the right ventricle and confirmed by intraoperative transesophageal echocardiography.

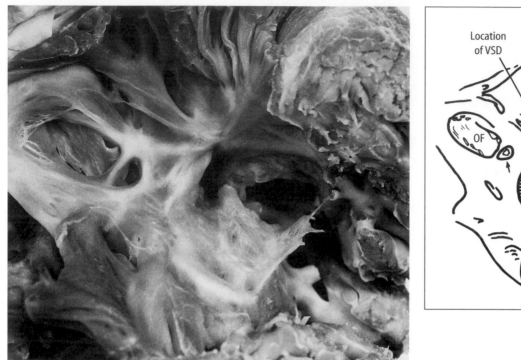

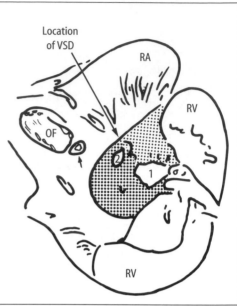

13.30 Double orifice tricuspid valve. The specimen has been opened across the right atrioventricular junction, with partial detachment of the tricuspid valvar leaflet from the annulus. The septal leaflet has an Ebstein-like malformation (dense stippling). The main orifice (1) in the valve leads to the right ventricle, as does a second orifice (2) between the septal and antero-superior leaflets. The second orifice is subjacent to a perimembranous ventricular septal defect (see Figure 13.31 below). There is a fenestrated atrial septal defect of the oval fossa, together with an unusual small "muscular" interatrial defect of the limbus (arrow) which abuts on to the atrioventricular septum.

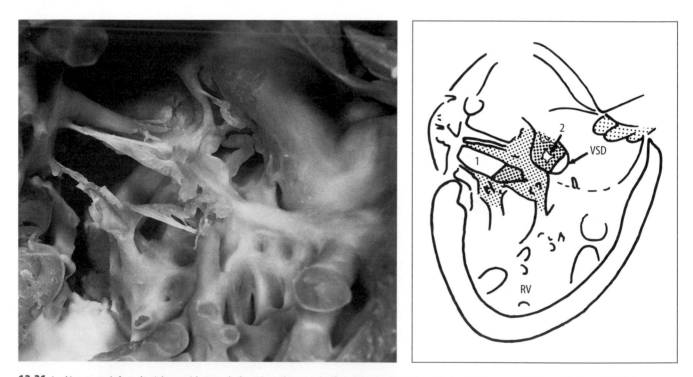

13.31 Looking upwards from the right ventricle towards the atrium, the second orifice of the dysplastic tricuspid valve (2) is seen next to the ventricular septal defect.

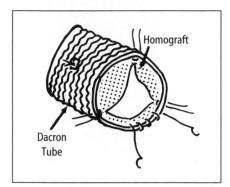

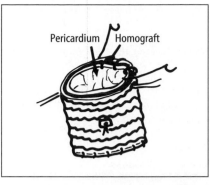

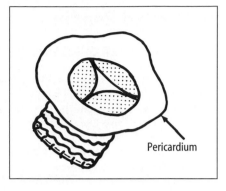

13.32 There is no obvious way to repair this valve, as the antero-superior leaflet is also abnormal with a second orifice. Tissue valves are preferred in the tricuspid position to avoid anticoagulation and, possibly, heart block. As the right atrium is usually enlarged in patients coming to valve replacement, an unstented homograft is one option. The homograft is mounted within a Dacron tube large enough to accommodated its sinuses. The excess diameter of the tube at the arterial end of the valve (which will become the ventricular end of the implant) is taken up in a continuous suture line.

13.33 A pericardial collar is attached to the ventricular end of the homograft which will lie within the right atrium. This is done with the pericardium inverted into the valve. The sinuses of the homograft are also attached to the Dacron graft with through-and-through mattress sutures, supported on both sides with pericardial pledgets.

13.34 Withdrawal of the pericardial collar shows the "top hat" appearance of the completed prosthesis, with a smooth inflow from the pericardium to the homograft.

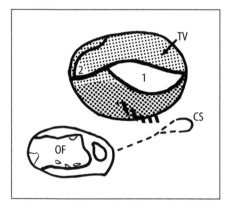

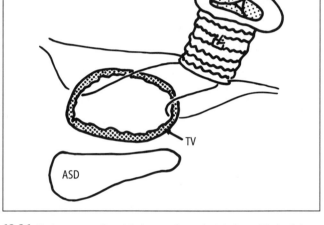

13.35 On cardiopulmonary bypass with moderate hypothermia, the ventricular septal defect is closed through the right atrium (see Chapter 11). The coronary sinus is then cut back to drain in the left atrium. In this heart, with an unusual type of "primum atrial septal defect," the safest way of doing this probably would be first to enlarge the atrial septal defects and then to connect them to the orifice of the coronary sinus (dashed line), giving good visualization of the wall of the coronary sinus within the left atrium.

13.36 The lower suture line of the homograft prosthesis is done with simple interrupted stitches at the anatomical tricuspid valvar annulus, incorporating the unresected leaflet tissue.

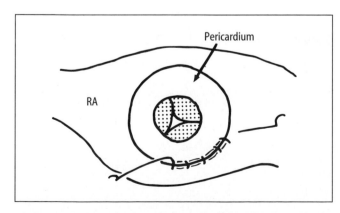

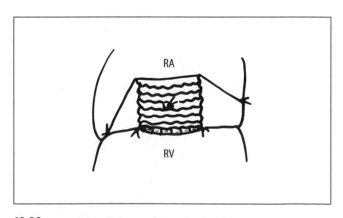

13.37 The upper suture line attaches the pericardial collar to the septum and free wall of the right atrium, leaving the coronary sinus orifice and atrial septal defect below the collar. It is important to neither rotate nor compress the homograft with this second suture line.

13.38 At completion, the homograft sits within the right atrium. There is a smooth inflow from the atrium across the valve and a widely patent orifice, such that anticoagulation is not necessary.

Suggested Reading

Anderson RH, Becker AE. Anomalies of the atrioventricular valves. In: Robertson WB (ed). Systemic Pathology, Vol 10. The Cardiovascular System: Part A. General Considerations and Congenital Malformations. Churchill Livingstone 1993. Chapter 9;137.

Becker AE, Becker MJ, Edwards JE. Pathologic spectrum of dysplasia of the tricuspid valve. Features in common with Ebstein's malformation. Arch Pathol 1971;91:167.

Carpentier A, Chauvraud S, Mace L, Relland J, Mihaileanu S, Marino JP Abry B, Guibourt P. A new reconstructive operation for Ebstein's anomaly of the tricuspid valve. J Thorac Cardiovasc Surg 1988; 96:92.

Danielson GK, Fuster V. Surgical repair of Ebstein's anomaly. Ann Surg 1982;196:499.

Frescura C, Angelini A, Daliento L, Thiene G. Morphological aspects of Ebstein's anomaly in adults. Thorac Cardiovasc Surg 2000; 48(4):203.

Hanley FL, Sade RM, Blackstone EM, Kirklin JW, Freedom RM, Nanda NC and the Congenital Heart Surgeons Society. The tricuspid valve and outcomes in pulmonary atresia and intact ventricular septum. J Thorac Cardiovasc Surg 1993;105:406.

Kanjuh VI, Stevenson JE, Amplatz K, Edwards JE. Congenitally unguarded tricuspid orifice with co-existing pulmonary atresia. Circulation 1964;30:911.

McKay R, Sono J, Arnold R. Tricuspid valve replacement using an unstented pulmonary homograft. Ann Thorac Surg 1988;46:58.

Milo S, Stark J, Macartney FJ, Anderson RH. Parachute deformity of the tricuspid valve (case report). Thorax 1979;34:543–6.

Quaegebeur JM, Sreeram N, Fraser AG, Bogers JJC, Stumper OF, Hess J, Bos E, Sutherland GR. Surgery for Ebstein's anomaly: The clinical and echocardiographic evaluation of a new technique. J Am Coll Cardiol 1991;17:722.

Starnes VA, Pitlick PT, Bernstein D, Griffin ML, Choy M, Shumway NE. Ebstein's anomaly appearing in the neonate. J Thorac Cardiovasc Surg 1991;101:1082.

Tourniaire A, Deyrieux F, Tartulier M. Maladie d'Ebstein: essai de diagnostic clinique. Arch Mal Coeur 1949;42:1211.

Wenink ACG, Gittenberger-de-Groot AC. Straddling mitral and tricuspid valves: morphological differences and developmental backgrounds. Am J Cardiol 1982;49:1959.

Zuberbuhler JR, Allwork SP, Anderson RH. The spectrum of Ebstein's anomaly of the tricuspid valve. J Thorac Cardiovasc Surg 1979; 77:202.

14 Mitral Valvar Anomalies

Introduction

The inlet of the morphologically left ventricle is guarded by the mitral valve. The normal mitral valve extends from the atrioventricular junction as far as the anterolateral and posteromedial papillary muscles. The valve has two leaflets – mural and aortic – of which the mural has a long, narrow shape and is attached to approximately two-thirds of the valvar circumference. It may be a single entity or composed of several scallops. The square-shaped aortic leaflet is attached to the remaining one-third of the valvar annulus and is in direct fibrous continuity with the aortic valve. The leaflets are sometimes called "posterior" (or "lateral") and "anterior" respectively, but the orientation of the valve is such that neither leaflet lies strictly in those positions. When the mural and aortic leaflets close, they coapt to form the zone of apposition, now regarded as a " commissure". Traditionally, the end points of this line of closure have been designated as two separate commissures, albeit that they are simply the two ends of one continuous line of junction. Each commissure is supported by a papillary muscle, one of which is situated anterolaterally and the other posteromedially in the ventricle, although the actual origins of the muscles are fairly close together.

Malformations of the atrioventricular valves need to be studied and described in terms of their component parts. These are the annulus, the leaflets, the tendinous cords, and the papillary muscles. The annulus of either of the atrioventricular valves can be congenitally dilated, although this lesion is usually acquired. Complete absence of the annulus, producing valvar atresia in the anticipated position of either the mitral or tricuspid valve, is considered separately in Chapters 24 and 25. A second malformation that may produce valvar atresia occurs when leaflet tissue is present as an imperforate membrane. The imperforate mitral valve is frequently found with an atretic aortic valve as part of hypoplastic left heart syndrome, but it can also be seen with

a patent aortic valve and concordant ventriculo-arterial connections. If any tension apparatus is present in this situation, it is usually hypoplastic.

The valvar annulus may override the septal crest in the presence of a ventricular septal defect. Frequently, when there is mitral valve overriding, the leaflets straddle the septum and in doing so their tension apparatus and papillary muscles come to occupy positions in both ventricles. When the mitral valve is straddling, the portion which crosses the crest of the septum usually comes to lie in the outlet portion of the right ventricle. Discordant or double outlet right ventriculo-arterial connections are commonly found in association with these lesions. Depending on the degree of straddling, the atrioventricular connection will vary between the extremes of concordant atrioventricular connection and double inlet right ventricle, in which, by definition, more than 50% of the mitral valve is connected to the right ventricle.

Considering the leaflet tissue in a dysplastic mitral valve, the papillary muscles may extend to the leading edge of the anterior leaflet, without differentiation into tendinous cords. The intercordal spaces are then obliterated. This forms the "arcade" lesion, which is sometimes described as a "hammock valve." Dual orifices can be seen in the mitral valvar leaflets, each being supported by its own papillary muscle, although these lesions are more frequently found in the left-sided portion of a common atrioventricular valve, along with deficient atrioventricular septation. The dual orifices are produced by an interconnection of either valvar or fibromuscular tissue dividing the valve into separate portions. Another variant of mitral valvar anomaly is the so-called "parachute valve." This is more of an abnormality of papillary muscles rather than the leaflets. All the tendinous cords from the mitral valvar leaflets converge into either a fused mass of the paired papillary muscles or, more strikingly, into a single papillary muscle which may or may not be accompanied by an extremely hypoplastic secondary muscle. A parachute mitral valve is usually found with coarctation of the aorta, but additionally may be accompanied by a supravalvar ring in the left atrium and subaortic fibrous obstruction, this being a complex known as Shone's syndrome. Parachute valves are commonly found with atrioventricular septal defects.

Proplapsing of the leaflets of the mitral valve is often associated with collagen vascular disease. It can affect either the whole of the valve or solitary scallops of the mural leaflet. The proplapsing portions of the leaflets balloon back into the left atrium across the atrioventricular junction and are often thickened and dysplastic ("floppy valve"). It is held that there are probably congenital origins for the proplapsing valve, such as poor support from the tendinous cords in early life.

The aortic leaflet is occasionally found to have a cleft as an isolated lesion. The axis of the cleft then points towards the subaortic outlet. This arrangement requires normal atrioventricular septation. Cleft aortic leaflet more frequently occurs with straddling mitral valve. It is a completely different lesion from the functional commissure which is seen between the bridging leaflets of the left-sided valve in atrioventricular septal defects and which points towards the atrial septum.

Very rarely with the usual atrial arrangement and concordant atrioventricular connections, the mitral valve may display some adherence of the mural leaflet to the ventricular wall with apical displacement of the hinge point, analogous to Ebstein's malformation of the tricuspid valve.

Malformations of the mitral valve, while uncommon in isolation, not infrequently influence the clinical course and surgical management of complex congenital heart lesions. In the context of decreased pulmonary blood-flow, procedures which augment the pulmonary circulation may reveal a previously unsuspected obstructive lesion; while, conversely, a large left-to-right shunt may exaggerate the hemodynamic importance of a mitral valvar anomaly. It is thus an area which requires both careful investigation and good clinical judgement to plan successful treatment.

Unlike the right side of the heart where a cavopulmonary anastomosis may be used to partially bypass a small tricuspid valve, there is no simple technique to circumvent a hypoplastic mitral valve. The first decision, therefore, is whether the mitral annulus is large enough to accommodate all the pulmonary venous return to the left heart. If not, the patient probably will need to enter some form of "hypoplastic left heart" management, leading to a Fontan circulation. This includes an adequate interatrial communication and relief of or protection of the lungs from pulmonary hypertension. When multiple levels of the systemic circulation are obstructed or hypoplastic, this may be the best option, even when only a borderline small mitral valve is present.

When the valvar annulus is within about one to two standard deviations of the normal for the size of the patient, the first preference is always conservative repair of the native mitral valve. This can often be accomplished with the variety of techniques available for valve repair and using echocardiographic guidance. In general, fused leaflets are opened at their commissures. Subvalvar obstruction at the level of the tendinous cords or papillary muscles is relieved by incision and/or resection of abnormal attachments. If the valve is incompetent, the annulus is revised to an appropriate size and the leaflets are brought into apposition by the resection of flail or redundant segments with shortening of elongated cords or papillary muscles as needed. While these maneuvers are technically more challenging in the small infant heart, acceptable, if not perfect valvar function can often be achieved, thus delaying valve replacement at an early age. Prosthetic rings are usually not implanted until the patient is fully grown. Operations before about three months of age are avoided because immature collagen in the very young heart makes valve repair extremely difficult.

While replacement of the mitral valve is possible at any age, it commits the patient either to long-term anticoagulation or reoperation, or both, and thus should not be advised when other options are available. In a very small heart, the currently available mechanical prostheses may be difficult to implant even in a supra-annular, left atrial position. An inverted aortic valve prosthesis is a possible solution in some cases. Biological valves have generally proved unsatisfactory because of early calcification and tissue failure in young patients. However, in patients with a large left atrium, the "top hat" homograft aortic valve, mounted within a Dacron cylinder, has been used with some success. A final option, with which there has been very limited experience, is to bypass the mitral valve with left atrial to left ventricular extracardiac conduit.

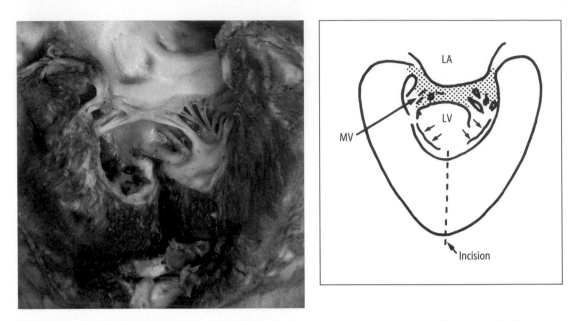

14.1 Mitral valvar stenosis. This posterior view shows a small cavity left ventricle with grossly thickened walls and endocardial fibroelastosis (arrows). The mitral valve has a small orifice and is stenotic as a result of the obliteration of intercordal spaces and attachment to multiple small papillary muscles which are implanted more posteriorly than normal. This produces the so-called "arcade" lesion or "hammock" mitral valve. In this heart, the major associated lesion is critical aortic stenosis. The arterial duct is widely patent and there is no abnormality of the aortic arch or coarctation.

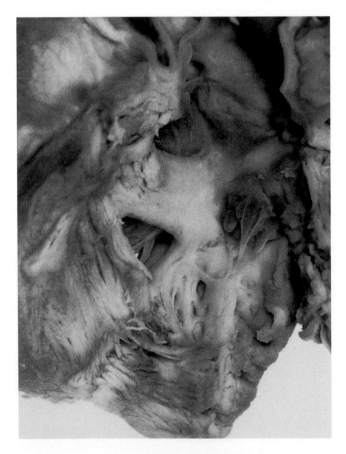

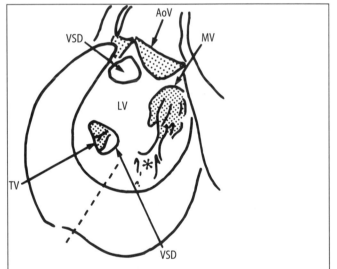

14.2 Mitral valvar stenosis. The tiny left ventricle has been opened in the plane indicated by the dashed line, for photography. The miniature mitral valve is supported by only a single papillary muscle (asterisk) and is thus a "parachute" type of valve. A small two-leaflet aortic valve lies above a perimembranous ventricular septal defect and there is a second large muscular trabecular defect through which leaflet material of the tricuspid valve is seen. This case also has a small atrial septal defect of the oval fossa and generalized hypoplasia of the aortic arch.

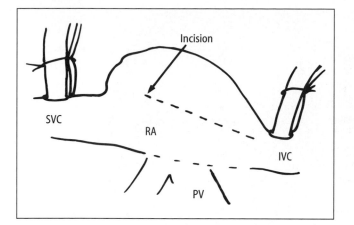

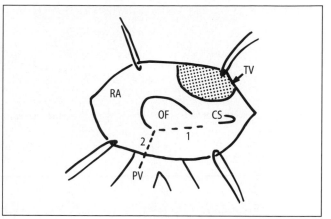

14.3 In older children, the mitral valve is approached, as in adults, directly through the left atrium. In small children and infants, however, even an enlarged left atrium gives limited access and a right atrial approach is usually employed. This is convenient also for the repair of associated atrial or ventricular septal defects. Two venous cannulas are used with moderately hypothermic cardiopulmonary bypass. The right atrium is opened with a long oblique incision anterior to the terminal crest.

14.4 To expose the left atrium, the floor of the oval fossa is incised on its rightward side (1) and rotated medially. If necessary, a second incision (2) is made across the right side of the septum and through the free walls of the right and left atriums into the upper lobe pulmonary vein.

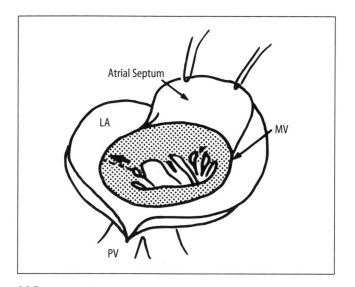

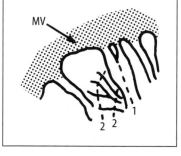

14.6 Fused subvalvar cords are divided (dashed line 1) and the intercordal spaces are opened up as much as possible. Accessory papillary muscles and cords which tether the body of the leaflet to the ventricular wall are excised (dashed line 2). Although these maneuvers may seem small, they can usually improve the effective orifice of the valve at the expense of some mitral regurgitation.

14.5 Upward traction of the septal flap generally gives excellent exposure of the mitral valve through either a midline sternal incision or a right thoracotomy. The "arcade" or "hammock" type of valve is difficult to repair and rarely gives a good long-term result. However, valvotomy may relieve the obstruction and delay valve replacement for several months or years. When it is possible to identify a fused commissure, this is incised to the valvar annulus (arrow).

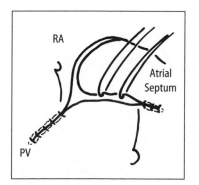

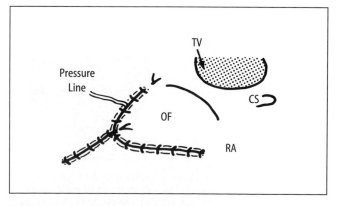

14.7 After testing the valve by infusion of saline into the left ventricle, the atrial septum and walls of the left and right atriums are reapproximated with continuous monofilament sutures.

14.8 A pressure monitoring line which has been placed percutaneously or through the innominate vein into the right atrium is positioned across the septum for left atrial pressure monitoring. This leaves a tiny residual interatrial communication after its removal, but minimizes the risk of hemorrhage, particularly if the left atrial pressure remains elevated post-operatively.

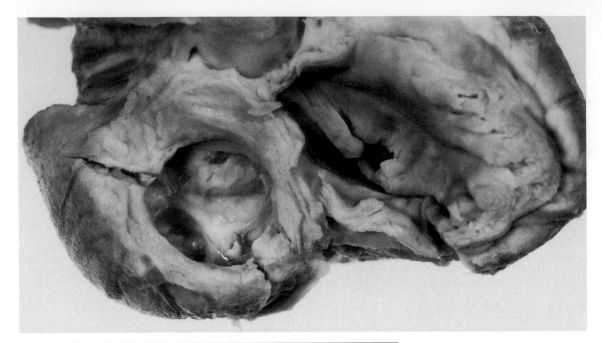

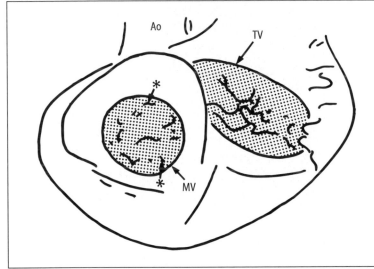

14.9 Mitral valvar stenosis. The atriums have been removed to show the mitral and tricuspid valves from above. The annulus of the mitral valve is relatively normal in size but the leaflets are grossly dysplastic and aneurysmal. Only a few pinhole orifices (asterisks) are present. This is an extreme "hammock" lesion. The tricuspid valve is normal. See also the view shown on the opposite page (Figure 14.10).

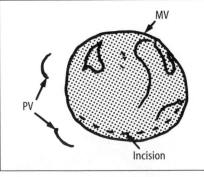

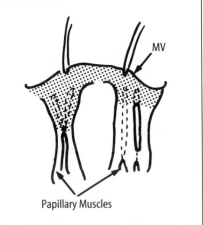

14.11 From the atrial view, this mitral valve appears very unfavorable for repair and valve replacement may, indeed, be necessary. However, preoperative echocardiography will have demonstrated mobile leaflet tissue and the two relatively normal-sized papillary muscles, and there is a normal-sized annulus, so it is worth inspecting the subvalvar area. This is done by making an incision along the base of the lateral leaflet (dashed line).

14.12 Elevating the lateral (mural) leaflet with fine stay-sutures, it is possible to open up the intercordal spaces and divide the fused papillary muscles (dashed lines).

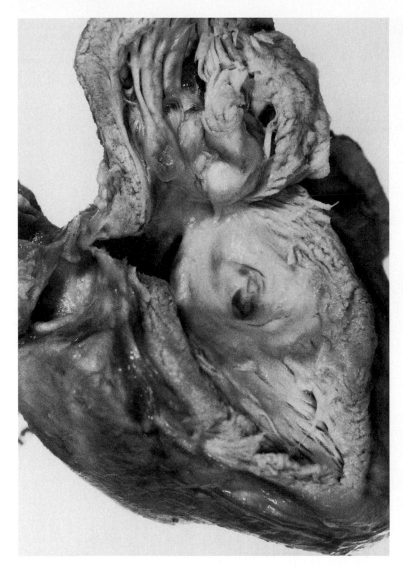

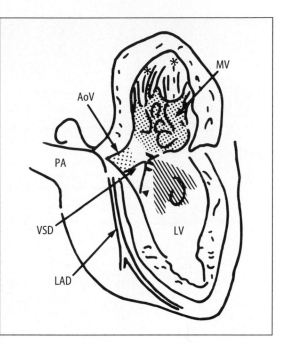

14.10 The left ventricular aspect of this heart again shows the aneurysmal leaflets of the mitral valve which has been rotated upwards. They are supported by two papillary muscles (asterisks) which are somewhat joined together but not hypoplastic. Intercordal spaces at the edge of the leaflet have been obliterated. A depression on the ventricular septum, in the area of the left bundle branches, lies in apposition to the dysplastic anterior leaflet. A small aortic trunk overrides a perimembranous malalignment ventricular septal defect, which potentially obstructs the left ventricular outflow by a muscle bar along its lower edge (triangle). Coarctation of the aorta is also present in this patient.

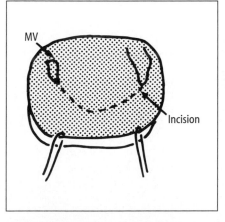

14.13 With knowledge of the underlying support, the leaflet tissue is incised to join the small pinhole orifices into a single opening, or so-called "commissure".

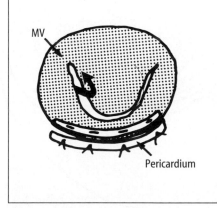

14.14 After reattachment of the lateral leaflet over pericardial strips, the valve is tested by injection of saline into the left ventricle and, subsequently by transesophageal echocardiography. If the repair is not acceptable, the valve is replaced.

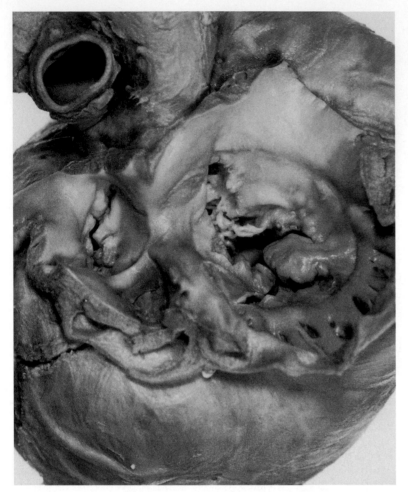

14.15 Mitral valvar stenosis. Double orifice. Both the left and right atriums have been removed and the atrioventricular valves are seen from above, at the back of the heart. The mitral valve annulus is slightly small and is partitioned by a fibromuscular ridge (asterisk), producing two orifices. The valve is supported by two complete sets of papillary muscles (not seen) which crowd the left ventricular inflow. This heart also has a perimembranous ventricular septal defect, small aortic root, and coarctation of the aorta.

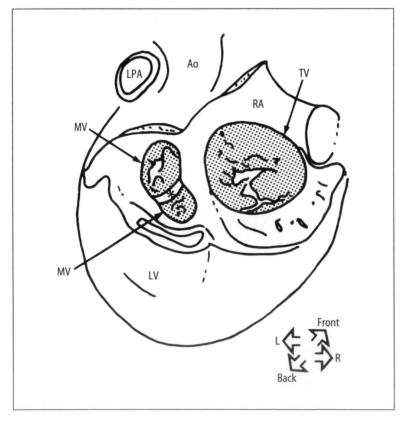

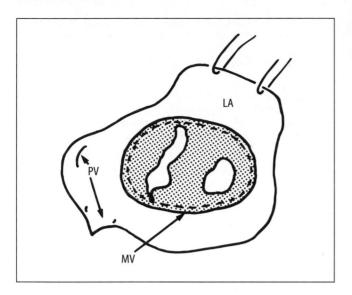

14.16 The mitral valve in this heart is unlikely to be salvageable because the papillary muscles are obstructing the left ventricle. For this reason, it is also inadvisable to leave the subvalvar apparatus *in situ* as is usually done to enhance left ventricular function following mitral valve replacement. Using a trans-septal approach (see Figures 14.3–14.5), the leaflets and subvalvar apparatus are excised (dashed line).

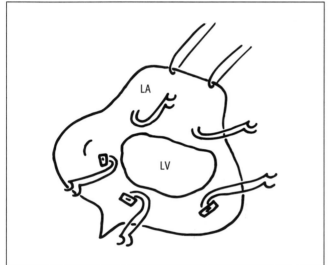

14.17 When there is a small left ventricular cavity, the prosthetic valve is often implanted in the left atrium in a "supra-annular" position to avoid narrowing in the left ventricular outflow. The suture line is mapped out with everting, pledgeted mattress sutures. These lie below the entrance of the pulmonary veins, but pass up on to the interatrial septum where stitches are placed through the septum.

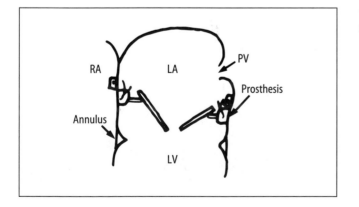

14.18 Diagrammed in cross-section, the prosthesis lies in the left atrium, above the native mitral valvar annulus and below the entrance of the pulmonary veins.

Suggested Reading

Angelini A, Becker AE, Anderson RH, Davies MJ. Mitral valve morphology: normal and mitral valve prolapse. In: Boudoulas H, Wooley CF (eds). Mitral valve proplapse and the mitral valve prolapse syndrome. Futura, New York,1988:13.

Bolling SF, Iannettoni MD, Dick II, Rosenthal A, Bove EL. Shone's anomaly: Operative results and late outcome. Ann Thorac Surg 1990;49:887.

Carpentier A. Mitral valve reconstruction in children. In: Anderson RH, Macartney FJ, Shinebourne EA, Tynan M (eds). Paediatric Cardiology, Vol 5. Churchill Livingstone 1983. 361.

Carpentier A, Branchini B, Cour JC et al. Congenital malformations of the mitral valve in children. Pathology and surgical treatment. J Thorac Cardiovasc Surg 1976;72:854.

Chauvaud S, Fuzellier JF, Houel R, Berrebi A, Mihaileanu S, Carpentier A. Reconstructive surgery in congenital mitral valve insufficiency (Carpentier's techniques): long-term results. J Thorac Cardiovasc Surg 1998;115:84.

Layman TE, Edwards JE. Anomalous mitral arcade: a type of congenital mitral insufficiency. Circulation 1967;35;389.

Leung M, Rigby ML, Anderson RH, Wyse RKH, Macartney FJ. Reversed off-setting of the septal attachments of the atrioventricular valves and Ebstein's malformation of the morphologically mitral valve. Br Heart J 1987;57:184.

Mazzera E, Corno A, Di Donato R, Ballerini L, Marino B, Catena G, Marcelleti C. Surgical bypass of the systemic atrioventricular valve in children by means of a valved conduit. J Thorac Cardiovasc Surg 1988;96:321.

Okita Y, Miki S, Dusuhara K, Ueda Y, Tahata T, Tsukamoto Y, Komeda M, Xamanaka K, Shiraishi S, Tamura T, Tatsuta N, Koic H. Early and late results of reconstructive operation for congenital mitral regurgitation in pediatric age group. J Thorac Cardiovasc Surg 1988;96:294.

Prifti E, Vanini V , Bonacchi M, Frati G, Bernabei M, Giunti G, Crucean A, Luisi SV, Murzi B. Repair of congenital malformations of the mitral valve: early and midterm results. Ann Thorac Surg 2002;73:614.

Ruckman RN, Van Praagh R. Anatomic types of congenital mitral stenosis: report of 49 cases with consideration of diagnosis and surgical implications. Am J Cardiol 1978;42:592.

Ruschapt DG, Bharati S, Lev M. Mitral valve malformation of Ebstein type in absence of corrected transposition. Am J Cardiol 1976; 38:109.

Shone JD, Sellers RD, Anderson RC, Adams PJ, Lillehei CW, Edwards JE. The developmental complex of "parachute mitral valve," supravalvular ring of left atrium, subaortic stenosis, and coarctation of the aorta. Am J Cardiol 1963;11:714.

Wenink ACG, Gittenberger-de Groot AC. Straddling mitral and tricuspid valves: morphological differences and developmental backgrounds. Am J Cardiol 1982;49:1959.

Williams WG. Valve surgery in children. Can J Cardiol 1988;4:311.

15 Pulmonary Valvar Anomalies with Intact Ventricular Septum

Introduction

The normal pulmonary valve has three semilunar, pocket-like sinuses of approximately equal size. The semilunar-shaped hinge points of the valvar leaflets are attached partly to the muscular subpulmonary infundibulum of the right ventricle and partly to the root of the pulmonary trunk. In the centre of the free edge of each leaflet is a thickened nodule. The nodules of each leaflet coapt with each other within the pulmonary trunk when the valve is closed. In contrast with the aortic valve, which is in fibrous continuity with the mitral valve, the normal pulmonary valve is separated from the tricuspid valve by the muscle of the right ventriculo-infundibular fold.

In pulmonary stenosis with intact ventricular septum, there is usually incomplete obstruction to blood-flow from the right ventricle to the pulmonary circulation at valvar level. Less frequently, the obstruction may be found at the infundibular level or among the trabeculations of the right ventricle. Rarely, stenosis is present within the pulmonary arterial pathways. Tetralogy of Fallot, complete transposition or other anomalies may include morphologically similar lesions as part of more complex malformations.

Pulmonary stenosis is found in association with a number of syndromes and as a part of several systemic diseases. In Williams syndrome, both pulmonary stenosis and supravalvar aortic stenosis may occur together. Other systemic diseases, such as glycogen storage disease, may affect some or all of the cardiac valves. The rubella virus is well known as a causative agent for all types of pulmonary valvar stenosis and there are also many references in the literature to a genetic basis for these lesions. As in pulmonary valvar atresia, pulmonary stenosis has a major effect on the overall morphology of the heart, although little change in the clinical picture is seen if small muscular ventricular septal defects are present. Deficiency of the atrial septum is a common finding.

The most severe type of pulmonary stenosis is produced by fusion of all three valvar leaflets. The result is a smooth dome-shaped valve, usually with a central orifice. Alternatively, the orifice may have an eccentric position. Fusion of the three commissures is evident also at the periphery of the valve as supravalvar narrowing of the sinutubular junction. Stenotic pulmonary valves which have the rudiments of four commissures have been described, but stenosis is rarely found with two-leaflet valves. Although commissural fusion may be seen also at the periphery of less severely stenotic valves, the central portions of the leaflets are mobile and usually thickened. These valves may eventually become calcified. Another variant of pulmonary valvar stenosis is produced when the orifice of a three-leaflet pulmonary valve is narrowed at the level of the commissures and the sinuses. The commissures in these cases are not fused to each other, but rather are tethered at their apices to the arterial wall, reducing the size of the opening of the valvar sinuses. The sinuses become dilated, which produces an "hour-glass" malformation. Valvar stenosis is invariably accompanied by post-stenotic dilatation of the main pulmonary artery, after the age of about two months.

Pulmonary valvar stenosis, like pulmonary valvar atresia, is rarely seen without additional changes in the heart. There is usually hypertrophy of the right ventricular wall and, in these hearts, the size of the ventricular cavity is reduced. In extreme hypertrophy, the trabecular component of the right ventricle may even become obliterated, although this is more typical of pulmonary valvar atresia with intact septum. Infundibular stenosis with intact ventricular septum is extremely rare as an isolated lesion, and cases which appear to be such are likely previously to have had a ventricular septal defect which closed. The coexistence of infundibular and valvar stenosis without a ventricular septal defect is also very uncommon, as is a "two-chambered" right ventricle caused by hypertrophy of the septomarginal trabeculation within the right ventricle. With critical pulmonary stenosis, the tricuspid valvar tension apparatus may be thickened, together with fibrosis of the endocardium, suggesting that there has been ischaemia of the myocardium. Even the left side of the heart may be affected, frequent findings being hypertrophy of the ventricular walls and disarray at a microscopic level in both the arterial walls and the myocardium.

Other lesions which occasionally cause obstruction of the right ventricular outflow tract in the absence of valvar stenosis include aneurysmal tissue from the membranous septum, or even an aneurysmal valve of the inferior caval vein (Eustachian valve) passing through the tricuspid valve (spinnaker syndrome). Even more rarely, subvalvar obstruction may be caused by tumours.

Pulmonary atresia, which is complete obstruction to the pulmonary outflow tract, is produced by a number of mechanisms. Two variations tend to be associated with infundibular atresia. In one, there is an absence of pulmonary valvar leaflets, such that no sinuses are visible at the root of a tiny, blind-ending pulmonary trunk. In the second variation, prominent commissural ridges radiate towards the pulmonary trunk from the centre of a poorly formed atretic valve. Still another type of valvar anatomy is a smooth, formed but atretic valve projecting into the pulmonary root, with only peripheral commissural ridges. This variant is the thin, dome-shaped valve, which is more characteristic of critical pulmonary valvar stenosis. These latter variations tend to be associated with a patent subpulmonary infundibulum which extends to the undersurface of the valvar membrane.

Pulmonary valvar atresia is never an isolated lesion. It is invariably accompanied by anomalies of the right ventricle, the myocardium and the tricuspid valve. Because there is complete obstruction to the flow of blood into the pulmonary trunk, an alternative source of pulmonary blood-flow is necessary for the survival of the patient. In the presence of intact ventricular septum, this is usually a persistently patent arterial duct and it is extremely rare to find major systemic to pulmonary collateral arteries to the lungs. The pulmonary trunk may be of normal size, small, or atretic, and the size does not correlate with the capacity of the ventricle which is exceedingly variable.

The thickness of the right ventricular wall, however, does usually correlate with the size of the ventricular cavity. Although three different groups have been identified, depending on the proportions of the right ventricular cavity, there is a spectrum of cavity sizes. The groups correspond to the extent of myocardial hypertrophy which, in turn, is reflected in ventricular function. They range from extremes of dilatation to severe hypoplasia, with mild reduction in cavity volume in between. With severely hypoplastic right ventricular cavity, the mural hypertrophy may be excessive and obliterate the apical and/or outlet components, leaving only an identifiable inlet. With moderate cavitary hypoplasia, all components of the ventricle tend to be well represented. In grossly dilated ventricles with thin walls, which usually are found in the presence of an Ebstein anomaly of the tricuspid valve, all components of the ventricle are well visualized.

The myocardium of either or both ventricles in pulmonary atresia with intact septum may exhibit ischaemic changes or other abnormalities. When the right ventricular cavity is small and the ventricular wall is very thick, fistulous communications between the cavity and the coronary arteries are to be expected. In this way, the myocardium harbours a network of ventriculo-coronary arterial connections, even to the extent of producing a "spongy" myocardium. In ventricles of near to normal size, these communications are rarely found. In the extremely rare situation of the complete absence of proximal coronary arteries, all the coronary blood of necessity flows to the myocardium via such fistulous communications. Endocardial fibrosis is commonly found in the right ventricle and may be present throughout the spectrum of cavity sizes. It is less common in the left ventricle of these hearts, but, when present, may herald a dysplastic mitral valve. Also, there may be a convex bulging of the ventricular septum into the left ventricular outflow tract. Uhl's anomaly, i.e. profound hypoplasia of the right ventricular myocardium and a paucity of trabeculations, has been seen in association with pulmonary atresia and severe dysplasia of the tricuspid valve.

The tricuspid valvar annulus is usually small in hearts with pulmonary atresia and intact ventricular septum, and its size correlates well with the size of the right ventricular cavity and the degree of myocardial hypertrophy. The tricuspid valvar leaflets are also commonly dysplastic, but this feature, in contrast, has no correlation with the degree of ventricular hypoplasia. Ebstein's anomaly of the tricuspid valve is a frequent finding and often obstructive, even to the extent of subdividing the ventricle into inlet and trabecular/outlet portions.

Valvar pulmonary stenosis, including critical pulmonary stenosis in the newborn, is virtually always managed by initial balloon valvuloplasty. Patency of the arterial duct may be necessary for several days afterwards to maintain acceptable arterial saturation in neonates, and this is usually achieved with a continued infusion of prostaglandin. It is only cases with residual obstruction who come to operation, usually after several months and additional catheter interventions. These tend to be patients with dysplastic valves and/or subvalvar muscular obstruction, often with associated Noonan's syndrome. In virtually every case, excision of the thickened valvar leaflets with enlargement of the pulmonary annulus by means of a transannular patch will be necessary to relieve the obstruction. An atrial septal defect or patent oval fossa is usually present and this is closed at the same time, as is any persistently patent arterial duct.

The management of pulmonary atresia with intact ventricular septum is vastly more challenging, but can be resolved into basically three components. The first is to ensure long-term pulmonary blood-flow, after ductal patency has been established initially with prostaglandin. This virtually always means a systemic-pulmonary anastomosis, despite the appearance of a "good" right ventricle in some patients. The classical Blalock-Taussig shunt and Waterston anastomosis have been widely used in the past, but a modified Blalock shunt interposing a synthetic graft between a subclavian and a pulmonary artery is now preferred for its technical ease and flexibility. If it is clear at this time that the patient's right ventricle will not become useful and a Fontan-type of circulation will be the ultimate goal, the shunt is usually placed on the right side. If, however, simultaneous valvotomy is planned with a view to a two-ventricle circulation, the systemic-pulmonary anastomosis is done on the left side.

The second objective which, unlike the first and third, does not apply to all patients, is decompression of the right ventricle. Forward decompression through the pulmonary valve is done both to augment pulmonary blood-flow and to encourage development of the right ventricle as a useful pumping chamber. While "hot wire" or radiofrequency perforation of the valve followed by balloon valvuloplasty may accomplish this in the catheter laboratory, it is often necessary to open the valve surgically. The available technical options are transpulmonary or transventricular "valvotomy," with or without inflow occlusion or cardiopulmonary bypass. Given the capacity for subsequent interventional dilatation once continuity is established between the right ventricle and pulmonary arteries, it no longer appears justified to carry out an extensive procedure to open up the right ventricular outflow in the neonatal period. Therefore, usually a closed transventricular or transpulmonary operation is done. If ventricular decompression remains suboptimal after several months and usually several interventional, balloon dilations, it is then necessary to perform a transannular outflow patch on a cardiopulmonary bypass. "Backward" decompression of the right ventricle by removal of the tricuspid valve may be useful at the time of the Fontan operation in patients who do not have a right ventricular dependent coronary circulation.

The final goal is to separate the systemic and pulmonary circulations, either with a two-ventricle repair or with some type of Fontan procedure. At either extreme of the morphological spectrum, it is fairly clear which hearts are suitable for two-ventricle repair and which require management as a single ventricle, but decision-making in between may be difficult. Some cases require a "one-and-a-half" ventricle repair, using the right ventricle to pump the inferior caval blood to the lungs in combination with a bidirectional superior caval vein to pulmonary artery anastomosis. If the tricuspid valve is within about two standard deviations of the normal size, two-ventricle repair is usually possible. This consists of closure of the atrial septal defect, improvement of the tricuspid valvar function (if possible) and division of any obstructing muscle bundles within the right ventricle, with or without implantation of an orthotopic pulmonary homograft valve. A few of these patients return later for tricuspid valve replacement (see Chapter 13). As in other types of "single ventricle," the Fontan circulation may be established by a variety of techniques, either as a single procedure or staged palliation (see Chapter 24).

The patient with an extremely hypoplastic right ventricle which has decompressed itself to a degree, through the coronary circulation, constitutes a difficult problem. As proximal coronary arterial stenoses are not uncommon in such patients, coronary angiography is essential to plan their management. If this reveals significant proximal obstructions, the right ventricle is not decompressed and, at the time of the Fontan operation, the tricuspid valve is left in continuity with the pulmonary venous atrium (through an atrial septal defect) to maximize oxygen saturation in the coronary arterial blood.

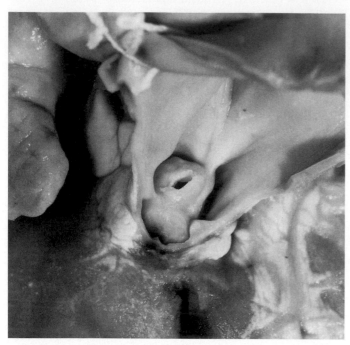

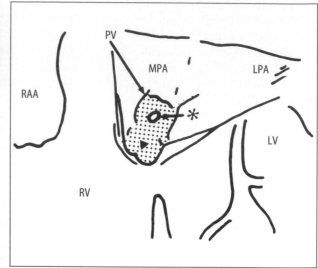

15.1 Pulmonary stenosis. The main pulmonary artery has been opened into the left branch, revealing a domed stenotic valve. The three interleaflet triangles have achieved a similar level at the origin of the pulmonary trunk and there are three well-defined sinuses. The valvar leaflets are thickened and aneurysmal (triangle). All three commissures are fused, leaving only a small eccentric orifice (asterisk). The subpulmonary right ventricular outflow is delineated by the anterior interventricular (left anterior descending) coronary artery.

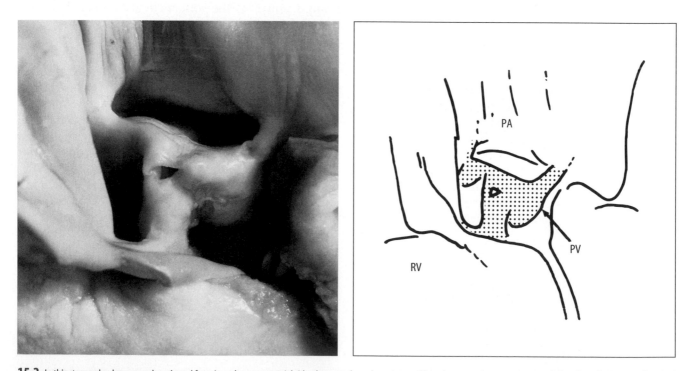

15.2 In this stenosed pulmonary valve, viewed from its pulmonary arterial side, there are three deep sinuses. The valvar commissures are extremely fused, producing a small central orifice. The valvar leaflets are thickened.

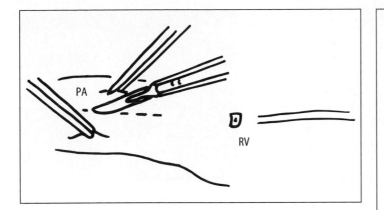

15.3 Stenotic pulmonary valves such as these are virtually always managed by balloon valvuloplasty in the cardiac catherization laboratory and thus rarely seen by the cardiac surgeon. Open surgical valvotomy, however, is also a well-described procedure with time-honoured efficacy. Cardiopulmonary bypass with mild hypothermia (30°–32° C) is established with two venous cannulas if the right atrium is to be opened for closure of an interatrial defect. A pledgeted stay-suture on the infundibulum of the right ventricle facilitates exposure of the pulmonary valve, as does positioning the operating table "head-up" and towards the surgeon. The pulmonary artery is opened vertically just distal to the valvar sinuses, with slight upward tension on the vessel from the surgeon's and assistant's forceps.

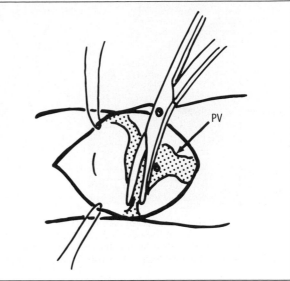

15.4 Each commissure is sharply dissected away from the wall of the pulmonary artery to the bottom of the valvar sinus.

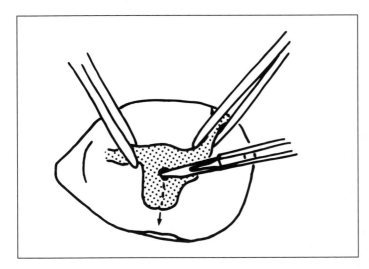

15.5 The mobilized commissure is incised from the valvar orifice outwards in its midpoint. Conversely, the incision may be carried from the pulmonary arterial wall to the lumen of the valve. Counter-traction is provided by the forceps of the surgeon and the assistant on the leaflets to either side of the commissure that is being opened.

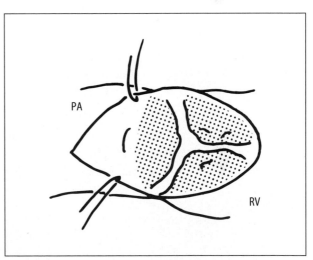

15.6 Each of the other two fused commissures is mobilized and incised, producing the maximal orifice with three mobile valvar leaflets. This will result also in a degree of pulmonary incompetence, which is usually well tolerated.

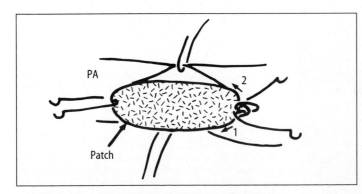

15.7 The pulmonary artery is closed with a small patch of autogenous pericardium to avoid any narrowing. The patch is positioned with fine double-ended monofilament sutures at each end. Beginning the closure at the valvar sinuses helps both to avoid damage to the leaflets and to place bites more accurately in the less accessible part of the anastomosis.

15.8 The suture line is completed with the second suture, working back down on either side from the top of the patch. The outflow patch does not cross the ventriculoarterial junction and hence is not "trans-annular".

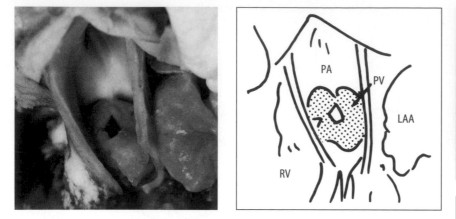

15.9 Pulmonary stenosis. The pulmonary valve in this heart has three sinuses, but the commissures are poorly defined and the leaflet tissue is extremely thickened. The leaflets "dome" to a central orifice which is nearly one-third the diameter of the ventriculo-arterial junction. The small lateral slits in the valvar orifice may be the result of an attempted balloon valvuloplasty as there is no evidence of a surgical procedure in this heart.

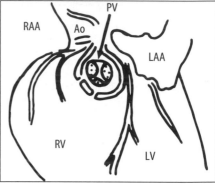

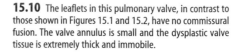

15.10 The leaflets in this pulmonary valve, in contrast to those shown in Figures 15.1 and 15.2, have no commissural fusion. The valve annulus is small and the dysplastic valve tissue is extremely thick and immobile.

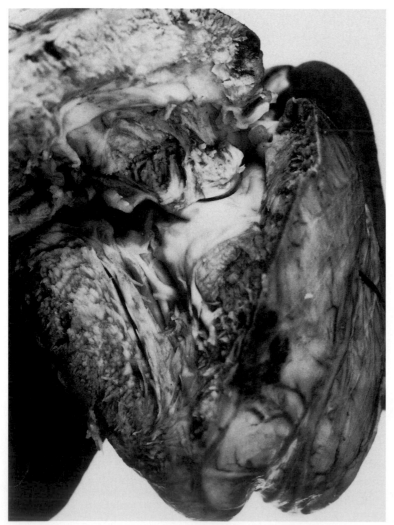

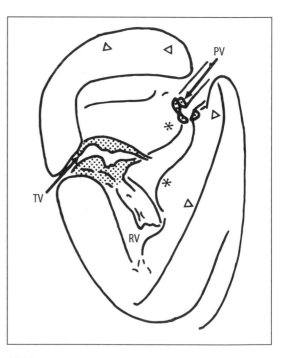

15.11 The right ventricle of the valve illustrated in Figure 15.10 is grossly hypertrophied with thickening of both the free wall and the septomarginal trabeculation which has been divided (asterisks). The tricuspid valve is also dysplastic with poorly formed papillary muscles. If the parietal wall, which has been lifted up, is closed down (open triangles), it is possible to appreciate the extensive subpulmonary muscular stenosis that is present, as well as the small volume of the right ventricular cavity.

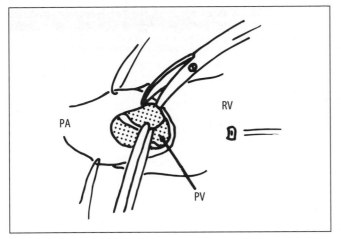

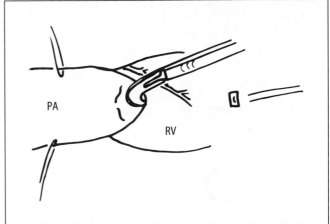

15.12 Simple commissurotomy or valvuloplasty is doomed to failure in hearts such as those shown here, firstly because the obstruction at valvar level is due to thickened immobile leaflet tissue and /or a hypoplastic annulus rather than commissural fusion, and secondly because there is also subpulmonary obstruction. At open operation, the valvar leaflets are first excised to permit assessment of the annulus and subpulmonary outflow.

15.13 On the rare occasion that the subvalvar muscular region is not obstructive, the incision in the pulmonary artery is closed with a small pericardial patch and, if the patient is a neonate, prostin is continued post-operatively awaiting recovery of right ventricular function. Nearly always, however, it is necessary to extend the incision onto the right ventricular infundibulum to relieve subvalvar obstruction. This is conveniently done with a no. 12 blade ("hook knife"), noting the more transverse orientation of the small right ventricle, as delimited externally by coronary arterial branches.

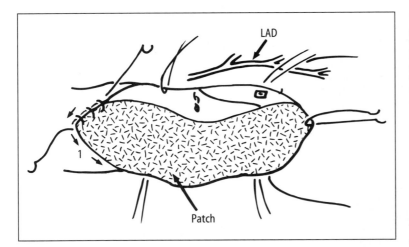

15.14 The sides of the ventriculotomy are retracted with pledgeted stay-sutures. Excessively hypertrophied muscles on the inner surface of the free wall and, in this case, also the hypertrophied septomarginal trabeculation are excised. The tricuspid valve should be visualized and its subvalvar apparatus, which may insert unusually close to the outflow tract, should be carefully conserved. The outflow is then enlarged with a patch of autogenous pericardium, starting distally at the apex of the pulmonary arterial incision.

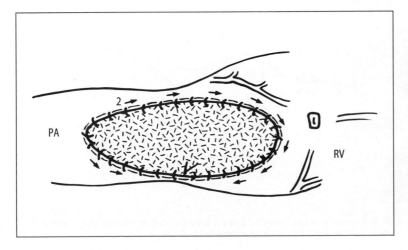

15.15 Over the ventriculotomy it is the epicardium that "holds the stitches" and no attempt is made to penetrate the full thickness of the massively hypertrophied free wall of the right ventricle. On completion, the patch often lies close to the left anterior descending coronary artery and major infundibular branches of the right coronary artery. If additional sutures are needed for hemostasis, it is important to avoid occluding major coronary branches.

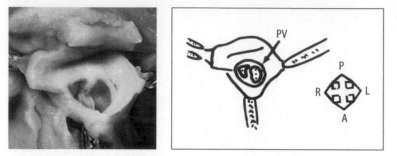

15.16 Pulmonary atresia (imperforate pulmonary valve). The pulmonary valve is seen from its arterial aspect, the walls of the pulmonary artery having been retracted to demonstrate the small valve. Two sinuses are seen, but the free edges of the leaflets are completely fused together.

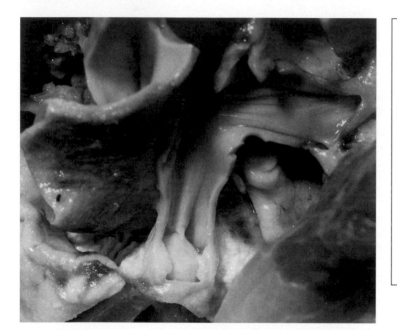

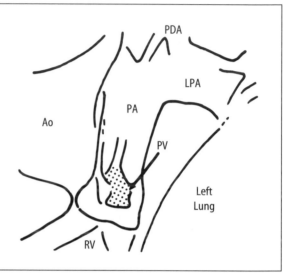

15.17 In this imperforate pulmonary valve, the leaflets are domed and the commissures are totally fused. Three sinuses are present. The left pulmonary artery and the retracted aorta are also seen.

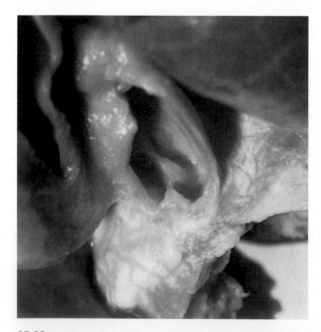

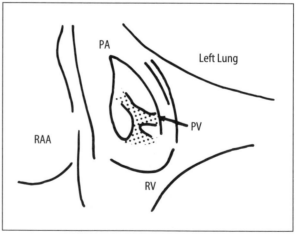

15.18 In a third example of pulmonary atresia, seen close up from above, the valvar leaflets are thinner but poorly developed and the commissures are again completely fused, resulting in an imperforate valve. There are three sinuses. The interventricular septum in each of these hearts is intact.

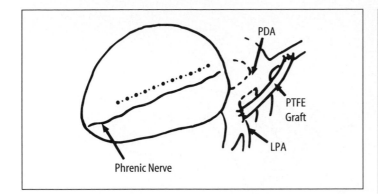

15.19 One protocol for the management of an imperforate pulmonary valve with a reasonably well-developed right ventricle is a combined transventricular valvuloplasty and systemic pulmonary anastomosis. The pulmonary blood-flow is first assured by a left modified Blalock-Taussig shunt. As pulmonary blood-flow is dependent on the arterial duct during the procedure, the position of the shunt is slightly more distal than usual. The pericardium is then opened at a distance of about 1 cm anterior to the phrenic nerve (dotted line). Good exposure of both posterior and anterior mediastinal fields is usually obtained through a long anterolateral thoracotomy in the fourth intercostal space.

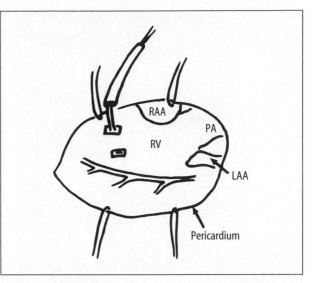

15.20 A double pledgeted mattress suture is placed low down on the right ventricle and passed through a snugger. The site of the suture is a compromise which is determined by the length of the cannula that will be inserted to perforate the valve (which is usually short) and the need for room to expand the dilatation balloon (which is always too long).

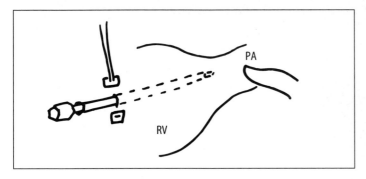

15.21 A needle and cannula (usually about 16G) are passed from the right ventricle into the pulmonary artery while palpating the main pulmonary artery. Often (but not invariably), there is a slight "give" or "pop" as the cannula perforates the valve. Also (but not invariably), blood coming from the cannula may become pinker. There is always significant blood loss during the procedure and this should be anticipated by the anesthetist.

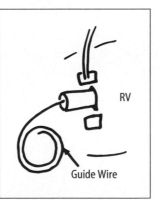

15.22 The needle is withdrawn, leaving the cannula across the pulmonary valve, and a guide wire is passed through the cannula.

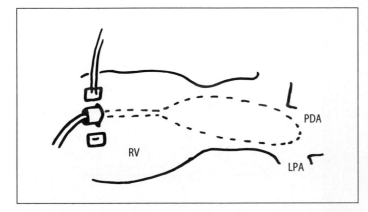

15.23 The cannula is withdrawn, using the pledgeted stay-suture to control hemorrhage, and the dilatation catheter is passed over the guide wire and across the pulmonary valve. The balloon generally "splits" the myocardium at the insertion site and a collar of hemostatic sponge may be helpful to control bleeding. Alternatively, a sheath may be placed over the guide wire for the introduction of a dilatation catheter, but this is usually stiff and awkward. The currently available balloons, which are designed for intravenous placement with fluoroscopic guidance, may enter either the duct or the left pulmonary artery. The balloon is inflated, usually causing a "cracking" sensation as the valvar leaflets are split. If arterial saturation drops dramatically, this usually indicates that the inflated balloon has occluded the arterial duct and the shunt, so it should be deflated rapidly.

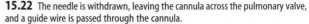
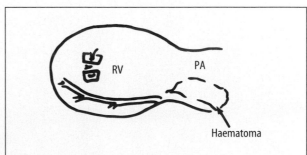

15.24 After the dilatation catheter is withdrawn, the stay-suture is tied down and additional stitches placed if needed to obtain hemostasis. If there is a hematoma over the pulmonary trunk, it is *not* explored because bleeding is very likely tracking back from the arterial duct or the shunt and will be controlled by the adventitia. The pericardium is loosely approximated with interrupted sutures, the shunt is checked for patency and the thoracotomy incision is closed.

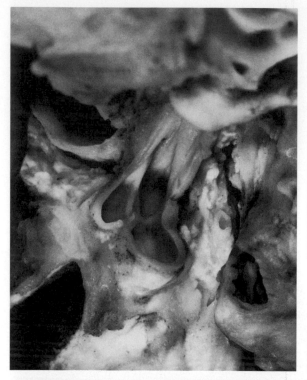

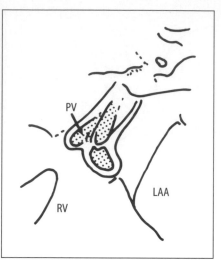

15.25 Pulmonary atresia with intact ventricular septum. Two of the three sinuses have been cut away to demonstrate three completely fused valvar leaflets. There is no orifice through the valve, but the body of the leaflets is relatively thin and mobile.

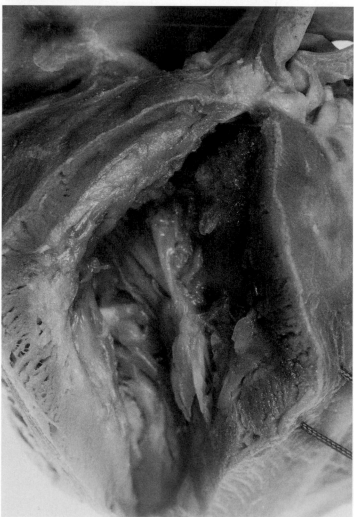

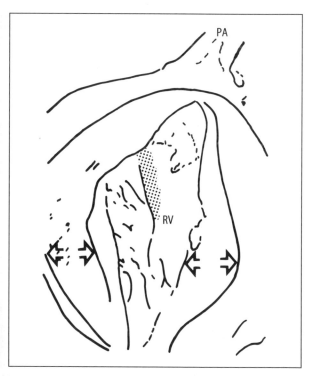

15.26 The right ventricular outflow tract in another heart with pulmonary atresia has been opened vertically below the valve to reveal a small volume muscle-bound cavity. There is massive hypertrophy of the free wall (arrows).

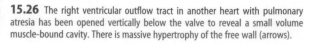

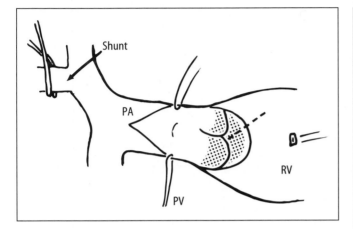

15.27 In hearts with pulmonary atresia and intact ventricular septum where decompression of the ventricle has otherwise been inadequate or not possible, a staged outflow patch may be employed. The systemic pulmonary shunt is left patent but temporarily occluded during cardiopulmonary bypass. When the valvar leaflets can be mobilized, it may be possible to leave one or two posteriorly as a functional cusp.

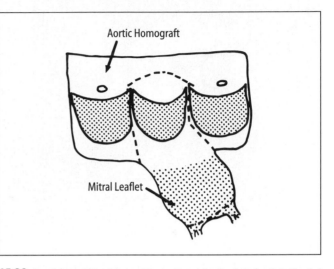

15.28 A monocusp patch, while providing a valve mechanism for only a limited period of time in most patients (weeks to months), may improve the early post-operative hemodynamics. Usually the non-coronary leaflet of an aortic homograft is trimmed (dashed line), retaining the attached anterior mitral leaflet. However, the ventriculotomy often angles leftward (Figure 15.27), whereas the mitral leaflet angles rightward and thus may be unsuitable. In that case, it is removed and replaced with a patch of homograft arterial wall, pericardium, or other prosthetic material.

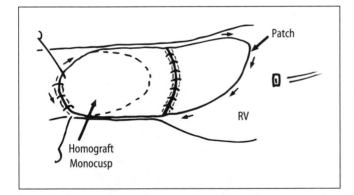

15.29 To provide any valve function, the monocusp anteriorly must coapt with something posteriorly. This is generally accomplished by siting the valve as far distally as possible, such that it abuts against the posterior pulmonary arterial wall or a retained leaflet. Again, resection of the anterior mitral leaflet when it is too short prevents the monocusp from being pulled down into the ventricle. Otherwise, its insertion does not differ from that of any other transannular right ventricular outflow patch (see Figures 15.13–15.15).

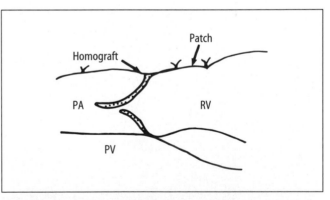

15.30 Shown in cross-section, the monocusp leaflet lies above the subpulmonary right ventricular infundibulum with a proximal patch of sufficient length to enlarge the outflow anteriorly. While such ventricles may develop remarkable function over time, they do not support the pulmonary circulation immediately after operation. Accordingly, the systemic pulmonary shunt is reopened to come off bypass.

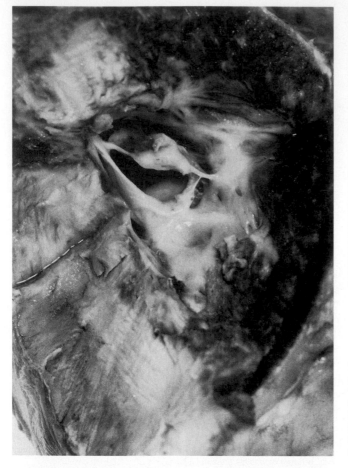

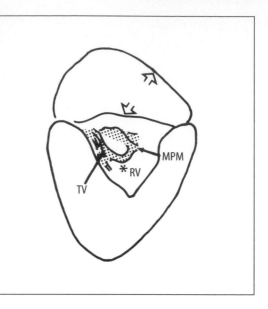

15.31 Pulmonary atresia, intact ventricular septum. Tricuspid valve. Right ventricle. The small right ventricle has been opened with a "fish mouth" incision around the apex, through which this view is up towards the tricuspid valve. The ventricular wall is extremely thick (arrows) and the cavity is lined by fibrosed endocardium. The small tricuspid valve has sparse cordal attachments and there are no papillary muscles. Most of the septal leaflet is adherent to the septum (asterisk) in an Ebstein-like fashion.

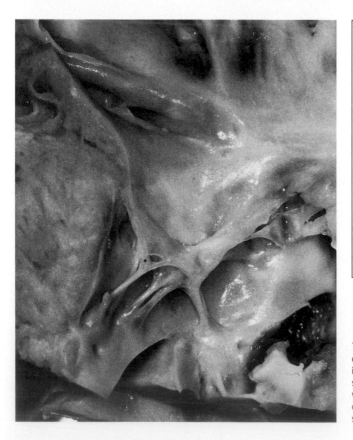

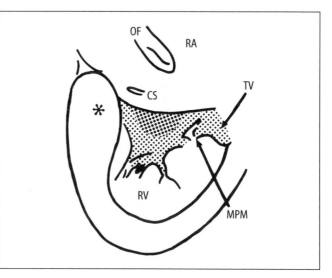

15.32 Another heart with pulmonary atresia and intact ventricular septum has been opened across the right atrioventricular junction. Most of the tricuspid valve septal leaflet is again adherent to the septum (dense stippling) and the free edge is thickened with support from only a few short cords. The papillary musculature is poorly developed. The ventricular walls are thickened (asterisk) and the small cavity is lined by thickened endocardium. The atrial septum contains a defect in the oval fossa. The orifice of the coronary sinus is in the normal position.

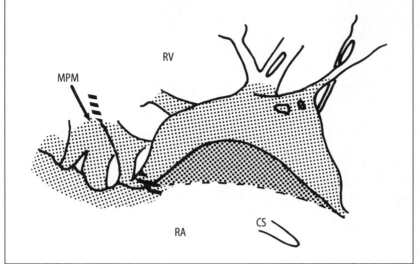

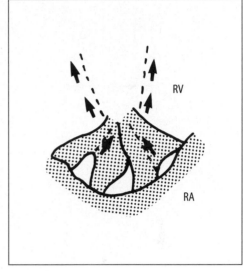

15.33 While a successful two-ventricle repair is highly unlikely in hearts such as these, it may be possible to salvage "half" a right ventricle, and this may be desirable in view of the uncertain long-term results of the Fontan circulation. To that end, function of the small tricuspid valve can nearly always be improved by a variety of techniques which must be individualized to each situation. Seen as the surgeon would view it from the right atrium, the valve shown in Figure 15.32 has little commissural fusion. However, it may be possible to liberate fused cords and develop papillary muscles from the ventricular endocardium. The conduction tissue will run under the area of leaflet adherence, with the right bundle branch near the poorly developed medial papillary muscle complex. Unlike a true Ebstein's malformation, there is no large anterior leaflet to fashion into a monocusp valve.

15.34 The cords attaching in the area of the medial papillary muscle are fenestrated and incisions are made deep into the thickened ventricular septum to "carve out" a papillary muscle. This should be wider at its base and will probably cause right bundle branch block.

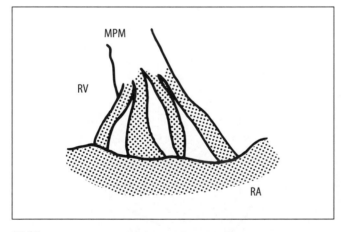

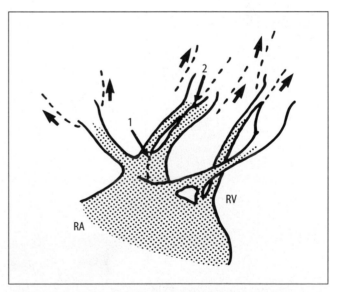

15.35 The resulting tricuspid valvar support, although far from normal, has an improved mobility and sub-leaflet opening.

15.36 The other group of cords has some fusion which also may be released by incisions towards both the leaflet (1) and the ventricular cavity (2). Again, papillary muscles are liberated by dissection into the thickened myocardium. It may be possible also to free some of the adherent leaflet from the septal endocardium.

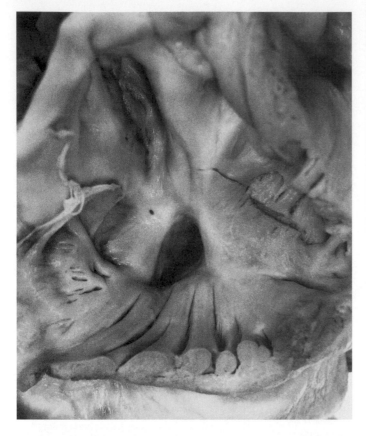

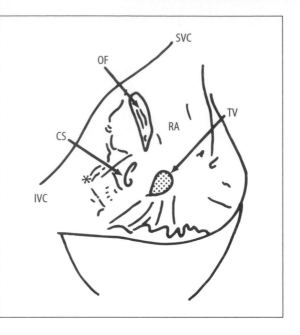

15.37 Pulmonary atresia, intact ventricular septum. Right atrium. Looking down on the right atrium shows a small stenotic tricuspid valve. The flap valve of the oval fossa is elongated, but the surrounding muscular limbus is clearly defined. Residual fibres from the embryonic venous valves (Chiari network) lie above the entrance of the inferior caval vein (asterisk). The right atrium also receives the superior caval vein and coronary sinus.

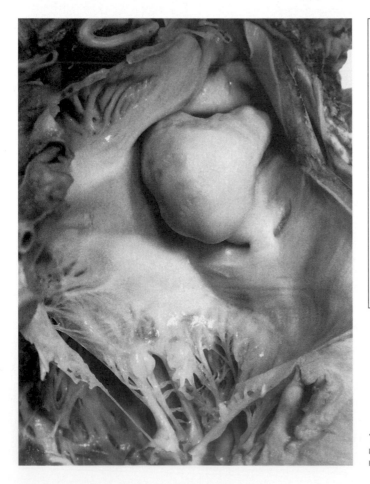

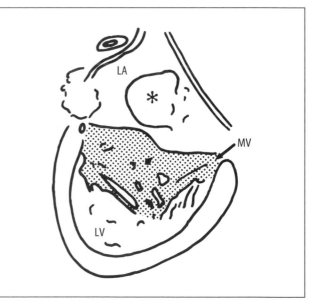

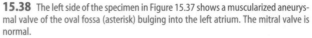

15.38 The left side of the specimen in Figure 15.37 shows a muscularized aneurysmal valve of the oval fossa (asterisk) bulging into the left atrium. The mitral valve is normal.

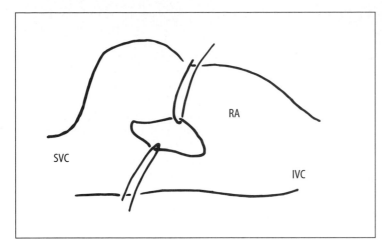

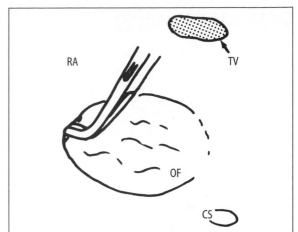

15.39 An atrial septal defect is essential in pulmonary atresia with intact ventricular septum, and the aneurysmal valve of the oval fossa completely obstructs the interatrial communication in this heart. Balloon septostomy would not be effective and the large muscular flap of tissue would be difficult to open by blade septectomy. Either closed (Blalock-Hanlon) or open surgical septectomy would therefore need to be carried out, probably as an emergency. Considering the resources available, septectomy on cardiopulmonary bypass would have the advantage of potentially resuscitating the patient, particularly if a systemic-pulmonary anastomosis is also required. For open atrial septectomy, only a small oblique incision is necessary in the right atrium.

15.40 The coronary sinus and caval orifices, as well as the tricuspid valve are identified. The latter may be difficult to differentiate from the oval fossa. A right-angled instrument is passed across the top of the flap valve and rotated 180° to hook the tissue into the right atrium.

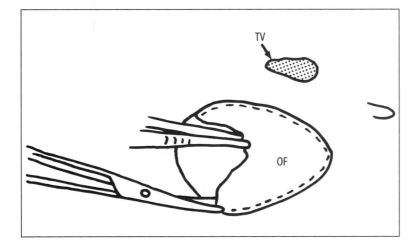

15.41 The valve of the oval fossa is then grasped with forceps and completely excised, staying within the muscular boundaries of the limbus to avoid injury to the conduction tissue and perforation of the heart.

15.42 On completion, there is an unrestrictive, widely patent interatrial communication. No attempt is made to enlarge the tricuspid valve at this time. The walls of the right atrium are inspected to be certain than they have not been "button-holed" and the atriotomy is closed with a running monofilament suture, taking care to evacuate air from the left side of the heart.

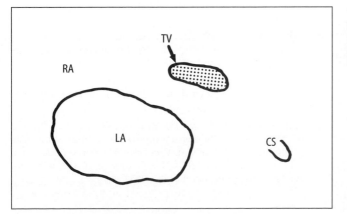

Suggested Reading

Anderson RH, Anderson C, Zuberbuhler JR. Further morphologic studies on hearts with pulmonary atresia and intact ventricular septum. Cardiol Young 1991;1:105.

Anderson RH, Ho SY. Pathologic substrates for $1^1/2$ ventricular repair. Ann Thorac Surg 1998;66:673.

Anderson RH, Macartney FJ, Shinebourne EA, Tynan MJ. Pulmonary stenosis. In: Paediatric Cardiology 1987, Vol 2. Chapter 39, p959. Churchill Livingstone.

Billingsley AM, Laks H, Boyce SW, George B, Santulli T, Williams RG. Definitive repair in patients with pulmonary atresia and intact ventricular septum. J Thorac Cardiovasc Surg 1989;97:746.

Becker AE. Quadricuspid pulmonary valve. Anatomical observations in 20 hearts. Acta Morphologica Neerlando-Scandinavia. 1972; 10:299.

Becu L, Somerville J, Gallo A. Isolated pulmonary valve stenosis as part of more widespread cardiovascular disease. Br Heart J 1976; 38:472.

Blount SG Jr, Van Elk J, Balchun OJ, Swan H. Valvular pulmonary stenosis with intact ventricular septum, clinical and physiological response to open valvotomy. Circulation 1957;15:814.

Bull C, DeLaval MR, Mercanti C, Macartney FJ, Anderson RH. Pulmonary atresia with intact septum: a revised classification. Circulation 1982;66: 266.

Chowdhury UK, Airan B, Sharma R, Kothari SS, Saxena A, Venugopal P. One and a half ventricle repair with pulsatile bidirectional Glenn: results and guidelines for patient selection. Ann Thorac Surg 2001;71:1995.

Cole RB, Muster AJ, Lev M, Paul MH. Pulmonary atresia with intact ventricular septum. Am J Cardiol 1968;21:23.

de Laval M, Bull C, Hopkins R, Rees P, Deanfield J, Taylor JFN, Gersony W, Stark J, Macartney FJ. Decision making in the definitive repair of the heart with a small right ventricle. Circulation 1985;72 (suppl II):II-52.

Freedom RM. Pulmonary atresia with intact ventricular septum – the significance of the coronary arterial circulation. In: Redington AN, Brawn WJ, Deanfield JE, Anderson RH (eds). The Right Heart in Congenital Heart Disease. Oxford University Press 1998; 6;p41.

Freedom RM, Dische MR, Rowe RD. The tricuspid valve in pulmonary atresia with intact ventricular septum. Arch Path Lab Med 1978;102:28.

Freedom RM, Harrington D. Contributions of intramyocardial sinusoids in pulmonary atresia and intact ventricular septum to a right-sided circular shunt. Br Heart J 1974;36:1061.

Freedom RM, Wilson GJ. Endomyocardial abnormalities. In: Freedom RM (ed). Pulmonary atresia with intact ventricular septum. Futura Publishing Company Inc., New York 1989;Chapter 7: p89.

Fricker FJ, Zuberbuhler JR. Pulmonary atresia with intact ventricular septum. In: Anderson RH, Macartney FJ, Shinebourne EA, Tynan M (eds). Paediatric Cardiology, Vol 2. Churchill Livingstone, Edinburgh, 1987, p711.

Fyfe DA, Edwards WD, Driscoll DJ. Myocardial ischaemia in patients with pulmonary atresia and intact ventricular septum. J Am Coll Cardiol 1986;8:402.

Hanley FL, Sade RM, Blackstone EH, Kirklin JW, Freedom RM, Nanda NC and the Congenital Heart Surgeon's Society. The tricuspid valve and outcomes in pulmonary atresia and intact septum. J Thorac Cardiovasc Surg 1993;105:406.

Harinck E, Becker AE, Gittenberger-de Groot AC, Oppenheimer-Dekker A, Versprille A. The left ventricle in congenital isolated pulmonary valve stenosis. Br Heart J 1977;39:429.

Koretzky ED, Moller JH, Korns ME, Schwartz CJ, Edwards JE. Congenital pulmonary stenosis resulting from dysplasia of the valve. Circulation 1969;40:43.

Lamy M, de Grouchy J, Schweisguth O. Genetic and non-genetic factors in the aetiology of congenital heart disease: a study of 1188 cases. Am J Hum Gen 1957;9:17.

Lenox CC, Briner J. Absent proximal coronary arteries associated with pulmonary atresia. Am J Cardiol 1972;30:666.

Miller GAH, Restifo M, Shinebourne EA, Paneth M, Joseph MC, Lennox SC, Kerr IH. Pulmonary atresia with intact ventricular septum and critical pulmonary stenosis presenting in the first months of life. Br Heart J 1973;35:9.

Milo S, Fiegl A, Shem-Tov A, Neufeld HN, Goor DA. Hour-glass deformity of the pulmonary valve: a third type of pulmonary stenosis. Br Heart J 1988;60;128.

Monibi AA, Neches WH, Lenox CC, Park SC, Mathews RA, Zuberbuhler JR. Left ventricular anomalies associated with Ebstein's malformation of the tricuspid valve. Circulation 1978;57: 303.

O'Connor WN, Cottrill CM, Johnson GL, Noonan JA, Todd EP. Pulmonary atresia with intact septum and ventriculocoronary communications: surgical significance. Circulation 1982;64:805.

Restivo A, Cameron AH, Anderson RH, Allwork SP. Divided right ventricle: a review of its anatomical varieties. Pediatric Cardiology 1984;5:197.

Rowe RD. Maternal rubella and pulmonary artery stenoses. Report of eleven cases. Pediatrics 1963;32:180.

Rowe RD. Pulmonary stenosis with normal aortic root. In: Keith JD, Rowe RD, Vlad P (eds). Heart disease in infancy and childhood. 3rd edn. Macmillan, New York, p761.

Shaddy RE, Startevant JE, Judd VE, McGough EC. Right ventricular growth after transventricular pulmonary valvotomy and central aortopulmonary shunt for pulmonary atresia and intact ventricular septum. Circulation 1990;82:157.

Simcha A, Wells BG, Tynan MJ, Waterston DJ. Primary cardiac tumours in infancy and childhood. Archives of Diseases in Childhood. 1971;46:508.

Uhl HMS. Previously undescribed congenital malformation of the heart: almost total absence of the myocardium of the right ventricle. Bull Hopkins Hosp 1953;91:197.

Zuberbuhler JR, Anderson RH. Morphological variations in pulmonary atresia with intact ventricular septum. Br Heart J 1979;41: 281.

Zuberbuhler JR, Fricker FJ, Park SC, Anderson RH, Lenox CC, Neches WH, Mathews RA. Pulmonary atresia with intact ventricular septum: Morbid anatomy. In: Goodman MJ, Marquis RM (eds). Paediatric Cardiology, Vol 2. Heart disease in the newborn. Churchill Livingstone, Edinburgh, p285.

16 Aortic Valvar Anomalies and Left Ventricular Outflow Tract Obstruction

Introduction

The left ventricular outflow tract extends from the tip of the anterior mitral valvar leaflet to the junction of the sinuses of Valsalva with the ascending aorta (the sinu-tubular bar) and thus occupies a central position, both structurally and functionally, in hearts with concordant ventriculo-arterial connections. The normal aortic valve has three leaflets which attach to the outflow along semicircular "hinge points", with intervening triangles separating their ventricular aspects. The top of each interleaflet triangle is the apex of a commissure where adjacent leaflets meet along the zone of coaptation during valvar closure. On their arterial side, the commissures separate three expansions in the aortic wall – the three sinuses of Valsalva – each of which is guarded by a leaflet that moves into the sinus during opening of the valve. Two of the three sinuses normally contain the origin of a coronary artery and are thus named the right and left coronary aortic sinuses, after their respective coronary arterial origins. The "intercoronary commissure" lies between them, while the non-coronary sinus is separated from the left sinus of Valsalva by the left non-coronary commissure and from the right sinus of Valsalva by the right non-coronary commissure. In the normal aortic valve, the leaflets – and hence the sinuses of Valsava – are usually of slightly unequal size.

The subvalvar left ventricular outflow contains both muscular and fibrous components, in contrast to the right ventricle which has a completely muscular subpulmonary infundibulum. The muscular portion is in part ventricular septum and in part the anterior parietal wall of the left ventricle. The latter includes a normally inconspicuous structure called the antero-lateral muscle bundle or "muscle bundle of Moulaert." Included among the fibrous components are the central fibrous body (containing the right fibrous trigone and membranous interventricular septum), the left fibrous trigone, the anterior (aortic) leaflet of the mitral valve, and the subaortic fibrous curtain (or "area of aortic/mitral fibrous continuity"). The bundle of His traverses the central fibrous body along the postero-inferior margin of the membranous septum, usually running slightly towards the left of the crest of the ventricular septum. The left bundle branch originates almost immediately and then fans out across the left ventricular septal surface. Very rarely, the aortic valvar leaflets are separated from the mitral valve by an intervening rim of muscle that produces a completely muscular subaortic outlet to the left ventricle (aortic/mitral fibrous discontinuity).

The fibrous and muscular components of the normal left ventricular outflow lie in exquisitely precise and functionally important relations to each other and to the leaflets of the aortic valve. While the base of each leaflet, and hence each interleaflet triangle rests on a muscular or fibrous portion of the left ventricular outflow, the apex is attached to the wall of the aortic sinus, beyond the ventricular cavity. This allows expansion of the aortic root during isovolemic left ventricular contraction, a mechanism that pulls the valvar leaflets apart and commences opening of the valve prior to any ejection of blood. Since the length of the free edge of each leaflet is approximately equal to the diameter of the aorta, it can fold back into the aortic sinus during left ventricular ejection, completely removing the valve from the orifice of the outflow tract. These two mechanisms not only minimize resistance to left ventricular emptying at the level of the valvar leaflets, but also reduce mechanical stress on the leaflets themselves. At subvalvar level, the right and left fibrous trigones anchor the subaortic fibrous curtain with its attached anterior mitral valvar leaflet to the muscular and membranous interventricular septums respectively. This constitutes a hinge mechanism by which the fibrous components of the outflow tract move backward and forward during muscular contraction, enlarging the left ventricular outflow during ventricular systole.

Malformations of the aortic valve or the constituent parts of the left ventricular outflow may produce in theory, obstruction, regurgitation, or a combination of both. In practice, however, congenital lesions that result in pure regurgitation are extremely rare and generally do not involve the valvar leaflets. These are a ruptured sinus of Valsava aneurysm or fistula (which begins in the aortic sinus and usually ends in the right atrium or right ventricle), and aorto left ventricular tunnel (which usually connects the left ventricular outflow with the ascending aorta distal to the sinutubular junction). "Congenital" aortic incompetence, therefore, is found more commonly as an acquired complication of bicuspid aortic valve, ventricular septal defect, subaortic obstruction, connective tissue disease, or inflammatory (rheumatic) heart disease.

Obstructive lesions of the left ventricular outflow tract span a broad spectrum of malformations which may involve any of the constituent parts, singly or in combination. Traditionally, they have been divided into supravalvar, valvar, and subvalvar categories, but most often, pathological changes occur at more than one level. In some instances, such as neonatal critical aortic stenosis, the abnormality is clearly a congenital malformation. Others, like discrete subaortic stenosis, are lesions acquired on a congenital predisposition. However, both have the end result of obstructing the systemic ventricle early in life. Abnormalities of a similar nature may be found also in hearts with discordant ventriculo-arterial connections (transposed great arteries) or other anomalous ventriculo-arterial connections, and they will be illustrated in the relevant chapters.

Supravalvar obstruction begins at the sinutubular junction, to which it may remain confined as a shelf of thickened intima or from which it may extend diffusely as far as the descending aorta. The increased fibrous and elastic tissue, along with thickening of the medial and intimal layers, constricts the sinutubular ridge, bringing the tops of the valvar leaflets and sinuses towards the aortic lumen. Potentially, this can block the entrance to a sinus of Valsalva and obstruct the orifice of the left or, less commonly, the right coronary artery. However, the coronary arteries are more often dilated and show atherosclerotic changes from perfusion at suprasystemic pressure because they otherwise lie below the level of the obstruction. Direct involvement of the valvar leaflets is unusual, but they often become thickened; the left coronary leaflet in particular tends to be smaller than normal. A well-documented association among supravalvar aortic stenosis – elfin facies, mental retardation, and a small stature (failure to thrive) – has been called Williams syndrome, but the identical cardiac lesion is found as a familial form (with autosomal dominant transmission and no impairment of intelligence), or sporadically in association with infantile hypercalcemia.

At the level of the valvar leaflets, obstruction during early infancy or the neonatal period usually results from a "unicusp" valve with an eccentric keyhole-shaped orifice between the left and non-coronary aortic sinuses. This is called "critical" or "neonatal" aortic stenosis and accounts for somewhere between 3% and 10% of all stenotic aortic valvar lesions. Such valves possess only a single fully developed interleaflet triangle which extends to the sinutubular junction above the mitral valve. The other two rudimentary triangles lie beneath ridges of thickened tissue on the arterial side of the leaflet and demarcate three aortic sinuses, but the triangles do not reach the sinutubular junction. As such, the dysplastic leaflet tissue spirals around the orifice as a continuous sheet of mucoid connective tissue with a greatly reduced hinge point or attachment to the left ventricular outflow. Its free edge measures less than the circumference of the combined sinuses, and the leaflet can thus open only by a limited flap valve mechanism. This type of morphology is usually accompanied by abnormalities of the mitral valve and a small cavity, hypertrophied left ventricle with endocardial fibroelastosis. At its extreme, critical aortic stenosis merges with the hypoplastic left heart syndrome. Occasionally, however, the ventricular cavity is dilated and thin-walled, with or without endocardial fibroelastosis.

Valvar anomalies that produce obstruction later in infancy or childhood tend to have two leaflets and two commissures orientated anteroposteriorly in the aortic root, with one coronary arterial orifice in each sinus. A rudimentary commissure or "raphe" can often be identified as a ridge of variable thickness and length in the leaflet that faces the pulmonary trunk, which is then larger than the other leaflet. This indicates developmentally a basically three sinus aortic root, with the facing leaflet subtending two rudimentary aortic sinuses, but the raphe does not lie above a fully developed interleaflet triangle. Alternatively, the two leaflets may be anterior and posterior, with both coronary arteries arising in the posterior sinus. Truly two-leaflet, two-sinus aortic valves are not unusual and not necessarily stenotic. Obstruction results from thickening of the leaflets themselves, with or without fusion of the commissures, and from a reduction in the length of the free edge (in comparison with the diameter of the aortic root), such that the leaflet tissue remains fixed across the outflow tract during ventricular ejection. Thickening, subsequent calcification, and loss of coaptation with leaflet prolapse results in the eventual incompetence of the valve. Aortic valves with two leaflets are frequently associated with coarctation of the aorta. Less often, in perhaps one-third of stenotic aortic valves, there are three leaflets, three aortic sinuses and three fused commissures, leaving a dome-shaped diaphragm with a central orifice, similar to that seen in pulmonary valvar stenosis. Obstruction in these cases depends on the extent of commissural fusion.

While subaortic obstruction of some degree nearly always accompanies valvar aortic stenosis as a result of secondary muscular hypertrophy, several distinct entities, in their own right, may cause severe obstruction to left ventricular outflow below the level of the valve. Most common among these is discrete or "fixed" subaortic stenosis due to a shelf of fibrous tissue. This always attaches to the muscular septum and then extends for a variable distance across the membranous septum and subaortic fibrous curtain, often completely encircling the outflow tract. It may be located immediately beneath the aortic valvar leaflets and extend to their ventricular surface, or it may lie low down in the ventricle with attachments to the ventricular aspect of the anterior mitral valve leaflet. Crossing both the membranous septum (with conduction tissue) and the fibrous trigones, the subaortric membrane, or ring, is thought to restrict both the normal movement of the mitral valve and the subaortic fibrous curtain during cardiac contraction, as well as blocking the outflow of blood from the ventricle. A complete ring, in extreme circumstances, may narrow the left ventricular outflow to an eccentric orifice of only a few millimetres in diameter. There is usually associated muscular hypertrophy, and the jet of blood accelerating through the subaortic obstruction against the under-surface of the aortic valve may lead to the thickening and incompetence of the valvar leaflets.

A second, less common type of fibrous obstruction results from aneurysmal tissue tags or accessory leaflet tissue derived from the membranous septum or mitral valve. These are often grape- or parachute-like structures that float into the subaortic area during ventricular systole. In the presence of a ventricular septal defect, such accessory tissue may originate also from the tricuspid valve. Moreover, anomalous attachment of a papillary muscle from either the mitral valve or from a tricuspid valve which straddles through a ventricular septal defect may anchor the subvalvar apparatus within the left ventricular outflow tract.

Obstructions of primary muscular origin result from hypertrophy and/or displacement of the various muscular components of the left ventricle. Enlargement of the anterolateral muscle bundle may be significant in isolation or, combined with even minimal thickening of the septal myocardium, it can contribute to the formation of a long, fibromuscular tunnel-type of obstruction. Malalignment of muscular septal components, which occurs in the context of a ventricular septal defect, can bring the outlet septum leftward between the defect and the aortic valve, with resultant narrowing of the left ventricular outflow. Such "malalignment ventricular septal defects" are strongly associated with coarctation of the aorta and interrupted

aortic arch. Even in the rare event of the complete absence of an outlet septum ("doubly committed subarterial ventricular septal defect"), the medial end of a muscular right ventriculo-infundibular fold may bulge through the defect into the left ventricular outflow below the aortic valve.

In contrast with these so-called "fixed" types of subaortic obstruction, asymmetrical septal hypertrophy or idiopathic hypertrophic subaortic stenosis (IHSS) is considered to be a "dynamic" form of obstruction. The muscle hypertrophy in this entity, which has a well-established genetic basis, consists of extreme thickening of the entire ventricular septum from below the level of the mitral valve papillary muscles to the aortic valvar leaflets. As the obstruction evolves, however, fibrous tissue tends to accumulate on the subendocardial surface and, in some hearts, a ridge limited to the ventricular septum, appears to coapt with the free edge of the open mitral valve. This is not unlike the fibrous shelf seen in discrete subaortic stenosis and may have similar implications for left ventricular function.

While ideal management would undoubtedly be the restoration of both normal structure and function, interventions on the obstructed left ventricular outflow tract, whether they are done by surgery or at cardiac catheterization, remain primitive and of necessity largely palliative by comparison with the exquisite natural design of the aortic valve and its subaortic outflow. Treatment is therefore focused on the conservation of left ventricular function and the maintenance of optimal hemodynamics for the longest time possible, taking into consideration the age and size of the patient, what is known regarding the natural history of lesions in this part of the heart, and the limitations of prosthetic materials. Perhaps more than almost any other area of congenital heart disease, long-term outcome depends as much on decision-making as on technical skill. In this regard, both the surgeon and the interventional cardiologist may need to acknowledge occasions when the patient's best interest is better served by tools of another trade.

Supravalvar aortic stenosis is a progressive lesion with a small but definite incidence of sudden death. Repair is thus carried out at a gradient of about 50 mm Hg., regardless of the patient's age or absence of symptoms. The localized "hour-glass" obstruction at the sinutubular junction may be completely relieved with good long-term results by means of resection of the supravalvar ridge internally and pericardial patch aortoplasty into one, two, or three of the sinuses of Valsalva. For diffuse lesions, the patch is continued beyond the distal extent of the obstruction to the left subclavian artery or aortic isthmus, if necessary. Cannulation of the ascending aorta requires special care in this anomaly because a layer of thickened intima can be lifted up by a short cannula, producing acute aortic dissection.

Neonatal critical aortic stenosis in patients with an adequate mitral valve and left ventricle is generally treated by balloon valvuloplasty or surgical valvotomy after resuscitation of the patient with prostaglandin, if necessary. While there has been much debate regarding the number and extent to which the imperforate commissures should be divided, the results of balloon valvuloplasty (which often splits the leaflet body) suggests that this is of less importance than achieving the maximal outflow diameter. Most of these patients require further relief of left ventricular outflow obstruction at some point. When this is localized at valvar level and aortic incompetence is not present, balloon valvuloplasty is again a reasonable option. Otherwise, open operation is needed to repair or replace the valve and to deal with any subvalvar obstruction.

Beyond early infancy, an initial valvotomy is usually the procedure of choice for valvar obstruction, although a role for balloon dilatation may also be emerging in this subset of patients. Nearly all these patients come to reintervention within ten years of the initial procedure and, in general, the patient's own aortic valve should be conserved for as long as possible. This can often be achieved by repeat valvotomy and/or repair of aortic regurgitation. When the valve replacement becomes necessary, it is preferable to avoid anticoagulation in most teenage and young adult patients by the implantation of an aortic homograft or pulmonary autograft. While these procedures definitely commit a patient to further reoperations, the hemodynamic advantages of a completely unobstructed outflow may be important for long-term ventricular function, and many young patients are either non-compliant or find anticoagulation for a mechanical prosthesis incompatible with their life-style aspirations.

The management of subvalvar obstruction is more complex. Good relief of isolated, discrete subaortic stenosis is safely accomplished without damage to the conduction tissue or valves by blunt enucleation of the fibrous tissue, following its finger-like extensions on to the aortic and mitral valvar leaflets, and distally on the ventricular septum. Myectomy, with mobilization of the left and, to a limited extent, the right fibrous trigones is also necessary in most patients to restore mobility of the anterior mitral valve leaflet and ensure long-term patency of the outflow tract. Hypertrophied and malaligned muscle bundles can generally be resected, either working retrogradely through the aortic valve or from the right side of the heart through a ventricular septal defect. It should be recognized that the presence of a ventricular septal defect may completely mask the hemodynamic importance of left ventricular outflow obstruction, and the decision to enlarge this area must be made on its appearances at preoperative imaging and intraoperative inspection rather than any measured gradient. In that regard, inspection of the subaortic area routinely through any large perimembranous ventricular septal defect often reveals fibrous ridges of tissue or small muscle bars which can be removed, possibly avoiding later evolution into hemodynamically important obstructive lesions.

When there is tunnel-type or diffuse narrowing of the left ventricular outflow, simple excision, even on repeated occasions, is rarely sufficient to achieve complete or lasting relief of the obstruction. When the aortic valve is normal, ventricular septoplasty (or "modified Konno procedure") is then indicated to enlarge the subaortic outflow. If the aortic valve also needs replacement, this is done as a complete aortic root replacement with coronary artery reimplantation and enlargement of the subaortic area, using a pulmonary autograft or aortic homograft. In very young patients, the pulmonary autograft may offer the advantage of growth potential and possibly avoid later reoperations on the left side of the heart, although the homograft used to reconstruct the right ventricular outflow tract invariably needs eventual replacement.

Among the pediatric population, patients with hypertrophic cardiomyopathy and asymmetric septal hypertrophy come less often to operation. However, the principles of aggressive muscle excision with mobilization of the fibrous trigones is equally applicable to this group of patients. This can usually be accomplished through the aortic valve in the relaxed heart. In all procedures on the left ventricular outflow, patient size permitting, intraoperative transesophogeal echocardiography is worthwhile to monitor the early results of the intervention and avoid residual lesions.

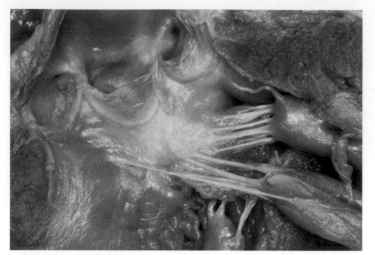

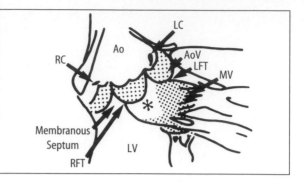

16.1 Left ventricular outflow tract. Normal aortic valve. The hearts in Figures 16.1, 16.2, and 16.3 have been opened from the left ventricle into the aorta, across the muscular outlet septum. The postero-medial papillary muscle of the mitral valve has been rotated to the left, allowing the outflow tract to be viewed from the front. The normal aortic valve shown here has three sinuses with three leaflets separated on their ventricular aspect by well-defined interleaflet triangles. The triangle between the right and non-coronary leaflets abuts onto the membranous septum and the right fibrous trigone. The full width of the non-coronary leaflet, as well as its two adjacent interleaflet triangles and part of the left coronary leaflet, lie in fibrous continuity with the mitral valve through the subaortic curtain (asterisk). The left fibrous trigone attaches the subaortic curtain to the muscular septum. The orifices of the left and right coronary arteries are located almost centrally within their respective sinuses, just below the sinutubular bar.

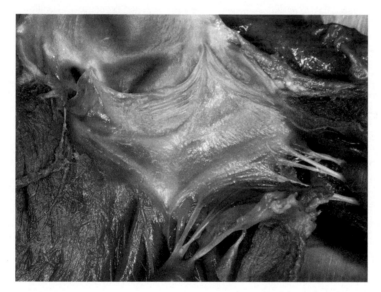

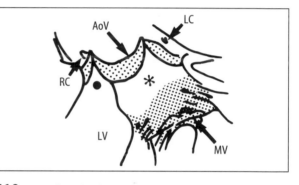

16.2 Aortic valve with only two leaflets and sinuses (bicuspid aortic valve) in an otherwise normal heart. The sinus of Valsalva which contains both coronary orifices, has been transected. Two well-developed interleaflet triangles are seen and a large membranous septum is present (black dot). The mitral and aortic valves have a large area of fibrous continuity (asterisk).

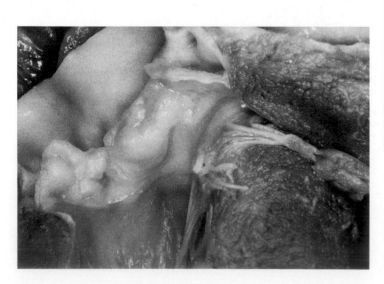

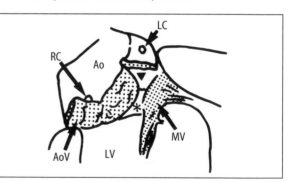

16.3 Critical aortic stenosis. The valvar leaflets are thickened and dysplastic, with knobbly excrescences on their ventricular aspect. There is a relatively normal interleaflet triangle between the left and non-coronary sinuses (triangle), but the other two are very rudimentary. On the aortic aspect, ridges of tissue above each interleaflet triangle define three aortic sinuses, but they do not extend to the free edge of the leaflet or reach the height of the sinutubular bar. The free edge of the leaflet tissue is thus continuous around the outflow tract as a unileaflet valve with a single commissure. The membranous septum is absent. A small subaortic curtain (asterisk) lies between the aortic and mitral valves.

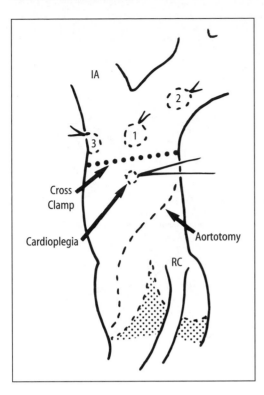

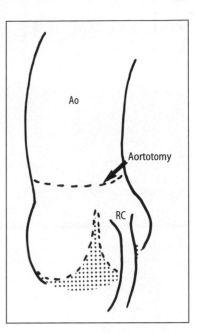

16.4 *(left)* The standard surgical approach to the aortic valve and subvalvar left ventricular outflow tract is through an incision in the ascending aorta. Arterial cannulation for cardiopulmonary bypass is done sufficiently high to permit application of the aortic cross-clamp and, if desirable, delivery of cardioplegia above the aortotomy. The usual site (1) is just below the origin of the innominate artery, but the right lateral side (3) or transverse aortic arch (2) may be used to gain more access to the ascending aorta or to cannulate distally to a previous cannulation site. A "hockey-stick" incision is one that spirals obliquely across the front of the aorta into the mid-portion of the non-coronary sinus of Valsalva (dashed line).

16.5 *(above right)* A transverse aortotomy lies just above the sinutubular junction and should always be sited several millimetres above the origin of the right coronary artery. This is the preferred incision when transection of the ascending aorta may be necessary as, for example, in aortic root replacement. It is also useful in young infants where the small diameter of the aorta may be compromised by the closure of an oblique incision.

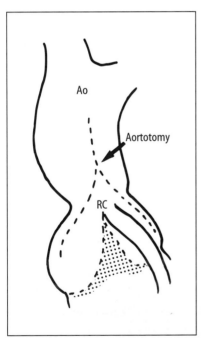

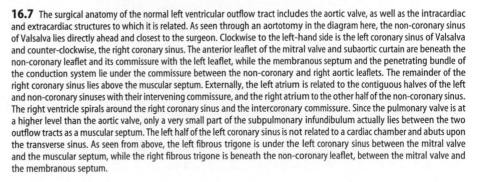

16.6 For supravalvar aortic stenosis, a "trouser-shaped" incision may be used to enlarge two of the aortic sinuses. This aortotomy begins vertically above the origin of the right coronary artery and diverges into the non-coronary sinus and the left part of the right coronary sinus, leaving the origin of the right coronary artery on a flap of sinus tissue which also supports the commissure between the right and non-coronary aortic leaflets.

16.7 The surgical anatomy of the normal left ventricular outflow tract includes the aortic valve, as well as the intracardiac and extracardiac structures to which it is related. As seen through an aortotomy in the diagram here, the non-coronary sinus of Valsalva lies directly ahead and closest to the surgeon. Clockwise to the left-hand side is the left coronary sinus of Valsalva and counter-clockwise, the right coronary sinus. The anterior leaflet of the mitral valve and subaortic curtain are beneath the non-coronary leaflet and its commissure with the left leaflet, while the membranous septum and the penetrating bundle of the conduction system lie under the commissure between the non-coronary and right aortic leaflets. The remainder of the right coronary sinus lies above the muscular septum. Externally, the left atrium is related to the contiguous halves of the left and non-coronary sinuses with their intervening commissure, and the right atrium to the other half of the non-coronary sinus. The right ventricle spirals around the right coronary sinus and the intercoronary commissure. Since the pulmonary valve is at a higher level than the aortic valve, only a very small part of the subpulmonary infundibulum actually lies between the two outflow tracts as a muscular septum. The left half of the left coronary sinus is not related to a cardiac chamber and abuts upon the transverse sinus. As seen from above, the left fibrous trigone is under the left coronary sinus between the mitral valve and the muscular septum, while the right fibrous trigone is beneath the non-coronary leaflet, between the mitral valve and the membranous septum.

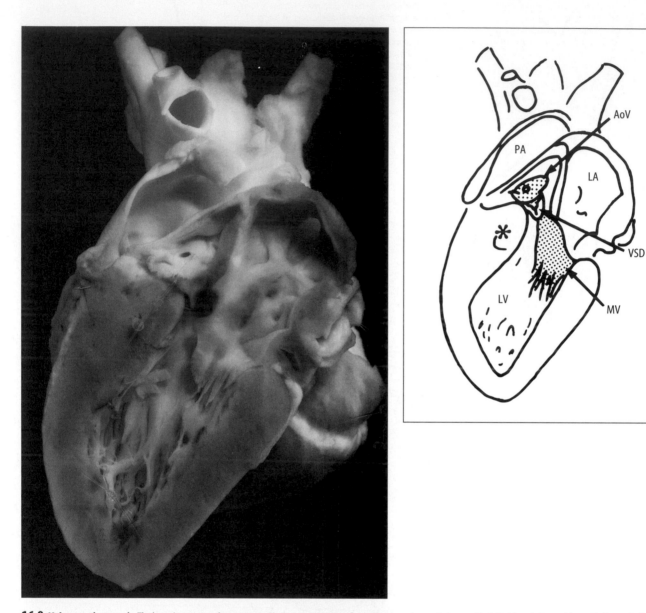

16.8 Valvar aortic stenosis. The heart is a mounted museum specimen in preservation fluid. It has been transected across the left atrium, left ventricle, and left ventricular outflow in a sagittal plane. Thickened ridges on the arterial side of the aortic valvar leaflets extend on to the wall of the aorta, indicating the sites of three completely fused commissures. This produces a "unicusp" aortic valve with a small central orifice. The linear dimensions of the left ventricle are normal, but the free wall is thickened and there is massive hypertrophy of the outlet septum (asterisk). A perimembranous ventricular septal defect is seen immediately below the aortic valve. The long segment of left ventricular hypertrophy contributes additional muscular outflow obstruction. The tension apparatus of the mitral valve has been removed.

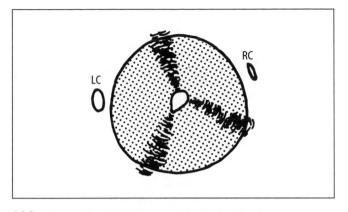

16.9 Looking at the arterial side of a stenosed aortic valve, the surgeon sees an irregular mass of thickened leaflet. It is the fibrous ridges, which extend up onto the aortic wall, that define the sites of the fused commissures and their underlying interleaflet triangles. The left coronary artery is dominant more often in hearts with valvar aortic stenosis, which is important to remember if delivery of cardioplegia directly into the coronary arterial orifice is used for myocardial management.

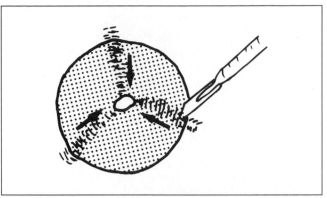

16.10 Commissurotomy is performed with a surgical knife (usually a no. 11 blade in older children or an opthalmology micro-blade in infants and neonates), cutting exactly in the middle of the fibrous ridge. The incision extends into the thickened area on the aortic wall to mobilize the hinge-point of the leaflet maximally. Working from the aortic wall to the valvar orifice facilitates an accurate valvotomy and, after the first commissure is opened, it may be necessary to stabilize the leaflet with forceps while the other two are incised. This leaves the largest area of coaptation to give leaflet support during subsequent closure of the valve.

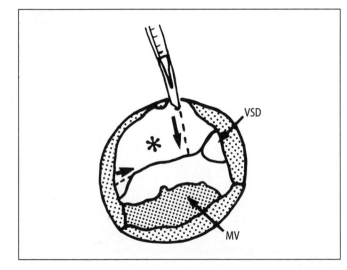

16.11 The hypertrophied subaortic muscle bar is excised, working through the aortic valve. Deep vertical incisions are made from just below the leaflet hinge points under the intercoronary commissure and under the left leaflet near the left fibrous trigone, leaving a rim of muscle beside the defect in the ventricular septum. These extend to the level of the papillary muscles of the mitral valve if necessary, and the muscle mass between the two incisions (asterisk) is excised with scissors. Orientating the knife blade towards the lumen of the left ventricular outflow tract or, in larger patients, carefully using a "hook knife" (no. 12 blade) may help to prevent damage to the valvar leaflets. It is important to carry the excision to the left fibrous trigone in order to liberate the subaortic fibrous curtain.

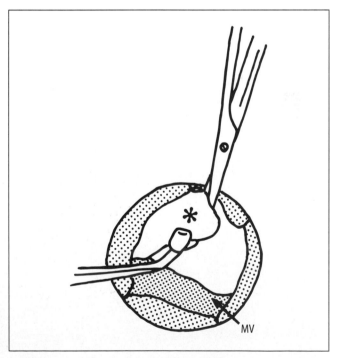

16.12 Because the endocardium holds the muscle together, it is easiest to remove the mass as a single piece. However, when this does not happen, grasping the remaining muscle fragments with a pituitary rongeur facilitates their retraction towards the surgeon and excision. The left ventricle is then irrigated extensively to remove tissue fragments and the outflow is calibrated with a Hegar dilator. The ventricular septal defect may be closed either through the aortic valve or through the right atrium and tricuspid valve (see Chapter 11).

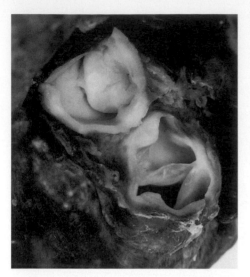

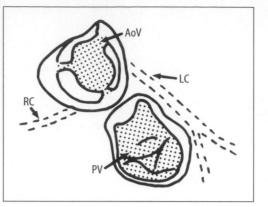

16.13 *(left)* **Critical aortic stenosis.** The aorta and the pulmonary trunk have been removed to show the arterial side of the valves. The aortic valve is slightly smaller than the pulmonary valve. Although its commissures are fused, producing a "unileaflet" valve, ridges of leaflet tissue extending on to the aortic wall clearly define the three aortic sinuses. The leaflet tissue is thickened with knobbly excrescences (not seen) on its ventricular surface.

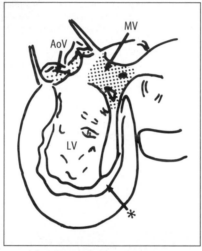

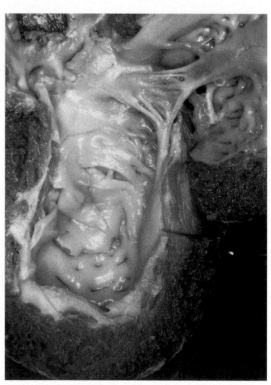

16.14 *(right)* The left ventricle in a different heart with critical aortic stenosis, showing a small cavity with thick walls. There is gross endocardial fibrosis (asterisk). The mitral valve is also small with fusion of its cords, producing an arcade lesion, similar to that seen on Figure 16.15.

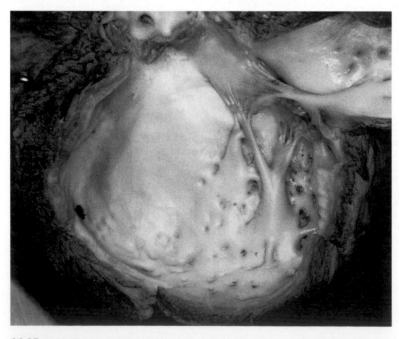

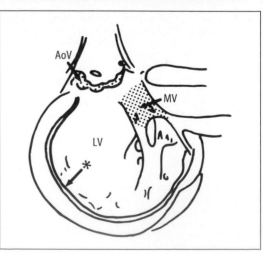

16.15 *(above)* The left ventricle in this heart with critical aortic stenosis is dilated and thin-walled with diffuse endocardial fibroelastosis (asterisk). A small mitral valve is attached to hypoplastic papillary muscles by tendinous cords which are short, thickened, and fused.

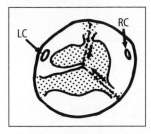

16.16 While critical valvar aortic stenosis is usually managed by balloon dilatation, this is occasionally unsuccessful, necessitating open surgical valvotomy. In the surgeon's view, the commissure between the left and non-coronary sinuses of Valsalva is usually patent, with the other two indicated by ridges of leaflet tissue. These are opened completely up (dashed lines) on to the aortic wall (see Figures 16.9–16.10).

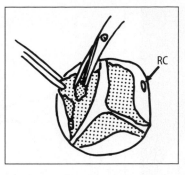

16.17 The leaflet is thinned by excision of the knobbly excrescences from its ventricular surface.

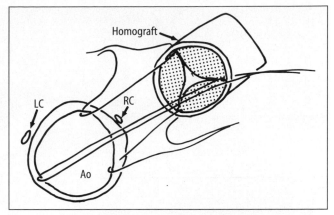

16.18 *(above right)* Valve replacement for critical aortic stenosis is virtually never required as a primary intervention in the neonatal period, but is frequently necessary later in life. When the subaortic area is widely open with an impaired left ventricle, the subcoronary homograft offers optimal relief of obstruction and the advantages of a tissue valve. Alternatively, a pulmonary autograft may be implanted, using essentially the same technique of insertion. The homograft is trimmed to about 2 mm below its leaflets and orientated by three initial sutures at each of the interleaflet triangles. This is to ensure that a sinus of the homograft ends up over the left coronary artery orifice.

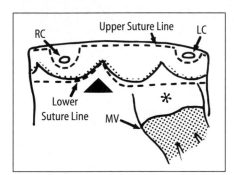

16.19 Since the critically stenotic aortic valve has poorly developed interleaflet triangles and shallow sinuses, the lower suture line must generally go below the hinge point of the native valvar leaflet (dashed line) to accommodate the homograft below the coronary orifice. It may thus be attached to the subaortic curtain (asterisk) in the area of the aortic-mitral continuity, but must rise above the membranous septum and conduction tissue (triangle) between the right and non-coronary aortic sinuses. The lower suture line is circular rather than scalloped.

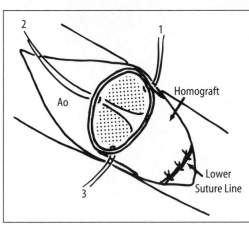

16.20 *(left)* After the lower suture line is completed, either with simple interrupted stitches or a running suture, the homograft is seated down into the left ventricular outflow tract. A mattress suture is then placed above each commissure of the homograft and brought through the aortic wall directly above the native commissure, placing the valve under slight tension to maintain coaptation of its leaflets.

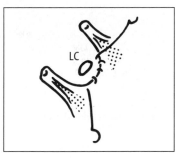

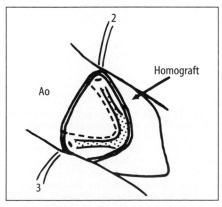

16.21 The left coronary sinus of the homograft is excised (dashed line), taking care to avoid injury to the valve leaflet. Because of the shallow sinuses of the native valve, the left coronary orifice usually lies low down, such that the sinus must be removed nearly to the hinge point of the homograft leaflet.

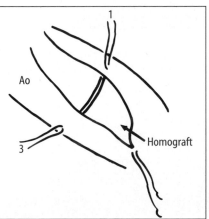

16.23 *(above)* The non-coronary sinus of the homograft is left intact and incorporated into the aortotomy closure. Additional mattress sutures passed through the homograft and aorta are used to obliterate any potential dead space, where hematoma could accumulate and distort the outflow tract.

16.24 *(right)* Seen in cross-section, it is important that this final suture line does not plicate the non-coronary sinus and cause prolapse of the non-coronary valvar leaflet.

16.22 *(above)* The upper suture line begins with a running monofilament stitch under the orifice of the left coronary artery and continues along the free edge of the valve, with homograft commissures held under tension. Similarly, the homograft sinus is excised over the right coronary orifice. At the top of each commissure, the two continuous sutures are passed through the wall of the aorta and tied over a pericardial pledget.

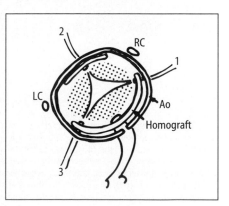

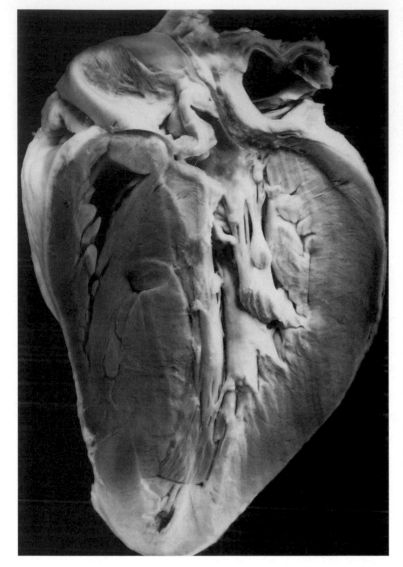

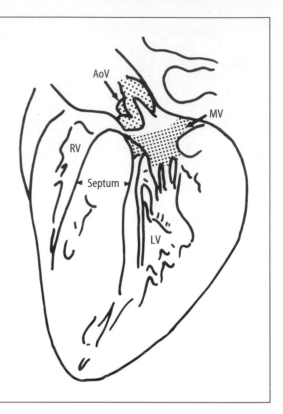

16.25 Valvar aortic stenosis. Mounted museum specimen in preservation fluid. The leaflets of the aortic valve are extremely thickened and dysplastic, and both the septum and the free wall of the left ventricle are massively hypertrophied. There is also fibrosis of the mitral valvar leaflets and tendinous cords.

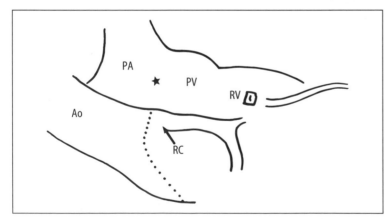

16.26 When left ventricular function is sufficiently good and only the aortic valve needs replacement, transfer of the patient's own pulmonary valve to the aortic position (Ross procedure) is a reasonable option for young patients. This can be done as a subcoronary implant (see Figures 16.16–16.24) or a complete root replacement. In preparation for the removal of the pulmonary valve, a pledgeted traction suture is placed on the right ventricular infundibulum. The top of the valvar sinuses are marked (star) prior to the commencement of cardiopulmonary bypass. The aortotomy (dotted line) will begin as a transverse incision several millimetres above the right coronary artery and then angle into the non-coronary aortic sinus in order to conserve as much length of ascending aorta as possible. Accordingly, the aortic cannulation is high on the ascending aorta.

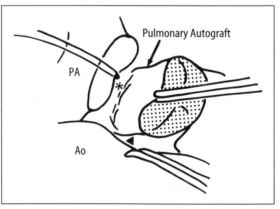

16.27 On cardiopulmonary bypass with moderate hypothermia and the heart still beating, either by means of aortic root perfusion or through direct cannulation and perfusion of the coronary arterial orifices, the main pulmonary artery is divided a few millimeters distally to the top of the valvar commissures. This incision begins at the marking suture and is completed looking inside the vessel. The pulmonary valve is then freed from the aorta and fibrous tissue in the transverse sinus, working backwards towards the heart with sharp dissection (scissors) or diathermy. There are usually dense fibrous bands between the aortic sinuses and the pulmonary trunk (triangle), and damage to the pulmonary autograft must be avoided even, if necessary, at the expense of entering the aorta (which subsequently will be removed) in this area. The right coronary artery is also vulnerable in this part of the dissection, particularly in reoperations. Posteriorly, the dissection is carried down to muscle, staying close to the pulmonary valve to prevent injury to the left main coronary artery (asterisk).

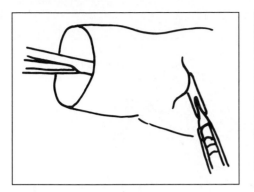

16.28 When the pulmonary trunk has been mobilized to the right ventricular epicardium on both sides, a right-angled instrument is passed retrogradely into the right ventricle about half a centimeter below the valvar leaflet. A no. 10 knife is used to cut down directly on to the tip of the instrument and initiate a transverse ventriculotomy. Coronary perfusion is interrupted at this time to facilitate a dry field.

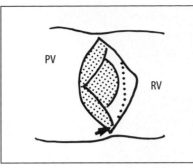

16.29 The ventriculotomy is carefully extended with scissors, taking care to identify the valvar leaflets and to leave at least 3–4 mm of muscle attached below them. As the right ventricular outflow is perpendicular to the left, the leaflet closest to the surgeon is the one most easily damaged (arrow). Within the right ventricle, a knife is used to mark the line of dissection by an incision into the posterior wall of the endocardium (dotted line).

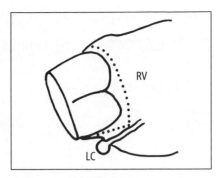

16.30 The dissection angles more superficially (towards the cavity of the right ventricle) as it proceeds upward along the septum, in order to avoid damage to the anterior interventricular coronary artery and its first large septal branch. Only epicardium remains on the pulmonary valve where this dissection meets that which was done in the transverse sinus. Nonetheless, post-operative echocardiography nearly always demonstrates impaired contractility of the upper interventricular septum. Coronary perfusion is re-established to check the bed of the pulmonary valve for hemostasis and to reconstruct the right ventricular outflow with a pulmonary homograft. The autograft is inspected for integrity and trimmed of excess fat and muscle. It is then placed in the pericardial space beside the heart (usually in blood) until it is inserted.

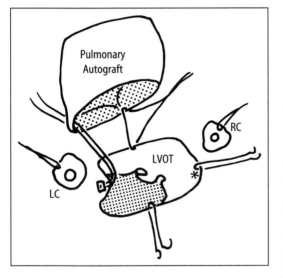

16.31 After opening the aorta, the coronary arterial orifices are excised with their surrounding sinuses, mobilized for several millimeters, and retracted with stay-sutures. The aortic valve is removed. In the region of the conduction tissue (asterisk), a rim of aortic sinus is left above the hinge point of the native leaflet. If needed, the outflow tract is enlarged with a vertical incision directly under the position of the left coronary orifice. This leaves the septal surface (which may have been dissected already on its right ventricular side to remove the autograft) with intact endocardium to hold the valve sutures. The autograft is orientated with its longer anterior aspect at the back and its thin area at the front, using four sutures to divide the outflow and the valve equally. Hemostasis is aided by a mattress suture supported by autogenous pericardium at the apex of the outflow-enlarging incision above the left atrium.

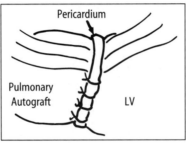

16.32 When all the simple interrupted sutures have been placed between the left ventricle and the pulmonary autograft, they are tied down over a collar of pericardium or other hemostatic material. Since the autograft is living tissue, this should be done gently with the minimal number of sutures.

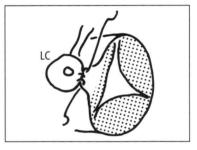

16.33 The button containing the left coronary orifice is trimmed and connected to the autograft with a running monofilament suture. Not infrequently in congenital aortic stenosis, the autograft sits down into the enlarged left ventricular outflow, such that the coronary artery comes to lie partly in the suture line above the valve.

16.34 *(right)* The ascending aorta is anastomosed to the pulmonary autograft with a continuous monofilament suture, accommodating the left coronary artery as needed. Cardioplegia is infused into the aortic root prior to completion of the suture line anteriorly to evacuate air. At this time, the integrity of the left coronary ostium is confirmed by observing cardioplegia passing into the anterior descending and circumflex branches of the left coronary artery. Usually, it will also fill the right coronary artery retrogradely from the left.

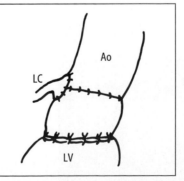

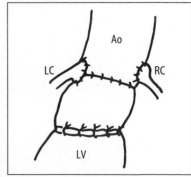

16.35 *(above right)* Further infusion of cardioplegia distends the autograft and ascending aorta for the accurate siting of the right coronary arterial orifice, which also may come to lie above the valve. A period of controlled root perfusion with the left atrial vent draining on the venous line is often useful to check the suture lines for hemostasis and resuscitate the heart. When the tissues are friable, it may be helpful to leave a small rim of aorta attached to the heart and then to stitch this superficially to the adventitia of the pulmonary autograft to cover most of the proximal suture line.

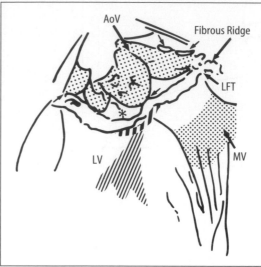

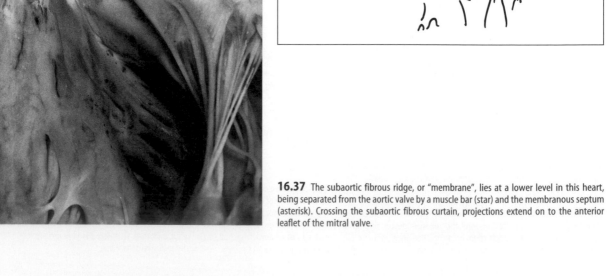

16.36 Discrete subaortic stenosis. A ridge of fibrous tissue encircles the left ventricular outflow immediately beneath the aortic valve and extends onto the ventricular surface of all three aortic leaflets (small arrows). The "membrane" passes across the subaortic fibrous curtain, fixing the left and right fibrous trigones to the muscular ventricular septum. It also bisects the membranous septum (asterisk) and lies over the conduction tissue.

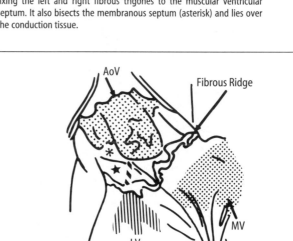

16.37 The subaortic fibrous ridge, or "membrane", lies at a lower level in this heart, being separated from the aortic valve by a muscle bar (star) and the membranous septum (asterisk). Crossing the subaortic fibrous curtain, projections extend on to the anterior leaflet of the mitral valve.

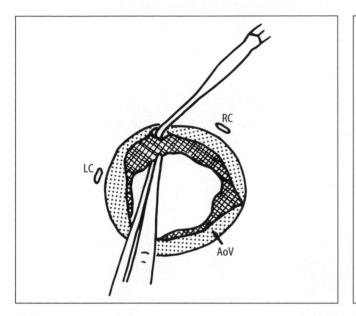

16.38 The fibrous component of subaortic obstruction is an acquired malformation and, as such, can be "peeled" away from the heart by blunt dissection. The "membrane" extends around the left ventricular outflow for a variable portion of its circumference, but always involves the muscular septum beneath the intercoronary commissure. The leaflets of the aortic valve are pushed back, and dissection is started in this area to find the plane between the endocardium and fibrous ring.

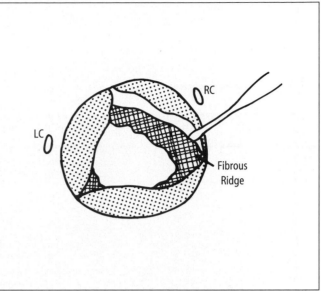

16.39 Enucleation of the fibrous ridge continues clockwise across the membranous septum. This technique avoids damage to the conduction tissue. The fibrous tissue is followed down onto the ventricular endocardium.

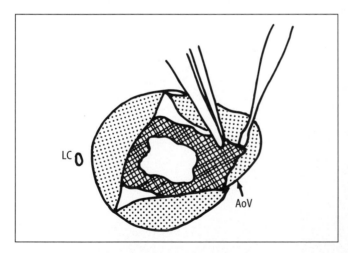

16.40 Extensions onto the ventricular surface of the aortic valvar leaflets are similarly removed, taking care not to tear the body of the leaflet or detach its hinge point.

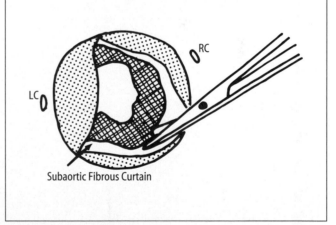

16.41 The fibrous ridge, if it extends to the anterior mitral valve leaflet or area of aortic/mitral fibrous continuity ("subaortic fibrous curtain"), is often more densely adherent in this area and requires sharp dissection with scissors or a knife blade for removal without injury to the mitral valve. The procedure is completed by muscle excision, as appropriate, mobilizing the fibrous trigones (see Figures 16.11–16.12).

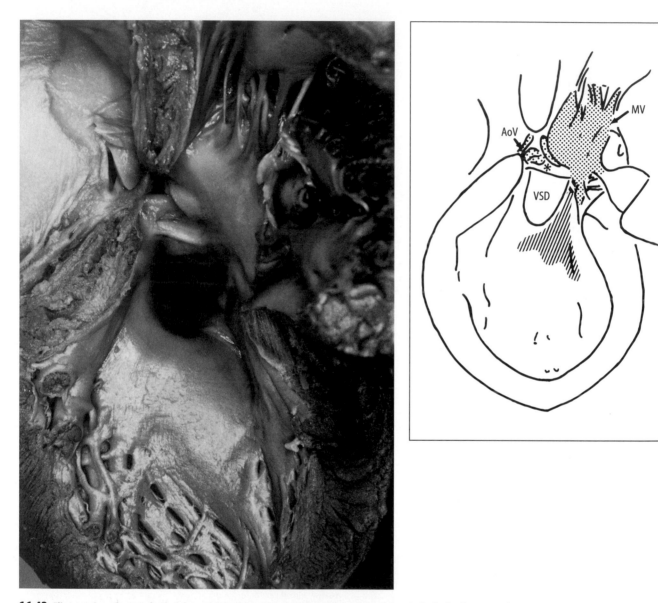

16.42 Fibrous subaortic stenosis. The left ventricle has been opened parallel to the septum and the mitral valve has been rotated upwards to the left. This demonstrates a large perimembranous ventricular septal defect which is separated from the aortic valve by a well-defined fibrous ridge (asterisk). The fibrous ridge produces obstruction below the aortic valve which is smaller than normal. In this case, there is also hypoplasia of the ascending aorta and transverse aortic arch.

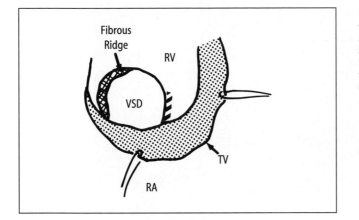

16.43 It is imperative to remove the subaortic fibrous ridge at the time of closure of the ventricular septal defect, as the left ventricle will rarely tolerate fixed obstruction in addition to the increased afterload resulting from closure of the defect and a borderline aortic valve. With a large perimembranous ventricular septal defect, the subaortic area is accessible through the right atrium and tricuspid valve. The conduction tissue lies to the right hand side of the defect and is not very closely related to the membrane in this case.

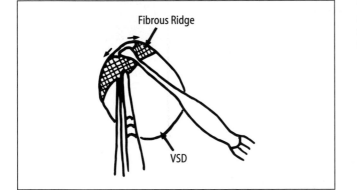

16.44 The fibrous ridge is grasped with forceps and enucleated from the endocardium by blunt dissection (see Figures 16.38–16.40) starting in its mid-portion and working in both directions. The aortic valvar leaflets are gently pushed away from the membrane.

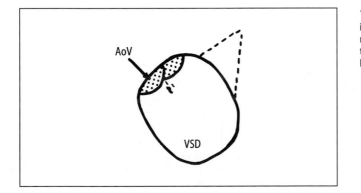

16.45 Following removal of the fibrous tissue, the aortic valve is tested by the infusion of cardioplegia into the aortic root. If the subaortic outflow still appears to be restrictive, it can be enlarged by the resection of muscle on the left ventricular side of the septum, working through the ventricular septal defect (dashed line). The ventricular septal defect is then closed with a patch (see Chapter 11).

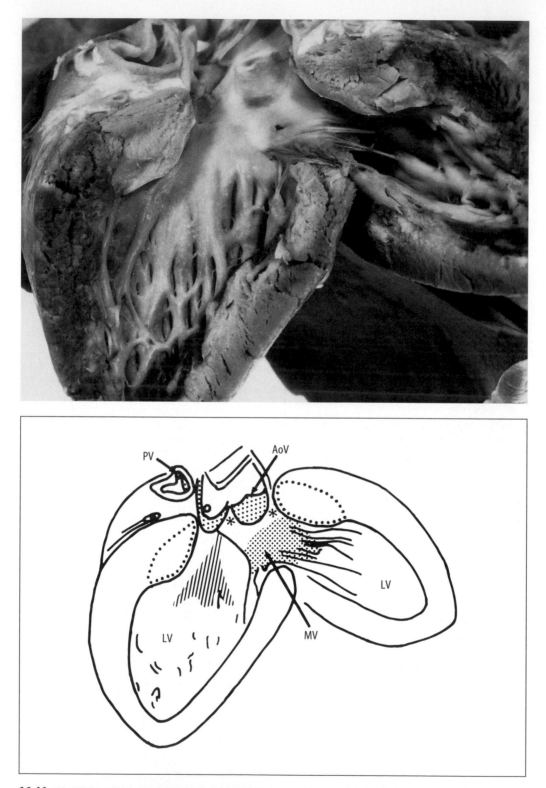

16.46 Subaortic muscle bar. The outflow of the left ventricle is obstructed by a massively enlarged anterolateral muscle bar (encircled by dots), which has been divided in opening the heart. The aortic valve has two well-developed interleaflet triangles between the leaflets (asterisks). The coronary arterial-bearing sinuses are separated by only a rudimentary commissure ("raphe"), producing a "bicuspid " or two-leaflet aortic valve. The interventricular septum is intact. The left ventricle is hypertrophied but comparatively healthy and without endocardial fibrosis. This patient also has coarctation of the aorta.

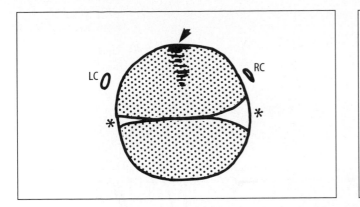

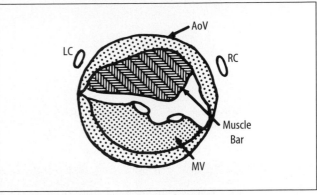

16.47 Since each of the fully developed commissures lies above a normal interleaflet triangle (asterisks), the aortic valve itself is not producing an obstruction at this point in time. The rudimentary commissure (arrow) does not lie above a well-developed interleaflet triangle and accordingly should not be incised.

16.48 The subaortic muscle bar is exposed through the aortic valve. Conduction tissue will be under the surgeon's right hand, approximately beneath the valvar commissure.

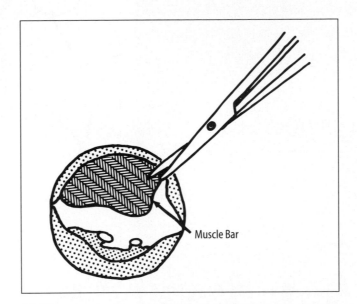

16.49 The mass of muscle is extensively resected, with or without prior sharp incision. The resection is carried around the overhanging "ledge" of the muscle bar and to the depth of the papillary muscles of the mitral valve.

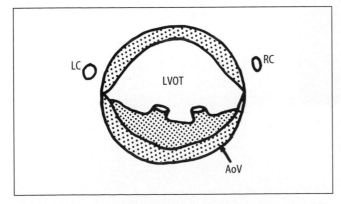

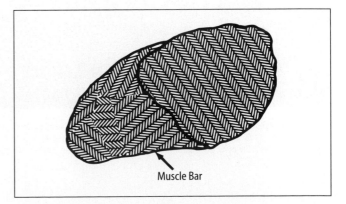

16.50 On completion, the outflow of the left ventricle is widely patent. The ventricular cavity is irrigated with saline to remove any fragments of muscle, and the aortotomy is closed after confirming the integrity of the mitral and aortic valves. Adequate muscle resection and relief of the outflow obstruction are confirmed by intraoperative transesophageal echocardiography.

16.51 The specimen of excised muscle is generally very large, both in absolute terms and in relation to the size of the aortic valve. In that regard, this situation is similar to that of idiopathic hypertrophic cardiomyopathy, although the patient here has coarctation of the aorta and a two-leaflet aortic valve.

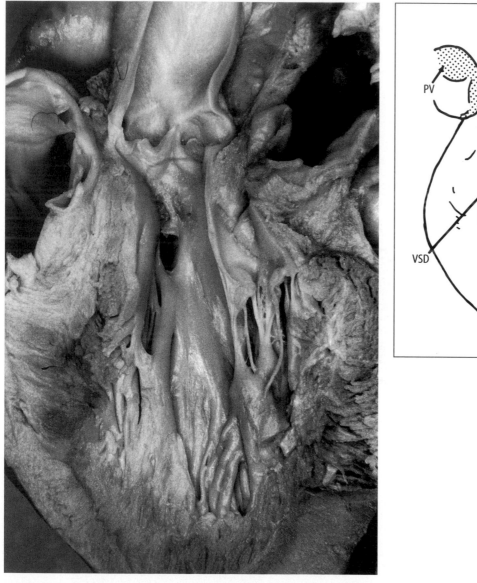

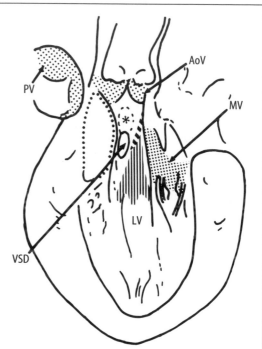

16.52 Muscular subaortic obstruction. A large muscular bulge (enclosed by dots) on the anterior wall of the left ventricle obstructs the left ventricular outflow from the mid-portion of the cavity to the subaortic area (tunnel obstruction). There is a small perimembranous ventricular septal defect, the distal portion of which is closed off by a fibrous membrane (asterisk). The aortic and mitral valves are normal. This patient also has coarctation of the aorta.

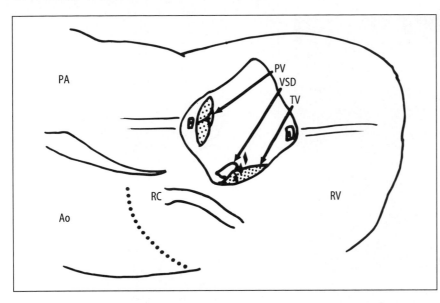

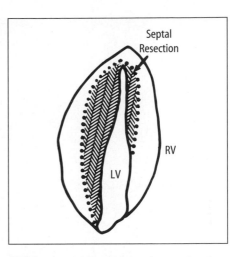

16.53 The aortic valve is essentially normal in this heart, so the first preference for management of the muscular subaortic obstruction would be resection through the aortic valve (see Figures 16.11–16.12 and 16.47–16.51). Failing to achieve an adequate outflow for the left ventricle by that method, the obstruction can be relieved by a "modified Konno procedure" or "ventricular septoplasty." On the cardiopulmonary bypass with bicaval cannulation and moderate hypothermia, the right ventricle is opened with a transverse incision below the free-standing subpulmonary infundibulum. In this heart, the small ventricular septal defect is a good guide to the septal incision. Otherwise, a right-angled instrument is passed retrogradely through the aortic valve and palpated through the septum. The conduction tissue lies along the posterior margin of the ventricular septal defect.

16.54 Since the left and right ventricular outflows leave the heart at right angles to each other, a transverse incision in the floor of the right ventricle will be a vertical incision in the outflow of the left ventricle. This is extended distally beyond the lowest part of the obstruction and proximally to just below the aortic valvar leaflet (into the fibrous membrane in this case), monitoring the incision on the left side by looking through the aortic valve. Muscle is resected from the left ventricular side of the septum. This resection should not extend to the medial papillary muscle complex on the right side in order to leave a margin of tissue above the conduction tissue.

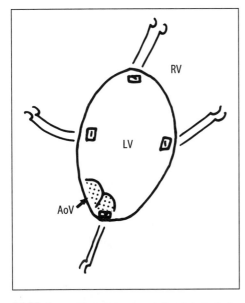

16.56 *(right)* An appropriately sized patch of Dacron or other material is anchored in the right ventricle with the four mattress sutures and then oversewn with a continuous monofilament stitch on the right ventricular side of the septum. The ventriculotomy is then closed directly or, if the patch on the ventricular septal defect appears to have narrowed the right ventricular outflow tract, it is closed with a second patch. The left ventricular outflow and valve are inspected on the left side through the aortotomy which is then closed in the usual manner.

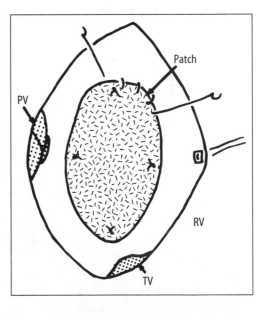

16.55 Four mattress sutures supported by pledgets of autologous pericardium are placed from the left ventricle to the right ventricle for positioning of the patch on the greatly enlarged ventricular septal defect.

16.57 *(right)* When the ventricular septum is intact and extremely hypertrophied, it may be difficult to make the initial incision accurately in the floor of the right ventricle. An alternative is to divide the aortic valve precisely through the interleaflet triangle between the right and left coronary sinuses, taking care not to damage either leaflet. This incision is then extended into the ventricular septum below the free-standing subpulmonary infundibulum which supports the pulmonary valve. Accurate repair of the incision at the conclusion of the septoplasty is imperative to conserve aortic valve competence, prevent hemorrhage, and achieve hemostasis.

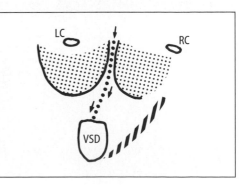

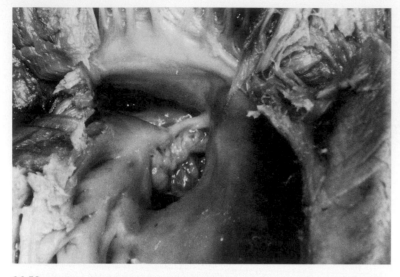

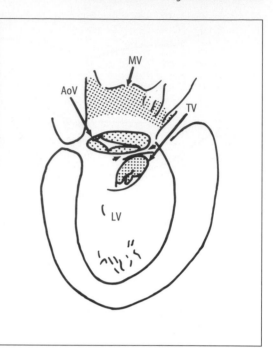

16.58 Subaortic obstruction by the tricuspid valve. The septal surface of the ventricle is exposed to show a perimembranous ventricular septal defect, the main axis of which extends into the trabecular portion of the septum. Leaflet tissue of the tricuspid valve is attached to the margin of the defect and protrudes into the subaortic region below a fibrous ridge (small arrows). The aortic arch is interrupted in this patient.

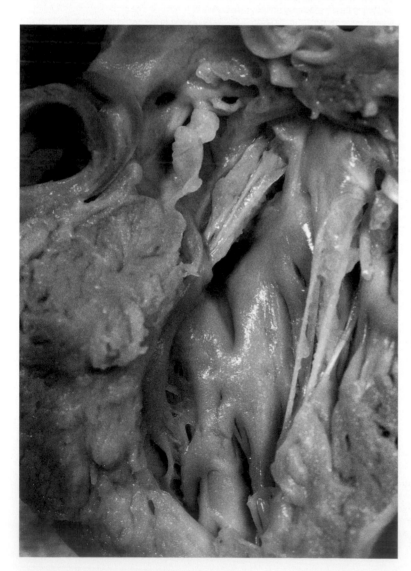

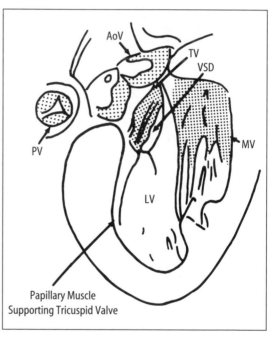

16.59 In this heart, seen on the left ventricular side of the septum, the perimembranous ventricular septal defect is confluent, extending into both inlet and trabecular portions of the right ventricle. A leaflet of the tricuspid valve straddles through the defect and is attached to a papillary muscle within the left ventricle, causing obstruction to the left ventricular outflow tract below a slightly nodular aortic valve. The mitral valve has elongated tendinous cords. Associated coarctation of the aorta is present.

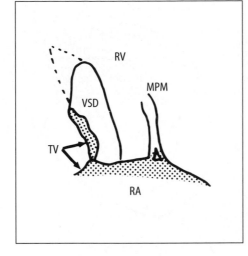

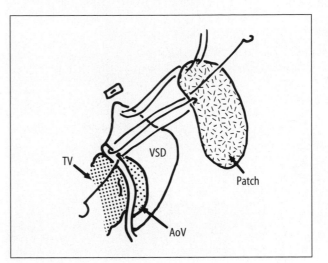

16.60 At the time of closing the ventricular septal defect through a right atrial approach, the tissue tags of tricuspid leaflet (Figure 16.58) can easily be visualized in the subaortic area. While resecting them and reattaching the leaflet would be one option, it is also possible to achieve a good outflow for the left ventricle by enlargement of the ventricular septal defect (dashed line).

16.61 The tricuspid valvar tissue is then retracted into the right ventricle, and the patch for closure of the ventricular septal defect is sutured to the fibrous ridge, pulling it away from the left ventricular outflow and taking care to avoid damage to the nearby aortic valve leaflet. The apex of the ventricular septal defect enlargement is a weak spot in the suture line and should be reinforced with a pledgeted mattress stitch when a continuous technique is used for closure of the ventricular septal defect.

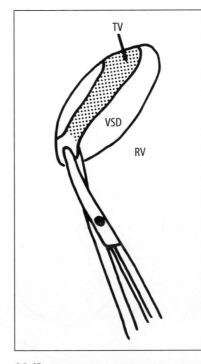

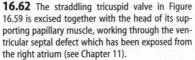

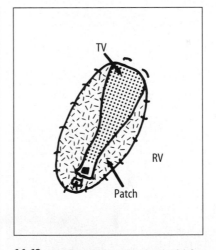

16.63 After closure of the ventricular septal defect on the right ventricular side of the septum, the papillary muscle is reattached to the patch or to the right ventricle if this a more appropriate position. There is usually some residual tricuspid valvar regurgitation following the procedure, but it is rarely of hemodynamic importance.

16.62 The straddling tricuspid valve in Figure 16.59 is excised together with the head of its supporting papillary muscle, working through the ventricular septal defect which has been exposed from the right atrium (see Chapter 11).

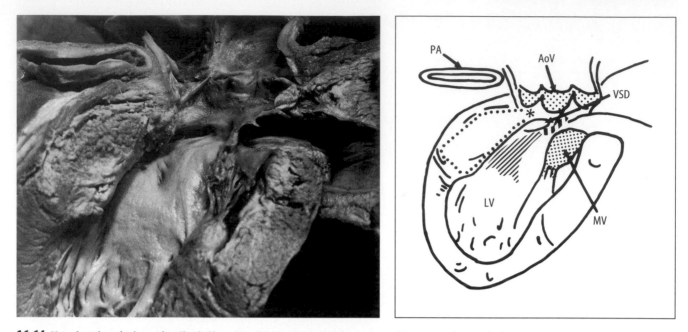

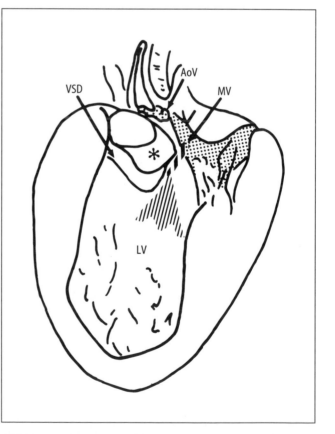

16.64 Muscular subaortic obstruction. The slit-like perimembranous ventricular defect is separated from a normal aortic valve by muscular outlet septum which is malaligned over the left ventricular outflow. The subaortic region is obstructed by a long antero-lateral muscle bundle which extends from the outlet septum (asterisk) onto the anterior wall of the left ventricular outflow (enclosed by dots). Associated coarctation of the aorta is present in this case.

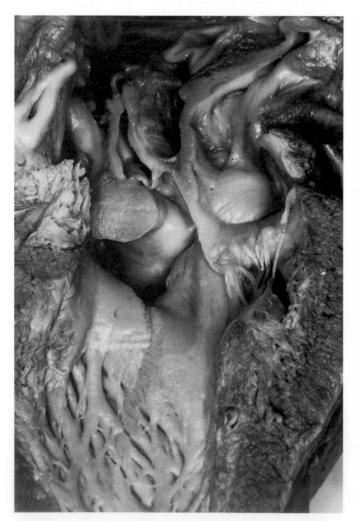

16.65 Subaortic obstruction in this heart is due to a bizarre muscular structure which is composed of malaligned outlet septum (asterisk) running through a muscular ventricular septal defect to the right ventriculo-infundibular fold. The aortic valve is dysplastic and both the valve and aortic root are hypoplastic. Interruption of the aortic arch is also present in this case. While muscular subaortic obstruction is not uncommon with an interrupted aortic arch, it is unusual to find associated valvar aortic stenosis.

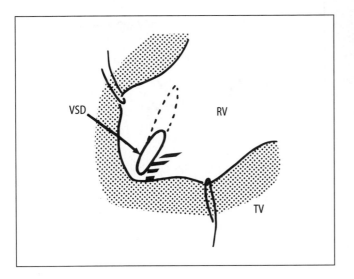

16.66 While the small aortic valve in the second heart (Figure 16.65) would necessitate management with a Damus-Kaye-Stensel or Norwood type procedure (see Figures 27.3–27.7), it is usually possible to relieve directly a muscular obstruction, such as that shown in the first specimen (Figure 16.64) through the ventricular septal defect. Exposure is set up through the right atrium and tricuspid valve (see Chapter 11), and the ventricular septal defect is incised towards the outlet septum at about 12 o'clock as seen by the surgeon (dashed line).

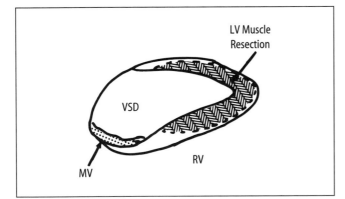

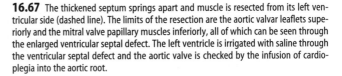

16.67 The thickened septum springs apart and muscle is resected from its left ventricular side (dashed line). The limits of the resection are the aortic valvar leaflets superiorly and the mitral valve papillary muscles inferiorly, all of which can be seen through the enlarged ventricular septal defect. The left ventricle is irrigated with saline through the ventricular septal defect and the aortic valve is checked by the infusion of cardioplegia into the aortic root.

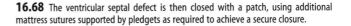

16.68 The ventricular septal defect is then closed with a patch, using additional mattress sutures supported by pledgets as required to achieve a secure closure.

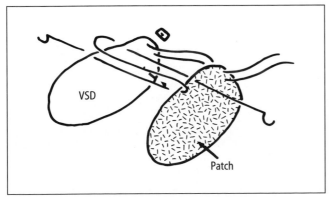

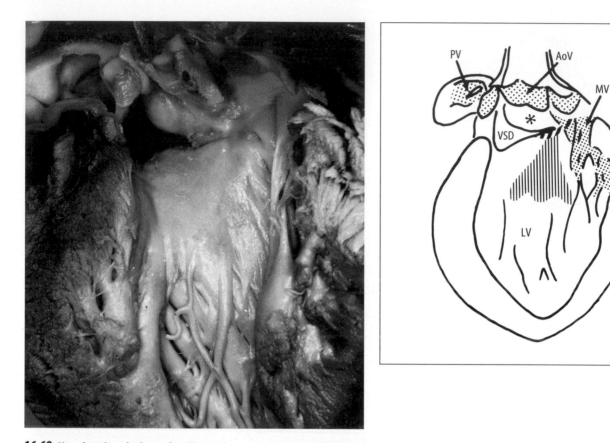

16.69 Muscular subaortic obstruction. There is a large perimembranous ventricular septal defect, viewed on the left ventricular side of the septum, and which is roofed by the aortic and pulmonary valves (doubly committed subarterial ventricular septal defect). The right ventriculo-infundibular fold (asterisk) is seen from the left side through the septal defect and potentially bulges into the subaortic area. The outlet ("infundibular") septum is completely absent. Associated interruption of the aortic arch is present.

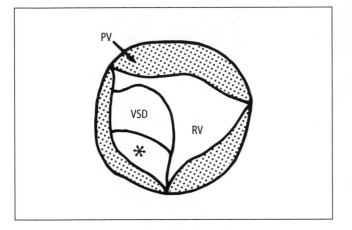

16.70 At the time of arch repair via a mid-line sternotomy, a ventricular septal defect immediately beneath the semilunar valves is approached in the first instance through a transverse incision in the main pulmonary artery (see Chapter 11). As the pulmonary trunk is large, it should be possible to expose the entire defect and the muscle bar (asterisk) by retraction of the pulmonary valvar leaflets in this case.

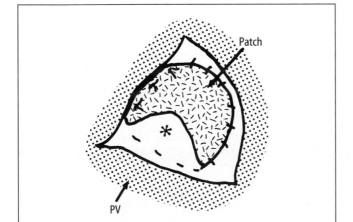

16.71 Since part of the aortic valve is supported by the right ventriculo-infundibular fold (asterisk) in this heart, rather than completely resect the muscle, it is elevated and rotated towards the right side of the heart with a stay stitch. This brings another leaflet of the aortic valve into view. Limited muscle resection is then possible with full visualization of the aortic leaflet

16.72 The defect is closed with a patch which passes to the base of the aortic valve, leaving the muscle bundle on the right ventricular side. Sutures between the aortic and pulmonary valves are placed from the pulmonary artery, through the base of the pulmonary valvar leaflet and into the patch in the right ventricle. The lower margin of the patch is attached to the base of the tricuspid valvar leaflet if the defect extends to the tricuspid valve, or to the right ventricular side of the septum if there is a muscular margin. The former may be difficult to see through even a greatly enlarged pulmonary valve, in which case a right atrial incision is also employed.

Suggested Reading

Anderson RH, Devine WA, Ho SY, Smith A, McKay R. The myth of the aortic annulus: The anatomy of the subaortic outflow tract. Ann Thorac Surg 1991;52:640.

Anderson RH. Clinical anatomy of the aortic root. Heart 2000;86:670.

Angelini A, Ho SY, Anderson RH, Devine WE, Zuberbuhler JR, Becker AE, Davies MJ. The morphology of the normal as compared with the aortic valve having two leaflets. J Thorac Cardiovasc Surg 1989;98(3):363.

Arnold R, Kitchiner D. Left ventricular outflow obstruction. Archives of Disease in Childhood 1995;72:180.

Cassidy SC, Van Hare GF, Silverman NH. The probability of detection of a subaortic ridge in children with ventricular septal defect or coarctation of the aorta. Am J Cardiol 1990;66:505.

Choi JY, Sullivan ID. Fixed subaortic stenosis: anatomical spectrum and nature of progression. Br Heart J 1991;65:280.

Doty DB, Polansky DB, Jenson CB. Supravalvar aortic stenosis. Repair by extended aortoplasty. J Thorac Cardiovasc 1977;74:362.

Duran C, Kumar N, Gometza B, Al Halees Z. Indications and limitations of aortic valve reconstruction. Ann Thorac Surg 1991;52:447.

Edwards JE. Pathology of left ventricular outflow tract obstruction. Circulation 1965;31:586.

Freedom RM, Pelech A, Brand A, Vogel M, Olley PM, Smallhorn JF, Rowe RD. The progressive nature of subaortic stenosis in congenital heart disease. Int J Cardiol 1985;8:137.

Gerosa G, McKay R, Davies J, Ross DN. Comparison of the aortic homograft and the pulmonary autograft for aortic valve or root replacement in children. J Thorac Cardiovasc Surg 1991;102:51.

Ho SY, Muriago M, Cook AC, Thiene G, Anderson RH. Surgical anatomy of aorto-left ventricular tunnel. Ann Thorac Surg 1998; 65:509.

Kirklin JW, Barratt-Boyes BG. Cardiac Surgery, Morphology, Diagnostic Criteria, Natural History, Techniques, Results and Indications. 2nd edn. Churchill Livingstone, New York 1993.

Kitchiner D, Jackson M, Malaiya N, Walsh K, Peart I, Arnold R, Smith A. Morphology of left ventricular outflow tract structures in patients with subaortic stenosis and a ventricular septal defect. Br Heart J 1994;72:251.

Konno S, Imai Y, Tida Y, Wakajima M, Tatsuho K. A new method for prosthetic valve replacement in congenital aortic stenosis associated with hypoplasia of the aortic valve ring. J Thorac Cardiovasc Surg 1975;70:909.

Leung MP, McKay R, Smith A, Anderson RH, Arnold R. Critical aortic stenosis in early infancy. Anatomic and echocardiographic substrates of successful open valvotomy. J Thorac Cardiovasc Surg 1991;101:526.

McKay R, Ross DN. Technique for the relief of discrete subaortic stenosis. J Thorac Cardiovasc Surg 1982;84:917.

McKay R, Smith A, Leung MP, Arnold R, Anderson RH. Morphology of the ventriculoaortic junction in critical aortic stenosis. Implications for hemodynamic function and clinical management. J Thorac Cardiovasc Surg 1992;104(2):434.

Merrick AF, Yacoub MH, Ho SY, Anderson RH. Anatomy of the subpulmonary infundibulum with regard to the Ross Procedure. Ann Thorac Surg 2000;69 (2):556.

Moulaert AJ, Oppenheimer-Dekker A. Anterolateral muscle bundle of the left ventricle, bulboventricular flange and subaortic stenosis. Am J Cardiol 1976;37:78.

Ross DN. Homograft replacement of the aortic valve. Lancet 1962; 2:487.

Shone JD, Sellers RD, Anderson RC. Adams P Jr, Lillehei CW, Edwards JE. The developmental complex of "parachute mitral valve," supravalvar ring of the left atrium, subaortic stenosis and coarctation of the aorta. Am J Cardiol 1963;11:714.

Smallhorn JF, Anderson RH, Macartney FS. Morphological characterisation of ventricular septal defects associated with coarctation of the aorta by cross-sectional echocardiography. Br Heart J 1983; 49:485.

Somerville J, Ross DN. Homograft replacement of aortic root with re-implantation of coronary arteries. Br Heart J 1982;47:473.

Somerville J. Aortic stenosis and incompetence. In: Anderson RH, Macartney FJ, Shinebourne EA, Tynan M. (eds). Paediatric Cardiology 1987;Vol 2: 40, p977. Churchill Livingstone. Edinburgh, London, Melbourne and New York.

Sono J, McKay R, Arnold R. Accessory mitral valve leaflet causing aortic regurgitation and left ventricular outflow obstruction. Case report and review of published reports. Br Heart J 1988;59:491.

Vouhé PR, Poulain H, Bloch G, Loisance DY, Gamain J, Lombaert M, Quiret J, Lesbre J, Bernasconi P, Pietri J, Cachera J. Aortoseptal approach for optimal resection of diffuse subvalvar aortic stenosis. J Thorac Cardiovasc Surg 1984;87:887.

Vouhé PR, Neveux JY. Surgical management of diffuse subaortic stenosis: an integrated approach. Ann Thorac Surg 1991;52:654.

Williams JCP, Barratt-Boyes BG, Lowe JB. Supravalvar aortic stenosis. Circulation 1961;24:1311.

Yacoub MH, Onuzo O, Riedel B, Radley-Smith R. Mobilization of the left and right fibrous trigones for relief of severe left ventricular outflow obstruction. J Thorac Cardiovasc Surg 1999;117:126.

Zielinsky P, Rossi M, Haertel JC, Vitola D, Lucchese FA, Rodrigues R. Subaortic fibrous ridge and ventricular septal defect: role of septal malalignment. Circulation 1987;75:1124.

17 Tetralogy of Fallot

Introduction

The constellation of anomalies observed first by Stensen and described subsequently as a tetralogy by Fallot includes obstruction of the right ventricular outflow, a large ventricular septal defect, overriding of the aortic valve, and hypertrophy of the right ventricle. It is now recognized that the hallmark of this malformation is anterior deviation of the outlet (infundibular) septum, which produces malalignment with the trabecular septum and the resulting malalignment ventricular septal defect. The defect usually (in 80% of cases) reaches the tricuspid valve with fibrous continuity between aortic and tricuspid valves in this area and is thus "perimembranous". In the remaining hearts the posterior limb of the septomarginal trabeculation fuses with the ventriculo-infundibular fold, separating the tricuspid from the aortic valve and resulting in a "muscular" ventricular septal defect. Rarely, the outlet septum is completely absent. This produces a doubly committed, subarterial (juxta-arterial) defect, in which the posterior margin may be composed of either muscle or tissue of the fibrous continuity area. Additional muscular defects in the trabecular septum are not uncommon. While the ventricular septal defect in Fallot's tetralogy is large by definition, restriction may be produced by an extension of fibrous tissue from the tricuspid valve or a remnant of membranous septum, a so-called "flap valve ventricular septal defect." This results in a suprasystemic pressure in the right ventricle.

The axis of the conduction tissue passes from the atrioventricular node in the apex of the triangle of Koch, to the postero-inferior margin of a perimembranous ventricular septal defect, behind the fibrous tissue (or "frap") which connects the aortic, mitral, and tricuspid valvar leaflets. From here, the non-branching bundle usually runs to the left side of the septum, several millimeters from the margin of the ventricular septal defect. However, this is not invariable and the non-branching bundle may lie on the crest of the septum. With a muscular ventricular septal defect, the posterior limb of the septomarginal trabeculation lies between the crest of the septum and the axis of the conduction tissue. The right bundle branch passes on the right ventricular side of the septum in close proximity to the medial papillary muscle complex, notwithstanding that this complex may be displaced and hypoplastic in tetralogy.

In addition to hypertrophy and displacement of the outlet septum, right ventricular outflow obstruction may result from enlarged, free-standing septoparietal muscle bundles in the subpulmonary area, valvar obstruction, supravalvar narrowing in the main pulmonary artery, and branch or bifurcation stenosis of the more distal pulmonary arterial tree. Complete obstruction at infundibular or valvar level produces tetralogy with pulmonary atresia. Depending on the length of the outlet septum and the degree of muscular obstruction, the right ventricle may become partitioned into a main chamber and a subpulmonary chamber, connected through an infundibular orifice. Externally, a large infundibular branch of the right coronary artery often indicates the site of this muscular structure. Occasionally, the level of obstruction lies further down within the ventricle, as the result of an enlarged septomarginal trabeculation and parietal extensions which cross the ventricular chamber. This produces the so-called "tetralogy with low-lying infundibular stenosis." Another uncommon variant is "tetralogy with absent pulmonary valve." In these patients, the pulmonary valve is represented by a ridge of thick fibrous tissue which produces both stenosis and incompetence. The resulting post-stenotic dilatation of the branch pulmonary arteries, along with intrinsic pulmonary abnormalities, often leads to severe respiratory compromise early in life among this subset of patients.

The extent of aortic overriding is variable in tetralogy of Fallot. When more than half the aortic valve is committed to the right ventricle, the defect can be regarded strictly as that of "double outlet right ventricle," and may be described as "tetralogy with double outlet right ventricle." In most hearts, and in distinction to the classic double outlet right ventricle in which both great arteries have a muscular infundibulum, aortic-mitral continuity, however, is maintained. In general, the aortic outflow is larger than normal and obstruction to the systemic circulation is almost never associated with Fallot's tetralogy. Important but infrequent variations in the coronary arteries include the anomalous origin of the left anterior descending artery from the right coronary artery and the origin of the right coronary artery as a branch of the anterior descending artery. In both cases, the anomalous coronary artery crosses the right ventricular outflow tract.

Management of the tetralogy of Fallot is often used as a measure of expertise in congenital heart surgery. This is not without good reason. Careful decision-making, meticulous surgical technique and impeccable post-operative care can achieve near-perfect survival rates, as well as excellent long-term results. However, the ideal of normal systemic and pulmonary circulation is probably rarely attained, even with the secure closure of the ventricular septal defect, relief of all obstruction to right ventricular outflow, and optimal conservation of myocardial function. Early repair to prevent right ventricular dysfunction often involves a transannular patch, which invariably results in some degree of pulmonary incompetence, while delayed or secondary correction after a systemic-pulmonary shunt carries a greater likelihood of arrythmias, residual right ventricular hypertrophy, and/or pulmonary arterial problems.

Decision-making begins with an evaluation of the patient's pulmonary arteries. If these are of sufficient calibre to accept the entire cardiac output, closure of the ventricular septal defect will be tolerated. The next consideration regards relief of the right ventricular outflow obstruction, and in particular whether the pulmonary annulus is so small that it requires a trans-annular patch. If a ventriculotomy is necessary, closure of the ventricular septal defect may be done by this route. Alternatively, a "transatrial/transpulmonary" approach may be used for both the repair of the ventricular septal defect and muscle resection, with only very limited or no ventriculotomy. In general, very young patients (neonates to about three or four months) have little cardiac hypertrophy and require less muscle resection than older patients. It may be useful in this group to leave a patent oval fossa to decompress the right heart early after operation. Associated defects, such as additional muscular ventricular septal defects, are treated on their own merits.

When pulmonary arterial development is inadequate for primary repair or other considerations make this inadvisable, symptomatic patients may be palliated with a systemic-to-pulmonary artery shunt. This will bring about the growth of pulmonary arteries and improved oxygenation, such that complete correction can be carried out later with lower operative risk. The type and position of the shunt is determined by both anatomical considerations and surgeon/institution preference. When one pulmonary artery branch is smaller than the other or is disconnected from a source of blood-flow, the anastomosis is constructed to this vessel. When the patient has a duct-dependent pulmonary circulation, the shunt is generally placed on the opposite side (usually right) to avoid interruption of pulmonary blood-flow during the construction of the anastomosis. When there are no other compelling factors, it is generally placed on that side opposite to the aortic arch to facilitate closure at the time of sternotomy. Central shunts (via a mid-line sternotomy) and balloon pulmonary valvuloplasty have also been employed effectively for palliation. As most patients will now come to correction within the first few years of life, a modified Blalock procedure using a prosthetic graft generally provides adequate palliation without the sacrifice of systemic arteries, major risk of pulmonary arterial distortion, or development of pulmonary hypertension.

The increase in long-term survival has now created a new population of adults with repaired cyanotic heart disease, the great majority of whom have had surgery for tetralogy of Fallot. Reoperations are not uncommon for residual lesions (atrial and ventricular septal defects, right ventricular outflow obstruction) or pulmonary valve incompetence and, in the future, may become necessary for arteriosclerotic coronary artery disease. A thorough understanding of the underlying malformation and previous operative interventions is thus essential for the ongoing management of this group of patients.

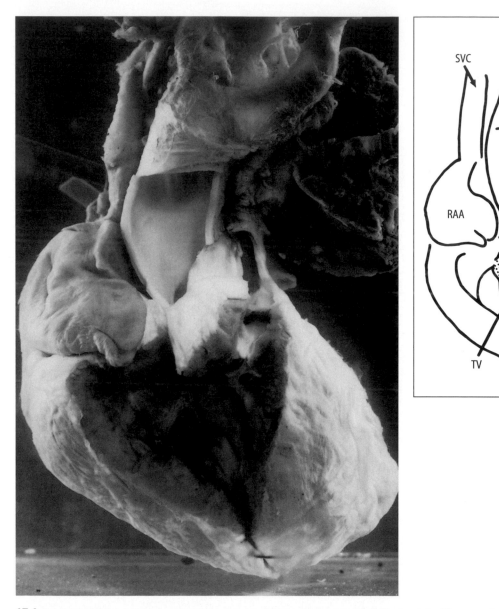

17.1 Tetralogy of Fallot. Anterior view of a window dissection which has been mounted to display the relationships among the dextroposed aorta, the small pulmonary artery and the right ventricle. Anterior deviation of the outlet (infundibular) septum (asterisk) separating the subaortic outflow from the subpulmonary outflow produces subpulmonary stenosis. The pulmonary valve is also small and dysplastic. The aorta overrides the ventricular septal defect, which is not seen clearly because of the angle from which the specimen has been photographed. There is severe hypertrophy of the right ventricular free wall.

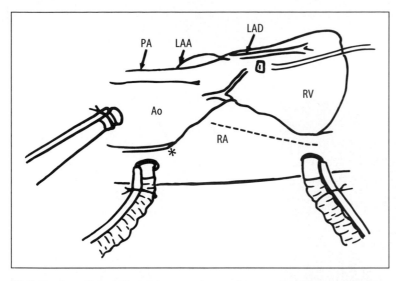

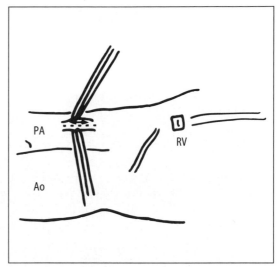

17.2 Bicaval cannulation with arterial return to the ascending aorta gives optimal flexibility for the complete repair of Fallot's tetralogy. To compensate collateral flow with increased perfusion, an oversized cannula is easily accommodated by the large ascending aorta, if this is desirable. Cannulation of the inferior caval vein as far lateral as possible leaves room to extend inferiorly the right atrial incision for transatrial access to the right ventricle (dashed line). The superior caval vein is cannulated above the site of the sinus node (asterisk) and its blood supply. A stay-suture on the right ventricle facilitates exposure of the pulmonary artery. This is usually placed just below the large infundibular branch of the right coronary artery which runs to the area of muscular infundibular obstruction.

17.3 From a surgeon's view, the main pulmonary artery may appear very small as a result of lying partly behind a large ascending aorta. Rotation of the operating table towards the surgeon and traction on the stay-suture help to expose the vessel. The main pulmonary artery is opened with a knife vertically between the assistant's and surgeon's forceps, above the valve sinuses. Elevation of the vessel (which collapses on bypass) prevents injury to its posterior wall.

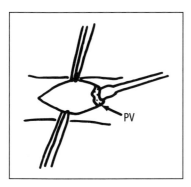

17.4 *(left)* The right and left branch pulmonary arteries are calibrated with Hegar dilators to exclude any proximal stenosis, especially if repair is being done based upon non-invasive preoperative imaging. A small retractor (such as a nerve root retractor) at the cardiac end of the incision exposes the pulmonary valve. The pulmonary artery is held open either with forceps or fine stay-sutures.

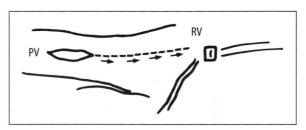

17.5 The size of the pulmonary annulus is measured with Hegar dilators after any leaflet fusion is relieved by the incision of each commissure to the pulmonary arterial wall (see Figures 15.4–15.6). If this is smaller than about two standard deviations below the average normal size for the patient's body surface area, the incision is carried on to the right ventricle, if possible conserving the large infundibular coronary artery.

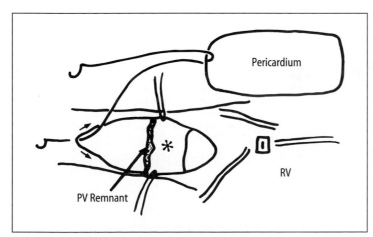

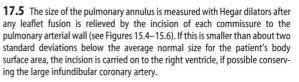

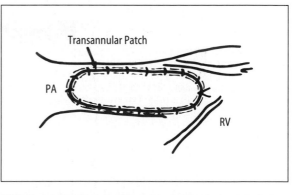

17.6 The extent of the ventricular incision depends on the length of the outlet (infundibular) septum (asterisk). The ventriculotomy usually runs a few millimeters below the lower margin of the infundibular septum. Remnants of leaflet of the pulmonary valve serve no useful purpose in the absence of a coapting surface anteriorly and are thus excised to reduce turbulence in the outflow tract. Following muscle resection and closure of the ventricular septal defect, a rectangular patch is placed to enlarge the outflow and main pulmonary artery. This can be done in the beating heart with a fine pump-sucker positioned in the distal main pulmonary artery.

17.7 The completed transannular patch is slightly redundant in both directions and should achieve an outflow which is slightly larger than normal. An excessively large patch or residual distal obstruction may predispose to aneurysm formation. Placement of a transannular patch leaves the patient with free pulmonary regurgitation, tolerance of which in both the short and long term is variable and dependent on a number of factors. It should thus be reserved for cases where measurements of the pulmonary valve indicate a definite need.

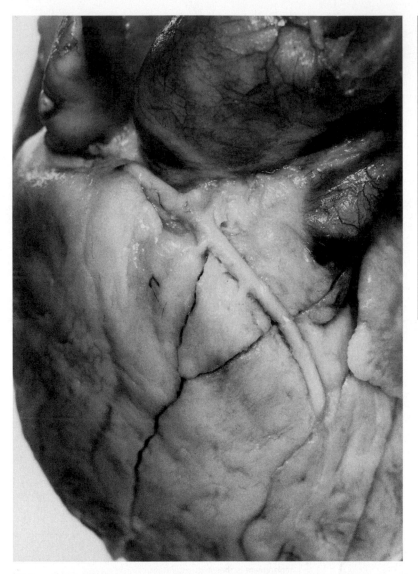

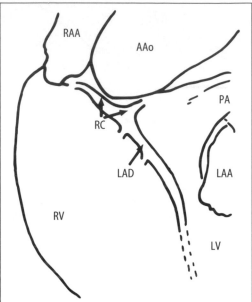

17.8 Tetralogy of Fallot. Anomalous origin of the entire left anterior descending coronary artery from the right coronary artery. The heart is viewed externally from the left and anteriorly. A large right coronary artery divides into two equal branches shortly beyond its origin. The left anterior descending coronary artery passes across the outflow of the right ventricle, angling slightly downwards to the anterior interventricular groove. There is no anterior descending branch from the left coronary artery in this heart, although sometimes such a vessel supplies the upper portion of the interventricular septum and the distal left anterior descending artery arises lower down from an infundibular branch of the right coronary artery. The anomalous origin of the anterior descending coronary artery is found in about 5% of hearts with Fallot's tetralogy.

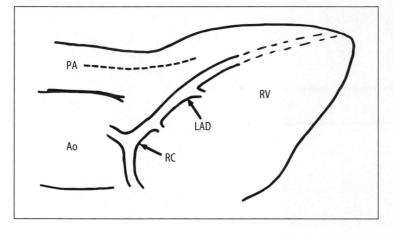

17.9 The anomalous origin of the left anterior descending coronary artery precludes the usual incision across the right ventricular infundibulum for a transannular outflow patch. However, such a coronary artery always deviates slightly towards the apex of the heart, leaving a small corner of subarterial right ventricular outflow tract between the pulmonary valve and upper margin of the artery. The incision from the pulmonary artery may be safely extended into this area (dashed line).

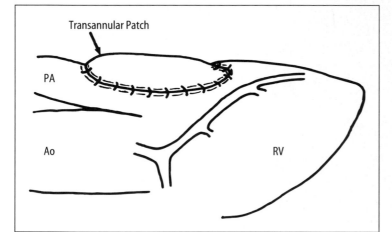

17.10 Even though the distance between the pulmonary valvar annulus and anomalous coronary artery may be only a few millimeters, a transannular patch combined with transatrial muscle resection inside the right ventricle achieves sufficient relief of the outflow obstruction. The transannular patch lies slightly more towards the left side of the pulmonary artery than usual and angles towards the interventricular septum. Its proximal extent on the right ventricle comes very close to the coronary artery.

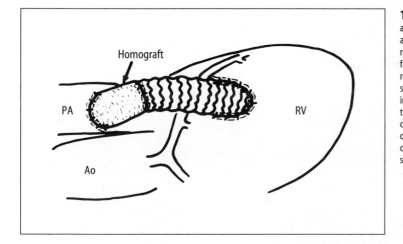

17.11 Alternatively, the traditional management of a small outflow tract associated with the anomalous origin of the anterior descending coronary artery has been the placement of a valved extracardiac conduit between the right ventricle and the pulmonary artery over the vessel. This is a less satisfactory solution because it commits the patient to reoperation for conduit replacement in the future and frequently results in a preliminary palliative systemic-pulmonary anastomosis, awaiting patient growth for conduit implantation. The course of the coronary artery also necessitates a lower-than-ideal incision on the body of the right ventricle which tends to place the conduit directly on the front of the heart and behind the sternum, rather than over the left shoulder of the heart. In this position it is more vulnerable to compression by the sternum and at greater risk of damage during re-sternotomy.

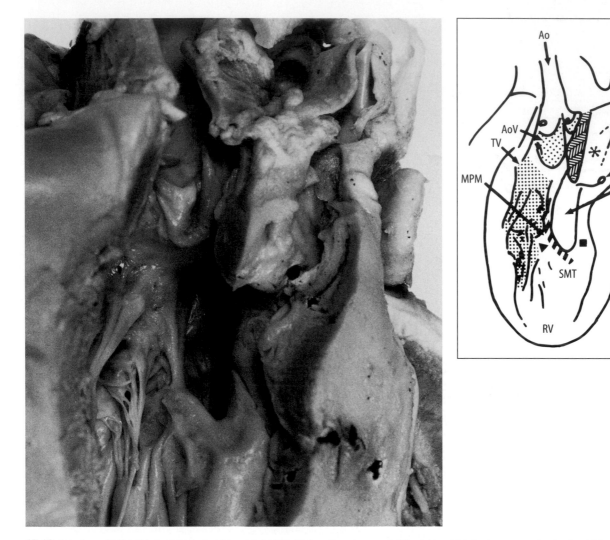

17.12 Tetralogy of Fallot. Tubular hypoplastic right ventricular infundibulum. The anterior wall of the right ventricle has been removed, as has the rightward half of the outlet septum. This shows extreme anterior displacement of a long hypertrophied infundibular septum (asterisk). The anterior limb of the septomarginal trabeculation (square) runs on to the free wall of the hypertrophied right ventricle, where its fusion with the infundibular septum produces a severely restricted infundibular orifice. The posterior limb (triangle) supports the medial papillary muscle of the tricuspid valve. A very large ventricular septal defect extends to the tricuspid valve and there is extreme overriding of the aortic valve, such that the lesion could be described as "tetralogy-type double outlet right ventricle." The pulmonary valvar leaflets are small and dysplastic. The conduction tissue lies along the posterior margin of the perimembranous ventricular septal defect where fibrous continuity between the tricuspid and aortic valves is clearly shown.

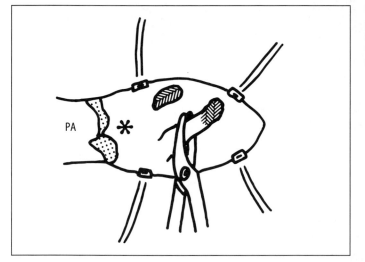

17.13 A long tubular infundibulum necessitates a ventriculotomy and outflow patch which in this heart would extend across the hypoplastic pulmonary valve (transannular patch), because only part of the obstruction can be relieved by muscle resection. The infundibular orifice guides the division of the first large septal extension, identification of which is facilitated by the passage of a right-angled instrument beneath the muscle bundle. It is then possible to remove any small bundles within the infundibular chamber (directly below the pulmonary valve) and any further septal extensions, mobilizing the infundibular septum (asterisk) from the septomarginal trabeculation.

17.14 The parietal extensions of the infundibular septum (asterisk), which anchor it to the ventriculo-infundibular fold, are also divided downwards from above. This is done in an oblique direction to avoid damage to the aortic valve or perforation of the heart. Again, each muscle bundle is defined by lifting it away from the septum prior to incision.

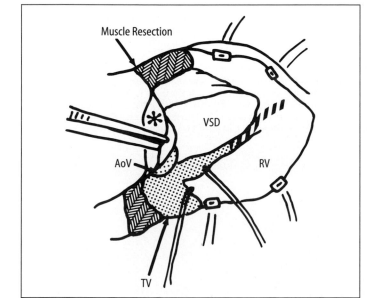

17.15 Sufficient muscle is divided or resected to give access to the ventricular septal defect, and achieve an adequate pathway between the main right ventricle and subpulmonary infundibular area. The infundibular septum itself (asterisk) is now mobile and can be elevated towards the pulmonary valve, assisting in exposure of the defect. It is not resected, however, because this muscle supports the aortic valve on the side away from the surgeon and serves for secure attachment of the patch. The placement of stay-sutures in the anterior and septal leaflets of the tricuspid valve also facilitates the exposure of the ventricular septal defect by elevating the lower margin towards the ventriculotomy. The conduction tissue lies towards the surgeon and passes on the right-hand margin of the defect, as seen through a right ventriculotomy.

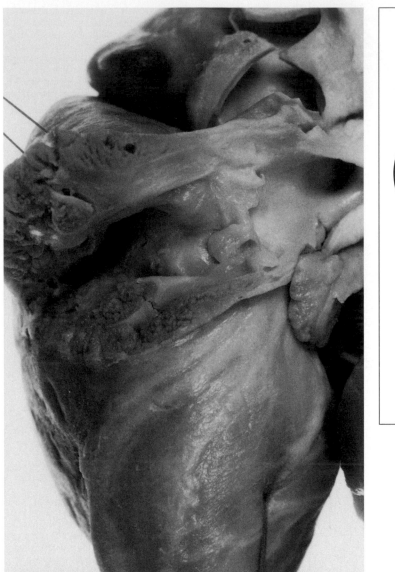

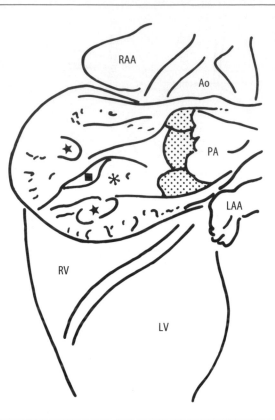

17.16 Tetralogy of Fallot. The right ventricular outflow tract has been opened vertically across the infundibular chamber and pulmonary valve into the pulmonary artery. The pulmonary valve has three leaflets which are thickened and slightly dysplastic. The valve and main pulmonary artery are smaller than normal but not severely hypoplastic. A subpulmonary (infundibular) chamber is narrowed by hypertrophy and anterior deviation of the outlet septum (asterisk). It connects to the main cavity of the right ventricle through a small aperture, the "infundibular orifice" (square). This orifice is further compromised by hypertrophied parietal extensions of the infundibular (outlet) septum which have been transected in this specimen (stars), as well as septoparietal trabeculations in the lower portion of the ventricle (unseen). The long axis of the infundibulum lies at right angles to the plane of the infundibular orifice. This is unusual in tetralogy of Fallot. The main part of the right ventricle is of normal size but is not seen.

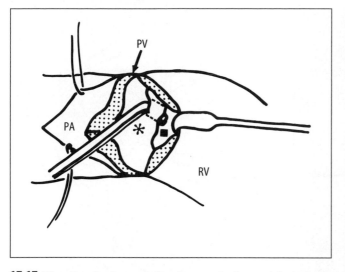

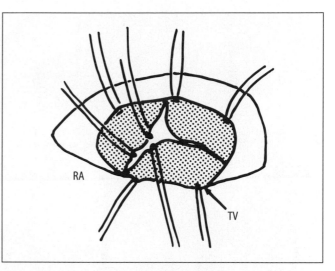

17.17 When attempting to conserve the pulmonary valve (in general, that is when its diameter measures within two standard deviations of the mean normal value), a vertical incision is first made in the main pulmonary artery and extended proximally into the valvar sinus. From this route, the branch pulmonary arteries are measured, any fusion of the valvar commissures is released, and the pulmonary annulus is calibrated with a Hegar dilator. Retraction of the valve leaflets then exposes the infundibular septum (asterisk) and the infundibular orifice (square). After its identification with a right-angled instrument, at least the first septal extension is divided to help orientate subsequent muscle resection through the right atrial approach.

17.18 The right atrium is opened with a long oblique incision (see Figure 17.2) and exposure is set up with stay-sutures at approximately 10 o'clock, 12 o'clock, and 2 o'clock on the tricuspid valvar annulus. This rotates the right ventricle about 90° away from the surgeon, such that the structures which formerly lay parallel to the operating table are now perpendicular to it. Additional fine stay-sutures on the anterior and septal tricuspid valvar leaflets retract them to expose the cavity of the right ventricle.

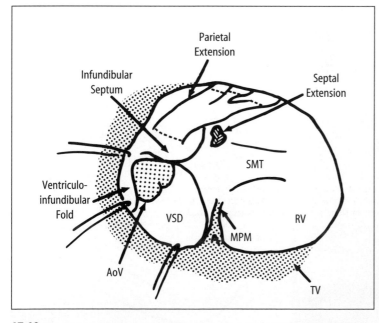

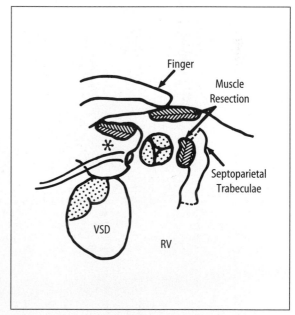

17.19 The surgeon's view through the tricuspid valve places the ventricular septal defect to the left with leaflets of the aortic valve seen through the defect. The septal muscle bundle, which was divided when working through the pulmonary valve, is now on the far (leftward) side of the ventricle and slightly towards the surgeon's left hand. It helps to indicate the position of the right ventricular outflow. The parietal extensions of the infundibular (outlet) septum remain to be resected (dashed lines) and pass from the infundibular septum away from the surgeon, around the outflow to the free right ventricular wall.

17.20 Following the removal of the hypertrophied parietal bundles, a stay-suture in the infundibular septum (asterisk) facilitates retraction of this structure, which has been liberated by the division of its septal and parietal extensions. This exposes the subpulmonary chamber and pulmonary valve, where further septoparietal muscle bundles are removed as needed to achieve an unobstructed outflow. Gentle digital pressure on the right ventricular free wall guides the depth of muscle resection and also improves exposure. In general, more extensive resection is necessary in older patients and also when a transannular patch is not used.

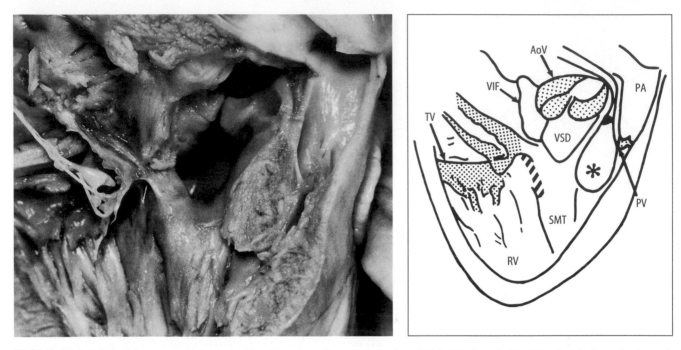

17.21 Tetralogy of Fallot. Extreme anterior displacement of the outlet septum and muscular ventricular septal defect. The free wall of the right ventricle has been rotated upwards to display the septal surface after opening the heart from the right atrium, to the apex, to the outflow tract. The hypertrophied outlet septum (asterisk) fuses with the anterior limb of the septomarginal trabeculation and produces near atresia of the subpulmonary outflow. A tiny remnant of pulmonary valve is patent. The posterior limb of the septomarginal trabeculation is continuous with the ventriculo-infundibular fold, such that the ventricular septal defect does not reach the tricuspid valve and is thus muscular, with the conduction tissue being remote from the lower margin. A normal aortic valve overrides the defect by at least 50%. The pulmonary valve lies at a much lower level than does the aortic valve.

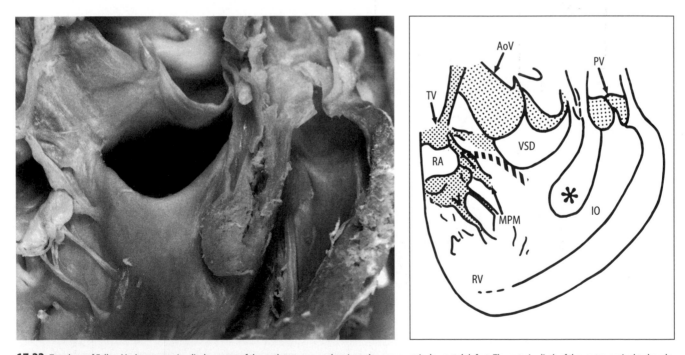

17.22 Tetralogy of Fallot. Moderate anterior displacement of the outlet septum and perimembranous ventricular septal defect. The anterior limb of the septomarginal trabeculation is fused with the enlarged outlet septum (asterisk), while the posterior limb supports the medial papillary muscle complex. The tricuspid valve is in fibrous continuity, through the aortic valve, with the mitral valve in the back of the defect. The aortic valve overrides the ventricular septal defect by about 50% and is at approximately the same level as the pulmonary valve. A well-defined subpulmonary chamber connects with the main right ventricular cavity through a wide infundibular orifice, most of the outflow obstruction resulting from the fusion of the pulmonary valvar leaflets.

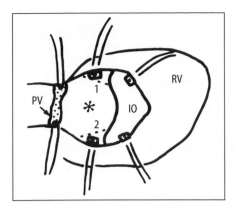

17.23 The first heart (see Figure 17.21) clearly requires a ventriculotomy for a transannular patch. Closure of the ventricular septal defect is also conveniently done by this route. After the placement of stay-sutures on the margins of the ventriculotomy, the infundibular septum (asterisk) is mobilized by the division of the septal (1) and parietal (2) extensions (dashed line).

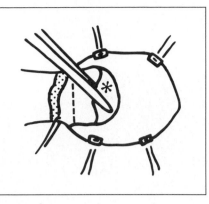

17.24 In this heart, the pulmonary valve is lower than the aortic valve, such that cautious, partial removal (dashed line) of infundibular septal muscle (asterisk) is both possible and desirable to enlarge the right ventricular outflow and provide access to the ventricular septal defect.

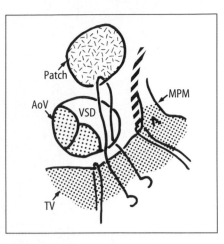

17.25 The ventricular septal defect and the tricuspid valve are visualized after resection of the muscle. As the defect does not extend to the tricuspid valve sutures may be safely placed entirely along its muscular margin. The conduction tissue will then lie between the patch and the medial papillary muscle complex.

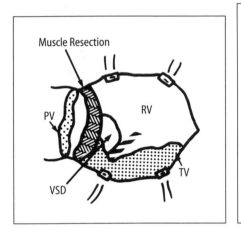

17.26 In the second specimen (see Figure 17.22), the ventricular septal defect extends to the tricuspid valve and the conduction tissue runs along its margin towards the medial papillary muscle complex.

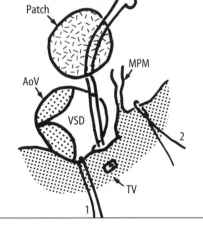

17.27 The first suture for the ventricular septal defect patch is placed on the base of the tricuspid valve at the deepest part of the suture line, which is usually at the commissure between the anterior (1) and septal (2) leaflets. Stay-sutures elevate the valve (and the defect) into the ventriculotomy for exposure. When the commissure extends to the annulus, there is usually still a small flap of fibrous tissue (the so-called "frap") where this stitch may be safely placed.

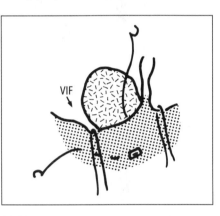

17.28 The patch is brought to the base of the anterior leaflet of the tricuspid valve with a continuous mattress suture, working clockwise towards the ventriculo-infundibular fold (which is also towards the surgeon).

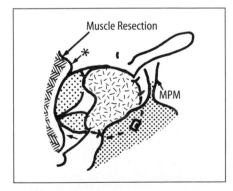

17.29 At the ventriculo-infundibular fold, a transition bite from valve leaflet is made back on to the muscle, and stitches are then placed radially around to the aortic valve, working towards the infundibular septum (asterisk). The second arm of the suture continues counter-clockwise towards the medial papillary muscle complex with stitches parallel to and about 3–5 mm away from the margin of the ventricular septal defect. Displacement of the patch into the left ventricle through the defect facilitates exposure at this time.

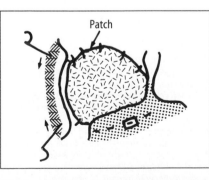

17.30 Small "valleys" are often found within trabeculations at the edges of the infundibular septum. Sutures are placed in such a manner as to obliterate residual ventricular septal defects at this site, and the patch attachment is completed to the infundibular septum with bites through its full thickness, radially to the aortic valve.

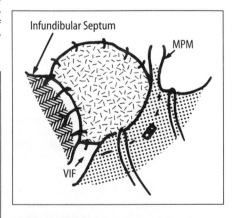

17.31 The final position of the patch is flat, as the generous systemic outflow needs no enlargement. It crosses the conduction tissue at the medial papillary muscle in the region of the right bundle branch and after the penetrating bundle has passed to the left side of the septum. If there has been resection of the infundibular septal muscle, potentially weak areas in the suture line may need additional mattress sutures supported by pledgets.

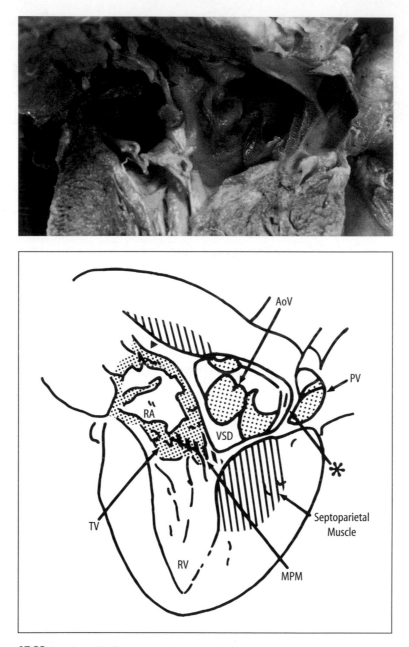

17.32 Tetralogy of Fallot. Absent outlet septum (doubly committed subarterial ventricular septal defect). The specimen has been opened from the apex across the outflow of the right ventricle, and the free wall is rotated to the right upwards to display the septal surface. A very large confluent perimembranous ventricular septal defect extends beneath the medial papillary muscle complex into the inlet septum and to both the aortic and pulmonary valves. The outlet septum is completely absent, such that only a ridge of fibrous tissue (asterisk) separates aortic and pulmonary valvar leaflets. The ventriculoinfundibular fold (triangle) is hypoplastic and does not join the septomarginal trabeculation, the anterior limb of which is fused with hypertophied septoparietal muscle. The pulmonary valve itself is small and atretic as a result of imperforate joined leaflets. The axis of the conduction tissue passes along the posterior margin of the ventricular septal defect towards the medial papillary muscle complex which attaches to the posterior limb of the septomarginal trabeculation.

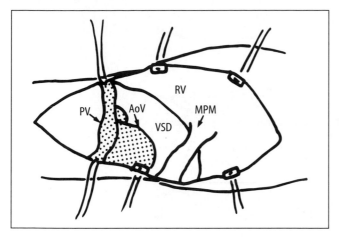

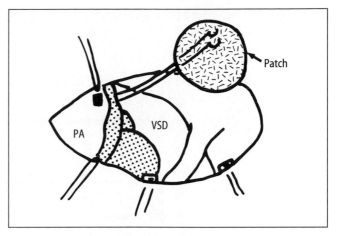

17.33 Closure of an isolated doubly committed subarterial ventricular septal defect which extends to the inlet septum can be done through the pulmonary and tricuspid valves, but the co-existence of imperforate pulmonary valve and subpulmonary muscular obstruction in this heart necessitates a ventriculotomy. This is done with the surgeon's and the assistant's forceps elevating the pulmonary artery/right ventricle to prevent injury to the aortic valve (which lies immediately posteriorly). There is little muscle which requires resection. Good exposure is obtained with stay-sutures on the edges of the ventriculotomy.

17.34 Interrupted mattress sutures are placed initially from the pulmonary artery through the fibrous ridge between the ventriculo-arterial valves and into the ventricular septal defect patch.

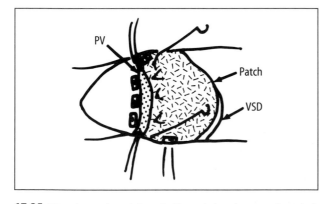

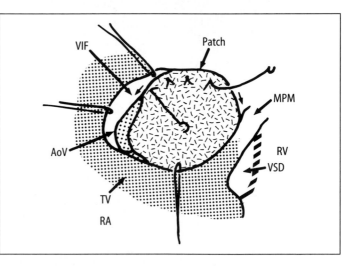

17.35 When the septal muscle is reached beneath the pulmonary valve on both sides of the ventricular septal defect, the patch is lowered and these sutures are tied. One end of each final double-ended suture is left long and passed into the right ventricle. The lower margin of the defect will be more easily seen through the tricuspid valve.

17.36 Exposure is then set up through the right atrium and tricuspid valve (see Figure 17.4). Suturing progresses continuously counter-clockwise towards the surgeon along the right ventriculo-infundibular fold, with bites taken radially to the aortic valve. A transition suture brings this arm through the base of the tricuspid valvar leaflet where it is held with a suture snap in the right atrium. At this point, the patch is elevated and cardioplegia is infused into the aortic root to exclude injury or distortion of the aortic valve. The second arm of the suture continues clockwise towards the medial papillary muscle complex. Conduction tissue will lie to the surgeon's right hand along the lower margin of the defect.

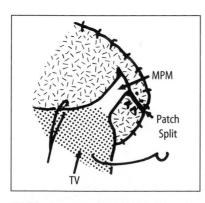

17.37 The patch is split to pass around the medial papillary muscle and beyond the conduction tissue. In this area, it is repaired with a few interrupted sutures. Suturing then progresses the base of the leaflet of the tricuspid valve with bites parallel to the ventricular septal defect (and hence conduction tissue).

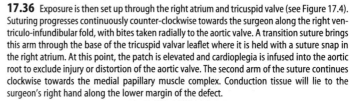

17.38 *(right)* Continuous mattress sutures through the base of both the septal and anterior leaflets of the tricuspid valve are supported by a strip of pericardium, working clockwise from the surgeon's right hand towards the left hand. Additional mattress sutures are placed as needed to reinforce any potentially weak areas of closure of the ventricular septal defect. The competence of the tricuspid valve is verified by the injection of saline into the right ventricle. A transannular patch is then used to reconstruct the right ventricular outflow (see Figures 17.6–17.7).

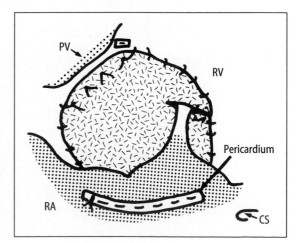

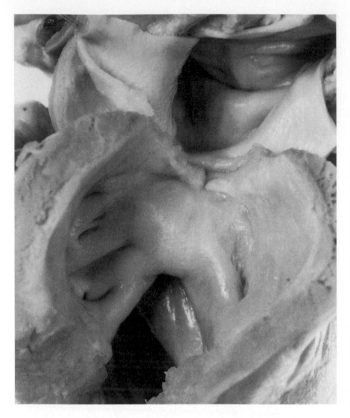

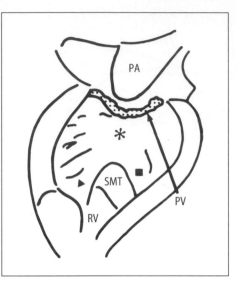

17.39 Tetralogy of Fallot with absent pulmonary valve. The right ventricular outflow has been transected vertically across the free wall of the infundibulum and separated to display the small aperture between the main portion of the right ventricle and the subpulmonary chamber. The outlet septum (asterisk) is hypertrophied and deviated, as are its septal (square) and parietal (triangle) extensions. The septomarginal trabeculation is partially visualized behind the septoparietal muscle bar (square). A ridge of fibrous tissue represents the pulmonary valve which lacks true sinuses. The main and branch pulmonary arteries show aneurysmal dilatation.

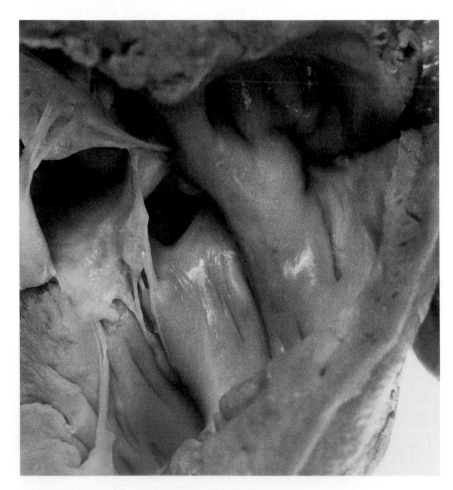

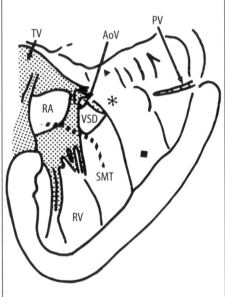

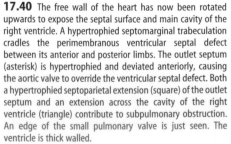

17.40 The free wall of the heart has now been rotated upwards to expose the septal surface and main cavity of the right ventricle. A hypertrophied septomarginal trabeculation cradles the perimembranous ventricular septal defect between its anterior and posterior limbs. The outlet septum (asterisk) is hypertrophied and deviated anteriorly, causing the aortic valve to override the ventricular septal defect. Both a hypertrophied septoparietal extension (square) of the outlet septum and an extension across the cavity of the right ventricle (triangle) contribute to subpulmonary obstruction. An edge of the small pulmonary valve is just seen. The ventricle is thick walled.

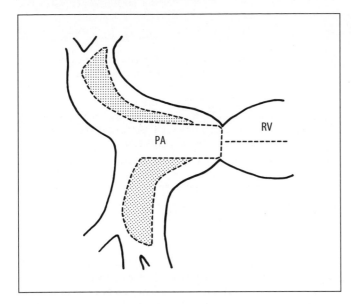

17.41 Muscle resection and closure of the ventricular septal defect in tetralogy of Fallot with absent pulmonary valve are essentially the same as in classic Fallot's tetralogy (see Figures 17.13–15, 17.17–20, and 17.26–31). It is generally accepted that the reduction of the aneurysmal pulmonary arteries with or without implantation of a homograft or other type of valvar mechanism helps to relieve accompanying bronchial compression. In this heart, a transannular incision is needed to enlarge the outflow, so the right ventricle is first opened vertically (dashed line). To retain tissue for a transannular patch, the pulmonary artery is opened transversely at the level of the rudimentary valve. Further incisions are then carried bilaterally into the main and lower lobe branch pulmonary arteries, with or without division of the ascending aorta for access. The shaded area is resected.

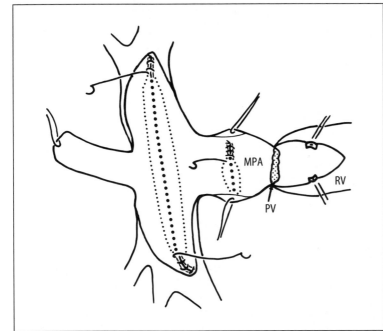

17.42 Working inside the pulmonary arteries, the posterior walls (dotted lines) of the right and left branches are plicated with a running suture from lung hilum to hilum, leaving a vessel which will be a few millimeters larger than normal for the patient's body surface area. A separate transverse plication of the main pulmonary artery helps to retract the bifurcation away from the trachea and prevent obstruction of the right branch.

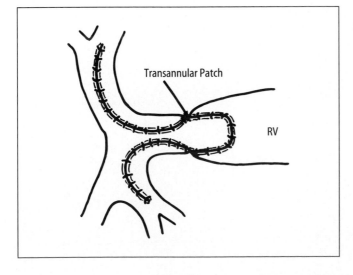

17.43 The anterior wall of the pulmonary arteries are repaired by direct suture with a fine running monofilament stitch. The tongue of the excess main pulmonary artery, thus produced by reduction in the size of the branches and the length of the main pulmonary artery, is continued over the ventriculotomy as a transannular outflow patch.

Suggested Reading

Alexiou C, Chen Q, Galogavrou M, Gnanapragasam J, Salmon AP, Keeton BR, Haw MP, Monro JL. Repair of tetralogy of Fallot in infancy with a transventricular or a transatrial approach. Eur J Cardiothorac Surg 2002;22:174.

Anderson RH, Allwork SP, Ho SY, Lenox SC, Zuberbuhler JR. Surgical anatomy of tetralogy of Fallot. J. Thorac Cardiovasc Surg 1981;81:887.

Blackstone EH, Kirklin JW, Bertranou EG, Labrosse CJ, Soto B, Bergeron LM, Jr. Preoperative prediction from cineangiograms of post-repair right ventricular pressure in tetralogy of Fallot. J Thorac Cardiovasc Surg 1979;78:542.

Brizard CPR, Mas C, Sohn Y-S, Cochrane AD, Karl TR. Transatrial-transpulmonary tetralogy of Fallot repair is effective in the presence of anomalous coronary arteries. J Thorac Cardiovasc Surg 1998;116:770.

Cobanoglu A, Schultz JM. Total correction of tetralogy of Fallot in the first year of life: late results. Ann Thorac Surg 2002;74:133.

de Leval MR, McKay R, Jones M, Stark J, Macartney FJ. Modified Blalock-Taussig shunt. Use of subclavian artery orifice as flow regulator in prosthetic systemic-pulmonary artery shunts. J Thorac Cardiovasc Surg 1981;81:112.

Dickinson DF, Wilkinson JL, Smith A, Hamilton DI, Anderson RH. Variations in the morphology of ventricular septal defect and disposition of atrioventricular conduction tissues in tetralogy of Fallot. J Thorac Cardiovasc Surg 1982;30:243.

Di Donato RM, Jones RA, Lang P, Rome JJ, Mayer JE Jr, Castaneda AR. Neonatal repair of tetralogy of Fallot with and without pulmonary atresia. J Thorac Cardiovasc Surg 1991;101:126.

Fraser CD Jr, McKenzie ED, Cooley DA. Tetralogy of Fallot: surgical management individualized to the patient. Ann Thorac Surg 2001;71:1556.

Gatzoulis MA, Shore D, Yacoub M, Shinebourne EA. Complete atrio-ventricular septal defect with tetralogy of Fallot: diagnosis and management. Br Heart J 1994;71(6):579.

Gerlis LM, Smith CE, Somerville J. The Brock procedure (closed infundibular resection) for Fallot's tetralogy: 43 years later. Cardiol Young 1998;8(3):408.

Ilbawi MN, Idriss FS, DeLeon SY, Muster AJ, Gidding SS, Berry TE, Paul MH. Factors that exaggerate the deleterious effects of pulmonary insufficiency on the right ventricle after tetralogy repair. Surgical implications. J Thorac Cardiovasc Surg 1987;93:36.

Kawashima Y, Kitamura S, Nakano S, Yagihara T. Corrective surgery for tetralogy of Fallot without or with minimal right ventriculotomy and with repair of the pulmonary valve. Circulation 1981;64:11.

Kirklin JW, Blackstone EH, Kirklin JK, Pacifico AD, Aremendi J, Bargeron LM Jr. Surgical results and protocols in the spectrum of tetralogy of Fallot. Ann Surg 1983;198:251.

Kirklin JW, Barratt-Boyes BG. Cardiac Surgery, Morphology, Diagnostic Criteria, Natural History, Techniques, Results and Indications. 2nd edn, Churchill Livingstone, New York. 1993, p 863.

Kurasawa H, Imai Y, Becker AE, Surgical anatomy of the atrioventricular conduction bundle in tetralogy of Fallot. New findings relevant to the position of the sutures. J Thorac Cardiovasc Surg 1988;95:586.

Nakata S, Imai Y, Takanashi Y, Kurosawa H, Tezuka M, Nakazawa M, Ando M, Takao A. A new method for the quantitative standardisation of cross-sectional areas of the pulmonary arteries in congenital heart disease with decreased pulmonary flow. J Thorac Cardiovasc Surg 1984;88:610.

Neirotti R, Galindez E, Kreutzer G, Coronel AR, Pedrini M, Becu L. Tetralogy of Fallot with subpulmonary ventricular septal defect. Ann Thorac Surg 1978;25:51.

Pacifico AD. In: Cowgill LD (ed.). Surgical considerations in repair of classical tetralogy of Fallot. Cardiac Surgery. Cynotic Congenital Heart Disease. Hanley and Belfus, Philadelphia, 1989, p 63.

Stellin G, Jonas RA, Goh TH, Brawn WJ, Venables AW, Mee RBB. Surgical treatment of absent pulmonary valve syndrome in infants: Relief of bronchial obstruction. Ann Thorac Surg 1983;36:468.

Stensen N. In: Bartelin T. (1671–72) (ed.), Willins FA (trans). Acta Medica et Philosophica Hafniencia, p 202. An unusually early description of tetralogy of Fallot. Proc Staff Meet Mayo Clin 1948;23:316.

Soto B, Pacifico AD, Cellabos R, Bargeron LM Jr. Tetralogy of Fallot: An angiographic-pathologic correlative study. Circulation 1981; 64:558.

Wessel HU, Cunningham WJ, Paul MH, Bastanier CK, Muster AJ, Idriss FS. Exercise performance in tetralogy of Fallot after intracardiac repair. J Thorac Cardiovasc Surg. 1980;80:582.

Warden HE, DeWall RA, Cohen M, Varco RL, Lillehei CW. A surgical–pathological classification for isolated ventricular septal defects and for those in Fallot's tetralogy based on observations made on 120 patients during repair under direct vision. J Thorac Cardiovasc Surg 1957;33:21.

18 Pulmonary Atresia with Ventricular Septal Defect

Introduction

Hearts with pulmonary atresia and ventricular septal defect merge imperceptibly with tetralogy of Fallot and pulmonary atresia, such that they sometimes are considered together as a single malformation. However, the occasional absence of an identifiable outlet septum and frequency of complex pulmonary arterial arrangements in pulmonary atresia with ventricular septal defect argue for a separate classification. Moreover, in its extreme form, with the complete absence of intrapericardial pulmonary arteries, pulmonary atresia with ventricular septal defect becomes an example of solitary arterial trunk or single outlet of the heart. Undoubtedly, it is the complexity of the pulmonary blood supply rather than the intracardiac morphology that personifies this malformation.

Because there is no pathway for blood from the heart to flow directly to the lungs, another source of pulmonary blood-flow must exist. Usually, this is from a persistently patent arterial duct or from other large collateral vessels that arise directly from the aorta or its major branches, the so-called "major aortopulmonary collateral arteries" or "MAPCAs." On rare occasions, there are still other sources, such as an aortopulmonary window, a persistent fifth aortic arch, or a coronary-to-pulmonary artery fistula. There is no obvious or consistent correlation between the source of pulmonary blood-flow and the arrangement or morphology of the pulmonary arterial tree. When bilateral arterial ducts are present, the pulmonary arteries are usually non-confluent, the duct on the right side arising from either the brachiocephalic or right subclavian artery to supply the right lung and a duct in the usual position supplying the left lung. Although rare, it has been established that an arterial duct and MAPCAs can coexist, and there may or may not be a pulmonary trunk present in these cases. In the absence of a patent arterial duct, major aortopulmonary arteries from the descending aorta are generally the only source of pulmonary blood-flow and

usually number between two and six. When different parts of the lung have different sources of blood, the situation is described as "multifocal" pulmonary blood supply.

"True" or sixth-arch pulmonary arteries in their normal anatomical position (as opposed to the collateral vessels that usually enter the lung on its posterior aspect from the posterior mediastinum) are usually present in some arrangement in pulmonary atresia with ventricular septal defect. In its mildest form, they are well-developed, confluent vessels separated from the right ventricle by only an atretic valve; while at the other extreme, the "true" pulmonary artery may be represented by a tiny or atretic vessel connected to a solitary pulmonary segment. A recent study in a small series of hearts with collateral arteries has shown that nearly two-thirds of the pulmonary segments were connected to central pulmonary arteries and one-quarter to collateral arteries. The remainder had a dual supply from both sources.

Within the lung, vessels of different origins anastomose with each other as far distally as the segmental level, in addition to lobar and hilar connections in so-called "manifolds" or "arterial rings." Rarely, extrapulmonary junctions are also found. Although the collateral arteries have been previously described as bronchial arteries, it has been argued more recently that they represent persistent congenital communications between the descending aorta and the lungs. Certainly they serve an oxygenating role rather than a nutritive one but, nonetheless, their branching patterns and extrapulmonary course remain reminiscent of bronchial arteries. This controversy will be resolved only when it is established whether both bronchial and collateral arteries may exist together.

Within the heart, the major obstruction which prevents blood reaching the "true" pulmonary artery, if one is present, may be at valvar or subvalvar level. Valvar obstruction is an imperforate membrane with the underlying infundibulum extending to its undersurface. When there is complete absence of the valve, the right ventricular infundibular cavity is crowded by hypertrophied muscle, such that the ventricular mass ends blindly without any potential communication to a pulmonary trunk. This is "infundibular" atresia and may represent extreme deviation or malalignment of the outlet septum which has fused with the parietal wall of the right ventricle. Rarely, the outlet septum cannot be identified and the aortic valve connects directly with the right ventricular parietal wall, analogous to what is seen in common arterial trunk.

The ventricular septal defect is usually subaortic and cradled in the angle of the septomarginal trabeculation. It may either be perimembranous, in which case there is likely to be substantial overriding of the aorta, or it may have a muscular postero-inferior margin because the posterior limb of the septomarginal trabeculation has fused with the right ventriculo-infundibular fold. In the perimembranous defect, the conduction tissue runs close to the margin of the ventricular septal defect and on the crest of the septum, thus being more vulnerable than in the muscular defect. With regard to the morphology of the ventricular septal defect and the course of the conduction tissue, these hearts are directly comparable with tetralogy of Fallot (Chapter 17). Also, as in Fallot's tetralogy, the ventricular septal defect is occluded rarely by fibrous tissue tags derived from the tricuspid valve.

The management of pulmonary atresia and ventricular septal defect has evolved steadily over many years, such that there now exists a formidable armamentarium of techniques and procedures that have been employed with varying degrees of success. However, the results of surgical interventions combined with better appreciation of the morphology and natural history, have vastly improved the overall outlook for this group of patients. What is fundamental to the long-term outcome is the pulmonary vasculature, and it is thus important to define clearly the source of pulmonary blood-flow for each of the 20 lung segments, as well as the pressure in major collateral vessels and presence of true, sixth-arch pulmonary arteries.

When the patient has all the pulmonary segments connected to confluent central pulmonary arteries, management proceeds along the lines of that for tetralogy of Fallot, with complete correction or palliation guided by the size of the pulmonary arteries (see Chapter 17). An exception is the occasional patient who has excessive pulmonary blood-flow and elevated pulmonary arterial pressure, who may need early intervention to control heart failure or to prevent the development of obstructive pulmonary vascular disease.

In cases where different parts of the lung are supplied by different sources of pulmonary blood-flow ("multi-focal pulmonary blood supply"), it is now recognized that at least 10, and optimally all 20, pulmonary segments should be joined to the right ventricle for complete correction. Thus, some type of "unifocalization" is necessary, either as staged, preliminary palliation or at the time of complete repair. The advantages of single-stage unifocalization with complete repair through a mid-line sternotomy are: potentially a fewer number of operations, prevention of myointimal stenoses in the collateral vessels, and the early relief of cyanosis and left ventricular volume-overload. This must be balanced against a long operative procedure that is technically demanding and may require considerable post-operative support, including the expertise of diagnostic and interventional cardiac catheterization.

In the case of staged unifocalization, the options are to work "centrally-to-peripherally," or "peripherally-to-centrally." The concept in the former is to bring about enlargement of the "true" pulmonary artery first, followed by the later attachment of collateral arteries. This is usually done by means of an outflow patch, a central shunt or attaching the diminutive true pulmonary artery directly to the ascending aorta via a mid-line sternotomy. Separate left and right thoracotomies are done at subsequent operations to unifocalize each lung.

Many techniques have been described for "peripheral-to-central" unifocalization, which is the only option when "true" intrapericardial pulmonary arteries are completely absent. In general, each collateral vessel is identified in the posterior mediastinum and dissected to its entrance into the lung parenchyma. The collateral vessels are then divided and joined to each other or to the "true" pulmonary artery, which is then connected to the systemic circulation by means of a modified Blalock-Taussig shunt. An alternative is to connect the ligated in situ collateral vessels to a large tube of pericardium, to which the shunt is then constructed. This consolidates all the blood supply to a single source (unifocalization) which is easily accessible and controllable at the time of complete repair. Ideally, it also fosters the development of the pulmonary arterial tree.

The interim results of unifocalization are monitored by cardiac catheterization and angiography within about six months of the procedure to document development of the vessels, exclude pulmonary hypertension, and dilate any stenoses. The possible advantage of staged unifocalization is independence from cardiopulmonary bypass, although it is clearly a labor-intensive protocol, often involving three, four, or five operations to reach complete correction. Overall, however, at least two-thirds of patients presenting with pulmonary atresia and ventricular septal defect should now ultimately achieve two-ventricle separation of the circulations through one or another of these pathways.

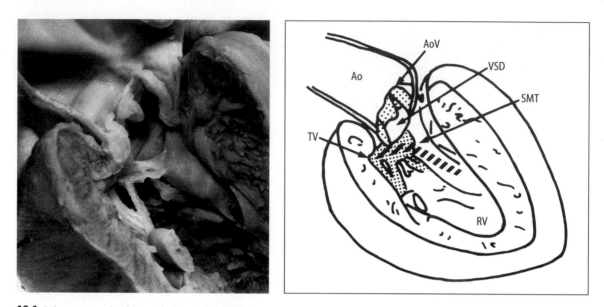

18.1 Pulmonary atresia with ventricular septal defect. The right ventricle has been opened vertically with an incision extended across the aortic valve. The aorta overrides a large perimembranous ventricular septal defect which has fibrous continuity among the tricuspid, aortic and mitral valves in its posterior margin. The wall of the right ventricle is very thick. There is no suggestion of any subpulmonary infundibulum, nor were pulmonary arteries found with the heart.

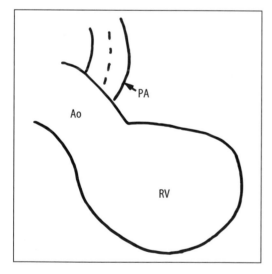

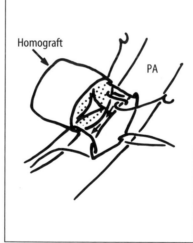

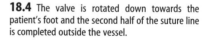

18.2 Complete repair is possible when a sufficient number of segments have been or can be recruited into pulmonary circulation. This involves connecting the pulmonary arteries to the right ventricle, usually with a valved extracardiac conduit. Having controlled all major sources of pulmonary blood-flow, the patient's temperature is reduced to about 30°C–32°C on cardiopulmonary bypass to maintain cardiac action, and a left atrial vent is allowed to drain on the venous line. When confluent, non-stenosed pulmonary arteries are present, an incision is made (without dissection) for the distal end of the conduit.

18.3 A pulmonary homograft is trimmed and joined to the pulmonary arteries with a fine continuous monofilament suture. The upper half of the anastomosis is done first with the valve held up towards the patient's head, working inside the artery. The suture line is interrupted in several places.

18.4 The valve is rotated down towards the patient's foot and the second half of the suture line is completed outside the vessel.

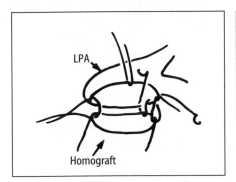

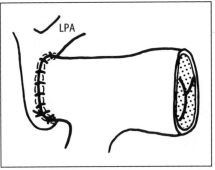

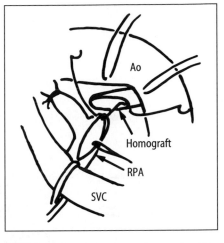

18.5 When the pulmonary arteries are not confluent, it is convenient to use a homograft pulmonary bifurcation to join them. The anastomosis to the left pulmonary artery is usually done first because it is the less accessible. Working inside the vessel (often at the lung hilum), the left branch of the homograft is sutured "end-to-side" to the pulmonary artery with a very fine continuous monofilament suture.

18.6 The anastomosis is completed outside the vessel and the right branch of the homograft is passed beneath the ascending aorta.

18.7 The right pulmonary artery is opened until its maximal diameter is reached, which is often just beyond a systemic pulmonary shunt or collateral vessel. The superior caval vein is retracted laterally and, if necessary, the anastomosis is continued to the lung hilum, working laterally to the caval vein. It is often helpful to suspend the large ascending aorta with heavy stay-sutures to the incision, taking care not to make the valve incompetent. Alternatively, the aorta can be transected for good exposure of the right pulmonary artery.

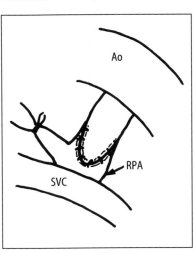

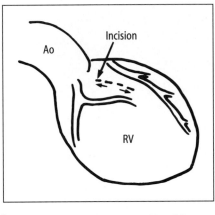

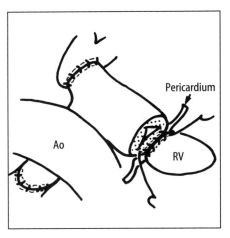

18.8 The completed anastomosis should neither rotate the homograft nor kink the native pulmonary artery. A line drawn on the anterior surface of the homograft prior to insertion will help to maintain its correct orientation.

18.9 *(above)* The ventriculotomy is positioned between major coronary arterial branches. As the aortic valvar leaflets may lie quite anteriorly, the incision is started low down and brought towards the base of the heart, looking inside the ventricle.

18.10 *(right)* After closure of the ventricular and any atrial septal defects, the proximal homograft is joined to the ventriculotomy just where the two lie in apposition. This suture line is started at its mid-point and supported posteriorly with a strip of pericardium. The homograft should not be distorted by pulling it down to the ventriculotomy.

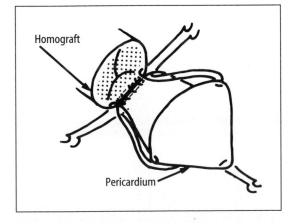

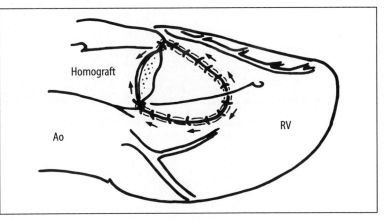

18.11 Anteriorly, a hood of pericardium is fashioned to complete the right ventricular outflow. This is usually more than half the circumference of the homograft. The corners are first anchored to the homograft and ventriculotomy with mattress sutures and the patch is anastomosed to the right ventricular epicardium.

18.12 *(below right)* The final suture line joins the homograft to the patch. When a complete bifurcation has been implanted, it is important to observe that the main pulmonary artery is not redundant and thus kinked. Should this occur, it is divided distally to the valvar sinuses, shortened and reattached to the homograft bifurcation.

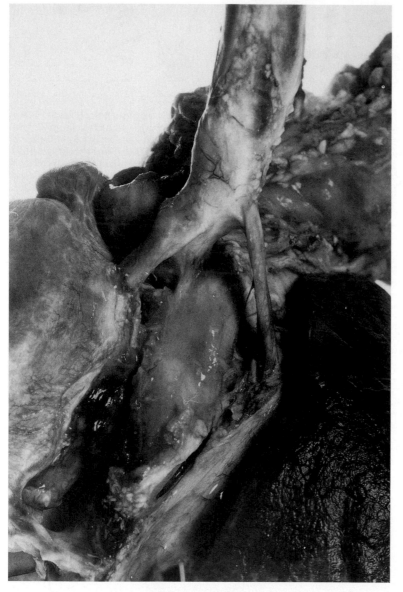

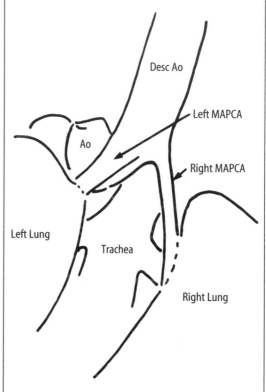

18.13 Pulmonary atresia with ventricular septal defect. Major aorto-pulmonary collateral arteries (MAPCAs). The heart is viewed from behind and the descending thoracic aorta has been lifted to show the collateral vessels to the left and right lungs. These lie behind the trachea and enter the posterior lung hilum. The pulmonary valve is atretic in this heart.

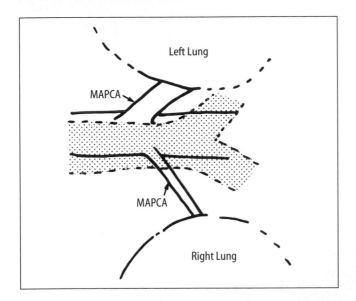

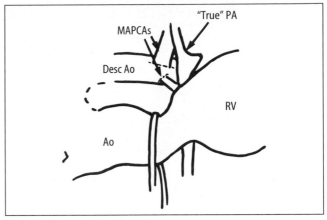

18.15 Alternatively, the descending aorta is exposed by dissecting through the back of the transverse sinus and pericardium. This is possible in pulmonary atresia because the "true" pulmonary arteries are generally small. The collaterals are then controlled at their origins (dashed lines), where they will be divided for unifocalization. The aorta tends to be slightly more accessible when there is a right aortic arch and right-sided descending aorta.

18.14 The anatomy of the preceding heart is shown as the surgeon would find it through a mid-line sternal incision for single-stage unifocalization and complete correction. The trachea and esophagus lie in front of the left-sided descending aorta. The collaterals must be controlled prior to commencement of cardiopulmonary bypass to prevent ventricular distension and systemic hypotension. This can be done by opening each pleural space, retracting the lung downward and towards the mediastinum, and encircling the vessel as it enters the posterior hilum of the lung.

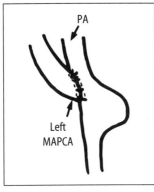

18.16 The left-sided MAPCA is divided with as much length as possible and anastomosed to the "true" pulmonary artery with a very fine suture. If the patient maintains adequate arterial saturation, this can be done without cardiopulmonary bypass. If bypass is needed for oxygenation, the patient is maintained at normothermia with a beating heart until unifocalization is completed.

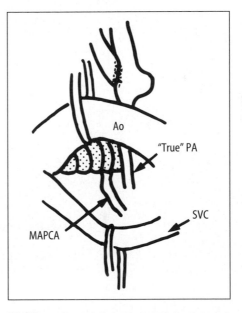

18.17 The right MAPCA is similarly divided at its origin but, in order to get a good anastomosis to the true right pulmonary artery, it is brought to the right side of the mediastinum. Here, the pericardium is opened posteriorly to the phrenic nerve, between the superior caval vein (retracted laterally) and the ascending aorta (retracted medially).

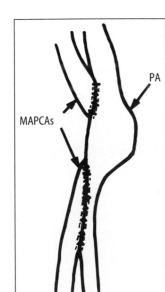

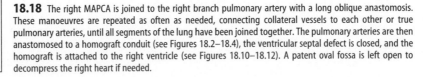

18.18 The right MAPCA is joined to the right branch pulmonary artery with a long oblique anastomosis. These manoeuvres are repeated as often as needed, connecting collateral vessels to each other or true pulmonary arteries, until all segments of the lung have been joined together. The pulmonary arteries are then anastomosed to a homograft conduit (see Figures 18.2–18.4), the ventricular septal defect is closed, and the homograft is attached to the right ventricle (see Figures 18.10–18.12). A patent oval fossa is left open to decompress the right heart if needed.

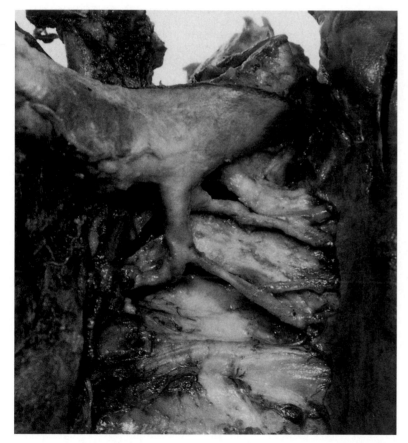

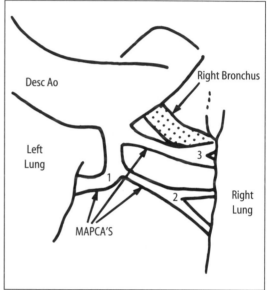

18.19 Pulmonary atresia with ventricular septal defect and MAPCAs. The specimen is viewed from behind with the descending thoracic aorta lifted upwards and to the left. Major aorto-pulmonary collateral vessels (MAPCAs) are given off to the left (1) and right lungs (2 and 3). The upper right collateral vessel enters the lung just posteriorly to the right bronchus, in contrast to a "true" pulmonary artery which would lie in front of the bronchus. The descending aorta is right-sided.

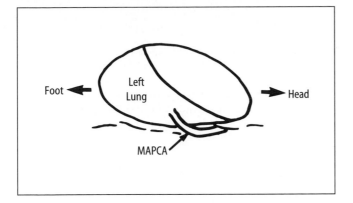

18.20 Staged unifocalization is planned according to the side of the aortic arch, and the origin and distribution of the pulmonary perfusion. In this case, the aortic arch and descending thoracic aorta are right-sided and the collateral to the left lung arises from the same MAPCA as the lower collateral to the right lung. It is likely that perfusion of the right lung will be adequate through its two MAPCAs if the left side is unifocalized first. Removing the left MAPCA should leave a long uncompromised segment of vessel of better caliber for subsequent right unifocalization. The MAPCA is found at the back of the left chest through a standard lateral thoracotomy. It is mobilized as far back into the mediastinum as possible, and the patient is heparinized prior to its division.

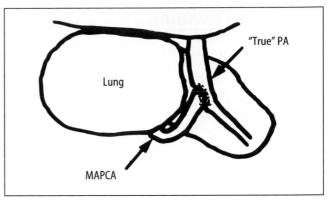

18.21 If a "true" pulmonary artery is present, the divided MAPCA is anastomosed to it (usually end-to-side) at its largest diameter with very fine monofilament sutures. In extremely small vessels, it may be an advantage to use interrupted stitches. When the "true" sixth arch pulmonary artery is too small or the MAPCA is too short to make such a connection, the vessels are joined within the hilum of the lung. Such an anastomosis may be necessary also if myointimal hyperplasia has caused a stenosis in the collateral vessel.

18.22 *(left)* A modified Blalock-Taussig shunt is interposed between the left subclavian artery and the pulmonary artery/ MAPCA as the sole blood supply to the unifocalized left lung.

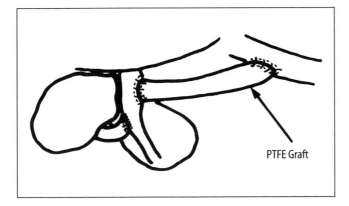

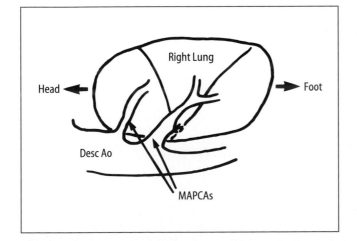

18.23 The right lung is unifocalized through a right thoracotomy at a separate procedure, either during the same hospitalization or at a later time. As the descending aorta is in the right chest, the collateral vessels are dissected to their origins. The aorta is usually decreased in size beyond major collaterals, which may aid their identification.

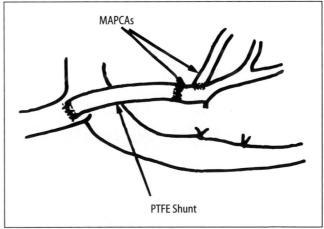

18.24 If a "true" pulmonary artery is not present, the MAPCAs are anastomosed to each other, taking care to relieve any stenotic areas, and then connected to the subclavian artery with a prosthetic tube graft. At the subsequent third-stage procedure through a mid-line sternal insertion, the left and right shunts are replaced with a graft between the arteries to each lung, and this is connected to the right ventricle, with or without complete closure of the ventricular septal defect.

Suggested Reading

Burczynski PL, McKay R, Arnold R, Mitchell DR, Sabino GP. Homograft replacement of the pulmonary artery bifurcation. J Thorac Cardiovasc Surg 1989;98:623.

Fisher EA, Thanopoulos BD, Eckner FAO, Hastreiter AR, DuBrow IW. Pulmonary atresia with obstructed ventricular septal defect. Pediatric Cardiology 1980;1:209.

Haworth SG, Macartney FJ. Growth and development of the pulmonary circulation in pulmonary atresia with ventricular septal defect and major aortopulmonary collateral arteries. Br Heart J 1980;44:14.

Haworth SG, Rees PG, Taylor JFN, Macartney FJ, de Laval M, Stark J. Pulmonary atresia with ventricular septal defect and major aortopulmonary collateral arteries. Effect of systemic pulmonary anastomosis. Br Heart J 1981;45:133.

Iyer KS, Mee RBB. Staged repair of pulmonary atresia with ventricular septal defect and major systemic to pulmonary artery collaterals Ann Thorac Surg 1991;51:65.

Krongrad E, Ritter DG, Hawe A, Kincaid OW, McGoon DC. Pulmonary atresia or severe stenosis and coronary artery – pulmonary artery fistula. Circulation 1972;46:1005.

Liao PK, Edwards WD, Julsrud PR, Puga FJ, Danielson GK, Feldt RH. Pulmonary blood supply in patients with pulmonary atresia and ventricular septal defect. J Am Coll Cardiol 1985;6:1343.

Macartney FJ, Scott O, Deverall PB. Hemodynamic and anatomical characteristics of pulmonary blood supply in pulmonary atresia with ventricular septal defect including a case of persistent fifth arch. Br Heart J 1974;36:1049.

McKay R, Stark J, de Laval M. Unusual vascular ring in infant with pulmonary atresia and ventricular septal defect. Br Heart J 1982; 48:180.

Rossi M, Rossi Filho R, Ho SY. Solitary arterial trunk with pulmonary atresia and arteries with supply to the left lung from both an arterial duct and systemic to pulmonary collateral arteries. Int J Cardiol 1988;20:145.

Rossi RN, Hislop A, Anderson RH, Martins FM, Cook AC. Systemic-to-pulmonary blood supply in tetralogy of Fallot with pulmonary atresia. Cardiol Young 2002;12:373.

Sawatari K, Imai Y, Kurosawa H, Ismatsu Y, Momma K. Staged operation for pulmonary atresia and ventricular septal defect with major aortopulmonary collateral arteries. New technique for complete unifocalisation. J Thorac Cardiovasc. Surg 1989;98;738.

Shimazaki Y, Tokuan Y, Iio M, Nakano S, Matsuda H, Blackstone EH, Kirklin JW, Shirakura R, Ogawa M, Kawashima Y. Pulmonary artery pressure and resistance late after repair of tetralogy of Fallot with pulmonary atresia. J Thorac Cardiovasc Surg 1990; 100:425.

Shore DF, Ho SY, Anderson RH, de Laval M, Lincoln C. Aorto-pulmonary septal defect coexisting with ventricular septal defect and pulmonary atresia. Annals of Thoracic Surgery 1983;35:132.

Thiene G, Frescura C, Bini RM, Valente ML, Galluci V. Histology of pulmonary atresia with ventricular septal defect. Circulation 1979; 60:1066.

Tynan MJ, Gleeson JA. Pulmonary atresia with bronchial arteries arising from the subclavian arteries. Br Heart J 1966;28:573.

19 Hypoplastic Left Heart Syndrome

Introduction

The constellation of anomalies that define the hypoplastic left heart syndrome is linked by the underdevelopment of those structures that enable the left ventricle to support the systemic circulation. Because this definition is, to a degree, a physiological one, the morphological characteristics of the hypoplastic left heart syndrome are diverse. Moreover, the anatomical concepts have often been explored and refined in response to a surgical intervention (mainly the Norwood operation), which has sometimes further blurred their understanding and application in both morphological research and clinical practice.

Historically, the terminology "hypoplastic left heart syndrome" was introduced to describe underdevelopment of the aorta, either as an isolated lesion or in combination with valvar aortic stenosis or atresia, or ventricular septal defect. At present, it is generally applied to hearts that have stenosis or atresia of the aortic valve, hypoplasia of the ascending aorta, and usually (but not invariably) an extremely small left ventricle. While these features may be found also in hearts with complete or congenitally corrected transposition of the great arteries, inclusion in hypoplastic left heart syndrome is limited to situations in which at least the pulmonary trunk arises from the morphologically right ventricle. Hearts with univentricular atrioventricular connection (so-called "single ventricle" with obstruction to the systemic outflow) are also excluded, although exceptions have been made in cases of complete atrioventricular septal defect with extreme malalignment of a common atrioventricular valve committed to the right ventricle. The differentiation of hypoplastic left heart syndrome from critical aortic stenosis remains arbitrary and is based more on features that predict a clinical outcome of successful biventricular repair than on strict anatomical criteria. However, overall, it requires more than just a small left ventricle to classify a malformation as hypoplastic left heart syndrome.

The aortic valve in hypoplastic left heart syndrome is either stenotic or atretic, the majority of hearts having the latter morphology. In the presence of aortic atresia, the ascending aorta functions merely as a long coronary artery to receive retrograde flow from the aortic arch and its lumen is correspondingly reduced to a diameter of 1–2 mm. Hearts with aortic stenosis, in contrast, tend to have a larger ascending aorta of about 2–3 times this width. The vessel is very thin-walled and fragile. Its narrowest diameter may be either at the sinutubular junction or at the junction with the innominate branch and transverse aortic arch. The transverse aortic arch is also, by definition, hypoplastic to a variable degree and may be completely interrupted. Coarctation of the aorta, when defined as a shelf of intimal tissue at the junction of the persistently patent arterial duct and the aortic isthmus, is present in about 80% of cases.

The mitral valve is also hypoplastic or atretic in this syndrome, and four subgroups may be categorized according to their respective combinations of aortic and mitral atresia (the most common) or stenosis. These groups correlate to a degree with other morphological findings. For instance, a smaller left ventricle is usually found in hearts with both aortic and mitral atresia, and a higher incidence of coronary artery anomalies in those with aortic atresia and mitral stenosis. However, these variations have not been found to influence surgical outcome. The mitral valve is said to be atretic even if it is indistinguishable (absent altogether), or otherwise when a dimple in the floor of the left atrium shows the only evidence of its position. On the other hand, it is also atretic if it is composed of imperforate valvar tissue. Stenotic valves usually have thickened leaflets with short thickened tendenous cords and short papillary muscles, but occasionally the leaflets are structurally normal and merely miniaturized.

The left ventricle is variable in size but usually extremely small and sometimes unidentifiable on gross dissection. Externally, it is usually delineated by the epicardial coronary arteries and does not reach the apex of the heart. When the mitral valve is patent, endocardial fibrosis is invariably present. Less extreme degrees of ventricular hypoplasia are found with the association with patency of either the inlet (mitral) or outlet (aortic) valve and atresia of the complementary outlet or inlet valve respectively. In the presence of a ventricular septal defect, the left ventricle may achieve normal or nearly normal dimensions, even when there is aortic atresia. This gives rise to the possibility of neonatal biventricular repair for the hypoplastic left heart syndrome, an oxymoron that has been addressed by renaming such cases "hypoplastic left heart complex." Interventricular communications, when present, are not infrequently multiple.

The left atrium, which nearly always (in 95% of cases) receives the pulmonary veins, is smaller than normal. This is often the consequence of leftward deviation of the atrial septum. The left atrial walls are usually hypertrophied and may be covered with endocardial fibrosis. The right atrium is enlarged and an atrial septal defect or persistently patent flap valve of the oval fossa usually provides an outlet to the left side of the heart. Restriction of this communication, however, may occur through premature closure of the flap valve of the oval fossa, a developmentally small foramen ovale, or an aneurysm of the flap valve. A mild degree of restriction may be hemodynamically beneficial after birth by elevating pulmonary venous pressure, which in turn favours the systemic circulation by decreasing pulmonary perfusion. However, severe obstruction results in profound hypoxia and marked elevation of pulmonary vascular resistance.

The right ventricle supports both the systemic and the pulmonary circulations. It always shows some degree of enlargement and constitutes the apex of the heart. The right ventricle is usually hypertrophied, although occasional thin-walled chambers have been encountered. When the ventricular septum is extremely hypoplastic, components of the septomarginal trabeculation are frequently detached from the ventricular wall, carrying the tension apparatus for the tricuspid valve into a free-standing arrangement. This occasionally produces abnormal anatomic spaces. Otherwise, when the septum is hypoplastic, the septomarginal trabeculation may be adherent either to the medial or even the superior wall of the right ventricle. The septum occasionally shows a pronounced curvature into the right ventricle. Whether these morphological variations in the components of the right ventricle, along with those in the thickness of the right ventricular walls, have implications for ventricular function is speculative at present. The tricuspid valvar orifice may be enlarged, but the leaflets themselves, with rare exceptions, are normally formed. Often, the tension apparatus shows

asymmetrical patterns. "Parachute"-type tricuspid valves have been reported, in which case the cavity of the right ventricle is frequently dilated.

The main pulmonary artery, like other parts of the right heart, is invariably enlarged to a considerable degree and continues into the descending aorta through an even larger persistently patent arterial duct. Its left and right branches, both arising from the posterior surface of the main pulmonary artery with the right more proximal than the left, however, tend to show less pronounced dilatation and have an extensive increase in smooth muscle throughout the arteriolar walls. The pulmonary valve occasionally has two sinuses and two leaflets which may be dysplastic, but the right ventricular outflow remains widely patent. Patency of the arterial duct is also essential for survival and, on occasion, this structure has been found to be tortuous or aneurysmally enlarged.

Although arising from the diminutive aortic root, the origins and the proximal course of the coronary arteries are usually normal. Frequently, however, portions of the coronary arterial walls are thickened, dilated, and tortuous. Fistulous communications with the left ventricle are well described. All the coronary arterial abnormalities occur more frequently in hearts with mitral stenosis and aortic atresia, as does endocardial fibroelastosis of the left ventricle. Again, this has not been documented to impact on clinical course or surgical outcome.

The management of hypoplastic left heart syndrome involves a tour de force of surgical technique, precise physiological regulation of the circulation, and teamwork among the cardiologist, anesthetist, intensivist, the family of the patient, and supporting technical and nursing staff. While some units decline this undertaking on the grounds that the results of treatment do not justify the extensive commitment of resources, there can be little remaining doubt at the present time that many patients with various forms of hypoplastic left heart syndrome now enjoy many years of life with good quality after either staged palliation to the Fontan circulation or cardiac transplantation. Moreover, the care of patients with hypoplastic left heart syndrome develops capabilities within a congenital heart programme which then benefit other patients with complex cardiac malformations, particularly of the single ventricle type.

Diagnosis of hypoplastic left heart syndrome is reliably established by echocardiography, often before birth, and there is no longer any place for diagnostic cardiac catheterization in this group of patients. At the end of the spectrums of critical aortic stenosis and mitral valvar stenosis, the morphology merges with that of the hypoplastic left heart syndrome, and the systemic circulation will not be supported adequately by the left heart. These cases need, in addition to precise and detailed echocardiographic measurements, good clinical judgement and careful decision-making as to whether a two-ventricle repair should be attempted or the patient should embark upon the Norwood–Fontan pathway. Additionally, there are a few patients with aortic valvar atresia – the hallmark of hypoplastic left heart syndrome – in whom the left ventricle is well developed by virtue of an associated ventricular septal defect. For them, a two-ventricle repair is appropriate. Given the higher risk of mortality in patients with other associated cardiac defects, genetic syndromes, or extracardiac malformations, it is imperative that the patient is fully investigated also for non-cardiac problems before planning the management of the heart anomaly.

Preoperative resuscitation and stabilization are essential prior to either the first stage Norwood procedure or cardiac transplantation. As systemic perfusion is through the arterial duct, its patency is maintained by prostaglandin infusion, avoidance of supplemental oxygen, and correction of acidosis. It is also essential that the patient has a minimally or unrestrictive interatrial communication. If this is not present, preliminary surgical septectomy or catheter dilation may be necessary to relieve hypoxia for successful resuscitation. Beyond this, systemic and pulmonary blood-flow is determined by the relative resistances in the respective circulations. Manoeuvres which decrease the pulmonary resistance (such as hyperventilation of the patient) will compromise the systemic perfusion, with resulting metabolic acidosis and impairment of organ function. These are strenuously avoided preoperatively. It is only when the patient has been physiologically and metabolically normalized that surgical intervention should proceed. In this regard it must be appreciated that, unlike an arterial switch operation for transposed great arteries or the correction of common arterial trunk, first-stage palliation of the hypoplastic left heart syndrome makes no improvement to the patient's circulation, but still adds all the damaging effects of cardiopulmonary bypass and surgical trauma to a sick neonate. Patients in whom right ventricular function remains impaired and/or for whom there is severe tricuspid valvar regurgitation despite the correction of all other metabolic disturbances should, therefore, possibly be considered for cardiac transplantation if this option is available, as ultimate attainment of a successful Fontan circulation is highly unlikely.

For those entering the Norwood–Fontan protocol, the traditional first stage involves reconstruction of the aortic arch with relief of any coarctation, connection of the main pulmonary artery to the aorta as the systemic outflow of the heart, atrial septectomy, and provision of pulmonary blood-flow by some type of systemic-pulmonary anastomosis. A variety of techniques have been employed to this end as so-called "modified"

Norwood procedures. Recently, a right ventricular to pulmonary artery shunt has been advocated with the theoretical advantages of making both the systemic (particularly the coronary) and the pulmonary blood-flow less dependent on the manipulation of pulmonary arterial resistance in the early post-operative period. These procedures are done through a mid-line sternotomy with either low-flow cardiopulmonary bypass, or profound hypothermia, and total circulatory arrest. While attempts have been made to use closed interventional techniques for palliation (such as ductal infiltration with formaldehyde or, more recently, stenting along with branch pulmonary artery banding), these have rarely produced survivors who were subsequently good candidates for the Fontan operation.

In the post-operative period following a first stage Norwood procedure, systemic and pulmonary blood-flow remain competitive and critically influenced by rapidly changing pulmonary vascular resistance, the manipulation of which demands constant and precise intervention. However, mechanical problems such as residual arch obstruction or a blocking systemic-pulmonary shunt must always be considered as potential sources of hemodynamic decompensation. These often require cardiac catheterization for the planning of surgical revision or interventional management. Early results suggest that the substitution of a right ventricular to pulmonary artery shunt for the systemic-pulmonary anastomosis, possibly in combination with the avoidance of total circulatory arrest, may alleviate much of the hemodynamic instability that has traditionally characterized the early post-operative course of these patients. Beyond the immediate post-operative period, the normal decline in pulmonary vascular resistance tends to favor increasing pulmonary blood-flow, which is generally more or less balanced by the somatic growth of the infant.

The Fontan circulation (see Chapter 24) constitutes definitive palliation for hypoplastic left heart syndrome and is usually achieved through a bidirectional cavopulmonary anastomosis or hemi-Fontan operation as an intermediate step. In general, patients who require additional procedures that are not amenable to techniques of interventional cardiology, such as the augmentation of branch pulmonary arteries or relief of recoarctation, will have this done at the time of a bidirectional cavopulmonary anastomosis. When the results of first stage palliation are truly optimal, occasional patients proceed directly to Fontan completion, with or without fenestration of the atrial baffle. In some cases, at the other extreme, there is impairment of ventricular function or worsening of tricuspid valvar regurgitation after the initial palliation. For these patients, cardiac transplantation remains an option and is preferable to a poor outcome with the Fontan circulation. Overall, about 60–70% of patients entering single ventricle treatment protocols eventually achieve successful separation of the circulations with a Fontan operation. While hypoplastic left heart syndrome thus remains among the highest risk groups for congenital heart surgery, there is now an encouraging degree of success with this malformation, which otherwise carries about a 95% mortality during the first month of life.

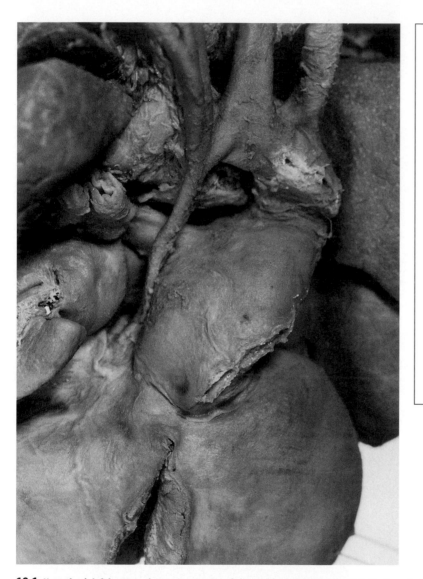

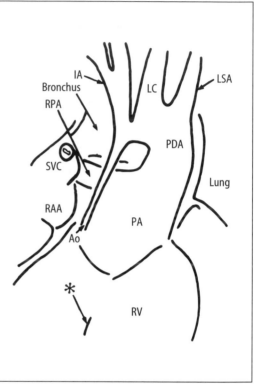

19.1 Hypoplastic left heart syndrome. Anterior view of a heart with atretic aortic valve and a tiny imperforate mitral valve, showing the roots of both the aorta and the pulmonary artery. The left ventricle (not seen) in this heart is extremely hypoplastic but does not have endocardial fibroelastosis. Both the large arterial duct and the oval fossa are widely patent, and the tricuspid valve is normal. A preductal coarctation shelf is present internally (not seen), and the left subclavian artery arises distally to the shelf, opposite the arterial duct. The right ventricle is dilated and its wall is thickened (asterisk).

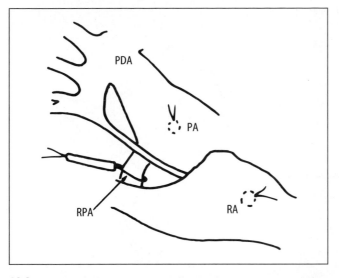

19.2 In preparation for the first stage Norwood procedure, the heart is exposed through a mid-line sternal incision, and purse-strings for cannulation are placed on the main pulmonary artery and the right atrium at its junction with the appendage. This site, in preference to the atrial appendage, facilitates later atrial septectomy through the cannulation site. The right pulmonary artery is encircled and, if needed to limit pulmonary blood-flow and support the systemic circulation, partially snared.

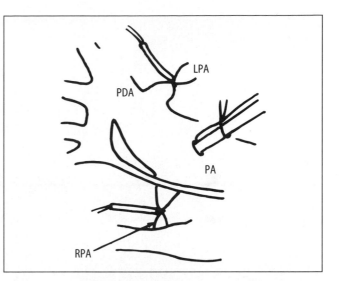

19.3 On cardiopulmonary bypass, the right pulmonary artery is occluded immediately and the left pulmonary artery is also encircled and snared. While the patient is cooled for profound hypothermia and total circulatory arrest, the branches of the aortic arch are dissected, as is the upper descending aorta.

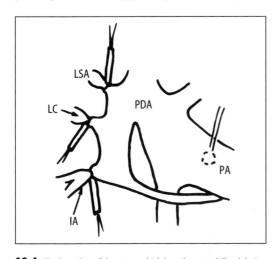

19.4 The branches of the aorta, which have been mobilized during cooling, are snared for total circulatory arrest. After clamping the aortic cannula cardioplegia is infused through the aortic cannula while the descending aorta is compressed with forceps and the venous side of the circulation is drained. The pulmonary arterial snares are then removed, as are the arterial and venous perfusion cannulas.

19.5 In order to avoid total circulatory arrest, a Gore-tex graft (which may be used later as the systemic- to pulmonary artery shunt) is first anastamosed to the innominate artery after heparinization of the patient.

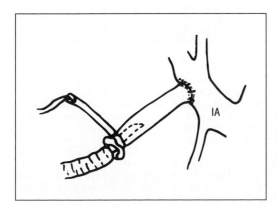

19.6 *(left)* The graft is deaired by allowing flow from the innominate artery down the PTFE tube, and then cannulated for arterial perfusion from the cardiopulmonary bypass machine. If the aortic arch is interrupted or extremely hypoplastic, it may be necessary to cannulate also either the arterial duct or the descending aorta to perfuse the lower half of the body.

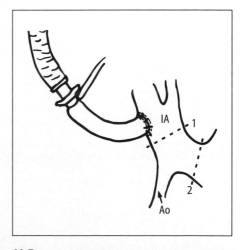

19.7 For reconstruction of the aortic arch in a classical Norwood procedure, the innominate artery is clamped (1) and flow is reduced appropriately for the patient's size. If a modification is used that does not involve opening the ascending aorta and proximal arch, the aorta may be clamped between the innominate and left carotid branches (2), which permits coronary as well as cerebral perfusion.

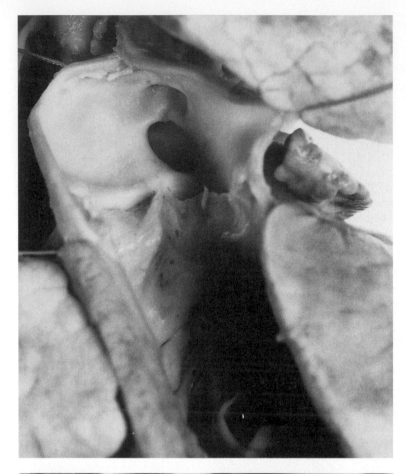

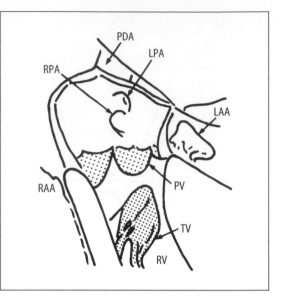

19.8 Hypoplastic left heart syndrome. Pulmonary arterial origins. This heart has absent left atrioventricular connection (mitral atresia), with a hypoplastic left ventricle and small dysplastic aortic valve overriding a perimembranous ventricular septal defect (potential double-outlet right ventricle). The subaortic outflow, however, is obstructed by aneurysmal tricuspid valvar tissue, and the tricuspid leaflets are slightly thickened on their edges. There is a patent arterial duct and an atrial septal defect of the oval fossa (not seen). The right and left branch pulmonary arteries originate from the back of the main pulmonary artery with the left pulmonary artery almost vertically distal to the right.

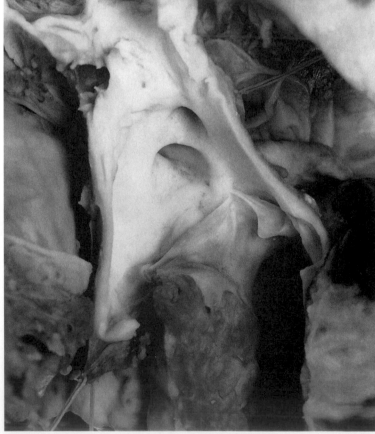

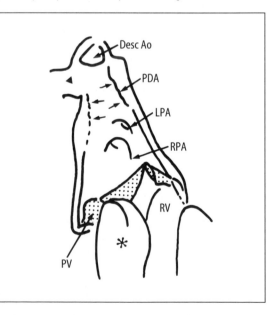

19.9 The right branch pulmonary artery in this heart arises from the right posterior aspect of the main pulmonary artery, just above the sinu-tubular junction. The left branch pulmonary artery is more distal, from the left posterior aspect. Their orifices are essentially in a superior–inferior relationship. The hypoplastic left ventricle (not seen) is associated with an atretic aortic valve and a miniaturized mitral valve. It has no endocardial fibrosis. The oval fossa is patent and the tricuspid valve normal (not seen). The right ventricle is thick (asterisk) and dilated. Ridges in the arterial duct (small arrows) indicate that it is closing and show the proximity of ductal tissue to the origins of the branch pulmonary arteries. A preductal coarctation shelf is present (triangle).

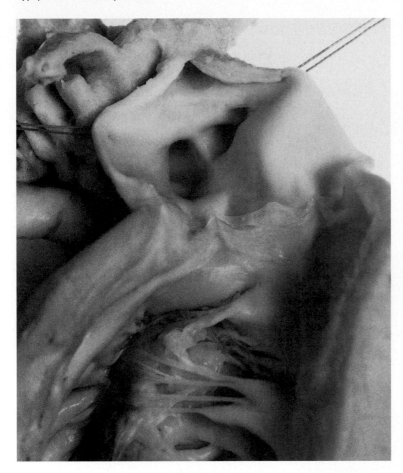

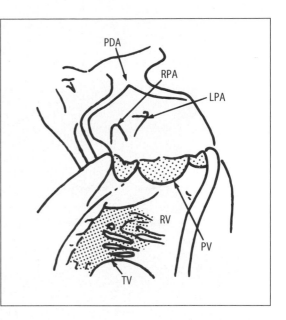

19.10 The right pulmonary artery is again given off just above the sinutubular junction, but the left branch is only slightly more distal than the right in its origin. Both orifices are on the posterior aspect of the main pulmonary artery, which continues to the descending aorta as a widely patent arterial duct. The aortic valve in this heart is atretic, and the mitral valve is miniaturized and dysplastic (none of these features are seen here). The tiny left ventricle has endocardial fibrosis. An atrial septal defect is present in the oval fossa. The right ventricular wall is slightly thickened, but the cavity is dilated. The tricuspid valve is normal.

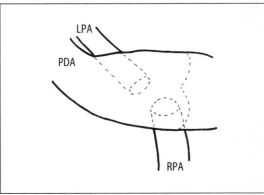

19.11 When the main pulmonary artery is divided, it should be remembered that its branches arise posteriorly, often one above the other, and the right is usually near the sinutubular junction.

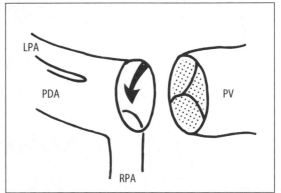

19.12 The main pulmonary artery (which will be augmented with a homograft patch) is divided just at or above the sinutubular junction to avoid stitching to the delicate sinus tissue, but as far below the origin of the right pulmonary artery as possible to avoid subsequent "bifurcation" stenosis.

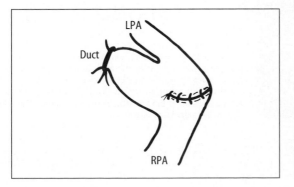

19.13 The excess pulmonary arterial wall on the anterior leftward side often permits direct closure of the distal segment with a fine continuous monofilament suture. Alternatively, the bifurcation is closed with a patch of pericardium or homograft pulmonary artery. The arterial duct is ligated at its junction with the descending aorta to avoid narrowing the origin of the left pulmonary artery.

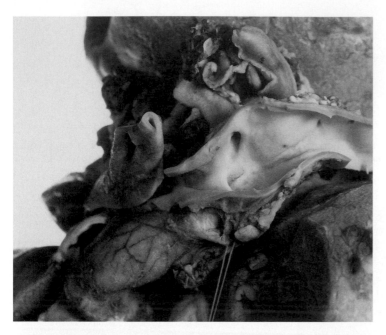

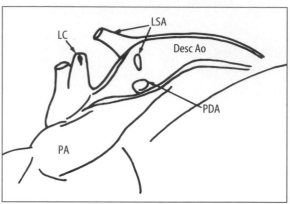

19.14 Hypoplastic left heart syndrome. Aortic arch and isthmus (left). The aortic arch has been opened across the isthmus into the descending aorta. The entry of the arterial duct is opposite the origin of the left subclavian artery. There is no coarctation of the aorta, although its diameter widens beyond the site of the arterial duct, and there is a slight protuberance of tissue above the entrance of the arterial duct.

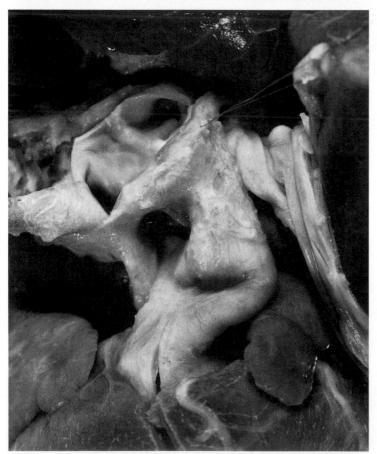

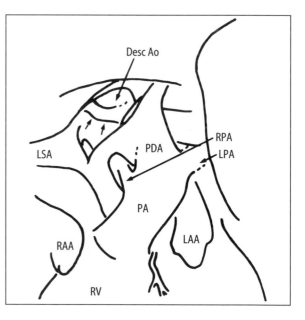

19.15 *(left)* The aortic isthmus, opposite a widely patent arterial duct in a different heart, is viewed from above, looking into the descending aorta. A well-defined, preductal coarctation shelf is present (small arrows). The main pulmonary artery (which has not been opened) gives off the right and left branch pulmonary arteries and then continues as the arterial duct. In this heart the oval fossa is patent, but its flap valve is aneurysmal (see Figure 19.42). The aortic valve is atretic and the mitral valve is miniaturized. The right ventricle is thick-walled and slightly dilated.

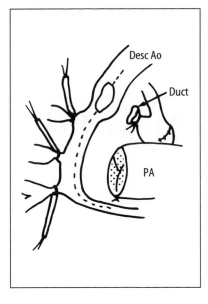

19.16 *(left)* After its ligation, the arterial duct is resected from the aorta, which provides an entrance into the aortic isthmus for reconstruction of the aorta. This incision is extended distally for about half a centimeter and proximally around the undersurface of the aortic arch, into the small ascending aorta to the level at which the pulmonary artery is divided. As the pulmonary artery is quite distensible, this point is usefully marked with fine stay-suture prior to circulatory arrest.

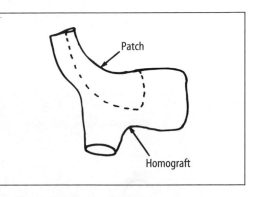

19.17 *(above)* A patch for the augmentation of the arch is cut, ideally, from a pulmonary homograft. The size and shape of the patch are critical to achieve an unobstructed systemic outflow and to avoid the distortion of the branch pulmonary arteries, which will lie behind it. The curve of the patch is approximated by the main and left branch pulmonary arteries of the homograft. Its length is that of the aortotomy and the base should equal the circumference of the native pulmonary trunk minus the circumference of the ascending aorta. In practice, the proximal portion of the patch, with the ascending aorta, may be conceptualized as a tube which replaces the arterial duct and moves it proximally on the aortic arch, while the distal part is a patch to enlarge the distal aorta and isthmus. As the homograft is also distensible, its size is made a little smaller than the native pulmonary trunk.

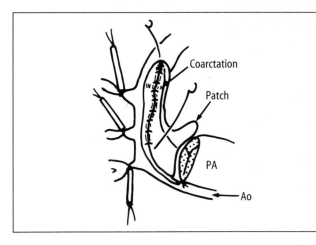

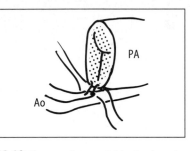

19.19 The ascending aorta is joined to the native pulmonary artery with at least three interrupted sutures to avoid kinking the small vessel.

19.18 Stitching the homograft patch to the aorta begins with the posterior wall of the descending aorta, working towards the surgeon inside the vessel and using a fine continuous monofilament suture. Any significant coarctation shelf is excised and the patch is carried well beyond the entrance of the arterial duct.

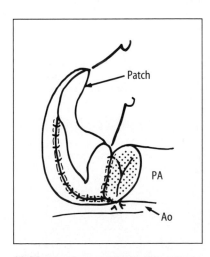

19.20 When the posterior suture line reaches the junction of the ascending aorta with the pulmonary artery, it continues around the pulmonary trunk.

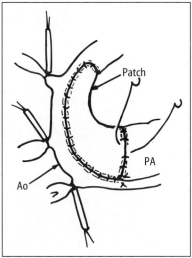

19.21 The reconstruction is completed anteriorly, running the second arm of the suture outside the vessels and homograft patch.

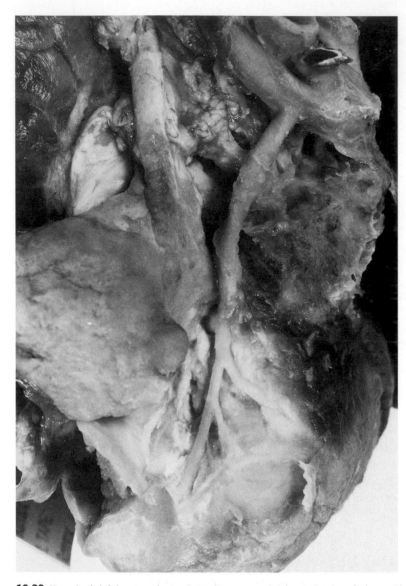

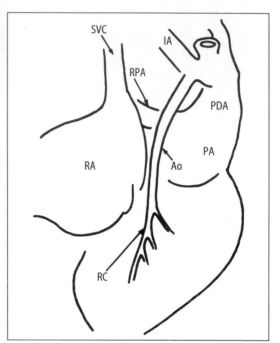

19.22 **Hypoplastic left heart syndrome.** External appearance. A right anterior view of a heart with atretic aortic valve shows a dissection of the ascending aorta and right coronary artery, which are of about equal size. In this heart, the slit-like left ventricle has no endocardial fibroelastosis, but fibrosis is present in the left atrium. The mitral valve (not seen) is represented by a dimple with a small orifice but no evidence of tension apparatus. The right ventricle is moderately hypertrophied and dilated, with delamination of the posterior edge of the septomarginal trabeculation from the septum (not seen). The arterial duct is patent. An atrial septostomy had been performed. This illustration emphasizes the function of the ascending aorta as a coronary artery.

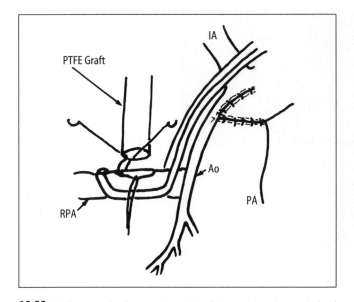

19.23 The first stage of palliation with a traditional Norwood procedure is completed by re-establishing a source of pulmonary blood-flow with a systemic pulmonary anastomosis. When a modified Blalock-Taussig shunt is done, it is usually placed between the right pulmonary artery and the distal innominate or proximal subclavian artery. If the proximal end has not already been done for cardiopulmonary perfusion (see Figures 19.5–19.7), both anastomoses may be done while the patient is rewarmed on cardiopulmonary bypass. Although the pulmonary artery is empty at this time, a side-biting clamp helps to expose the vessel. Care must be taken that this does not compress the small ascending aorta with resulting myocardial ischemia.

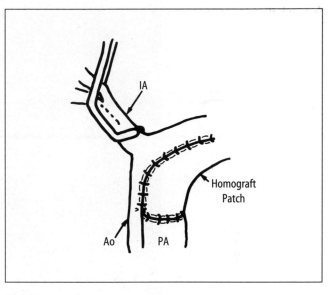

19.24 After the pulmonary anastomosis has been completed, a side-biting clamp is placed on the innominate artery and its branches. A longitudinal incision is made on the lower surface of the vessel, which can be rotated upward in the clamp if needed.

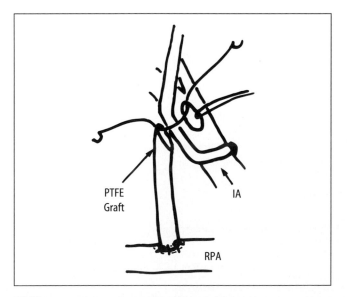

19.25 The proximal end of the graft is joined to the subclavian or innominate artery with a fine continuous monofilament suture.

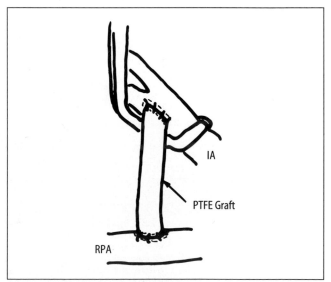

19.26 On completion, the graft takes a direct path to the right pulmonary artery or is angled slightly towards the left branch. The clamp is removed from the innominate artery and the shunt is occluded until the patient is ready to be weaned from cardiopulmonary bypass.

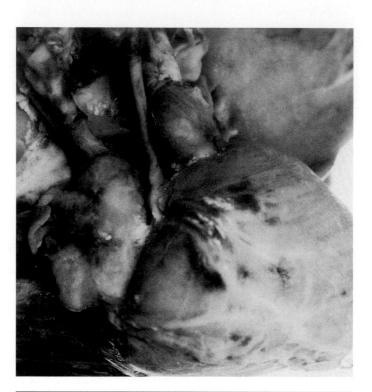

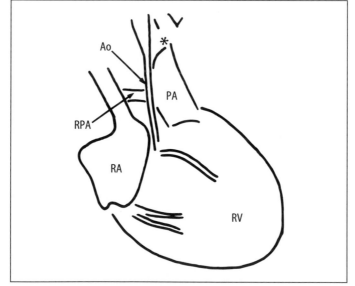

19.27 Hypoplastic left heart syndrome. Solitary ventricle, examined after a modified Norwood procedure. Neither a cavity nor an inlet valve of a second ventricle could be identified in the ventricular mass by blunt dissection. The aortic valve is also atretic, such that the coronary arteries are supplied retrogradely through the threadlike ascending aorta. A common atrium is present. The divided main pulmonary artery has been anastomosed to the junction of the left subclavian artery with the descending aorta (asterisk), and the pulmonary confluence is supplied through a posterior Waterston-type (aorto-pulmonary) anastomosis (not seen).

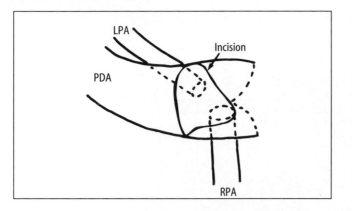

19.28 A number of technical modifications to the Norwood procedure have been described, mainly to avoid the implantation of prosthetic material and/or to reduce the length of the operation. In most of these, it is necessary to mobilize the descending aorta, such that it can be brought upwards towards the anterior mediastinum. The pulmonary artery is divided as far distally as possible to conserve the length on the proximal main pulmonary artery.

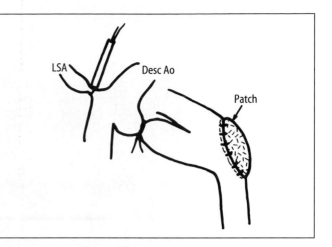

19.29 It then becomes necessary to close the distal pulmonary artery with a patch, usually of autogenous pericardium. The arterial duct is ligated at its junction with the aorta and all distal duct tissue is resected from the aorta.

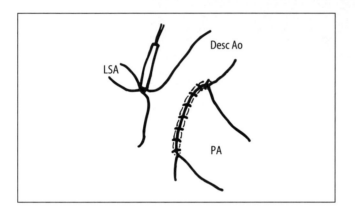

19.30 The pulmonary artery is anastomosed directly to the descending aorta, aortic isthmus and distal transverse aortic arch.

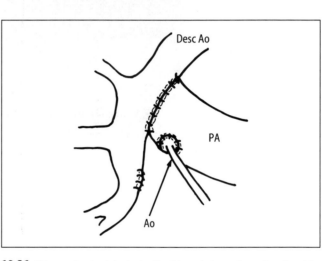

19.31 This procedure tends to shorten the distance between the aortic arch and the heart, particularly if a very wide main pulmonary artery reaches back to the undersurface of the transverse arch. Should this cause kinking of the ascending aorta, it is resected from the arch with a button of vessel wall and anastomosed to the pulmonary artery, analagous to a coronary artery anastomosis.

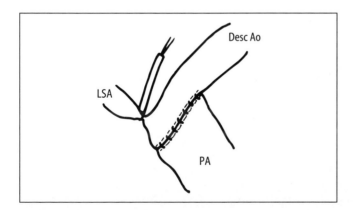

19.32 A variation on this technique is to divide the transverse aortic arch between the left common carotid and left subclavian arteries and create a long oblique "end-to-end" anastomosis with the main pulmonary artery.

19.33 *(right)* The proximal transverse aortic arch is then trimmed, if needed, and reattached to the side of the main pulmonary artery. All these techniques have the possible advantage of tissue-to-tissue apposition which conserves growth potential. However, there is a very definite risk of compression of the left pulmonary artery with subsequent stenosis and hypoplasia if the reconstruction is under any tension.

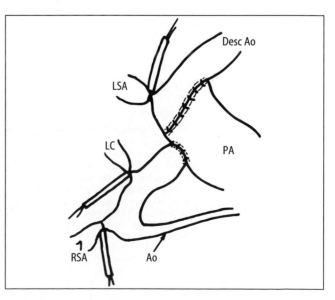

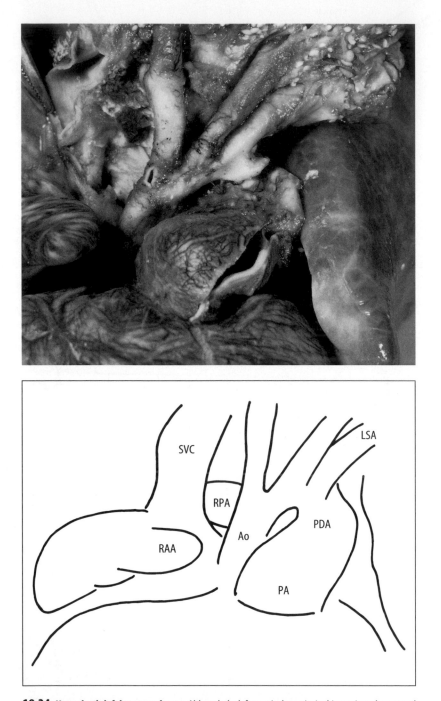

19.34 Hypoplastic left heart syndrome. Although the left ventricular cavity in this specimen has normal linear measurements, its walls are very thin by comparison with normal values, and the mitral valve is small, dysplastic, and stenotic. The aortic valve has three leaflets and three sinuses but is also small. The ascending aorta is of much better calibre than is usually seen in hypoplastic left heart syndrome, and, despite being inadequate to carry the entire systemic output, it probably does have significant antegrade flow. The pulmonary valve has three leaflets and sinuses, but the two facing the aorta are dysplastic. A tortuous arterial duct joins the descending aorta beyond a slightly hypoplastic aortic isthmus. The tricuspid valve is slightly dysplastic, and the right ventricle is thin-walled, dilated and covered with endocardial fibroelastosis. An atrial septal defect of the oval fossa is present, but the interventricular septum is intact. While arguably not a "hypoplastic left heart," hearts like this clearly fall into the Norwood-Fontan type of management.

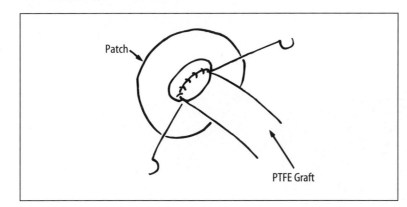

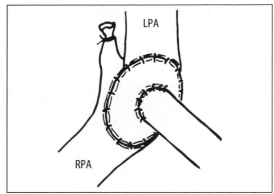

19.35 The management of this heart is particularly difficult because the mitral valve is stenotic on the left side and the right ventricle is poor on the other side of the circulation. If transplantation is not an option, the unusually large main pulmonary artery makes one of the modified Norwood procedures (see Figures 19.28–19.33) attractive to minimize or eliminate myocardial ischemic time. The use of a right ventricle to pulmonary artery shunt may also be advantageous to maintain diastolic perfusion pressure in the coronary arterial circulation post-operatively. In preparation for this, a cuff of Gore-tex patch is sewn to a 5 mm PTFE graft prior to the commencement of cardiopulmonary bypass.

19.36 The main pulmonary artery is divided as far distally as possible, and the graft carrying the PTFE shunt is anastamosed to the pulmonary bifurcation with a running monofilament suture. This can be done on bypass with the heart being perfused through a graft on the innominate artery (see Figures 19.5–19.7).

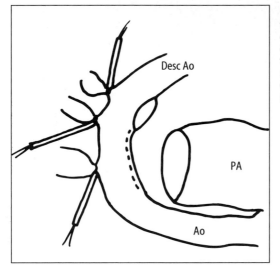

19.37 (*left*)The undersurface of the aortic arch is opened proximally and distally from the site where the arterial duct has been resected to match the diameter of the main pulmonary artery.

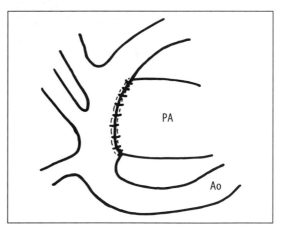

19.38 Since the ascending aorta is of good size, it is unlikely to become kinked and probably will continue to contribute forward flow after connection of the pulmonary artery to the aortic arch.

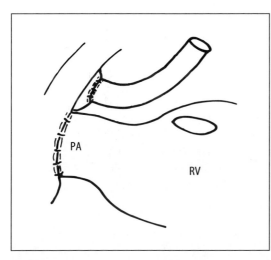

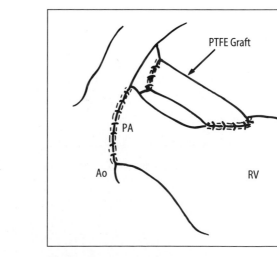

19.39 A right ventriculotomy is made as far leftward as possible and muscle is resected along the inner side of the incision. The incision is lower than that used in a right ventricular to pulmonary artery conduit for pulmonary atresia, for example, because the pulmonary valvar leaflets may be found further down on the subpulmonary infundibulum.

19.40 Anastomosis of the PTFE graft to the ventriculotomy completes the repair. The graft is carefully trimmed. If it is too short, it may compress the left anterior descending coronary artery, while a graft that is too long will kink as it passes from the anterior aspect of the ventricle back to the pulmonary artery.

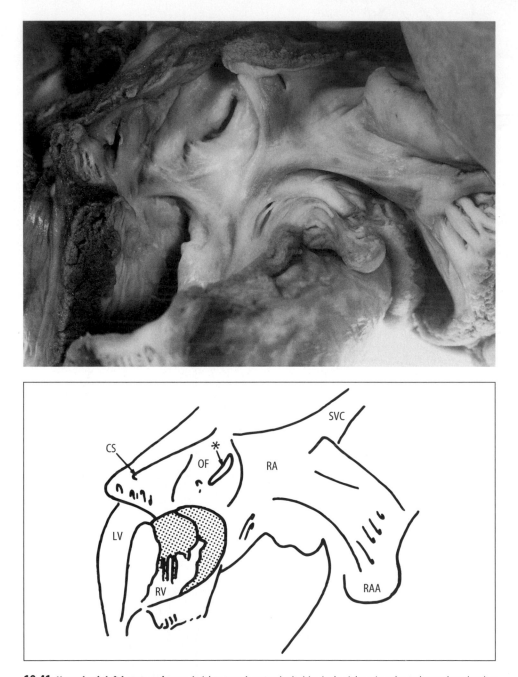

19.41 Hypoplastic left heart syndrome. Atrial septum. An extensive incision in the right atrium shows the patulous chamber with a slit-like defect (asterisk) in the oval fossa. This heart also has aortic atresia, a dysplastic miniaturized mitral valve, and endo-cardial fibroelastosis of the hypoplastic left ventricle. There is endocardial fibroelastosis in the moderately thick-walled right ventricle also, although the tricuspid valve (poorly seen) is normal. Coarctation of the aorta is present and the arterial duct is closed (not seen).

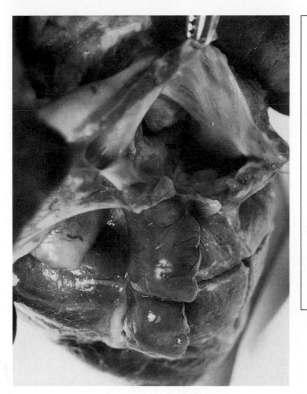

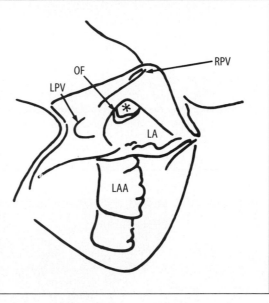

19.42 This left atrial view in a different heart with atretic aortic valve and miniaturized mitral valve shows a thickened aneurysmal flap valve (asterisk), virtually occluding the patent oval fossa. The left ventricle is extremely hypoplastic and the right ventricle is thick-walled. There is also generalized hypoplasia of the aortic arch. The arterial duct is patent and the tricuspid valve is normal.

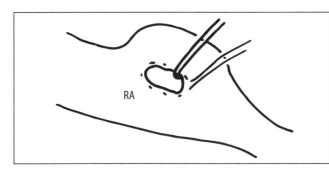

19.43 An unrestrictive interatrial communication is essential for pulmonary venous blood to return to the systemic circulation. Under total circulatory arrest or a brief period of myocardial ischemia if the heart is perfused, either before or after reconstruction of the aortic arch, the venous cannula is removed and the atrial septum is exposed through the cannulation site.

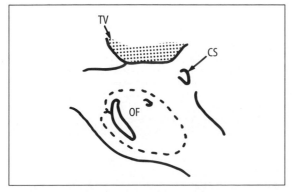

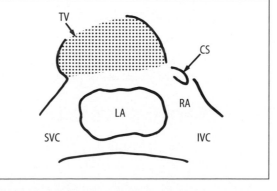

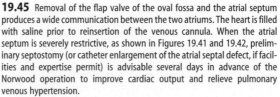

19.44 Having identified the oval fossa, the tricuspid valve, and the orifice of the coronary sinus, an incision is made to the top of the oval fossa. This is carried clockwise and counter-clockwise, beyond the oval fossa, to the bottom of the interatrial septum near the inferior caval vein (dashed line).

19.45 Removal of the flap valve of the oval fossa and the atrial septum produces a wide communication between the two atriums. The heart is filled with saline prior to reinsertion of the venous cannula. When the atrial septum is severely restrictive, as shown in Figures 19.41 and 19.42, preliminary septostomy (or catheter enlargement of the atrial septal defect, if facilities and expertise permit) is advisable several days in advance of the Norwood operation to improve cardiac output and relieve pulmonary venous hypertension.

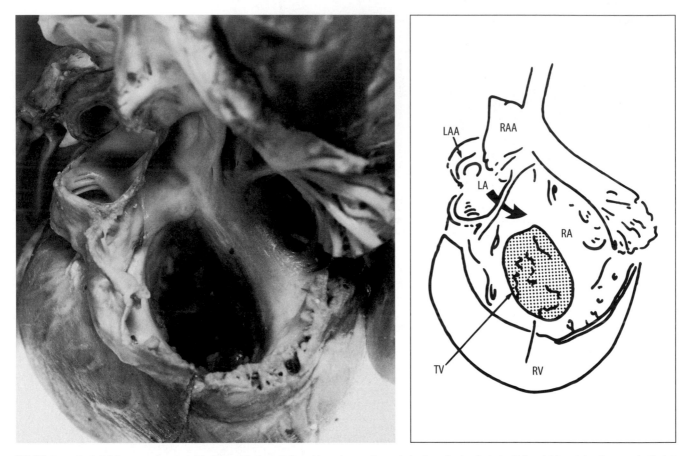

19.46 **Hypoplastic left heart syndrome.** Atrial relations. The heart is viewed from above and posteriorly after reflecting the incised left and right atrial walls anteriorly. The left atrioventricular connection is absent and the small left atrium drains through a large atrial septal defect of the oval fossa (arrow) into the much larger right atrium. The left ventricle is a slit-like cavity (not seen) and the right ventricle is a thin-walled dilated chamber. The septomarginal trabeculation is delaminated from the septal surface and thus is a free-standing structure between its points of attachment to the right ventricle. The potential ventriculo-arterial connection is a double-outlet right ventricle.

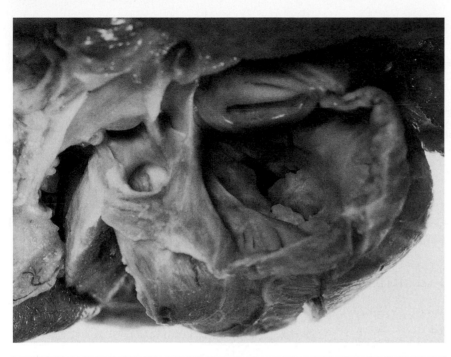

19.47 In a view similar to that of the previous specimen (Figure 19.46), the discrepancy between the large right atrium and small left atrium is again apparent. The mitral valve is miniaturized, while the tricuspid valve is normal. The two small arrows indicate the lower limbus of an atrial septal defect of the oval fossa. The endocardium of the left ventricle (not seen) is thick and fibrosed, while the right ventricle is thick-walled but not dilated. The arterial duct (not seen) is patent in this case.

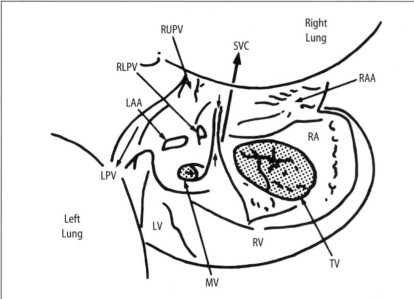

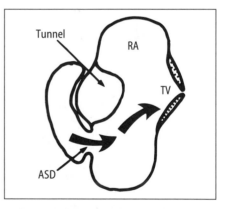

19.49 The relationship of a lateral tunnel to the atrial septal defect and tricuspid valve are shown diagrammatically in cross-section. Blood from the left atrium must drain around the tunnel (arrows) to the tricuspid valve.

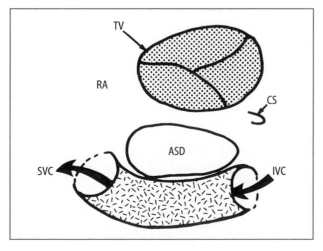

19.48 *(left)* Following successful first-stage palliation, patients with hypoplastic left heart syndrome become candidates for the Fontan circulation, either as a staged or single procedure (see Chapter 24). As illustrated in the above specimen and shown diagramatically here, the pathway routing blood from the inferior caval vein should be in a position that obstructs neither the interatrial communication nor the tricuspid valve. This is best achieved with a carefully positioned lateral tunnel or an extracardiac connection using an interposition graft.

Suggested Reading

Aiello VD, Ho SY, Anderson RH, Thiene G. Morphologic features of hypoplastic left heart syndrome – a reappraisal. Pediatric Pathology 1990;10:931.

Altmann K, Printz BF, Solowiejczyk DE, Gersony WM, Quaegebeur J, Apfel HD. Two-dimensional echocardiographic assessment of right ventricular function as a predictor of outcome in hypoplastic left heart syndrome. Am J Cardiol 2000;86;964–968

Anderson RH, Macartney FJ, Shinebourne EA, Tynan M (eds). Mitral valve anomalies and supravalvar ring. In: Paediatric Cardiology, Vol 2, Churchill Livingstone; Edinburgh, London, Melbourne, New York. 1987, Chapter 42:1023.

Asou T. Arch reconstruction without circulatory arrest: Historical perspectives and initial clinical results. Semin Thorac Cardiovasc Surg Pediatr Card Surg Annu 2002;5:89.

Bailey L, Concepion W, Shattuck H, Huang L. Method of heart transplantation for treatment of hypoplastic left heart syndrome. J Thorac Cardiovasc Surg 1986;92:1.

Bailey LL, Nehlsen-Cannarella SL, Doroshow RW, Jackobson JG, Martin RD, Allard MW, Hyde MR, Bui RHD, Petry EL. Cardiac allotransplantation in newborns as therapy for hypoplastic left heart syndrome. N Eng J Med 1986;315:949.

Barber G, Helton JG, Aglira BA, Chin AJ, Murphy JD, Pigott JD, Norwood WI. The significance of tricuspid regurgitation in hypoplastic left heart syndrome. Am Heart J 1988;116(6Pt I):1563.

Bartram U, Grunenfelder J, Van Praagh R. Causes of death after the modified Norwood procedure: a study of 122 postmortem cases. Ann Thorac Surg 1997;64 (6):1795.

Bharati S, Lev M. The surgical anatomy of hypoplasia of aortic tract complex. J Thorac Cardiovasc Surg 1984;88:97.

Chang AC, Farrell PE, Murdison KA, Baffa JM, Barber G, Norwood WI, Murphey JD. Hypoplastic left heart syndrome: Hemodynamic and angiographic assessment after initial reconstructive surgery and relevance to modified Fontan procedure. J Am Coll Cardiol 1991;17:1143.

Freedom RM. Atresia or hypoplasia of the atrioventricular and/or ventriculo-arterial junction. In: Anderson RH, Macartney FT, Shinebourne EA, Tynan M (eds). Paediatric Cardiology, Vol 2. Churchill Livingstone; Edinburgh, 1987, pp 737.

Gaynor JW, Mahle WT, Cohen MI, Ittenbach RF, DeCAmpli WM, Steven JM, Nicolson SC, Spray TL. Risk factors for mortality after the Norwood procedure. Eur J Cardiothorac Surg 2002;22:82.

Gittenberger-de Groot AC, Wenink ACG. Mitral atresia: morphological details. Br Heart J 1984;51:252.

Jonas RA, Lang P, Hansen D, Hickey P, Castaneda AR. First stage palliation of hypoplastic left heart syndrome. J Thorac Cardiovasc Surg 1986;92:6.

Lloyd TR, Evans TC, Marvin WJ Jr. Morphologic determinants of coronary blood-flow in the hypoplastic left heart syndrome. Am Heart J 1986;112(4):666.

Lloyd TR, Marvin WJ Jr. Age at death in the hypoplastic left heart syndrome: Multivariate analysis and importance of the coronary arteries. American Heart J 1989;117, 6:1337.

Mickell JJ, Mathews RA, Anderson RH, Zuberbuhler JR, Lenox CC, Neches WH, Park SC, Fricker FJ. The anatomical heterogeneity of hearts lacking a patent communication between the left atrium and the ventricular mass (mitral atresia) in presence of a patent aortic valve. European Heart J 1983;4:447.

Moodie DS, Gill CC, Sterba R, Stewart R, Ratliff NB. The hypoplastic left heart syndrome: evidence of preoperative myocardial and hepatic infarction in spite of prostaglandin therapy. Ann Thorac Surg 1986;42:307.

Norwood WI, Long P, Hansen D. Physiologic repair of aortic atresia – hypoplastic left heart syndrome. N Eng J Med 1983;308:23.

O'Connor WN, Cash JB, Cattril CM, Johnson GL, Noonan JA. Ventriculo-coronary connections in hypoplastic left hearts. An autposy microscopic study. Circulation 1982;66:1078.

Pigott JD, Murphy JD, Barber G, Norwood WI. Palliative reconstructive surgery for hypoplastic left heart syndrome. Ann Thorac Surg 1988;45:122.

Roberts WC, Perry LW, Chandra RS, Myers GE, Shapiro SR, Scott LP. Aortic valve atresia: a new classification based on necropsy study of 73 cases. Am J Cardiol 1976;37:753.

Ruschhaupt DG, Moshiree M, Lev M, Bharati S. Echocardiogram in mitral-aortic atresia. False identification of the ventricular septum and left ventricle. Pediatr Cardiol 1980;1:281.

Rychik J, Murdison KA, Chin AJ, Norwood WI. Surgical management of severe aortic outflow obstruction in lesions other than hypoplastic left heart syndrome. J Am Coll Cardiol 1991;18:809.

Sauer U, Gittenberger-de Groot AC, Geishauser M, Babic R, Buhlmeyer K. Coronary arteries in the hypoplastic left heart syndrome. Circulation 1989;80 (suppl I):I–168.

Starnes VA, Griffin ML, Pitlick PT, Bernstein D, Baum D, Ivens K, Shumway NE. Current approach to hypoplastic left heart syndrome. Palliation, transplantation, or both? J Thorac Cardiovasc Surg 1992;104:189.

Seliem MA, Chin AJ, Norwood WI. Patterns of anomalous pulmonary venous connection/drainage in hypoplastic left heart syndrome: diagnostic role of Doppler color flow mapping and surgical implications. J Am Coll Cardiol 1992;19:135.

Sinha SN, Rusnak SL, Sommers HM, Cole RB, Muster AJ, Paul MH. Hypoplastic left ventricle syndrome – analysis of thirty autopsy cases in infants with surgical considerations. Am J Cardiol 1978; 21:166.

4

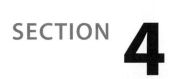

Four-chambered Hearts with Abnormal Ventriculo-arterial Connections

20 Common Arterial Trunk

Introduction

Common arterial trunk (persistent arterial trunk, truncus arteriosus) is the type of single cardiac outlet in which one vessel gives off the coronary, pulmonary, and systemic circulations within the pericardium. It is distinguished from aorto-pulmonary window by the presence of a single outlet valve, and also from pulmonary atresia with ventricular septal defect and major aortopulmonary collateral arteries (Collett's so-called "Type IV truncus arteriosus") by the origin of at least one pulmonary artery from the common arterial trunk. Variability occurs not only in the origins of the pulmonary arteries, which forms the basis of both anatomical and clinical classifications, but also in the morphology of the truncal valve, the coronary arteries, and the ventricular septal defect.

When the branch pulmonary arteries both arise from a common stem, the lesion is designated "Type I." The single orifice usually lies on the posterior leftward aspect of the common trunk, downstream from the valvar sinuses, and gives off left and right branches which pass to the lungs in the usual positions. Occasionally, the branches spiral around one another. In "Type II" common arterial trunk, the pulmonary arteries are given off by separate but adjacent orifices that also tend to lie on the posterior or leftward portion of the trunk. "Type III" malformations are much less common. In these, the two-branch pulmonary arteries arise from more widely separated orifices that may be on opposite sides of the trunk and/or at different levels. Occasionally, one pulmonary artery originates from the common trunk and the other (usually left), from a persistently patent arterial duct. "Type IV" truncus arteriosus is now recognized as a variant of pulmonary atresia with ventricular septal defect, in which true pulmonary arteries are completely absent and major collateral vessels from the descending aorta, as opposed to the trunk, supply the pulmonary blood-flow.

Although it is not structurally identical to a normal aortic valve, the truncal valve usually has three leaflets and retains fibrous continuity with the mitral valve. Less commonly, there are two leaflets or even four or more. The valve typically lies above the ventricular septal defect, arising from both ventricles, although it may be committed predominately to either the left or the right ventricle. When committed to the right ventricle, continuity with the mitral valve is occasionally lost, resulting in a completely muscular outflow and potential obstruction at the level of the ventricular septal defect. The spectrum of morphology of the valvar leaflets ranges from those that are grossly normal to valves that are severely deformed and thickened by myxomatous material. Clinically, the latter may result in truncal valvar stenosis and regurgitation.

Most ventricular septal defects in hearts with common arterial trunk lie between the two limbs of the septomarginal trabeculation and thus have a completely muscular lower margin. This shelters the conduction tissue from the edge of the defect. When the posterior limb of the septomarginal trabeculation fails to fuse with the right ventriculo-infundibular fold, there is continuity between the truncal and tricuspid valves which renders the defect perimembranous in its location. In these cases, the conduction tissue runs along the posterior margin of the defect. The defect is usually large and "subarterial," being roofed by the common truncal valve. However, restrictive ventricular septal defects have been described in common arterial trunk and, when the truncal valve attaches to the crest of the ventricular septum, this can virtually obliterate the interventricular communication. Multiple muscular defects are also an extremely rare but clinically important occurrence.

The coronary arteries generally arise from two orifices but may lie above the sinutubular junction. This occurs more often with the left coronary artery than with the right. Rarely, an orifice is found within a pulmonary arterial branch (usually the right). An important variation which is frequently seen is the presence of large infundibular branches arising from the right coronary artery. These supply the upper portion of the ventricular septum in hearts where the left anterior descending branch is small and displaced inferiorly, and must be respected in siting a right ventriculotomy.

A persistently patent arterial duct, contrary to former precepts, may be associated with common arterial trunk. When the ascending aorta is large and the aortic arch is well developed, a patent arterial duct is less likely to be present than when there is associated hypoplasia or coarctation of the aorta. Persistently patent arterial duct is invariable in common arterial trunk with interrupted aortic arch, and in these hearts, the left pulmonary artery may arise virtually within the arterial duct. Interruption of the aortic arch, which may be distal to the left subclavian artery (Celoria's Type A) or distal to the left common carotid artery (Type B), is found at post-mortem examination in about 20% of hearts with common arterial trunk. Other anomalies which are rarely associated with common arterial trunk include abnormal atrial arrangement or atrioventricular connections.

The circulatory implications of common arterial trunk are volume overloading of the left ventricle, coronary arterial insufficiency from rapid diastolic run-off into the lungs, and excessive pulmonary bloodflow. All these are exacerbated by a falling pulmonary vascular resistance after birth and may be compounded further by truncal valvar stenosis or regurgitation and/or obstruction of the aortic arch. Historically, because of the complexity of surgical repair, operation was either deferred or directed towards palliative procedures. As a result of established myocardial and pulmonary damage, such management rarely achieved widespread success. With the growing experience of neonatal open-heart surgery, it has become routine to carry out complete correction in the neonate at the first appearance of any signs of heart failure. In general, this is done either with profound hypothermia and circulatory arrest, or on cardiopulmonary bypass. The repair consists of detaching the pulmonary arteries from the common trunk; closing

the resulting defect in the trunk without injury to a coronary artery or distortion of the truncal valve; closing the ventricular septal defect, such that there is unobstructed flow from the left ventricle to the trunk; closing the persistent arterial duct when this is present and connecting the pulmonary arteries to the right ventricle without compromise of major coronary arterial branches. It may be useful to leave a patent oval fossa or to close only partially an interatrial defect to allow decompression of the right ventricle early post-operatively. These objectives have been met successfully by a variety of surgical techniques, each of which has its own merits and hazards, and must be individualized to the circumstances of a given patient. In all but the Type I common arterial trunk, most surgeons now completely divide the trunk for removal of the pulmonary arteries. Controversy remains regarding the necessity of a valved extracardiac conduit to connect the pulmonary arteries to the right ventricle, and many techniques of non-valved anastomoses have also given encouraging results. Stenotic and incompetent truncal valves are generally repaired at the time of complete primary correction.

In some cases, with severe associated cardiac malformations, limited infrastructure for neonatal open-heart surgery or extremely complex cardiac anatomy (such as severe truncal valvar stenosis with disconnected left pulmonary artery), staged palliation may still offer the best overall survival. Palliation in such a patient, for example, could include balloon valvuloplasty of the stenotic truncal valve with control of pulmonary bloodflow by some type of banding technique, followed later by a systemic-pulmonary anastomosis to the left pulmonary artery when the duct has become restrictive, and ultimate correction with truncal valve replacement and a pulmonary bifurcation homograft. For the vast majority of patients, however, complete primary correction in the neonatal period remains the management protocol of choice, recognizing that virtually all patients will require further operations to repair or replace the right ventricular outflow reconstruction.

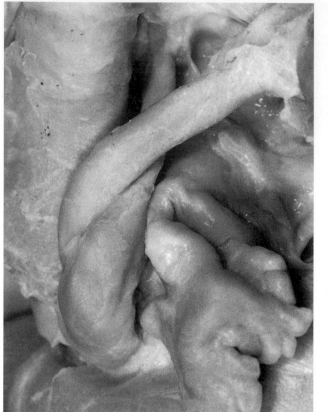

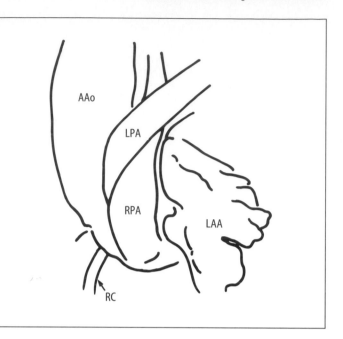

20.1 Common arterial trunk, Type I. External view from the left side showing the ascending aorta, the right coronary artery and the pulmonary arteries arising from the common arterial trunk. The pulmonary arteries spiral around each another.

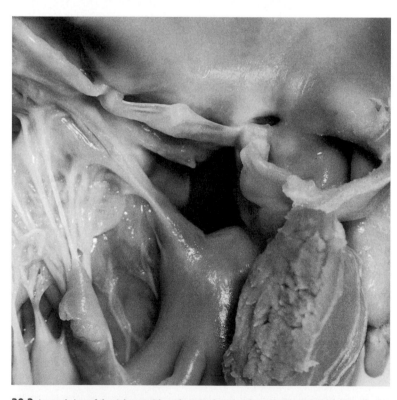

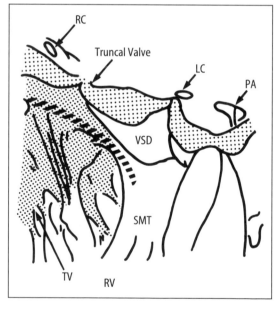

20.2 Internal view of the right ventricle and proximal trunk. A large ventricular septal defect lies between the limbs of the septomarginal trabeculation, the posterior division of which supports the medial papillary muscle complex and has not fused with the right ventriculo-infundibular fold. The defect is thus perimembranous, with a long area of continuity between the truncal and tricuspid valves. Conduction tissue passes along the lower margin of the defect. The truncal valve has three relatively normal leaflets. In the absence of an outlet septum, these form the upper margin of the ventricular septal defect, which is thus also a subarterial defect. About half of the truncal valve lies over each ventricle. The large right coronary artery arises within the sinus of Valsalva, but the left lies at the sinutubular junction, above a commissure of the valve and close to the origin of the pulmonary artery. The orifice of the pulmonary artery is unusually proximal, within the truncal valve sinus.

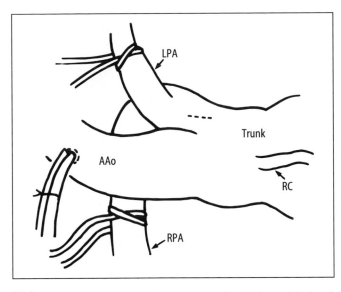

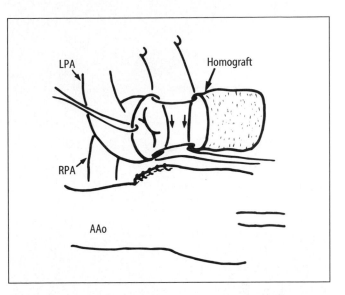

20.3 For complete repair, the ascending aorta is cannulated high up and the branch pulmonary arteries are encircled with vascular slings which occlude the vessels upon commencement of bypass. Limited constriction prior to that time will improve systemic and coronary arterial pressures. Although this is Type I trunk, the short main pulmonary artery arises unusually proximally, within the sinus of Valsalva. Its length is thus not obvious externally, so after cross-clamping the aorta, a short vertical incision is made (dashed line) anteriorly on the main pulmonary artery, to look inside the vessel. The positions of the valvar leaflets and coronary arterial origins are carefully noted, prior to extending this incision for the removal of the pulmonary arteries.

20.4 When there is sufficient length, the main pulmonary artery is divided a few millimeters beyond the truncal sinus. Its truncal end is closed primarily with a running suture in two layers. This will leave very little length before the origins of the branch pulmonary arteries, the orientation of which is maintained with stay-sutures to avoid rotation during attachment to the homograft valve. An end-to-end anastomosis is used to join the pulmonary arteries to a homograft or non-valved conduit.

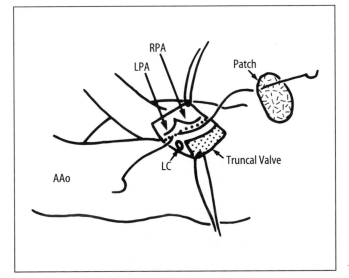

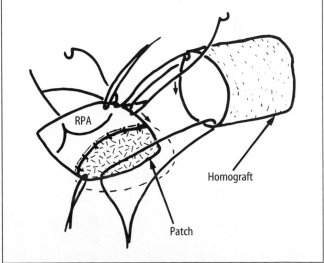

20.5 A useful alternative in this situation, which may avoid distortion of the truncal sinus of Valsalva, is to leave the short low pulmonary artery in situ and "septate" the trunk with a patch. The patch is sutured to the pulmonary arterial wall, below the origins of the branch pulmonary arteries. The coronary arteries and truncal valve remain on the aortic side of the patch. The first sutures are placed above the left coronary arterial orifice, such that good visualization ensures there is no injury to the vessel.

20.6 The homograft is then anastomosed to the incision in the main pulmonary artery with a fine continuous monofilament suture. The graft must be bevelled to arch gently towards the pulmonary artery. As the vessels are not mobilized, this technique should minimize the potential for kinking of the right or left pulmonary arterial branches. It is preferred over the excision of sinus tissue with a short main pulmonary artery, which then requires patch reconstruction of the sinus and may be complicated by bleeding from the delicate tissues or by truncal valve regurgitation from the distortion of the sinus. If a homograft valve is not available, the lower edge of the pulmonary arterial incision may be fashioned into a flap and turned down directly on to the right ventriculotomy. The outflow is then completed anteriorly with a pericardial or monocusp patch.

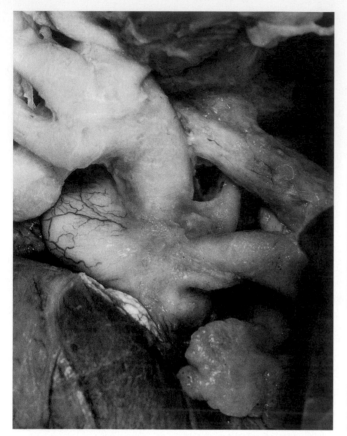

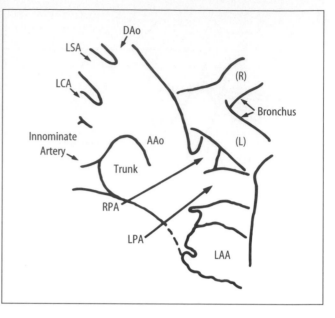

20.7 Common arterial trunk, Type II. Left anterior view in which the aortic arch has been retracted and rotated rightwards to demonstrate the relationships between the common trunk, the pulmonary arteries, and the bronchi. The pulmonary arteries arise adjacently to each other from the posterior leftward aspect of the trunk.

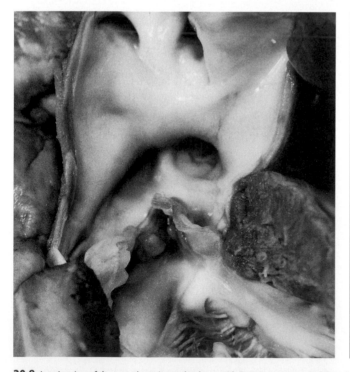

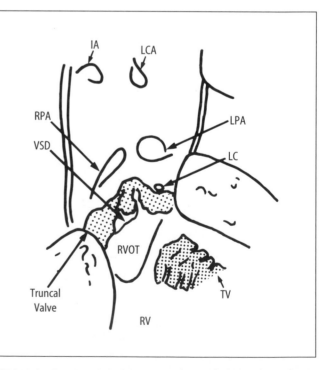

20.8 Interior view of the truncal root in another heart with Type II common arterial trunk. This heart has discordant atrioventricular connections, which is extremely rare in association with common arterial trunk. The branch pulmonary arteries stem from adjacent origins distally to the truncal valve. The left coronary artery, which supplies the left-sided morphologically right ventricle, is within the truncal sinus and the truncal valve is mildly dysplastic. The origins of the innominate and left common carotid vessels are visualized a short distance beyond the pulmonary branches. The trunk is connected predominantly to the left-sided morphologically right ventricle, such that only a corner of the muscular ventricular septal defect and some tricuspid valvar leaflet are seen.

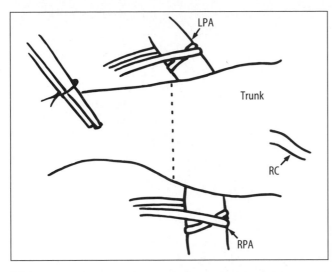

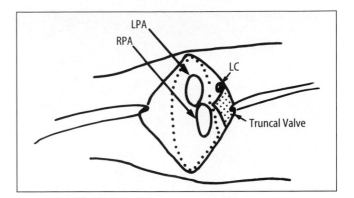

20.9 Complete primary repair of Type II common arterial trunk is performed through a vertical mid-line sternotomy, using profound hypothermia with circulatory arrest or periods of low pump flow. The ascending aorta is cannulated as high as possible above the pulmonary arterial origins to leave room for its division (dashed line) below a cross-clamp. Alternatively, if circulatory arrest is employed, the cross-clamp may be placed beyond a slightly more proximal aortic cannula. The branch pulmonary arteries are occluded during perfusion until the aorta has been clamped and cardioplegia infused.

20.10 Through a transverse incision above the truncal valvar sinuses, the positions of the coronary arterial orifices, truncal valvar leaflets, and branch pulmonary arteries are carefully inspected. The incision is then extended around the back of the trunk/ascending aorta to excise the pulmonary arteries with as much surrounding vessel wall as possible (dotted line). It is imperative to avoid injury to a coronary artery or truncal valve. This may dictate favoring these structures and leaving less tissue on some areas of the pulmonary arterial patch.

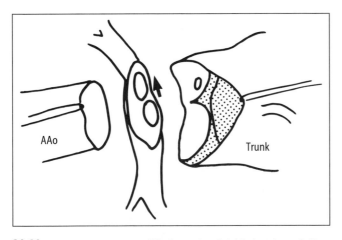

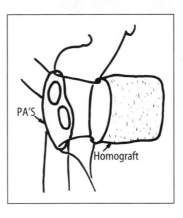

20.12 While aortic reconstruction is often done first, exposure for the distal homograft to pulmonary artery anastomosis is also optimal at this time, particularly if the origin of the right pulmonary artery is to the right side of the trunk. The homograft is trimmed slightly larger than the vessel patch and sutured continuously with a fine monofilament suture, taking care to avoid twisting or purse-stringing the pulmonary arteries.

20.11 The pulmonary arteries are fully dissected to their hilar branches to facilitate moving them leftward without kinking. Mobilization of the ascending aorta is completed to allow end-to-end anastomosis to the trunk without tension. At this point, it is convenient to inspect the ventricular septal defect through the truncal valve and plan the site of the ventriculotomy.

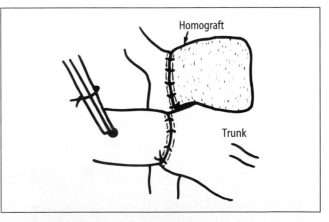

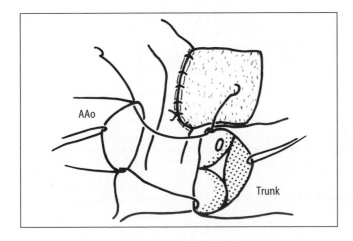

20.14 *(above)* In the completed reconstruction, the distal homograft-pulmonary artery anastomosis usually retracts slightly behind the trunk-to-ascending aorta connection, while anteriorly, the homograft wraps around the trunk slightly towards the right coronary artery to reach the ventriculotomy. An appreciation of these relationships guides trimming of the homograft at the time of primary repair and also its removal at subsequent reoperation for conduit replacement.

20.13 *(left)* The homograft is gently retracted to the left, while an end-to-end anastomosis is constructed between the distal ascending aorta and proximal arterial trunk. The considerable disparity in diameters is taken up symmetrically around the circumference of the anastomosis to avoid distortion of the truncal root. Meticulous attention to the coronary arterial orifices is important, as these often lie very close to the suture line.

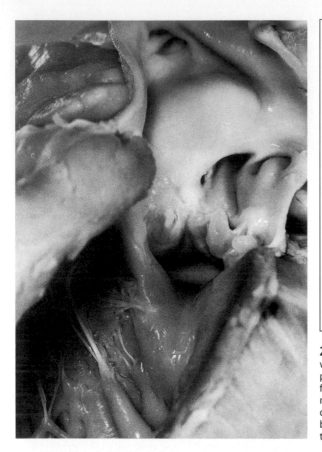

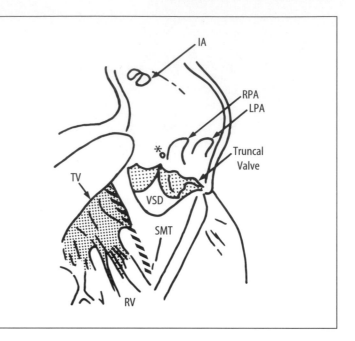

20.15 Common arterial trunk, Type III. This anterior view of the heart opened from the right ventricle across the trunk into the ascending aorta shows a muscular ventricular septal defect. The posterior limb of the septomarginal trabeculation is fused with the right ventriculo-infundibular fold, producing discontinuity between the truncal and tricuspid valves (and hence, a muscular margin to the ventricular septal defect). The conduction tissue is remote from the margin of the defect. The pulmonary arteries arise separately, distally to a four-leaflet truncal valve. The artefact beside the right pulmonary artery (asterisk) is not a coronary artery, the origins of which are within the sinuses of Valsalva (not seen).

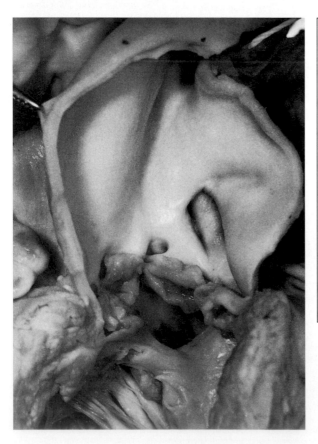

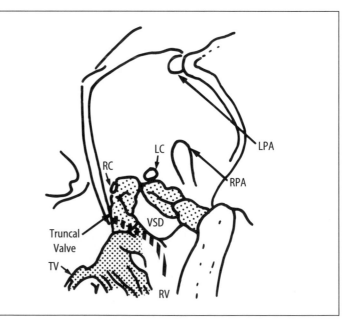

20.16 Common arterial trunk, Type III with perimembranous ventricular septal defect. Fibrous continuity is present between the truncal and tricuspid valves. The proximal conduction tissue runs along the margin of the defect. The truncal valve has four leaflets which are thickened and dysplastic but not fused together. The orifice of the left coronary artery lies above the valvar sinus. The right pulmonary artery arises proximally, but the stenotic left pulmonary artery is located distally, making this an extreme example of Type III common arterial trunk.

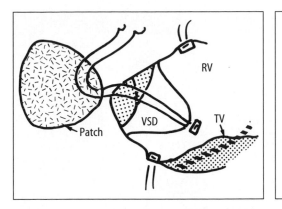

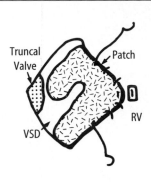

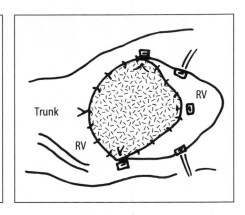

20.17 Closure of the ventricular septal defect in common arterial trunk is done through a vertical incision in the anterior wall of the right ventricle, carefully placed below the truncal valvar attachment. When there is a muscular margin, it is convenient initially to anchor the patch in the arms of the septomarginal trabeculation with a pledgeted mattress suture.

20.18 With the patch displaced to the left ventricular side of the septum, suturing continues along the anterior and posterior limbs of the septomarginal trabeculation.

20.19 As the roof of the defect is truncal valve, the suture line passes from the ventricular septum to the free right ventricular wall along the edge of the ventriculotomy. At the points of transition, additional mattress sutures supported by pledgets of pericardium are useful to reinforce the attachment of the patch to the myocardium.

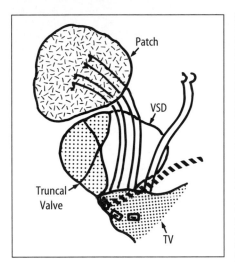

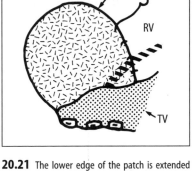

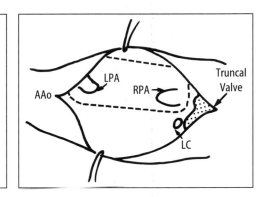

20.20 When the ventricular septal defect extends to the tricuspid valve, the conduction tissue is along the margin which lies under the surgeon's right hand. Sutures are initially placed through the base of the tricuspid valvar leaflet to avoid injury to the conduction system.

20.21 The lower edge of the patch is extended about 5 mm beyond the margin of the defect, which should bring it to pass posteriorly to the non-branching bundle. Working towards the ventriculotomy, the suture line usually crosses the right bundle branch and not uncommonly results in post-operative right bundle branch block.

20.22 When both pulmonary arteries arise at approximately the same level in a Type III trunk (upper specimen), they are managed similarly to Type II malformation (see Figures 20.9–20.14). More divergent origins (lower specimen) are treated on their individual merits. Here, an oblong segment is removed from the side and back of the aorta to include the pulmonary arterial branches (dashed line).

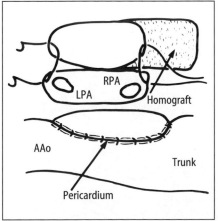

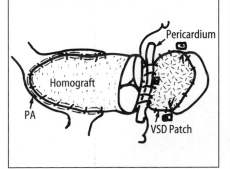

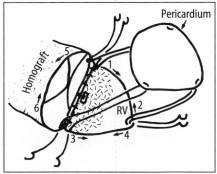

20.24 As the ventricular septal defect patch comes to the edge of the ventriculotomy, anastomosis of the posterior wall of the homograft to the right ventricle incorporates this patch. Hemostasis is facilitated by reinforcement of this suture line with a strip of autogenous pericardium.

20.25 The position of the homograft is checked by occluding the left atrial vent or injecting saline into the homograft. It usually lies nearly at a right angle to the right ventricle. A triangular hood of pericardium is used to complete the right ventricular outflow anteriorly. The length of its base is equal to the portion of the homograft which is not attached to the right ventricle. Its sides approximate the length of the ventriculotomy. Anchoring each corner of the pericardial hood maintains correct orientation of the patch and aids suturing the pericardium, firstly to the ventriculotomy and finally to the homograft.

20.23 The aorta is reconstructed with a patch of pericardium, Gore-tex, or homograft, being careful to avoid distortion of the truncal valve or compromise of a coronary artery. The patch of aorta containing the pulmonary arteries is anastomosed to an appropriately trimmed homograft with minimal mobilization to prevent kinking of the branches.

20.26 Common arterial trunk, Type III, with Type B interrupted aortic arch. The specimen has been opened vertically across the right ventricular outflow tract and trunk into the persistently patent arterial duct. This frontal view shows a three-leaflet truncal valve overriding the ventricular septal defect. The right pulmonary artery arises from the left side of the ascending aorta and the left pulmonary artery more distally, as a slit-like orifice just below the arterial duct. The descending aorta has been lifted upwards over the left atrial appendage.

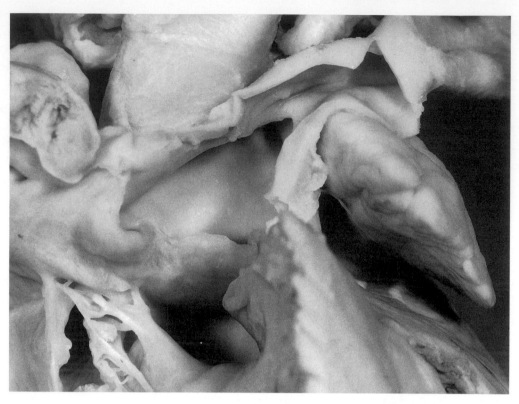

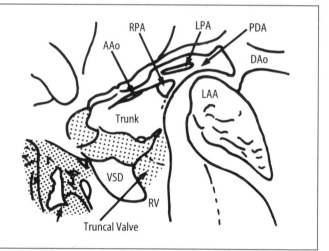

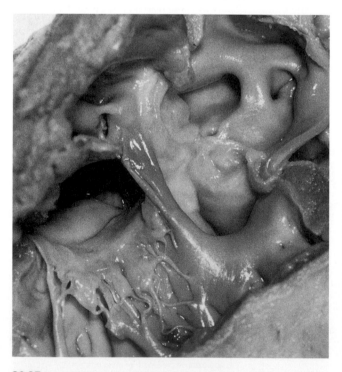

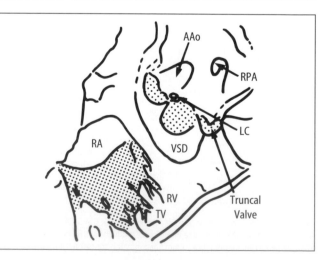

20.27 The same heart has been rotated to display the origins of the ascending aorta and right pulmonary artery. A coronary artery arises above the truncal valvar sinus. The ventricular septal defect has a completely muscular margin.

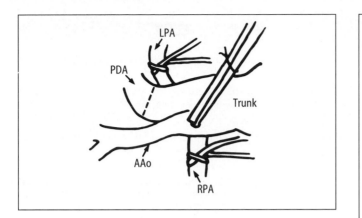

20.28 Common arterial trunk with interrupted aortic arch is corrected through a midline sternal incision. The branch pulmonary arteries are partially snared to enhance systemic blood-flow and to protect the lungs. A single arterial cannula at the base of the ascending aorta perfuses both the upper and lower body, while a single venous cannula permits core cooling. Under total circulatory arrest or with reduced perfusion to the upper body, the arterial duct is divided distally to the origin of the left pulmonary artery (dashed line). If this is not obvious externally, the duct may be opened with a short vertical incision and the positions of the pulmonary arterial orifices confirmed internally. Although it appears that the duct lies beyond the origin of the pulmonary arteries, in reality they all arise from the trunk, and this incision will be continued to remove the branch pulmonary arteries from the trunk.

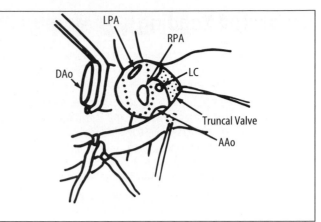

20.29 Ductal tissue is excised completely and the descending aorta, which has been extensively mobilized, is drawn into the anterior mediastinum with a C-clamp. Looking inside the trunk, the position of the ascending aorta, truncal valve, coronary arteries, and pulmonary arteries is identified with certainty. The pulmonary arteries are mobilized to the hilum of each lung, analogous to dissection for the arterial switch operation, and then excised from the trunk (dotted line). Their origin may be very close to that of a coronary artery, leaving only a small rim of surrounding tissue.

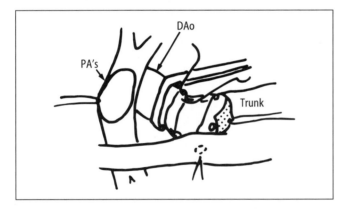

20.30 With the pulmonary arteries retracted towards the patient's head, the descending aorta is brought underneath them and is connected to the opening in the trunk, which has been created by removal of the pulmonary arteries, with a fine continuous monofilament suture. It is important to avoid damage to a coronary artery and distortion of the truncal valve, which is accomplished by adequate mobilization of the descending aorta and favoring the trunk during excision of the pulmonary artery.

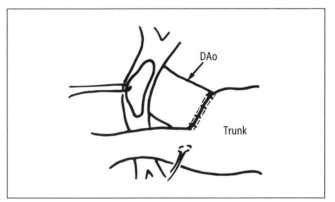

20.31 The completed arch reconstruction lies behind the bifurcation of the pulmonary artery and crosses the left main bronchus (see Figure 20.7). As this anastomosis becomes very inaccessible, it is useful to support at least the posterior portion with a strip of autogenous pericardium.

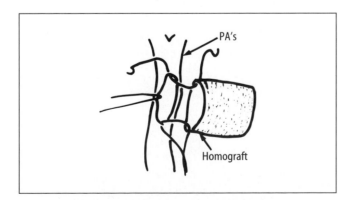

20.32 The distal end of a homograft valve is connected to the pulmonary arterial branches. The size of the homograft is chosen conservatively according to the patient's body size, as there is limited space in the mediastinum. It will need to be replaced in the future, anyway. Usually a 10–13 mm valve is satisfactory for a 3 kg neonate.

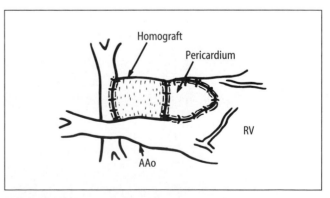

20.33 After closure of the ventricular septal defect through the ventriculotomy, the homograft is attached to the right ventricle (see Figures 20.24–20.25). If an aortic homograft is used, the anterior mitral valve leaflet may be sufficient to replace the anterior pericardial hood, but the valve should not be distorted by pulling it down to the ventricle. A large infundibular branch of the right coronary artery often crosses the outflow and should be preserved.

Suggested Reading

Alexiou C, Keeton BR, Salmon AP, Monro JL. Repair of truncus arteriosus in early infancy with antibiotic sterilized aortic homografts. Ann Thorac Surg 2001;71(5 Suppl):S371.

Barbero-Marcial M, Riso A, Atik E, Jatene A. A technique for correction of truncus arteriosus types I and II without extracardiac conduits. J Thorac Cardovasc Surg 1990;99:364.

Bove EL, Beckman III RH, Snider AR, Callow LB, Underhill DJ, Rocchini AP, Dick M, Rosenthal A. Repair of truncus arteriosus in the neonate and young infant. Ann Thorac Surg. 1989;47:499.

Bove EL, Lupinetti FM, Pridjian AK, Beckman RH III, Callow LB, Snider AR, Rosenthal A. Results of a policy of primary repair of truncus arteriosus in the neonate. J Thorac Cardiovasc Surg 1993;105:1057.

Carr I, Bharati S, Kusnoor VS, Lev M. Truncus arteriosus communis with intact ventricular septum. Br Heart J 1979;42:97.

Celoria GC, Patton RB. Congenital absence of the aortic arch. Am Heart J 1959;56:407.

Collett RW, Edwards JE. Persistent truncus arteriosus. A classification according to anatomic types. Surgical Clinics of North America 1949;29:1245.

Crupi G, Macartney FJ, Anderson RH. Persistent truncus arteriosus. A study of 66 autopsy cases with special reference to definition and morphogenesis. Am J Cardiol 1977;40:569.

Danton MH, Barron DJ, Stumper O, Wright JG, De Giovanni J, Silove ED, Brawn WJ. Repair of truncus arteriosus: a considered approach to right ventricular outflow tract reconstruction. Eur J Cardiothorac Surg 2001;20:95.

Kakadekar AP, Tyrrell MJ, McKay R. Aortogram after repair of common arterial trunk with interrupted aortic arch. Cardiol Young 1998;8:136.

Lenox CC, Debich DE, Zuberbuhler JR. The role of coronary artery abnormalities in the prognosis of truncus arteriosus. J Thorac Cardiovasc Surg 1992;104:1728.

Mavroudis C, Backer CL. Surgical management of severe truncal insufficiency: experience with truncal valve remodelling techniques. Ann Thorac Surg 2001;72:396.

McKay R, Miyamoto S, Peart I, Battistessa SA, Wren C, Cunliffe M, Robles A. Truncus arteriosus with interrupted aortic arch: Successful correction in a neonate. Ann Thorac Surg 1989;48:587.

Rodefeld MD, Hanley FL. Neonatal truncus arteriosus repair: Surgical techniques and clinical management. Semin Thorac Cardiovasc Surg Pediatr Card Surg Annu 2002;5:212.

Smith A, McKay R. Common arterial trunk with discordant atrioventricular connections. Cardiol Young 2000;10:145.

Suzuki A, Ho SY, Anderson RH, Deanfield JE. Coronary arterial and sinusal anatomy in hearts with a common arterial trunk. Ann Thorac Surg 1989;48:792.

Van Praagh R, Van Praagh S. The anatomy of common aortopulmonary trunk (truncus arteriosus communis) and its embryologic implications. A study of 57 necropsy cases. Am J Cardiol 1965;16:406.

21 Complete Transposition of the Great Arteries (Discordant Ventriculo-arterial Connections)

Introduction

Transposition of the great arteries defines a ventriculo-arterial connection which is discordant. In this arrangement, the aorta arises from the morphologically right ventricle and pulmonary artery from the morphologically left ventricle. Although this situation also occurs with the full spectrum of anomalies involving the atrioventricular junction (double inlet, left or right atrioventricular valve atresia, discordant atrioventricular connections), "complete transposition" refers only to hearts in which a morphologically right atrium is connected to a morphologically right ventricle and the morphologically left atrium is connected to the morphologically left ventricle (concordant atrioventricular connections). These chamber connections may exist with either the usual atrial arrangement (situs solitus) or with mirror-image atrial arrangement (situs inversus). Complete transposition is found with intact ventricular septum ("simple" transposition) in about three-quarters of cases. The remaining hearts have major associated malformations, such as large persistently patent arterial duct, subpulmonary or subaortic obstruction, and/or ventricular septal defect ("complex" transposition). Coarctation of the aorta may occur with either simple or complex complete transposition, but is much more frequent in the latter group.

The arterial trunks assume a variety of spatial relationships in complete transposition, but most commonly, the aorta lies anteriorly and slightly to the right of the pulmonary artery. With usual atrial arrangement, however, the aortic root may be anywhere in relation to the pulmonary root, from left anterior, anterior, right anterior, right lateral (side by side), to right posterior. These variations have implications for the ventricular outflow tracts and the central fibrous body, the morphology of which is frequently abnormal. Nonetheless, the atrial septum and inlet portion of the ventricular septum are usually aligned normally, meeting at the crux of the heart. Consequently, the course of

the conduction tissue in simple complete transposition is comparable with that of the normal heart.

Defects in the ventricular septum of hearts with complete transposition may be perimembranous or muscular. They are found in all the sites where ventricular septal defects occur in normally connected hearts (see Chapter 11) and, thus, the main axis of the conduction tissue is comparable in this regard. However, a frequent finding in transposition is malalignment between different components of the ventricular septum. This may produce additional types of defects, especially of the outlet of the heart which, by definition, cannot be found with concordant ventriculo-arterial connections. Such examples are those which fall into the "Taussig-Bing" subpulmonary type of defect. Another example is the so-called "inlet–outlet" muscular ventricular septal defect. This lies under the septal tricuspid valvar leaflet on the right side of the septum but does not extend to the posterior wall of the heart, and thus opens into the subpulmonary outflow of the left ventricle. In several cases of transposition, the conduction tissue has been found to pass posteriorly in these "inlet–outlet" muscular defects, in contrast with the "muscular inlet" ventricular septal defect which generally extends to the posterior wall of the heart in both ventricles and therefore has the axis of the conduction tissue passing anteriorly.

In most hearts with simple complete transposition, the aortic valve is supported completely by muscle and the pulmonary valve has fibrous continuity with the mitral valve. A variety of mechanisms may produce the obstruction of the left ventricular outflow, including stenosis of the pulmonary valvar leaflets, abnormal mitral valve attachments, aneurysmal fibrous tissue from the membranous septum or atrioventricular valves, and fixed or dynamic muscular obstruction. In the presence of a ventricular septal defect, malalignment of the outlet septum to the left or right also results in obstruction to the respective ventricular outflow. Associated coarctation of the aorta or interruption of the aortic arch is frequently present when the obstruction is subaortic (right ventricular outflow obstruction).

The coronary arteries in complete transposition arise from either or both of the two aortic sinuses which face the pulmonary valve. Several classifications have evolved to describe them. The convention used herein places an observer in the non-facing sinus of the aorta, looking towards the pulmonary valve. The aortic sinus, which falls under the observer's right hand, is the "right-hand facing sinus" and that under the left hand is the "left-hand facing sinus." As most individuals are right-handed, it is easy to remember that the right-hand facing sinus is also called "sinus 1." "Sinus 2" is the left-hand facing sinus. An alternative system places the observer in the non-facing pulmonary valvar sinus looking towards the aorta, which then reverses the right- and left-hand positions. All these classifications lose precision in the presence of a two-sinus (bicuspid) aortic valve or in extreme malalignment between aortic and pulmonary valve commissures. The five coronary artery configurations described originally by Yacoub are sometimes also referred to as types A–E, the most common being Type A (left anterior descending and circumflex arteries from sinus 1; right coronary artery from sinus 2) and Type D (left anterior descending artery from sinus 1; right coronary and circumflex arteries from sinus 2). A sinus may contain more than one coronary arterial orifice. Alternatively, a single coronary arterial orifice may supply all the coronary arteries. Externally, a coronary artery which arises in one sinus may appear to leave the aorta from another sinus (usually sinus 1), having passed around the aorta within the vessel wall. This is called an intramural coronary artery and has important implications for surgical management.

Complete transposition accounts for approximately 5% of all congenital cardiac malformations and usually presents with cyanosis soon after birth. Surgical management has evolved over many years and now offers a high probability of both survival and good late cardiac function for patients with simple transposition and, to a lesser degree, for those with complex associated malformations. Treatment is based primarily on cardiac morphology in complete transposition, but additional factors such as prematurity, non-cardiac anomalies, experience and expertise of the surgical infrastructure (anesthesia, perfusion, intensive care), and social circumstances (children of Jehovah's Witness faith) sometimes profoundly influence patient care. Optimal surgical management of simple complete transposition

is an arterial switch operation performed while the left ventricle is still capable of supporting the systemic circulation (generally during the first two weeks of life). While some coronary arterial patterns may complicate this procedure, techniques have been described for the successful management of all types of coronary anatomy in the neonatal arterial switch. When primary anatomical correction (arterial switch operation) is not done, the patient can undergo either a two-stage arterial switch procedure after preparation of the left ventricle by pulmonary arterial banding (or with post-operative left ventricular assist), or atrial redirection using a Mustard or Senning operation. Very rarely, associated left ventricular outflow obstruction, which is not amenable to surgical relief, complicates transposition with intact ventricular septum and precludes anatomical correction. For these patients, atrial redirection, usually with a left ventricle-to pulmonary artery extracardiac conduit, is appropriate.

Decision-making becomes more complex in the presence of a ventricular septal defect, particularly if there are associated anomalies of the atrioventricular valves or ventricular outflow tracts. Having determined that both ventricles are of adequate size, the next consideration is whether the left ventricular outflow is unobstructed (or can be made so) for the systemic circulation. If so, closure of the ventricular septal defect with an arterial switch procedure before the onset of pulmonary vascular disease is usually the operation of choice. When coarctation or hypoplasia of the aorta is present, this may be relieved at a preliminary operation (usually with pulmonary artery banding) or at the time of complete primary correction. In the presence of severe unresectable left ventricular outflow obstruction, attention is directed towards tunnelling the left ventricle to the aorta through the ventricular septal defect (Rastelli or REV operations). The size and position of the ventricular septal defect, insertion of tricuspid or mitral valvar apparatus within the pathway, size and position of the outlet septum, and position of the aorta, are all important additional considerations. Usually a right ventricle to pulmonary artery conduit or repositioning of the pulmonary artery is necessary in such cases. Patients not infrequently require augmentation of pulmonary blood-flow with a systemic-pulmonary shunt, while growing large enough to undergo these procedures. Rarely, ventricular imbalance, usually with straddling of an atrioventricular valve and/or multiple ventricular septal defects, precludes a two-ventricle repair. Management of such patients is then directed towards the Fontan circulation (see Section 5).

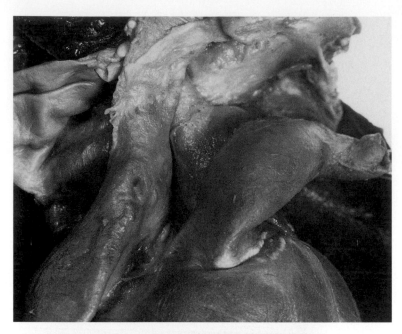

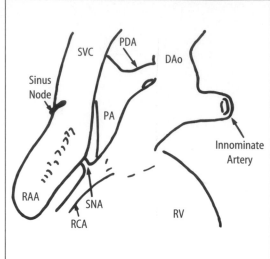

21.1 Simple complete transposition of the great arteries. External view, slightly to the right, showing the origin of the right coronary artery, which gives a small branch to the sinus node. The innominate artery and ascending aorta have been rotated leftward to show the main and right pulmonary arteries. A large persistently patent arterial duct connects the origin of the left pulmonary artery (not seen) to the aorta.

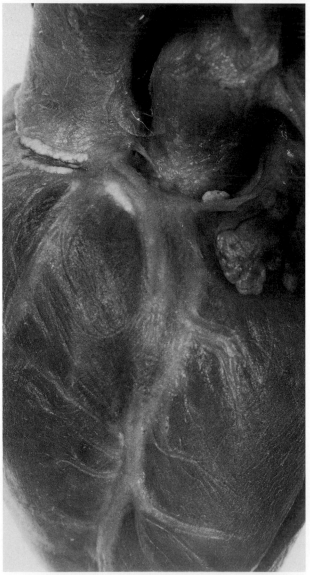

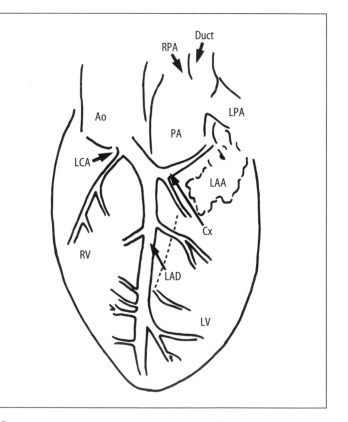

21.2 External view from the left side of the same heart, showing the origin of the left coronary artery. This vessel gives off a large infundibular branch, the anterior descending (interventricular) and the circumflex arteries. This is the most common arterial pattern in transposition. The aorta is anterior and to the right of the pulmonary artery, and the great arteries are of nearly equal size. The dashed line indicates the position of a coronary vein.

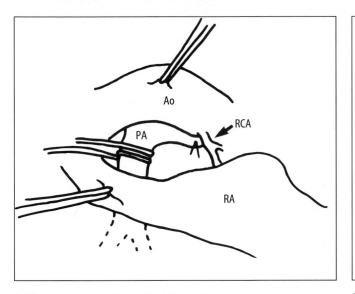

21.3 In preparation for the arterial switch operation, the ascending aorta and pulmonary artery are extensively dissected above the sinutubular junctions, and the right pulmonary artery is encircled with a vessel loop between the aorta and the superior caval vein. Eventually, it will be fully mobilized to the lung hilum. The probable site of reimplantation of the right coronary artery in the neo-aorta (proximal pulmonary artery) is marked with a suture. This is generally the closest point to the origin of the coronary artery and above the sinus of the neo-aorta.

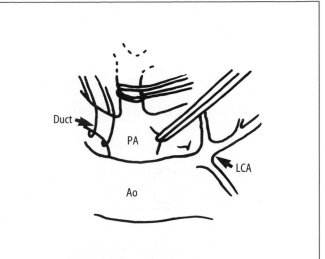

21.4 The arterial duct, which is often larger than the branch pulmonary arteries in the neonate on prostin, is dissected by retracting the main pulmonary artery down towards the heart and the ascending aorta gently leftward. As the duct will be divided, it is encircled with two silk ligatures. If convenient, the left pulmonary artery is encircled with a vessel loop at this time. Its dissection may be more difficult, however, and full mobilization to the lobar branches is generally done after vascular transection. A marking suture is placed on the neo-aorta at its closest point to the left coronary artery to guide subsequent coronary translocation.

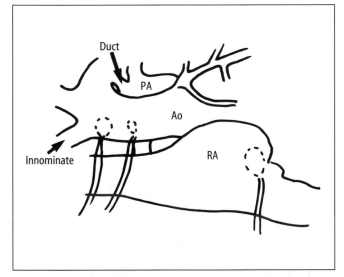

21.5 Purse-strings for cannulation are placed high on the ascending aorta, just below its innominate branch. The cardioplegia purse-string will be used to retract and orientate the distal aorta after transection and is thus carefully sited in the middle of the vessel anteriorly, with room for the cross-clamp between it and the aortic cannula. When a single straight venous cannula is used, the right atrial purse-string is placed at the junction of the atrium and its appendage.

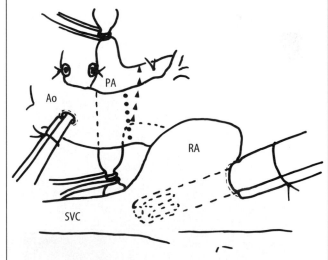

21.6 Immediately after the commencement of cardiopulmonary bypass, the pulmonary arteries are snared to prevent flooding of the lungs and cardiac distension. The ductal ligatures are tied and the duct divided. The aortic or both ends are generally oversewn. The venous cannula is stabilized by positioning its tip just within the orifice of the superior caval vein. It is essential to have excellent venous drainage at this point, as ligation of the arterial duct with occlusion of the branch pulmonary arteries gives no other way for blood to leave the right heart. Usually, a venous cannula in this position will also drain the left atrium through the septostomy defect. Failing that, the tip of the cannula can alternatively be passed across the atrial septum into the left atrium. Large black dots indicate the approximate site of the aortic transection, which is about 2–3 mm above the sinutubular junction in the neonate. Pulmonary artery transection (arrow heads) starts just below the origin of the right branch and is angled slightly towards the heart on the left side. This leaves a cuff of main pulmonary artery below the left branch, which helps to compensate for the rightward position of the neo-pulmonary artery (proximal aorta) and may reduce the risk of left pulmonary artery stenosis.

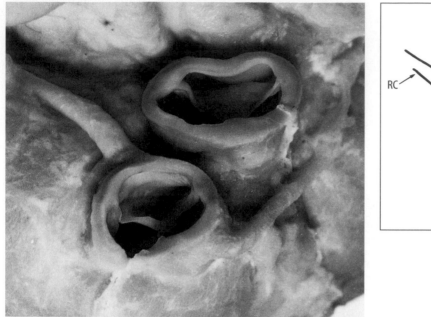

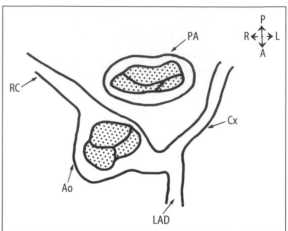

21.7 Coronary arterial patterns in TGA. Dual sinus origin with the right coronary artery from the left-hand facing sinus (sinus 2) and the left, from the right-hand facing sinus (sinus 1), bifurcating into left anterior descending and circumflex arteries. The aorta is anterior and to the right of the pulmonary artery. This is the most common situation in transposition (Yacoub Type A).

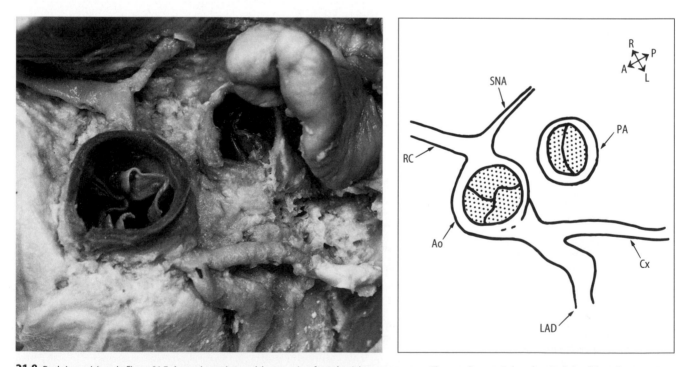

21.8 Dual sinus origin as in Figure 21.7. A prominent sinus nodal artery arises from the right coronary artery. The aorta lies anteriorly and to the right of the pulmonary artery. The pulmonary valve has two leaflets which are otherwise normal and accordingly would be acceptable for the systemic outflow (neoaortic valve). The left atrial appendage is immediately posterior to the pulmonary artery.

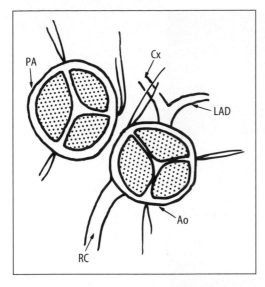

21.9 *(above)* Coronary artery translocation generally follows arterial transection in the arterial switch operation. Adventitial stay-sutures at each commissure help to expose the aortic and pulmonary sinuses. The ostium of each coronary artery is probed gently to exclude an intramural course and determine the direction of the vessel.

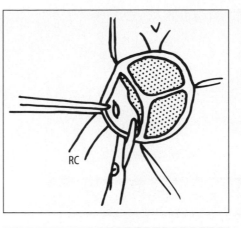

21.10 *(left)* The right coronary arterial ostium is excised first with a button of surrounding sinus tissue. This opens up the aorta for subsequent excision of the left coronary artery. In neonates, virtually the entire sinus is removed, leaving about 1 mm at the base.

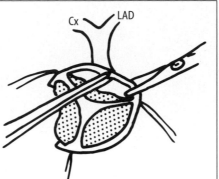

21.11 *(left)* Excision of the left coronary artery and its sinus is done with traction on the stay-sutures to facilitate exposure. Both blades of the scissors are kept close to the vessel wall to avoid damage to the valve leaflet or, near the bottom of the sinus, to the coronary artery itself. The right ventricular outflow tract is now inspected retrogradely through the valve and relieved of any obstructing muscle bundles.

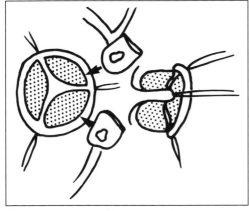

21.12 *(left)* Retraction of the aorta forward allows the coronary buttons to fall back towards the pulmonary artery. This, along with previously placed marking sutures, is a good guide to their new position. Occasionally, both coronary arteries will fit best into the same sinus, but locating them directly between the great vessels may risk compression if there is subsequent vascular distension (for example, from pulmonary hypertension) in the postoperative period.

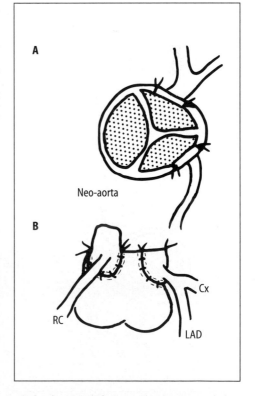

21.13 *(left)* Several types of incision in the pulmonary artery have been described to accommodate the coronary buttons without sinus distortion. Usually, however, they are implanted above the sinutubular junction, such that a simple vertical incision is adequate. The left (A) is implanted first. Suturing from the centre of the button upward minimizes the risk of rotation. The right coronary anastomosis (B) is also done working inside the vessel.

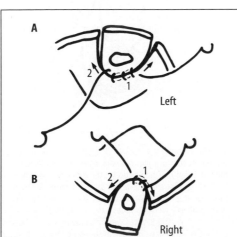

21.14 *(above right)* The coronary arteries are sited at the point which gives neither distortion nor kinking (A). This is not necessarily above the mid-portion of the sinus. A 1 mm probe is passed again gently into the orifice to confirm a good positon. In general, the right coronary artery tends to lie higher than does the left (B) and the upper portion of its button may need to be accommodated by a slit-incision in the distal aorta. If both buttons lie close together above a sinus of the neoaorta, they may be joined to each other above the inter-coronary commissure.

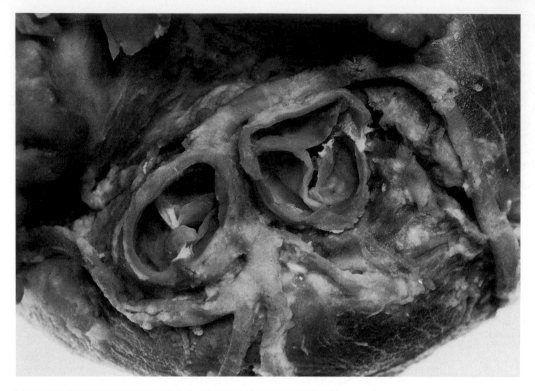

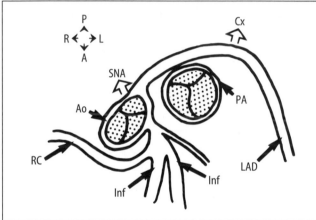

21.15 Coronary arterial patterns in TGA. Dual sinus origin with side-by-side great arteries. The right coronary artery arises from the right-hand facing sinus (sinus 1) and follows an anteroaortic course, giving off three large infundibular branches. The left coronary artery comes from the left-hand facing sinus (sinus 2) and takes a retropulmonary course. The sinus nodal branch (virtually at the origin of the left coronary artery) and circumflex branch are present but not easily seen in the photograph. There is poor alignment of the intercoronary commissure with the facing commissure of the pulmonary valve.

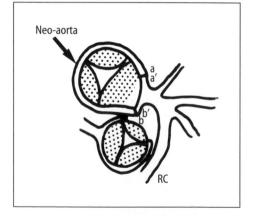

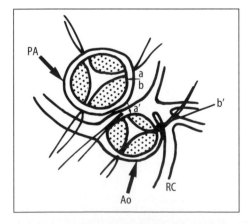

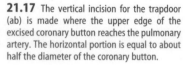

21.16 In the situation of an anteroaortic right coronary artery with early infundibular branches, extensive mobilization of the vessel (using the diathermy) and a trapdoor technique of reimplantation will permit the ostium to reach the neoaorta with minimal tension or displacement.

21.17 The vertical incision for the trapdoor (ab) is made where the upper edge of the excised coronary button reaches the pulmonary artery. The horizontal portion is equal to about half the diameter of the coronary button.

21.18 To prevent excessive enlargement of the neoaorta, the trapdoor flap is sutured back from "bb'" for about one-third of its length. The position of the coronary is usually sufficiently high above the valve that there is minimal distortion of the sinus itself. Translocation of the left coronary artery in this heart probably would be above the aortic/neoaortic anastomosis and the same sinus as the right coronary artery, also with a medially based flap hinged in the opposite direction to avoid kinking, particularly of the sinus nodal branch.

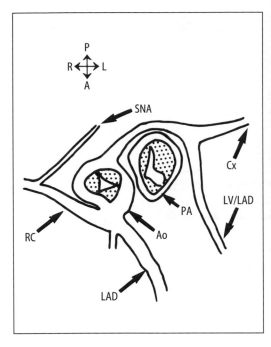

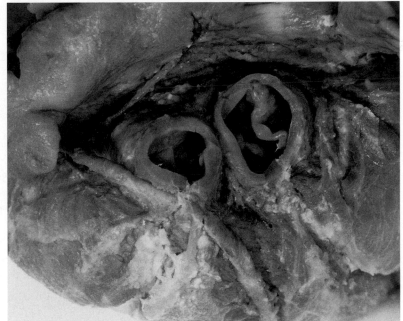

21.19 *(above left and right)* Dual sinus origin with side-by-side great vessels. The right coronary artery from the right-hand facing sinus (sinus 1) bifurcates into the anterior descending and right coronary arteries, the latter running an anteroaortic course. The left coronary artery arises from the left-hand facing sinus (sinus 2). It takes a retropulmonary course and gives off two well-developed branches to the left ventricle. One of these is the circumflex coronary and the other simulates an accessory anterior descending artery.

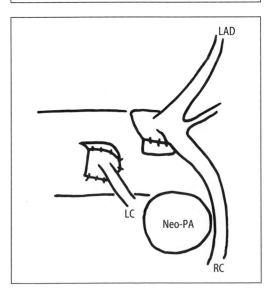

21.20 The presence of major branches running in opposite directions, as illustrated by the left anterior descending and right coronary arteries in this heart, is considered a contraindication to translocation by some surgeons. In that case a tunnel is constructed to the orifice (see single sinus origins). However, mobilization and the use of the trapdoor technique (see Figures 21.16–21.18) usually will achieve satisfactory transfer to the neoaorta. A medially based flap also facilitates translocation of the left coronary artery.

21.21 As a result of side-by-side great arteries and a retropulmonary course, the left coronary artery will be excessively long when it is moved to the neoaorta. Kinking is prevented by two manoeuvres – namely, the use of a medially based trapdoor and implantation at a more distal and medial position on the ascending aorta. In this situation, sinuses of the neopulmonary artery are generously reconstructed prior to the coronary anastomosis to prevent coronary distortion when the Lecompte maneuver is used. Alternatively, the pulmonary bifurcation is moved rightward by closing the distal main pulmonary artery and anastomosing the neopulmonary artery to a separate incision in the right branch. The presence of an anteroaortic right coronary artery would contraindicate the use of a transannular patch for right ventricular outflow obstruction. If present, it must be relieved by intracardiac resection or bypassed with an extracardiac conduit.

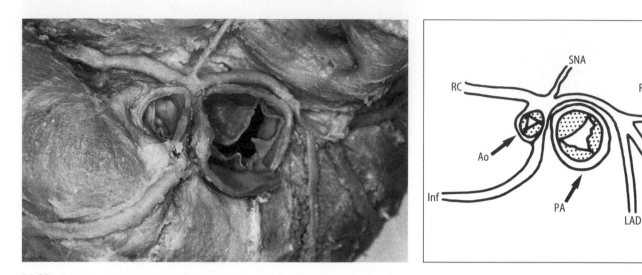

21.22 Coronary arterial patterns in TGA. Single sinus origin. The left main, sinus nodal, right coronary arteries, and a well-developed accessory infundibular branch originate from a single orifice in the left-hand facing sinus (sinus 2). The left main coronary artery trifurcates into circumflex, anterior descending (interventricular), and left ventricular branches. The infundibular branch to the right ventricle passes between the aorta and pulmonary artery. A less common situation is that the accessory infundibular artery arises separately from the right hand facing sinus (sinus 1), in which case the orifices in sinus 2 are treated as a "single sinus origin" (see Figures 21.24–21.27) and that in sinus 1, is translocated to the neoaorta (see Figures 21.9–21.14).The aortic valve lies to the right of the pulmonary valve (side-by-side great arteries) and is hypoplastic, although the discrepancy in the size of the vessels is not dissimilar to that encountered at any time with transposed great arteries and ventricular septal defect.

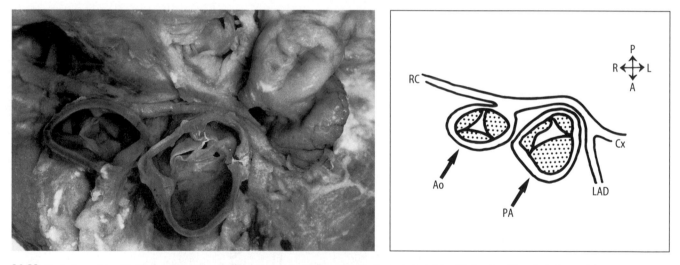

21.23 Single sinus origin with side-by-side great vessels. The right and left coronary arteries both arise in the left-hand facing sinus (sinus 2), the latter taking a retropulmonary course and bifurcating into anterior descending and circumflex arteries. The sinus nodal artery was not identified in this heart.

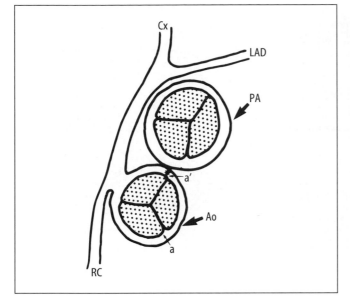

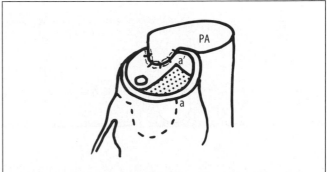

21.24 Because of the single sinus origin with proximal coronary arteries lying in opposite directions, translocation of the coronary ostia without distortion is not possible. Several techniques may be used to create a tunnel to the orifice of the coronary artery, provided this is not rotated more than 90° in any direction. The technique illustrated uses an aortopulmonary connection and flap of aortic sinus tissue. The facing sinuses that include the coronary artery origin are first joined together (a´), and a tunnel is created using tissue from the adjoining non-facing sinuses (a).

21.25 Part of the facing aortic and pulmonary sinuses are excised to a depth of about 1 mm above the coronary arterial orifice. Slightly more tissue is left on the pulmonary arterial side and the cut edges are joined with a fine running monofilament suture. A flap of tissue from the non-facing sinus is fashioned (dashed line), leaving it hinged above the commissure with the sinus which contains the coronary artery.

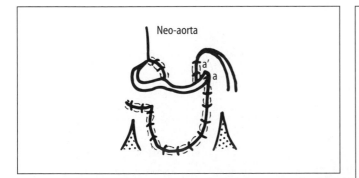

21.26 The flap is rotated into the sinus and sutured below the coronary arterial orifice, leaving the aortic valve leaflet outside, and the entrance to the coronary artery inside the recess. Both the aorto-pulmonary connection and the pocket of sinus wall should be as large as possible.

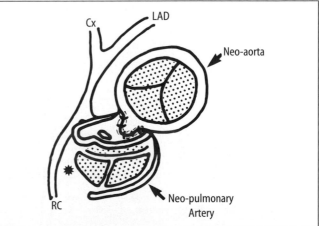

21.27 The completed tunnel leaves the coronary ostium in situ with unobstructed flow from the neoaorta. The distal ascending aorta is anastomosed to the neoaorta and the upper edge of the turned-in sinus flap. The deficiency in the neopulmonary arterial sinus (star) is repaired with a piece of autogenous pericardium. For the final anastomosis of the distal pulmonary artery to neopulmonary artery and pericardium, the outside wall of the pocket serves as the back wall of the facing neopulmonary arterial sinus.

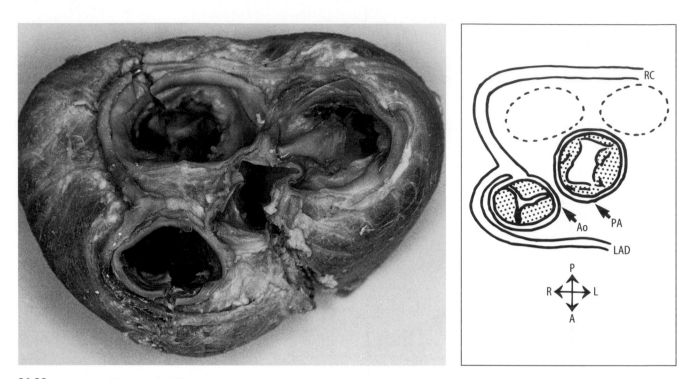

21.28 Coronary arterial patterns in TGA. Single sinus origin. There is a single orifice in the left-hand facing aortic sinus (sinus 2). The right coronary artery gives off an anterior descending branch and then continues in the atrioventricular sulcus to supply the posterior wall of the left ventricle. The left anterior descending (or anterior interventricular) coronary passes around the right side of the aortic root. The sinus nodal artery is difficult to identify in this specimen. It arises distally from the right coronary artery and passes across the diaphragmatic surface of the right atrium towards the sinus node. The aortic valve lies anteriorly and to the right of the pulmonary valve.

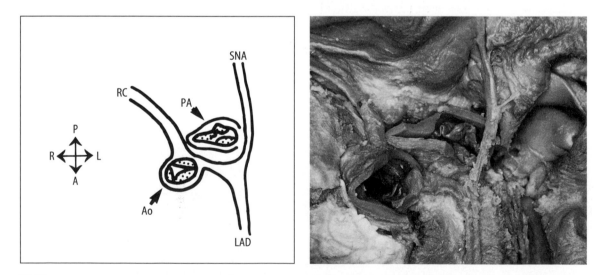

21.29 Single sinus origin from separate orifices in the left-hand facing sinus (sinus 2). The right coronary artery passes in the atrioventricular sulcus to supply the left ventricle distally. The anterior descending coronary artery, which also arises in sinus 2, runs between the aortic and pulmonary roots, and gives off a large sinus nodal artery which courses around the left side of the pulmonary root. The aortic valve lies to the right of and anterior to the pulmonary valve.

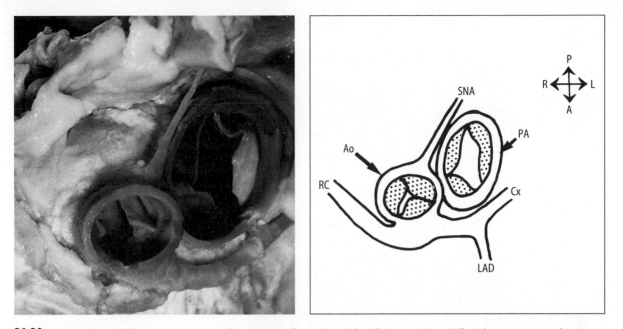

21.30 Single sinus origin of the main coronary arteries from separate orifices in the right-hand facing sinus (sinus 1). The right coronary artery takes a course anteriorly to the aortic root to reach the right atrioventricular sulcus. The main left coronary artery passes anteriorly around the pulmonary root and bifurcates into anterior descending and circumflex branches. The sinus nodal artery originates separately from the left-hand facing sinus (sinus 2). The aortic valve is anterior and to the right of the pulmonary valve.

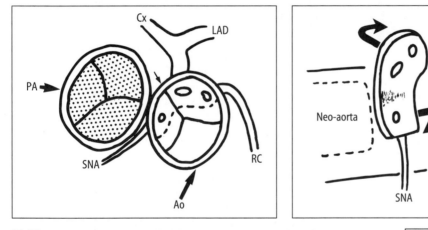

21.32 *(left)* The aortic button is rotated upwards approximately 90° to bring the upper edge perpendicular to the neoaorta. A flap of neoaorta is lifted at the level of the coronary button (dotted line), which will be above the valvar sinuses.

21.31 *(above)* There is poor alignment of the facing sinuses (see also Figure 21.29) and the major coronary arteries pass in opposite directions, making direct translocation to the neoaorta inadvisable. One technique in this situation is to treat all three orifices as a single button. The facing commissure (small arrow) between the right- and left-hand facing sinuses (sinus 1 and sinus 2) is detached from the aortic wall and retracted towards the surgeon. A large button of aortic sinuses 1 and 2 containing all the coronary arterial origins is removed (dotted line).

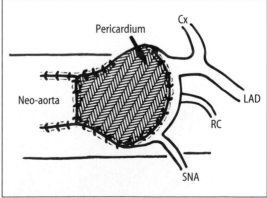

21.33 *(left)* The adjacent neoaortic wall and coronary artery button are joined with a running monofilament suture. Care is taken not to displace or rotate the coronary button.

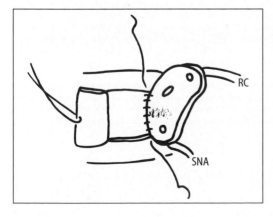

21.34 *(above)* A generous patch of autogenous pericardium is used to augment the flap of neoaorta and construct a hood over the coronary button. The neopulmonary sinuses are reconstructed with a rectangular-shaped patch of pericardium, to which the valve commissure is resuspended. This technique is applicable also to the management of intramural coronary arteries, although in that situation the ostium of the coronary artery is often stenotic and must be enlarged.

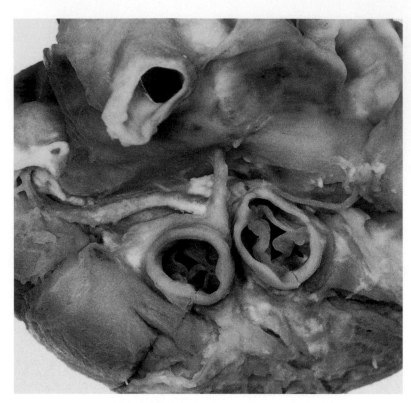

21.35 Coronary arterial patterns in TGA. Dual sinus origin. The circumflex and right coronary arteries arise from the left-hand facing sinus (sinus 2) and the left anterior descending artery from the right-hand facing sinus (sinus 1). The circumflex branch takes a retropulmonary course. This is the second most common coronary arterial pattern in TGA. A large sinus nodal branch originates with the right and circumflex arteries. A well-developed infundibular branch arises from the anterior descending artery and passes to the right ventricle. The aortic valve lies slightly anteriorly to and to the right of the pulmonary valve, with poor alignment of the commissures.

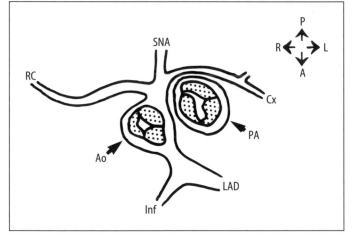

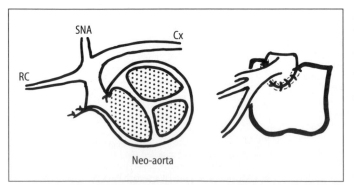

21.36 Two technical manoeuvres will facilitate the transfer of the right coronary artery to the neoaorta without kinking the circumflex branch. A medially based flap incision (see also Figures 21.20 and 21.21) in the neoaorta limits the degree of rotation of the coronary button, while implantation at a more distal level (partially or completely above the aortic suture line) accommodates the surplus length of the circumflex branch which is produced by moving its origin back to the neoaorta. Despite malalignment of the commissures/sinuses, the closest point on the neoaorta is used for coronary arterial transfer. In this example, both coronary arterial orifices would end up above the facing sinus of the neoaorta, the right being above the left. It is then necessary to augment the neopulmonary artery with a generous pericardial reconstruction to ensure that it moves forward away from the coronary arteries.

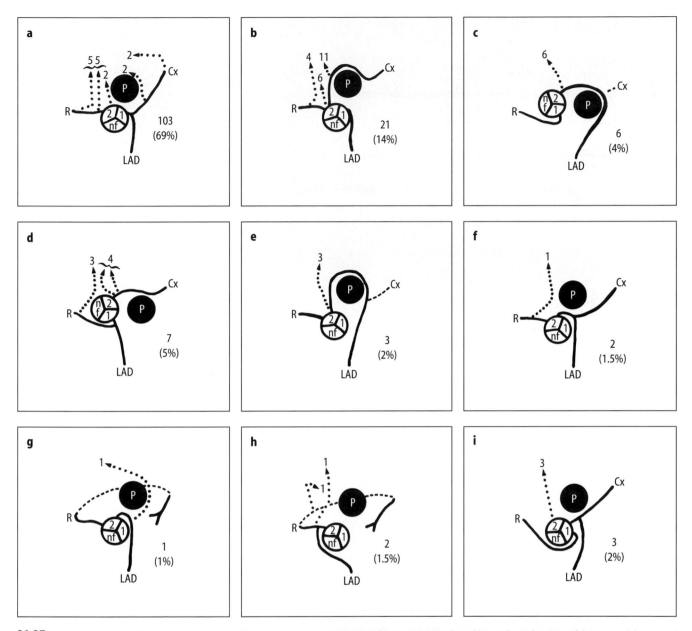

21.37 Summary of coronary arterial patterns found in 148 hearts with complete transposition of the great arteries. Dotted lines indicate the origins of the sinus nodal artery and numbers indicate the frequency with which each pattern was found. Dashed lines represent a continuation of the right coronary artery to the circumflex territory at the back of the heart. All relationships are orientated anatomically, as shown on the preceding page. In 87 hearts, the ventricular septum was intact, while 61 had a ventricular septal defect. Patterns shown in the diagrams referenced "a–e" were present both in hearts with and without ventricular septal defects, while those referenced "f–h" occurred only in hearts with an intact ventricular septum, and "i" only in those with a ventricular septal defect. Diagrams "a" and "b" account for the two most common patterns, which were found in about 83% of cases. However, the most common pattern (diagram "a") was not observed with side-by-side great arteries in this series. Single sinus origin (diagrams "e–i") occurred in 8% of the hearts, frequently with multiple orifices.

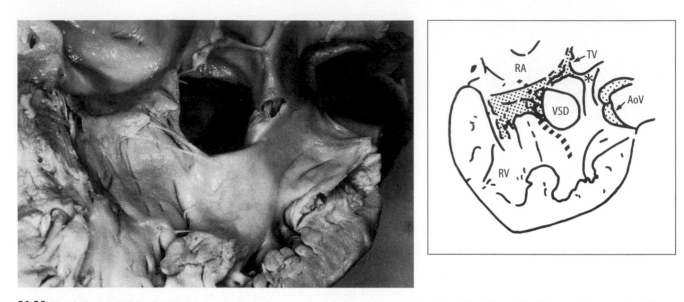

21.38 Ventricular septal defect in TGA. Perimembranous defect extending into the trabecular and outlet portions of the right ventricle: right ventricular aspect. The defect reaches the tricuspid valve and there is tricuspid-pulmonary valvar continuity through it, meeting the definition of a perimembranous defect. The lower margin extends distally to the insertion of the tricuspid valve, while the upper (anterior) margin is above the insertion of most of the medial papillary muscle complex and hence into the outlet septum (asterisk). This is hypoplastic but not displaced. Tension apparatus for the anteroseptal tricuspid valvar commissure inserts in both the apical and antero-superior sides of the defect. The conduction tissue runs along its posterior margin.

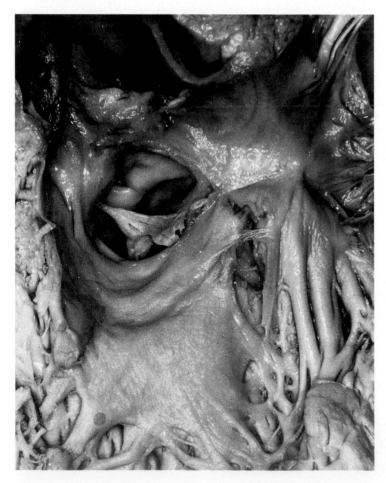

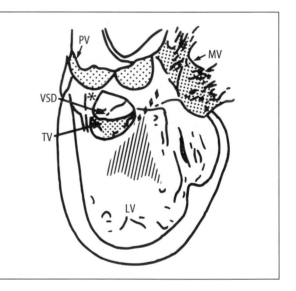

21.39 Left ventricular aspect. A small but clearly seen outlet septum (asterisk) separates the pulmonary and aortic valves. The tricuspid valve is attached to the anterior margin of the ventricular septal defect (on the outlet septum) and the leaflet is visualized through the defect. Because there is no displacement of the outlet septum, neither great artery overrides the defect. Externally the aorta is anterior and to the right of the pulmonary artery in this heart.

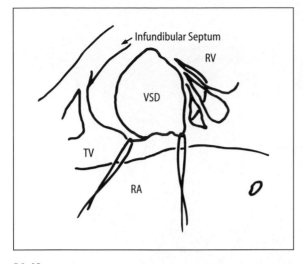

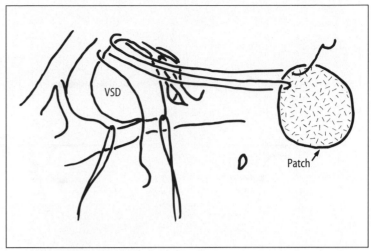

21.40 As neither outflow is obstructed and neither great artery overrides the ventricular septal defect, the preferred surgical management for this patient would be closure of the ventricular septal defect combined with arterial switch. The tricuspid valve in hearts with transposed great arteries, in contrast to those with normal ventriculo-arterial connections, is often just normal size, which may make exposure of the defect through the right atrium slightly difficult, particularly the upper extension towards the outlet septum. However, a right atrial approach is usually still employed. The conduction tissue will run along the posterior margin of the defect, on the surgeon's right-hand side, as viewed through the tricuspid valve.

21.41 Suturing along the left-hand margin of the defect with the patch held under slight tension towards the patient's feet will help to pull the upper portion (infundibular or outlet septum) into view. The tricuspid valvar leaflets and cords are retracted with stay-sutures.

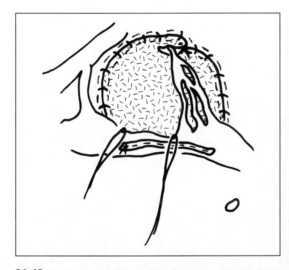

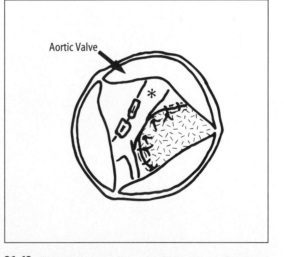

21.42 The tendinous cords inserting on the apical margin of the defect are near the conduction tissue and constitute important support for the antero-superior commissure. The patch is therefore split to pass around them and extend about half a centimeter beyond the posterior margin of the defect. In this area, it is repaired (patch-to-patch) with a few interrupted sutures. Sutures along the septal tricuspid valvar leaflet are supported with a small strip of autogenous pericardium. A small gap is left with the transition suture from the ventricular myocardium to tricuspid leaflet for the area of the penetrating bundle.

21.43 When the upper margin is not accessible through the tricuspid valve, it can be approached alternatively through the aorta after the great vessels have been divided and the coronary orifices have been removed. This is especially true when the infundibular septum is attenuated, as in this heart. Neither the conduction tissue nor the pulmonary (neoaortic) valve risk any injury by sutures passed through the outlet (infundibular) septum (asterisk).

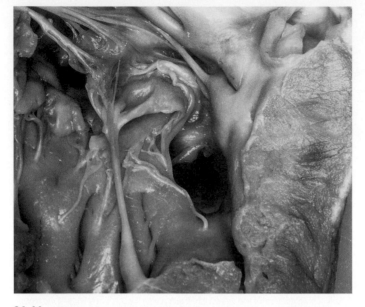

21.44 Ventricular septal defect in TGA. Right ventricular aspect showing a large peri-membranous defect extending into the trabecular portion of the right ventricle, in the angle of the septomarginal trabeculation. There is also a small area of fibrous continuity between the tricuspid valve and the mitral valve (seen through the defect and indicated on the diagram by stippling in a different direction). The outlet septum (asterisk) is malaligned and runs into the right infundibular fold. Additionally, there is an abnormal muscle bundle extending from the outlet septum and running towards the apex, anteriorly to the defect. The posterior basal limb of the septomarginal trabeculation supports a medial papillary muscle, while the apical portion is rotated on to the anterior wall of the right ventricle. The specialized conduction tissue passes along the posterior margin of the defect.

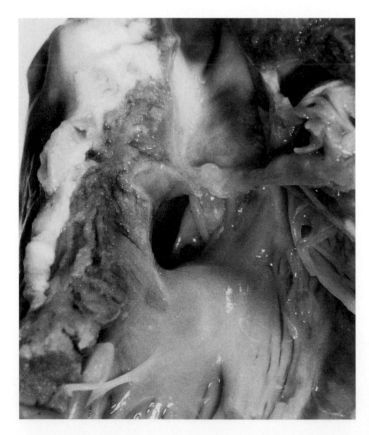

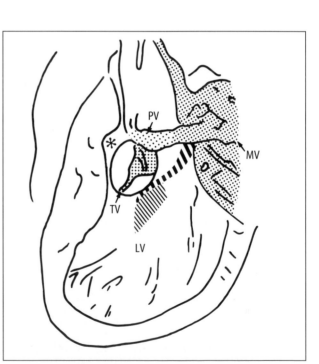

21.45 Left ventricular side, illustrating fibrous continuity between the pulmonary, mitral, and (seen through the defect) tricuspid valves. The pulmonary valve consists of a ridge of dysplastic tissue, analogous to that seen in "absent pulmonary valve syndrome" and is obstructive to the left ventricular outflow. The outlet septum (asterisk) is both displaced towards the left ventricle and rotated at an oblique angle relative to the trabecular septum. This also contributes to left ventricular outflow obstruction and causes the defect to lie in a slightly more subaortic than subpulmonary position. The common bundle and left bundle branch of the conduction tissue run posteriorly to the defect.

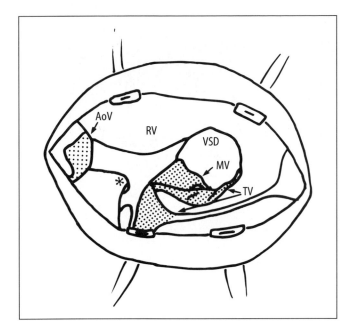

21.46 Left ventricular outflow obstruction, as a result of both the dysplastic pulmonary valve and displaced outlet septum, favors a surgical repair that directs the left ventricle to the anterior aorta in this heart (Rastelli or REV procedure). Enlargement of the ventricular septal defect by septal resection can improve both the size and geometry of the left ventricular to aortic pathway. The right ventricle is opened with a vertical or oblique incision. This is made low down to avoid injury to the aortic valve, which is typically located within the muscle of the right ventricular outflow. Retraction of the edges of the ventriculotomy with stay-sutures supported by pledgets gives clear exposure of the defect, the outlet septum (asterisk), the tricuspid valve and the subaortic area.

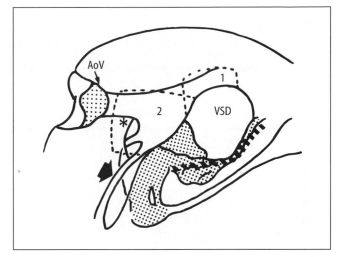

21.47 From the surgeon's perspective, the conduction tissue will pass along the right-hand margin of the defect. Traditionally, muscle has been removed anteriorly (1) to enlarge the ventricular septal defect. In this heart, however, rotation of an abnormal trabeculation on to the anterior wall of the right ventricle severely limits the amount of septum which can be removed in this area. Resection of this muscle does not, thus, improve greatly the left ventricular to aortic pathway. As described in the REV procedure, removal of the outlet septum (asterisk) between the defect and the aortic valve (2) will both enlarge the ventricular septal defect and create a direct route from left ventricle to aorta. The cords from the tricuspid valve to this area (arrow) are not supporting the leaflet and can be divided.

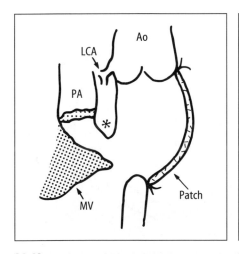

21.48 Seen in cross-section, the outlet septum (asterisk) lies between the posterior pulmonary artery and anterior aorta. When this is not resected, the tunnel patch must bulge into the right ventricle to obtain an unobstructed pathway from left ventricle to aorta. Potentially, this may compromise the outflow of the right ventricle as well as leave restriction to the left ventricular outflow.

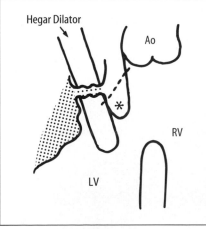

21.49 Resection of the outlet septum (asterisk) is guided by placement of a Hegar dilator backwards through the pulmonary valve. This also protects the mitral valve. Since the aorta lies at a higher level than the pulmonary artery, muscle is removed obliquely (dashed line) to avoid damage to the pulmonary valvar annulus and the left coronary artery.

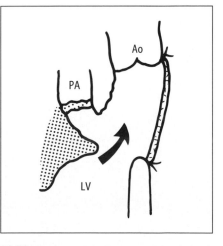

21.50 The left ventricular to aortic pathway (arrow) is now more direct and the patch is virtually flat. Depending upon the remainder of the procedure, the orifice of the pulmonary valve is closed, either from the right ventricle prior to completion of the left ventricular to aortic tunnel or from the pulmonary arterial side or both (see Figures 21.101–21.105).

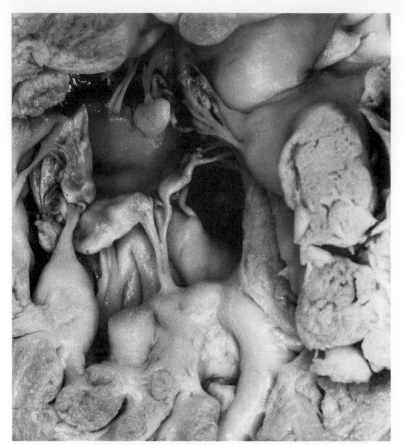

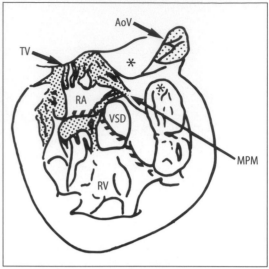

21.51 Ventricular septal defect in TGA. Right ventricular side exposed by removal of the anterior (free) wall, showing a perimembranous defect with inlet and trabecular extension. The subaortic area is severely narrowed by anterior displacement and hypertophy of the outlet septum (upper asterisk), as well as ramification of the septomarginal trabeculation onto the anterior wall of the ventricle (lower asterisk). The non-branching bundle lies on the postero-inferior margin of the defect. The medial papillary muscle complex inserts anteriorly and would lie within the long oblique pathway from the left ventricle to the aorta.

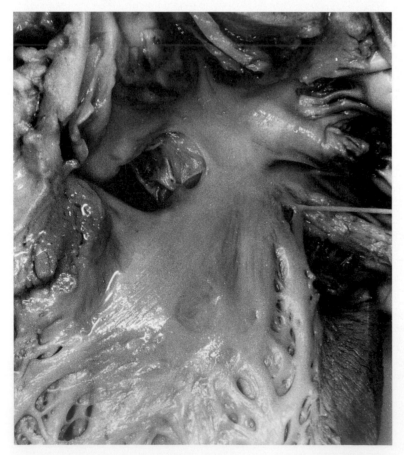

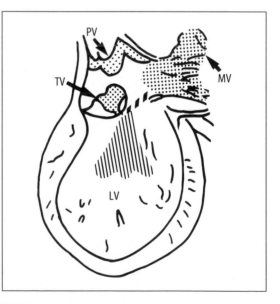

21.52 Left ventricular aspect of the above perimembranous inlet/trabecular defect, with the outlet septum, between the pulmonary valve and the upper margin of the defect, displaced anteriorly. This rightward or anterior malalignment of the outlet septum (away from the plane of the photograph), brings the pulmonary valve above the ventricular septal defect, which is thus "subpulmonary" and part of the spectrum of the so-called "Taussig-Bing" anomaly. However, pulmonary-mitral valvar continuity is retained. This is in distinction to the morphology described originally as the "Taussig-Bing" malformation where there was double outlet right ventricle and bilateral muscular infundibulum. The tricuspid valve is seen through the defect and inserts on its margin in proximity to the non-branching bundle and bifurcation of the conducting tissue.

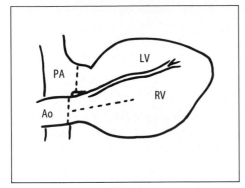

21.53 *(left)* Considering the right ventricular outflow obstruction, the insertion of the medial papillary muscle on the margin of the ventricular septal defect and the long distance between the defect and the aortic valve, tunnelling the left ventricle to the aorta is not a good option in this heart. Surgical management, therefore, consists of an arterial switch operation, closure of the ventricular septal defect, and enlargement of the right ventricular outflow by muscle resection and a transannular patch. The side-by-side great arteries are divided for the arterial switch and the neopulmonary artery is opened across the small aortic valve into the right ventricle (dashed lines).

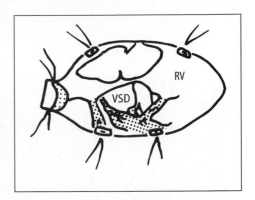

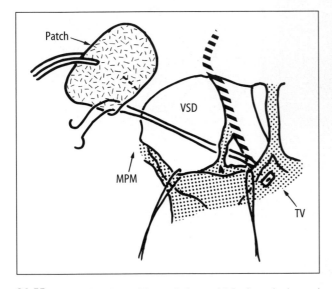

21.54 *(above right)* The ventriculotomy is held open with pledgeted stay-sutures. Division of the muscle bundles on the anterior free wall of the right ventricle facilitates exposure of the ventricular septal defect. However, its position in the inlet septum with an overlying papillary muscle and septal malalignment may make visualization of the posterior margin of the defect difficult. Alternatives would be to combine this approach with working either through the right atrium or backwards through the pulmonary (neoaortic) valve, remembering that a patch on the left side of the septum would cross the non-branching bundle and bifurcation of the conducting tissue.

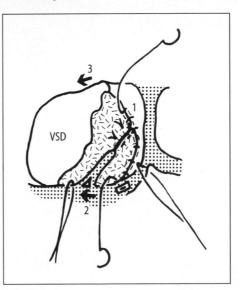

21.55 *(above)* Although part of the ventricular septal defect lies under the septal leaflet of the tricuspid valve, the defect does not extend to the posterior wall of the heart. The conducting tissue, therefore, runs along the posterior margin of the defect (to the surgeon's right hand). Retraction of the septal tricuspid valve leaflet exposes the posterior angle of the defect and elevates it into the right ventricle, where a pledgeted mattress suture is passed from the right atrial side through the base of the tricuspid valvar leaflet. This suture passes beneath the cords which insert on the crest of the defect and then through a patch held towards the patient's head.

21.56 *(above)* Having placed this initial suture, the patch is gently lowered into the heart and split to pass around the cords. Suturing continues (1) about 3–5 mm beyond the posterior margin of the defect to avoid injury to the conduction tissue. The split in the patch is repaired with interrupted sutures. Access to the margin of the defect at this time is improved by pushing the patch through the defect into the left ventricle. At approximately the junction of the trabecular septum with the outlet septum (3) it is convenient to return to the other arm of the suture along the tricuspid valvar leaflet (2) while mobility of the patch still permits good visibility. Alternatively, an interrupted suture technique may be employed throughout, with the patch held at a distance.

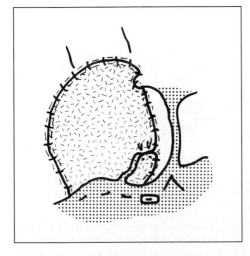

21.57 *(above)* Rightward displacement of the outlet septum and hypertrophy of muscle bundles tends to make the right ventricular cavity small. The completed patch should thus be flat to avoid further loss of right ventricular volume.

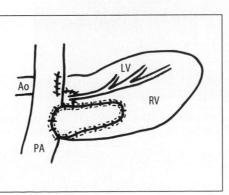

21.58 *(left)* With side-by-side great vessels the attachment of the neopulmonary artery to the pulmonary artery may lie more comfortably at a site other than the original pulmonary bifurcation. Moving it rightward in this heart helps to avoid compression of the left coronary artery which has been transferred to the neoaorta. A transannular patch enlarges the right ventricular outflow tract and closes the ventriculotomy.

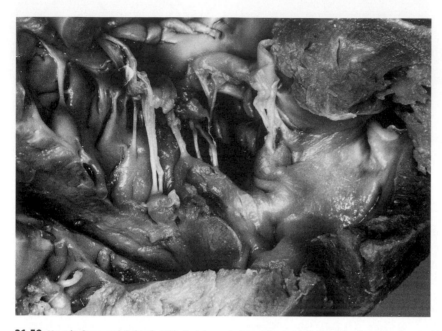

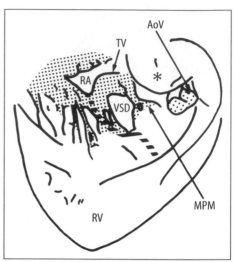

21.59 Ventricular septal defect in TGA. Septal aspect of the right ventricle. The defect lies under the septal leaflet of the tricuspid valve, posteriorly to the medial papillary muscle complex, which inserts on the outlet septum. The defect opens into the inlet of the right ventricle. The outlet septum is displaced rightward and hypertrophied. This malalignment (asterisk), together with hypertrophy of the ventriculo-infundibular fold, results in severe subaortic obstruction. The conduction tissue lies along the posterior margin of the defect.

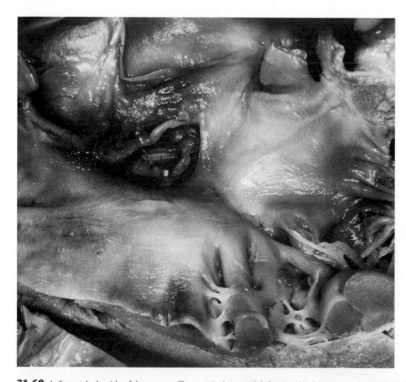

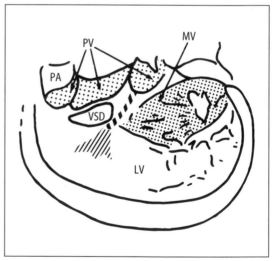

21.60 Left ventricular side of the septum. The ventricular septal defect is subpulmonary and extends to the area of fibrous continuity between the mitral, tricuspid, and pulmonary valves, in this way being also "perimembranous." The tricuspid valvar leaflet is seen through the defect. The papillary muscles of the mitral valve have been removed.

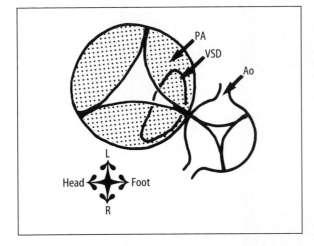

21.61 In this heart, rightward displacement of the outlet septum will necessitate enlargement of the right ventricular outflow tract with a transannular patch. Correction, therefore, requires an arterial switch procedure and closure of the ventricular septal defect. The defect lies beneath the pulmonary valve and, following division of the great arteries, may be approached retrogradely through the large pulmonary annulus.

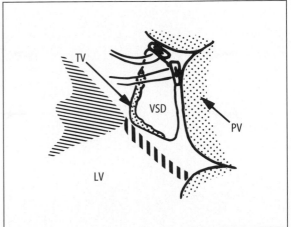

21.62 After retraction of the valvar leaflets, interrupted sutures are placed precisely along the upper margin of the defect, taking care to avoid damage to the neoaortic valve. The conduction system passes on the side of the defect which is closest to the surgeon in this exposure. The tricuspid valve is identified through the ventricular septal defect, on the right ventricular side of the septum in this area.

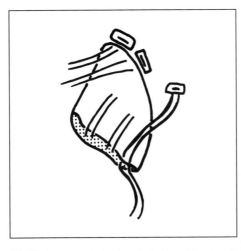

21.63 Sutures are deviated on to the base of the tricuspid valvar leaflet in order to avoid injury to the conduction system. By using interrupted sutures, each one may be placed accurately with good visualization of both the valvar leaflet and the left ventricular side of the septum.

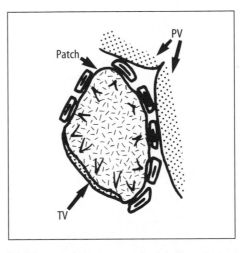

21.64 When all the sutures have been placed, they are passed through the patch and tied down. If there is a small leak at the transition between the sutures on the left side of the ventricular septum and those on the tricuspid valve, it is better to accept this than to risk heart block from additional stitches. The neoaortic valve leaflets are carefully inspected and the arterial switch part of the operation is then completed.

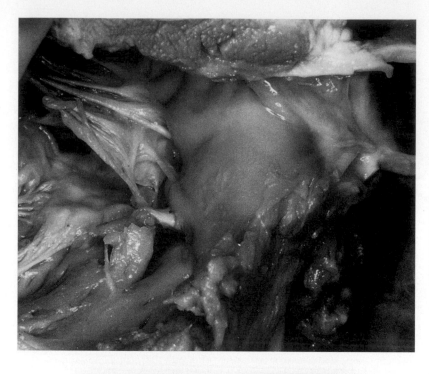

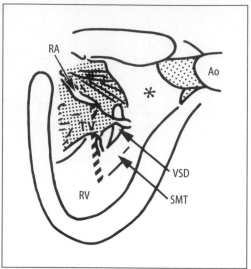

21.65 Ventricular septal defect in TGA. The anterior wall of the right ventricle has been retracted to show the tricuspid valve, aortic valve, and septum. The ventricular septal defect is muscular and lies along the posterior edge of the septomarginal trabeculation. The outlet septum (asterisk) is displaced (malaligned) towards the right ventricle and hypertrophied, producing subaortic obstruction. The aortic valve, however, is structurally normal. The conduction tissue runs posteriorly to the defect.

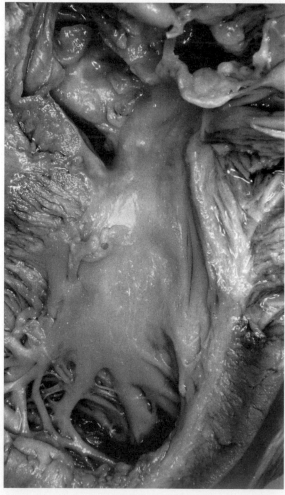

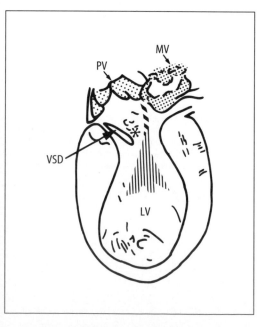

21.66 The septal aspect of the left ventricle in this heart shows the slit-like defect surrounded entirely by muscle. It is angled towards the outlet of the left ventricle with slight overriding of the pulmonary valve. Accessory fibrous tissue (asterisk) is intruding into the defect. The conduction tissue is separated from the margin of the defect by a rim of muscle.

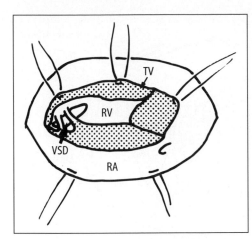

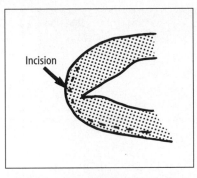

21.68 To improve exposure and avoid injury to cords, the septal and anterior leaflets of the tricuspid valve are detached in the area overlying the defect, about 3 mm from the base of the leaflet.

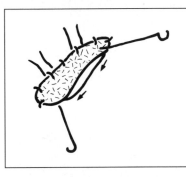

21.69 Retraction of the cut edge of the leaflets with fine stay-sutures now gives good access to the defect. The muscular margins are clearly identified. The conduction tissue lies to the surgeon's right hand and is separated from the posterior margin of the defect by a rim of muscle.

21.67 The arterial switch operation and closure of the defect would be the optimal repair for this heart. The neopulmonary valve is assessed intraoperatively after division of the aorta. The right ventricular outflow is enlarged, if necessary, with an infundibular or transannular patch. If an incision into the right ventricle is not needed, the defect would be approached through the right atrium. Stay-sutures at 10 o'clock, noon, and 2 o'clock on the tricuspid valvar annulus usually give good exposure, but, as major cords overlie the defect in this heart, access to the margins of the ventricular septal defect through the tricuspid valve may be somewhat limited.

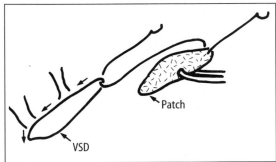

21.70 A continuous monofilament suture is started at the angle of the defect furthest away from the surgeon, with the patch held towards the patient's foot. Gentle traction on the suture then helps to pull the edge of the defect toward the surgeon.

21.71 The second arm of the suture is brought towards the surgeon along the posterior margin of the defect. Since the conduction tissue is remote, sutures may be safely placed entirely around the edge of the ventricular septal defect.

21.72 The tricuspid valve is repaired with interrupted mattress sutures supported by strips of pericardium. This slightly shortens the anterior and septal leaflets at their commissure. Taking slightly wider bites on the base of the leaflet compared with those on the cut edge will accomplish a limited annuloplasty and decrease the amount of tricuspid valvar incompetence.

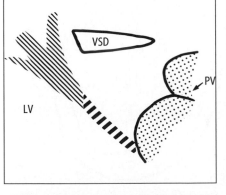

21.73 An alternative approach to the defect is to work retrogradely through the neoaortic valve on the left ventricular side of the septum, after division of the main pulmonary artery. Although the defect is not immediately adjacent to the valve, the large size and overriding of the valve still give good access. Looking into the left ventricle through the pulmonary (neoaortic) valve, the conduction tissue will run on the surgeon's side of the defect.

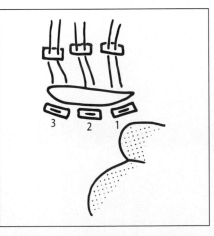

21.74 The defect is a slit which may be closed by direct suture without compromising the left ventricular outflow tract, or the mitral or neoaortic valves. This situation is *not* common. The first interrupted mattress suture is placed at the top of the defect and used to elevate the septum for placement of subsequent sutures.

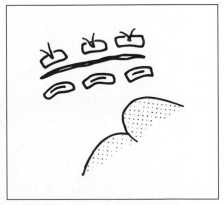

21.75 After all the sutures are placed, they are tied with just enough tension to approximate the edges of the defect. The last suture is kept close to the edge of the defect to avoid the conduction tissue. Care is taken also not to traumatize this area with instruments. The neoaortic valve is inspected finally for any signs of injury.

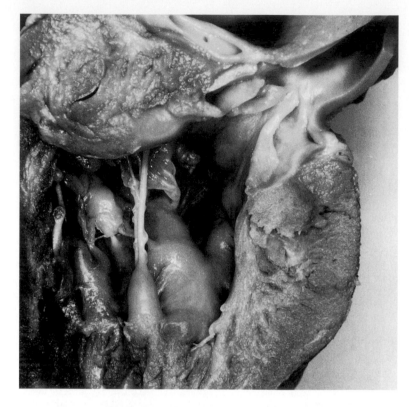

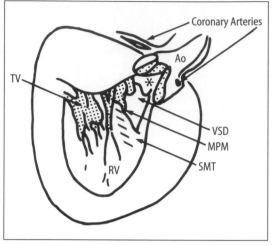

21.76 Ventricular septal defect in TGA. Perimembranous defect. The free wall of the right ventricle has been retracted upwards, exposing the septal surface and outflow tract. The defect is perimembranous, excavating into the trabecular septum in the angle of the septomarginal trabeculation. The medial papillary muscle complex is attached to the postero-inferior margin of the defect. The outlet septum (asterisk) lies in a plane displaced rightward (superficially into the right ventricle) in relation to the septomarginal trabeculation, thus producing gross malalignment. The aortic valve sinuses are set down into the muscular right ventricular outflow, such that the coronary arterial orifices and sinu-tubular junction lie at the epicardial surface of the heart. The conduction tissue passes along the postero-inferior margin of the ventricular septal defect subendocardially, until it reaches the medial papillary muscle, where the right bundle branch becomes intramyocardial. Nearer to the apex, it becomes subendocardial again.

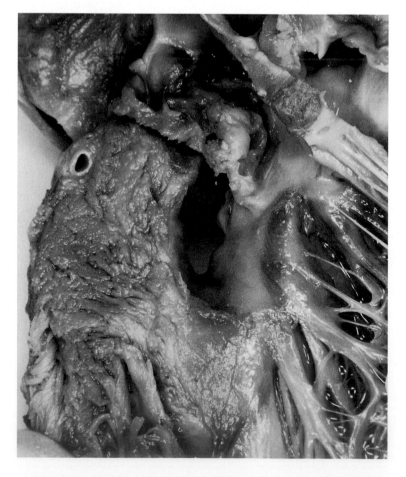

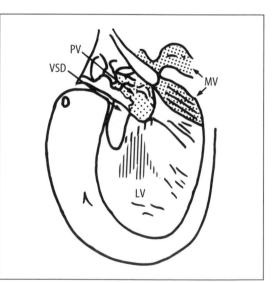

21.77 Left ventricular side of the septum, exposed by rotating the free wall upwards and to the right. The pulmonary valve is extremely dysplastic and the left ventricular outflow is obstructed by both the small stenotic valve and subpulmonary fibrous tissue extending to the area of fibrous continuity with the mitral valve. The right and left ventricles show equally severe hypertrophy and a large coronary arterial branch runs intramyocardially.

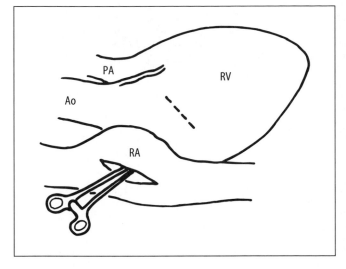

21.78 In view of the severe pulmonary obstruction, surgical management is planned to route the left ventricle through the defect to the aorta (Rastelli-type operation). The severe ventricular hypertrophy and downward displacement of the aortic valve into the right ventricle may complicate the ventriculotomy. The location of the defect and position of the aortic valve are first inspected through a right atriotomy. A right-angled instrument is then used to indicate the position of the right ventricular incision, which is kept very small until the interior of the right ventricle can be seen. Depending on the position of major coronary arterial branches, the ventriculotomy is either vertical or inclined obliquely up towards the left.

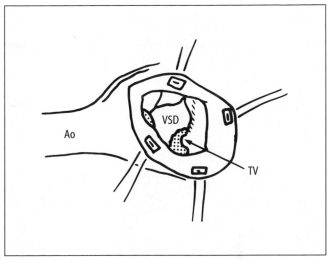

21.79 The thickened free wall of the right ventricle is held open with pledgeted stay-sutures, exposing the ventricular septal defect. The conduction tissue lies on the surgeon's right-hand margin of the defect. Thinning the endocardial side of the right ventricular free wall will improve access to the defect and outflow for the conduit without sacrifice of the coronary vessels or weakening the epicardial surface, which will later support the conduit to right ventricle anastomosis. The defect is equal in size to the aortic valve and does not need enlargement.

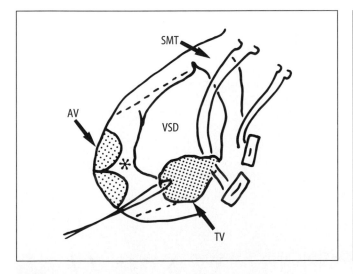

21.80 Since the conduction tissue runs along the edge of the defect, sutures are placed about 5 mm from its margin. Where the medial papillary muscle complex/tricuspid valve attach to the margin, the suture is passed through muscle and, leaving a gap, then through the tricuspid valvar tissue. It is important not to follow the muscular trabeculations onto the outlet (asterisk), which would create subaortic narrowing. From the septomarginal trabeculation and the tricuspid valve the suture lines pass outward on to the free wall of the ventricle (dashed lines).

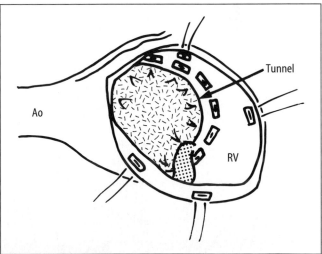

21.81 At the top of the ventriculotomy the Dacron patch comes around the aortic valve, often to the edge of the incision. Interrupted mattress sutures, supported by pericardial or Dacron pledgets, allow the path of the tunnel to be marked out accurately before the patch is inserted. The tunnel is slightly convex into the right ventricle and must be visualized in three dimensions. Closure of the pulmonary artery and connection of the right ventricle to the pulmonary artery with an extracardiac conduit completes the operation.

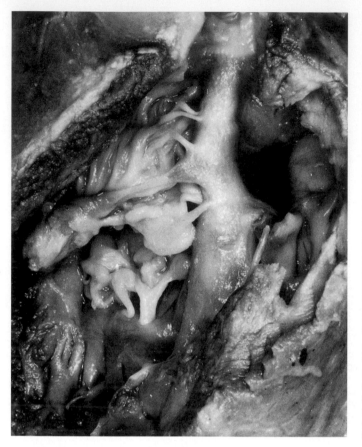

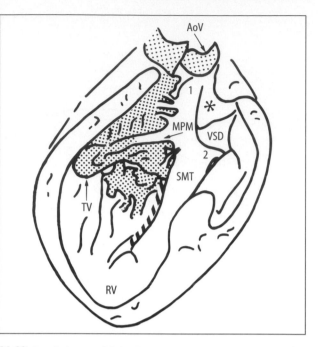

21.82 Ventricular septal defect in TGA. Right ventricular side of the septum. The muscular subaortic defect is produced by malalignment of the outlet septum (asterisk). The posterior limb of the septomarginal trabeculation extends to the right ventriculo-infundibular fold (1) and supports multiple cords from the tricuspid valve, while the anterior limb (2) passes through the ventricular septal defect. The aortic valve slightly overrides the defect. The tricuspid valve is grossly dysplastic. The conduction tissue is separated from the margin of the defect by the posterior limb of the septomarginal trabeculation.

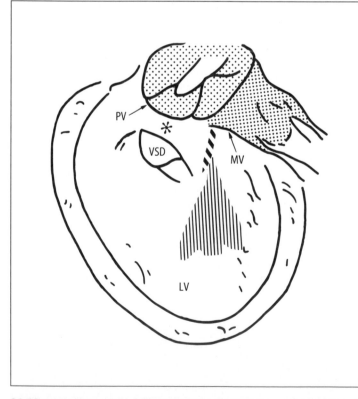

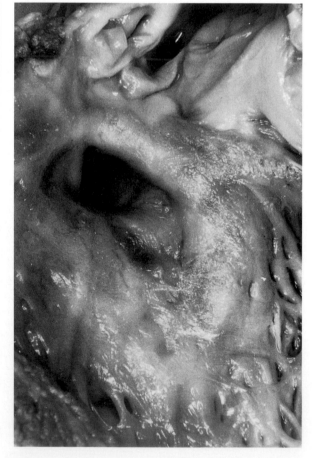

21.83 Left ventricular aspect of the muscular subaortic ventricular septal defect. The outlet septum (asterisk) is displaced into the left ventricle and produces mild subpulmonary obstruction. Conduction tissue is remote from the margin of the defect. In this heart the aorta lies anteriorly to the pulmonary artery and there is associated coarctation of the aorta.

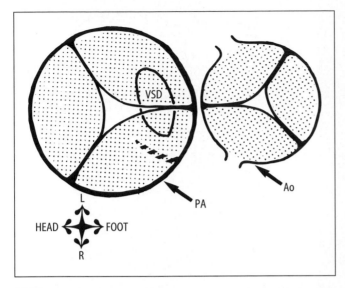

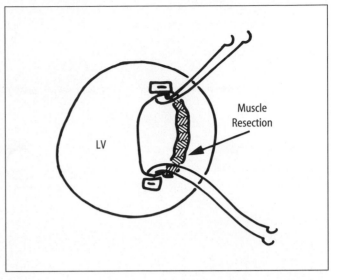

21.84 There are at least two surgical options in this case. The first possibility is to repair the coarctation and perform pulmonary artery banding with a view, ultimately, to a Fontan circulation, in consideration of the dysplastic tricuspid valve. The second option is repair of the coarctation, closure of the ventricular septal defect and arterial switch. In general, a circulation supported by two ventricles, whenever possible, is the preferred option. While the defect in this heart could be exposed through the tricuspid valve, its left-hand margin will be difficult to visualize. This is the result of short cordal attachments to the septomarginal trabeculation, and septal malalignment producing a deep crevice between the outlet septum and the posterior limb of the septomarginal trabeculation. Closure on the right ventricular side through the divided aorta is possible also, but again requires careful placement of sutures at junctions of the various muscle bundles. Given the comparatively remote position of the conduction tissue, the desirability of resecting the subpulmonary muscle bar (outlet septum) and the large size of the pulmonary valve, a transpulmonary approach would be preferred. From the surgeon's view, the conduction tissue will pass downwards on the left ventricular side of the septum, between the surgeon and the rightward margin of the ventricular septal defect.

21.85 Mattress sutures supported by pledgets at each side of the defect allow the septum to be gently rotated backwards and up towards the pulmonary valve. As the pulmonary valve lies at a deeper level than does the anterior aortic valve, the malaligned outlet septum can be removed from the subpulmonary area without much risk of injury to the aortic valvar leaflets.

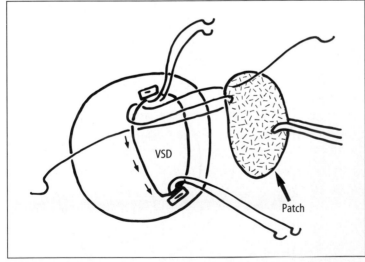

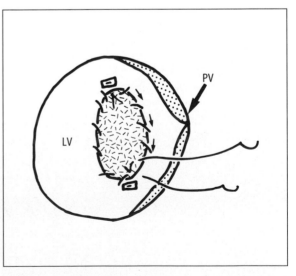

21.86 Sutures along the edge of the muscular ventricular septal defect are a safe distance from the conduction tissue. The retraction sutures are placed through the patch at the ends. Generally, the patch is lowered down to the septum after two or three bites to avoid tearing delicate myocardium.

21.87 The second arm of a continuous suture is used to complete the attachment of the patch to the septum, working forehand towards the surgeon. Stitches are placed between the area of muscle resection and the hinge-point of the pulmonary (neoaortic) valve. The completed patch is inspected and any areas of potential weakness are reinforced with additional pledgeted mattress sutures.

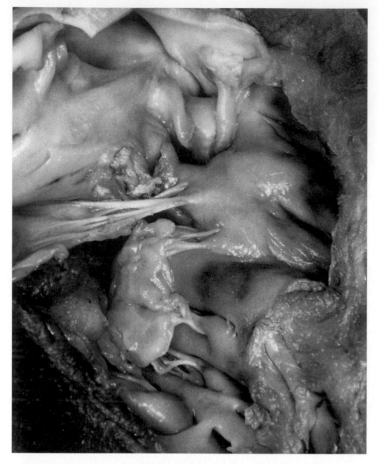

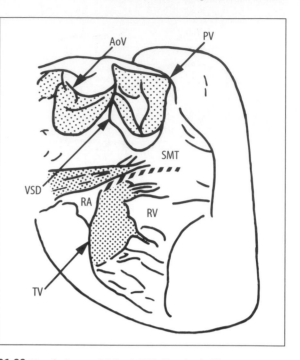

21.88 Ventricular septal defect in TGA. Muscular, doubly-committed sub-arterial defect. The right ventricle has been opened through its free wall to demonstrate the septal surface. The outlet septum is absent and the defect lies between the anterior and posterior limbs of the septomarginal trabeculation, of which the latter forms its muscular postero-inferior margin. The anterior aorta arises completely from the right ventricle and the pulmonary artery overrides the defect with fibrous continuity between the aortic and pulmonary valves. The conduction tissue is separated from the defect by the septomarginal trabeculation.

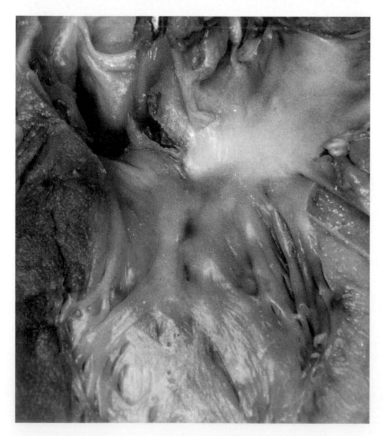

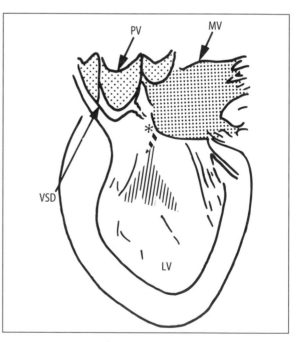

21.89 Left ventricular side of the septum, exposed by rotating the free wall upwards and to the left. The pulmonary valve overrides the ventricular septal defect but remains in continuity with the mitral valve. The membranous septum (asterisk) is intact. An "hour-glass" configuration narrows the left ventricular outflow at the level of the mitral valve and membranous septum.

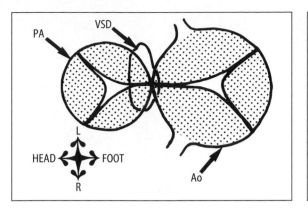

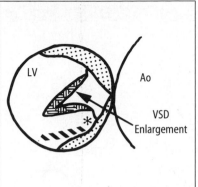

21.91 *(left)* After division of the great arteries and removal of the coronary orifices, scissors are used to incise the ventricular septum from the crest of the defect towards the apex of the left ventricle. The incision is made between the area of the conduction tissue/membranous septum (asterisk) and the hypertrophied free wall of the left ventricle (from which muscle also may be safely resected). Having positioned one blade of the scissors on the left side of the septum, the right ventricle is inspected through the aortic valve prior to making the incision, to avoid injury to the tricuspid valve.

21.90 *(above)* This heart is somewhat unusual in having a normal pulmonary valve which is, however, considerably smaller than the aortic valve. None the less, both ventricles are well developed and the atrioventricular valves are normal, so an arterial switch procedure with enlargement of the left ventricular outflow would be possible. From the surgeon's perspective, the doubly committed, subarterial defect gives access to left and right sides of the ventricular septum through the pulmonary and aortic valves respectively.

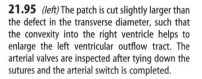

21.93 *(left)* The relation of the arterial valves to the ventricular septum is diagrammed in cross-section. The amount of fibrous tissue between the aortic and pulmonary valve leaflets is variable with doubly-committed subarterial defects. In this heart there is very little fibrous tissue and caution must be exercised to avoid catching the pulmonary leaflet (which will become the systemic arterial valve) in the suture.

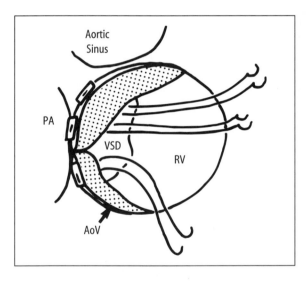

21.92 *(left)* The ventricular septal defect is approached through the anterior aortic (neopulmonary) valve. As the two arterial valves are in continuity, sutures pledgeted with autogenous pericardium are passed through the arterial wall into the ventricle immediately adjacent to the hinge-point of the valvar leaflet. When a coronary artery arises above the upper margin of the defect, it is important to leave sufficient sinus wall to support sutures for both closure of the defect and pericardial reconstruction of the sinus. Alternatively, the pledgeted sutures for closure of the ventricular septal defect may be passed first through the pericardial patch and then through the base of the sinus, sandwiching the rim of arterial wall between the Dacron and pericardial patches.

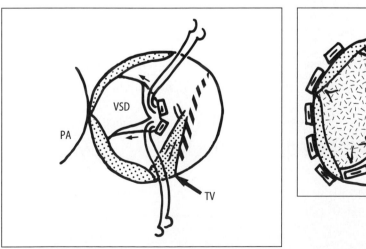

21.95 *(left)* The patch is cut slightly larger than the defect in the transverse diameter, such that the convexity into the right ventricle helps to enlarge the left ventricular outflow tract. The arterial valves are inspected after tying down the sutures and the arterial switch is completed.

21.94 *(above)* Because the defect has a muscular lower margin, sutures are placed on its edge, working from the apex of the enlargement (which may be a friable area of weakened tissue) back towards the aortic valve attachment. The medial papillary muscle complex lies between the edge of the defect and the conduction tissue. If the defect extends to the tricuspid valve, it is perimembranous and its lower portion is then approached through the tricuspid valve (see Figures11.50–11.53). In these cases, the conduction tissue will pass along the right-hand margin, as seen by the surgeon working through the right atrium.

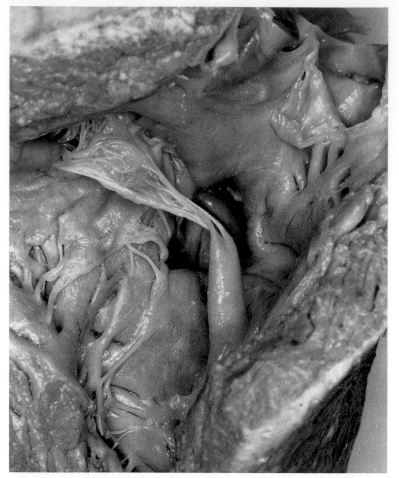

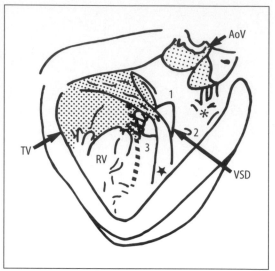

21.96 Ventricular septal defect in TGA. Right ventricular aspect of a muscular defect lying at the junction of the outlet (1), trabecular (2), and inlet (3) portions of the ventricle. Cords from the septal leaflet of the tricuspid valve attach to the postero-inferior margin of the defect but do not straddle into the left ventricle. Towards the apex of the heart, the septomarginal trabeculation, supporting the anterior papillary muscle of the tricuspid valve (star), rotates on to the anterior free wall of the right ventricle. The conduction system is separated from the edge of the defect by several millimeters of muscle. Muscular trabeculations extend to the hinge-point of the aortic valve leaflet (asterisk).

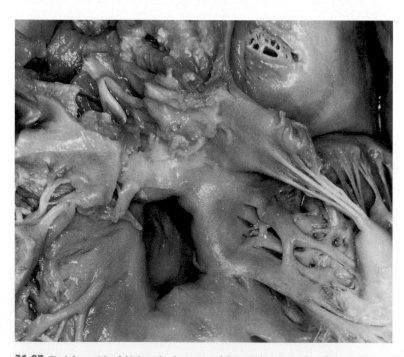

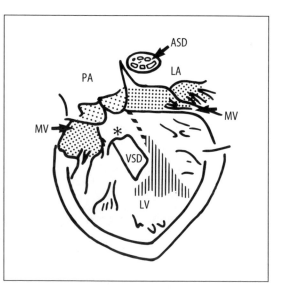

21.97 The left ventricle of this heart has been opened through the mitral valve which attaches to either side of the outlet septum (asterisk). The outlet septum is displaced into the left ventricle, producing muscular subpulmonary stenosis. The pulmonary valve is dysplastic. The defect has completely muscular margins and is not close to the conduction tissue. A fenestrated atrial septal defect of the oval fossa is seen from the left atrial side. In this heart the aorta is anterior and to the right of the pulmonary artery.

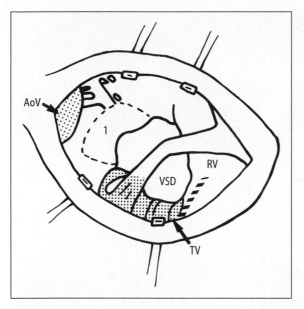

21.98 The presence of a dysplastic pulmonary valve and displacement of the outlet septum into the left ventricle eliminate the arterial switch operation as an option for this heart. However, resection of the outlet septum (1) is essential to connect the left ventricle to the aorta without obstruction in a Rastelli or REV procedure (see Figures 21.47–21.50). Exposed through an incision in the right ventricle, the conduction tissue will lie towards the surgeon's side of the defect, but separated from the right-hand margin by a rim of muscle under the cords from the tricuspid valve.

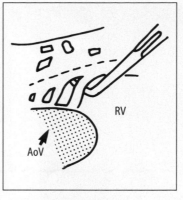

21.99 The suture line for the tunnel connecting the left ventricle to the aorta (dashed line) is brought up to the free wall of the right ventricle. It is important to ensure that no potential communications between the two ventricles remain behind muscle trabeculations. Muscle bundles attaching to the base of the aortic valvar leaflet are left intact if they are not obstructive, or divided as far away from the valve as possible to avoid loss of support for the sinus and subsequent aortic valve incompetence.

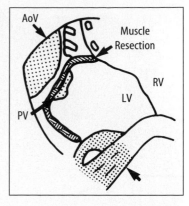

21.100 Following resection of the outlet portion of the septum and enlargement of the ventricular septal defect, the pulmonary valve will become accessible in the left ventricle. Secure closure of the pulmonary outflow is important in the Rastelli operation, both to avoid bleeding and to obliterate post-operative left-to-right shunting.

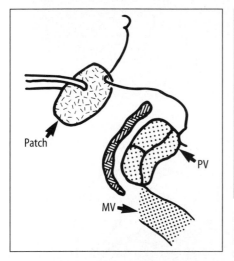

21.101 A patch of Dacron (or in cases of very small pulmonary valves, interrrupted mattress sutures supported by pledgets) is sutured to the ventriculoarterial junction of the pulmonary valve within the left ventricle. Stitches are placed within the valve "annulus" to avoid injury to the mitral valve or coronary arteries.

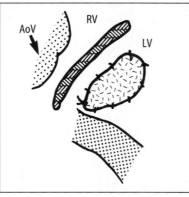

21.102 After completion of the patch, the pulmonary outflow falls back into the left ventricle. A small remnant of muscle supports the aortic valve and separates it from the Dacron patch closing the left ventricular outflow.

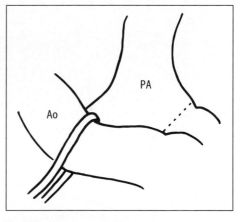

21.103 Externally, access to the pulmonary artery is achieved by dissecting it from the ascending aorta, which is encircled with a tape and retracted. The coronary arteries may arise fairly high on the aorta and pass close to the main pulmonary artery, thus placing them at risk of injury during this dissection. The pulmonary artery is transected just above the sinutubular junction (dotted line), taking care to avoid injury to a coronary vessel.

21.104 *(below left)* The distal main pulmonary artery will be used subsequently for the right ventricle to pulmonary artery conduit and is retracted upwards. A stay-stitch on the cardiac end of the vessel retracts it forwards and exposes the dysplastic valve leaflets. These are approximated with a continuous monofilament suture along the free margins.

21.105 *(right)* A purse-string is placed in the pulmonary arterial wall at the sinutubular junction. Before this it is tied, the valve sinuses are filled with hemostatic collagen felt and the suture is then gently tightened to avoid tearing the delicate arterial wall. Closing the left ventricular outflow at these three levels generally achieves hemostasis, but when additional sutures to the pulmonary artery are needed, these should be placed carefully in such a manner as to avoid compromise of any nearby coronary arteries.

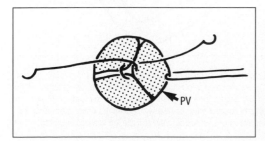

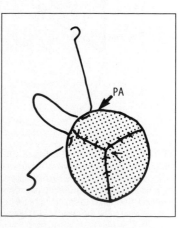

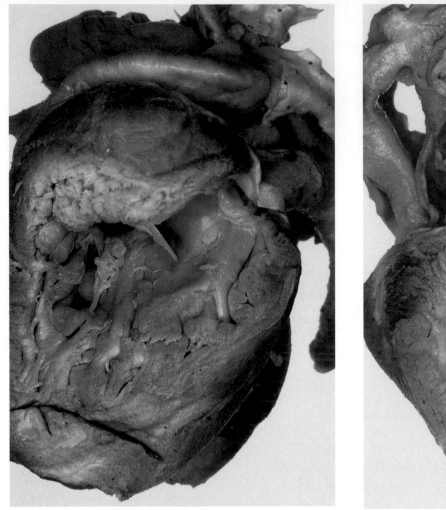

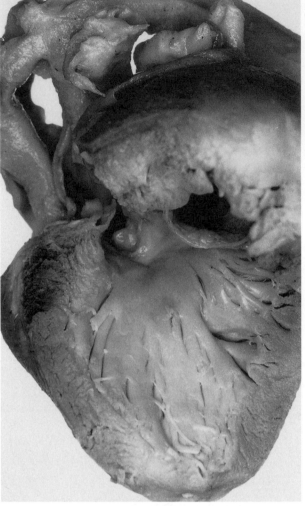

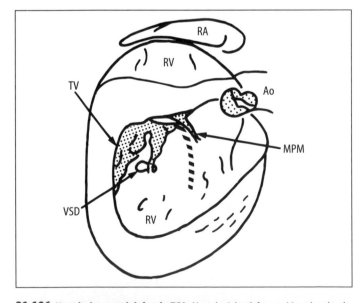

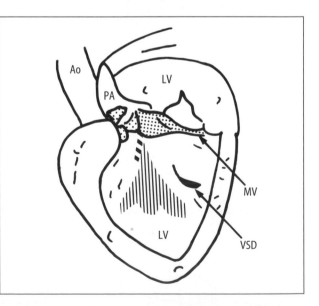

21.106 Ventricular septal defect in TGA. Muscular inlet defect positioned under the septal leaflet of the tricuspid valve. The defect lies posteriorly to the medial papillary muscle but is closely related to the posteroseptal papillary muscle and the posterior wall of the heart. The conduction system is anterior to and remote from the defect, having the usual relations to the intact membranous septum and medial papillary muscle. Proximally, it has a long intra-muscular course. The right ventricle has been opened from the apex like a clam shell.

21.107 Left ventricle, also opened from the apex with a clam-shell incision, showing the slit-like muscular ventricular septal defect. The defect abuts on the posterior wall of the heart, also in the inlet portion of the septum on the left ventricular side. This is in contrast with the next two specimens where the defects communicate between the right ventricular inlet and the left ventricular outlet.

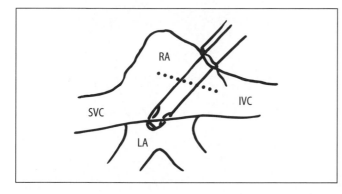

21.108 The ventricular septal defect in this heart is small and does not influence surgical management which, in the absence of ventricular outflow obstruction, is a neonatal arterial switch procedure. As closure of the ventricular septal defect can be done through the tricuspid valve and will not greatly prolong cardiopulmonary bypass or circulatory arrest times, a single venous cannula may be used for cardiopulmonary bypass. Inserting the cannula at the junction of the right atrium with its appendage leaves room for a standard atriotomy incision (dotted line) and facilitates positioning the tip across the atrial septum to drain the left side of the heart. After closure of the atrial septal defect, the tip is placed at the superior caval vein/right atrial junction which stabilizes the cannula and avoids trauma to the atrioventricular nodal area.

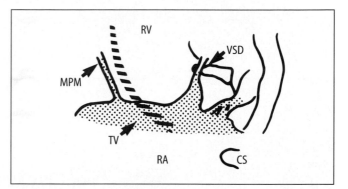

21.109 The ventricular septal defect is exposed through the right atrium and lies under the septal tricuspid valvar leaflet. Being surrounded by muscle, it is a muscular inlet defect. However, it lies posteriorly, with the right-hand margin extending virtually to the postero-medial papillary muscle and posterior wall of the heart. The conduction system will run in the usual position from the apex of the triangle of Koch towards the membranous septum and the medial papillary muscle, thus lying on the surgeon's left-hand side, remote from the defect.

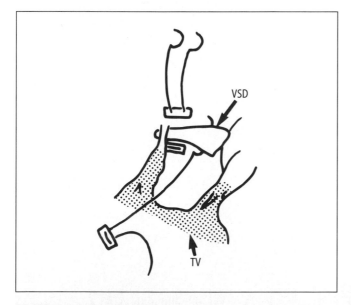

21.110 Identification of the ventricular septal defect within the right ventricular trabeculations may be difficult in the empty relaxed heart. In this event, a right-angled instrument passed through the interatrial communication and mitral valve can gently explore the left side of the septum until the tip appears through the defect. Interrupted mattress sutures supported by pledgets are then placed to approximate the muscular margins of the defect.

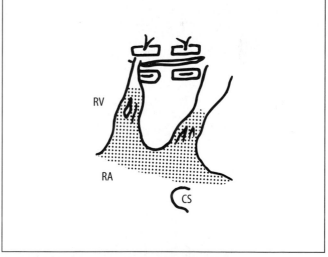

21.111 Appreciating the slit-like, horizontal orientation of the defect on the left side of the septum, the sutures are placed to bring the distal to the proximal margin of the defect. While closing the defect horizontally with forehand sutures may appear technically simpler from the right side, this would risk approximation of the trabeculations superficial to the margin of the defect and tension on the closure, both of which may predispose to a residual interventricular communication. Circulatory arrest time, if used, is minimized by placing a sucker through the right atrial cannulation site to re-establish perfusion while the atrial incision is closed.

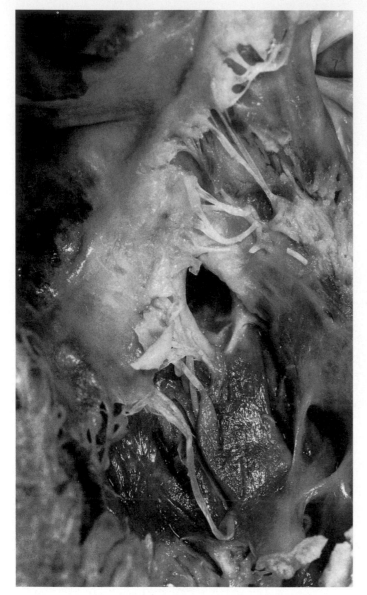

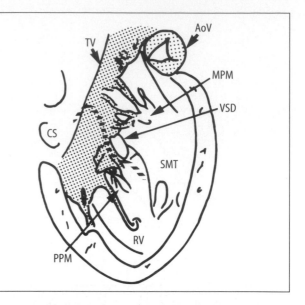

21.112 Ventricular septal defect in TGA. Septal surface of the right ventricle, showing a muscular defect which lies beneath the septal leaflet and subvalvar apparatus of the tricuspid valve (subtricuspid), but does not reach the posterior wall of the heart (contrast with Figure 21.106, which is also a muscular inlet defect). The axis of the conduction system runs posteriorly to the defect. The anterior margin of the defect is septomarginal trabeculation, which lies between the ventricular septal defect and the medial papillary muscle complex. Looking inside the defect, its oblique course through the malaligned septum is apparent and fibrosis is seen along the margins.

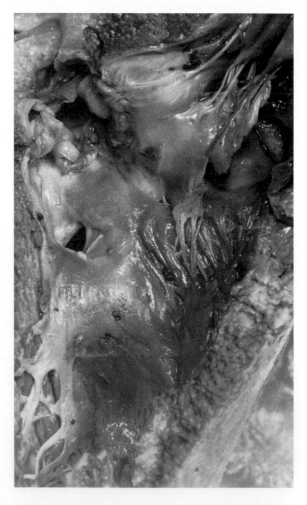

21.113 Left ventricular side, exposed by rotating the free wall upwards and to the left. The ventricular septal defect lies in a subpulmonary position on the left side, rather than reaching the posterior wall of the heart (asterisk). Its margins are malaligned, the side towards the apex being in a more superficial plane. The ventricular septal defect may be called an "inlet–outlet" defect because the right ventricular opening is in the inlet portion of the ventricle, while the left ventricular opening is in the outlet of the left ventricle. The proximal conduction system takes a long course.

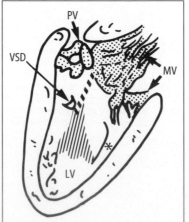

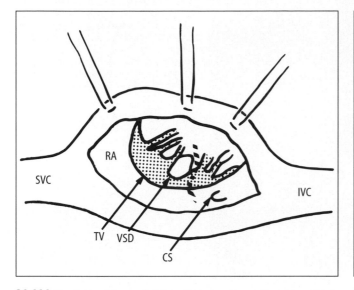

21.114 The slight malalignment of the outlet septum towards the right ventricle in this heart does not cause outflow obstruction. Both ventricles are well developed and the arterial valves are normal. An arterial switch operation with closure of the ventricular septal defect is thus the surgical correction of choice. The defect is approached through a standard right atrial incision and exposed by stay-sutures at 10 o'clock, noon, and 2 o'clock on the tricuspid valve annulus. Considering the time required for closure, bicaval cannulation and perfusion would be preferable to total circulatory arrest in patients of sufficient size. The conduction tissue lies subendocardially to the surgeon's right-hand side of the defect and is separated from its margin by a very narrow rim of muscle.

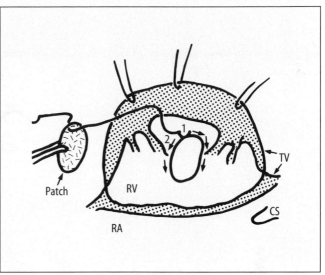

21.115 The cords of the tricuspid valve are attached along both sides of the defect, limiting access to the top margin. Access is achieved by detaching the septal tricuspid valvar leaflet a few millimeters from its base and retracting it towards the ventricle with fine stay-sutures (see Figures 21.68–21.72). Sutures for the patch are placed parallel to and directly on the right-hand margin of the defect to avoid conduction tissue. Suturing begins at the point furthest away from the surgeon (1) and progresses towards the "danger" area of the conduction tissue with the patch held away from the defect. The second arm of a continuous suture (2) is used to place stitches perpendicular to the margin after the patch has been lowered to the septum.

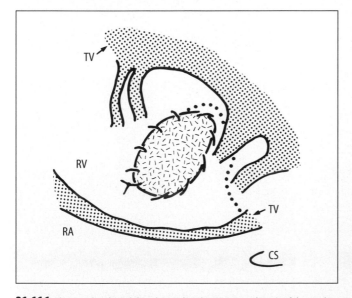

21.116 The completed patch lies close to but does not cross the axis of the conduction tissue with this technique. Alternatively, a much larger patch could be positioned over the conduction tissue and brought up to the base of the septal tricuspid leaflet, analogous to closure of a perimembranous ventricular septal defect (dotted line).

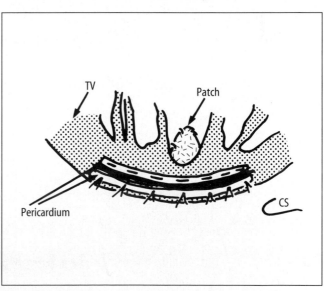

21.117 The tricuspid valve is repaired with fine interrupted mattress sutures supported on both sides by strips of pericardium. This shortens the septal leaflet by a small distance but does not cause major regurgitation through the valve. Following the arterial switch procedure, this valve remains on the low pressure right side of the heart, such that the mild tricuspid valvar regurgitation is well tolerated as the patient's pulmonary hypertension resolves.

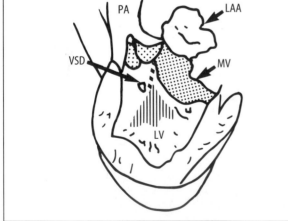

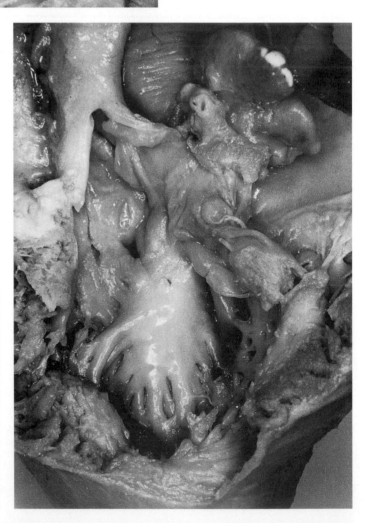

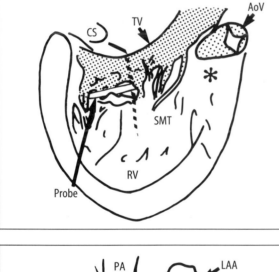

21.118 Ventricular septal defect in TGA. Subtricuspid, muscular defect in the inlet of the right ventricle. The defect is small and lies close to the medial papillary muscle complex which attaches to an enlarged septomarginal trabeculation. A probe has been passed through the defect to demonstrate its position. The axis of the conduction system runs posteriorly to the defect (surgeon's right-hand side looking through the tricuspid valve) and is not closely related to the margin of the ventricular septal defect. The outlet septum (asterisk) is enlarged also.

21.119 On the left side of the septum the defect opens into a subpulmonary position in the outlet of the ventricle and is thus another example of "inlet–outlet" defect in TGA. The conduction tissue runs towards the apex of the heart posteriorly to the defect. There is severe muscular hypertrophy which has reduced the left ventricle to a small cavity. While the pulmonary valve is normally formed and there is no discrete subpulmonary obstruction, the entire left ventricular outflow is hypoplastic.

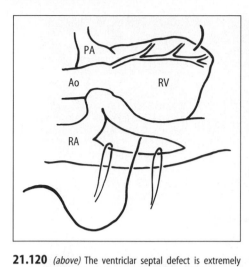

21.120 *(above)* The ventriclar septal defect is extremely small and, for purposes of surgical management, this heart may be considered an example of transposed great arteries with intact ventricular septum and left ventricular outflow obstruction. The defect may be closed through the tricuspid valve with interrupted mattress sutures (see Figures 21.108–21.111) at the time of atrial redirection (Mustard or Senning procedure). Because its cavity size is small and its outflow tract is diffusely hypoplastic without fibrous tissue or muscle that is amenable to resection, the severely hypertrophied left ventricle is decompressed with an extracardiac conduit to the pulmonary artery. The apical left ventriculotomy is facilitated by placement of a double-armed suture through the heart, working through the atrial septal defect and mitral valve.

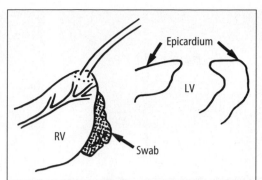

21.121 *(left)* With the apex of the heart supported by cold swabs and the table rotated towards the surgeon, traction is placed on the left ventricular suture. This rotates the apex towards the surgeon, such that a core of the thickened free wall (dotted line) can be excised with a no. 11 blade. Once the endocardium is identified, the edges of the ventriculotomy are undercut to improve outflow from the hypertrophied chamber. The epicardium is left intact to support the conduit anastomosis and ensure a good blood supply to this area.

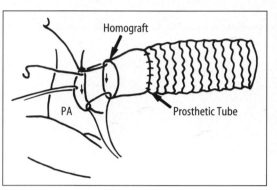

21.122 *(left)* A composite conduit is prepared by extending a homograft valve with a Dacron or Gore-tex tube graft. As there will be some flow through the native left ventricular outflow tract and limited space behind the left ventricle, the size of the conduit may be equal to or smaller than the diameter of the normal pulmonary artery. A longitudinal incision is made in the concavity of the left branch pulmonary artery and extended both proximally and distally into the lateral side of the main pulmonary artery. Generally, the posterior position of the pulmonary artery and this incision (compared with normally positioned great vessels) makes it easier to start with the posterior half of the anastomosis, working inside the pulmonary artery and valve, with the conduit positioned towards the patient's foot.

21.123 *(right)* The anterior half of the anastomosis is completed outside the vessel, again suturing forehand towards the surgeon. Visualization may be difficult in the not unusual situation of a large collateral pulmonary blood-flow. This can be managed by hypothermia and periods of reduced perfusion or, if the atrial repair is complete, allowing the heart to beat and empty the lungs. In either case, a sump-sucker (a feeding tube is convenient in small infants) passed through the conduit into the dependent pulmonary artery is helpful.

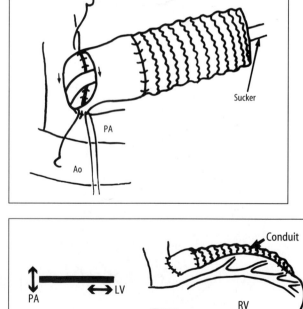

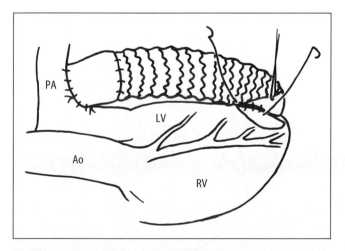

21.124 *(above)* The ventriculo-conduit anastomosis lies at an angle of approximately 90° to the homograft-pulmonary artery anastomosis (see Figure 21.125), and it is thus the medial side of the prosthetic graft which is trimmed to fit the ventriculotomy and avoid twisting the conduit. As the conduit is symmetrical, this geometry does not compromise hemodynamic function. The far side of the anastomosis is done inside the ventricle and the nearside is done outside, using a continuous monofilament suture (supported with strips of pericardium if the tissues are friable).

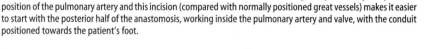

21.125 *(above)* When the heart is returned to the pericardium, the conduit lies posteriorly behind the left ventricle. Opening the posterior pericardium behind the phrenic nerve has been suggested to allow the conduit to fall into the left pleural space. However, this space is limited by the position of the pulmonary veins and will rarely accommodate an oversized or excessively long graft. Unlike a right ventricle-to-pulmonary artery conduit where the distal and proximal anastomoses are nearly in the same plane, those of the left ventricle-to-pulmonary artery conduit lie more or less at right angles to each other.

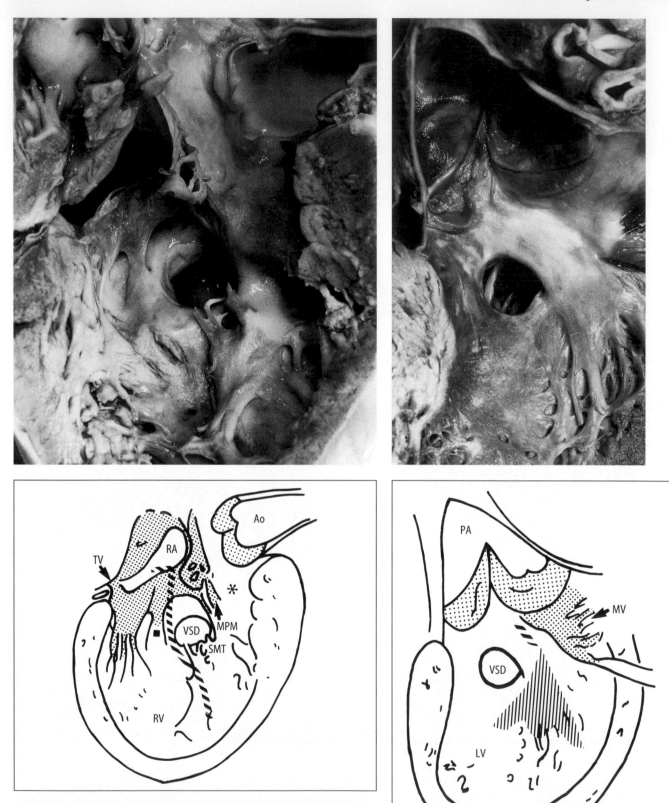

21.126 Ventricular septal defect in TGA. Large muscular defect. The right ventricle has been opened with the detachment of cords and papillary muscles to the anterior and posterior leaflets of the tricuspid valve which is rotated upwards. The defect is surrounded by muscle lying close to, but not under the septal leaflet of the tricuspid valve, and posteriorly to the medial papillary muscle complex. This inserts on the outlet septum (asterisk) antero-superiorly to the defect. Part of the subvalvar tricuspid mechanism is abnormal (square). This heart has not been studied histologically but, in consideration of the position of the ventricular septal defect in the left ventricular outflow tract, it is likely that the proximal conduction system takes a long course, bifurcating directly on or close to its posterior margin.

21.127 Left ventricular side of the septum. The ventricular septal defect is situated in a subpulmonary position, separated from the pulmonary valve by a short outlet septum which is not malaligned.

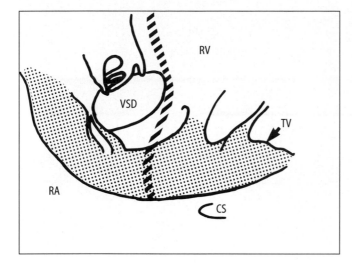

21.128 Both ventricles and their outlets are well developed in this heart, so that an arterial switch operation with closure of the defect would be the preferred surgical management. It is desirable also to leave the abnormal tricuspid valve on the low pressure, pulmonary side of the circulation. The ventricular septal defect will be readily accessible through the tricuspid valve. The conduction tissue, using this exposure, is likely to be related to the right-hand margin of the defect, from about 2 o'clock to 4 o'clock.

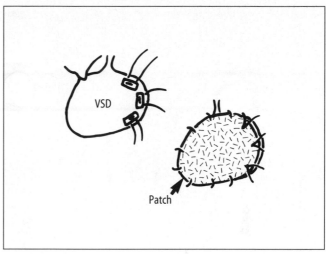

21.129 Closure of the defect on the right of the septum side can be accomplished by placing superficial sutures on the crest of the septum, or slightly towards the left ventricular side, through the defect in the areas of the conduction tissue and cordal attachments. Extension of the patch posteriorly to the defect and up to the base of the septal tricuspid leaflet is not a good option here, as the suture line would need to cross the conduction tissue in two places and would be limited posteriorly by the abnormal papillary muscle.

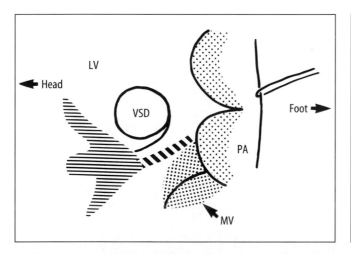

21.130 Alternatively, closure of the defect on the left side of the septum after division of the pulmonary artery for the arterial switch procedure would be an option also. The defect is fairly close to the large pulmonary valve and remote from the proximal conduction tissue. Exposure through the pulmonary valve is facilitated by a traction suture on the divided vessel which helps to rotate the outlet septum upwards and forwards (to the surgeon's right). The mitral valve and conduction system lie between the surgeon and the ventricular septal defect.

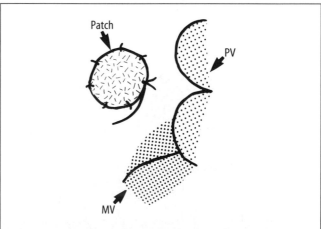

21.131 Sutures for the attachment of the patch are placed circumferentially around the muscular margin of the defect. This is facilitated by a half-circle needle of a size which can be comfortably passed through the pulmonary valve. Although transpulmonary exposure on the left side may be more difficult than through the tricuspid valve, in this particular ventricular septal defect there should be minimal risk of injury to the heart valves and conduction tissue with this approach.

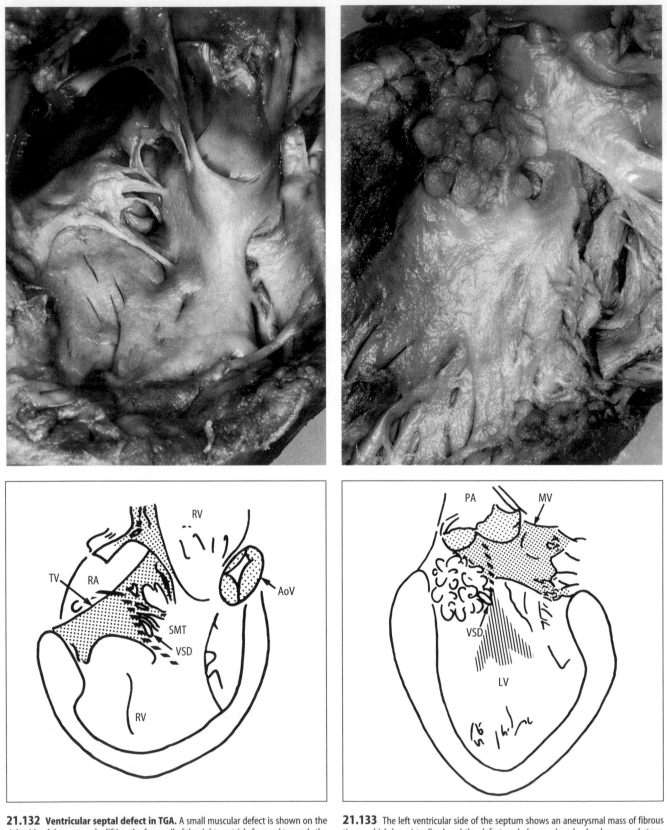

21.132 Ventricular septal defect in TGA. A small muscular defect is shown on the right side of the septum by lifting the free wall of the right ventricle forward towards the top of the picture. The defect lies under cords of the tricuspid valve, separated from the leaflet by a small rim of muscle (being thus a muscular inlet defect) and abuts on the posterior edge of the septomarginal trabeculation. The medial papillary muscle complex inserts at the lower edge of the outlet septum. The conduction tissue runs posteriorly to the defect.

21.133 The left ventricular side of the septum shows an aneurysmal mass of fibrous tissue which has virtually closed the defect and also produced subpulmonary obstruction. The pulmonary valve itself, however, is not restrictive. Conduction tissue lies close to the edge of the defect. In this heart, the aorta is anterior and to the right of the pulmonary artery.

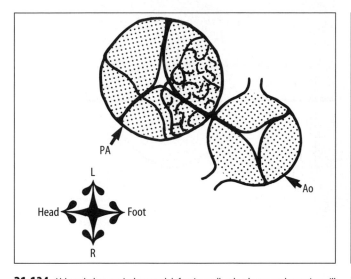

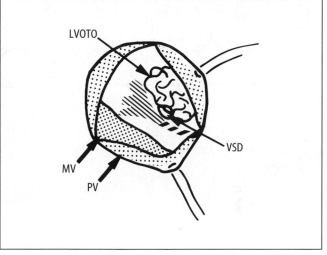

21.134 Although the ventricular septal defect is small, subpulmonary obstruction will have maintained elevated left ventricular pressure and the pulmonary valve is structurally normal, such that an arterial switch with closure of the defect will be possible even if the patient presents beyond the neonatal period. The outlet septum is not deviated significantly and resection of the fibrous excrescence can be done through the pulmonary (neoaortic) valve after division of the great arteries.

21.135 Stay-sutures above the pulmonary sinuses pull the valve forward and help to expose the obstructed posterior left ventricular outflow tract. The ventricular septal defect is a guide to the position of the conduction tissue which will lie towards the mitral valve between the surgeon and the defect.

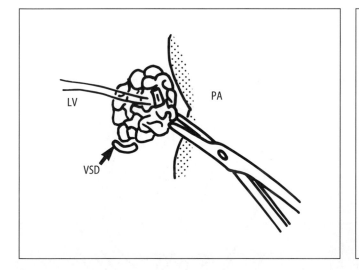

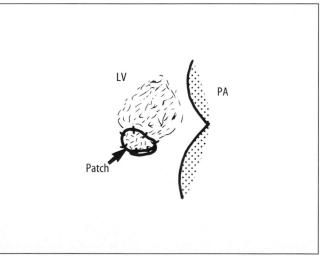

21.136 A stay-suture placed in the fibrous tissue is used to elevate it into the pulmonary valve. The fibrous mass is excised by sharp dissection, working downward from the pulmonary valve and staying on the far side of the ventricular septal defect.

21.137 The defect itself is small. However, it is likely to become enlarged if resection of the subpulmonary fibrous mass weakens the adjacent tissue. Closure with a patch is therefore prudent. If this is done on the left side of the septum, sutures are deviated towards the right ventricle in the area of the conduction tissue (see Figures 21.62–21.64).

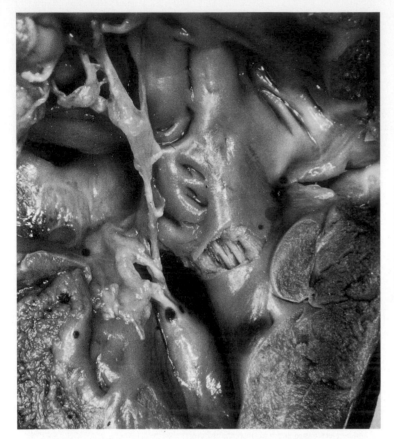

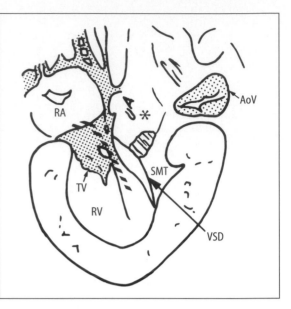

21.138 Ventricular septal defect in TGA. The right ventricular free wall has been rotated upward to demonstrate a long muscular defect which abuts onto the posterior edge of the septomarginal trabeculation. The body of the septomarginal trabeculation is rotated onto the wall of the right ventricle and contributes to outflow obstruction. The outlet septum (asterisk) is malaligned rightward, further narrowing the subaortic area. The tricuspid valve is abnormal, with poorly defined papillary muscles and short thick cords. The axis of the conduction tissue runs posteriorly to the ventricular septal defect but very close to its crest. This patient also has interruption of the aortic arch distal to the left subclavian artery.

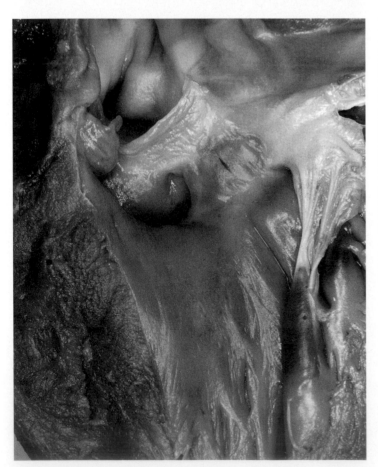

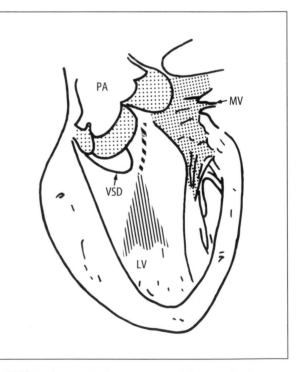

21.139 The left ventricular side of the septum shows malalignment of the outlet septum over the right ventricle, producing overriding of the pulmonary valve. The defect is thus "subpulmonary." This is also commonly called the 'Taussig-Bing' malformation where a subpulmonary ventricular septal defect occurs with transposed great arteries, although in reality it is a different malformation from the "true" Taussig-Bing malformation of subpulmonary defect with double outlet right ventricle.

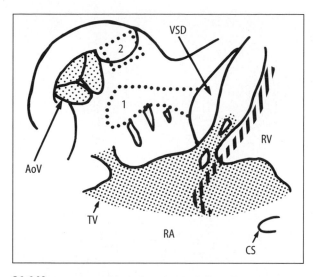

21.140 Compromise of both the right ventricular outflow and cavity is frequent in transposition of the great arteries with subpulmonary ventricular septal defect (Taussig-Bing malformation) as a result of the rightward deviation of the outlet septum. Anomalies of the tricuspid valve and aortic arch (coarctation or interrupted aortic arch) are also not uncommonly associated. The left ventricle is therefore used to support the systemic circulation by an arterial switch procedure with the closure of the defect, repair of any arch obstruction and relief of right ventricular outflow obstruction. The displaced outlet septum (1) may be carefully resected working from the right side, remembering that the pulmonary valve lies at a lower level than the aortic valve. Alternatively, a skin hook or stay-suture may be used to evert the outlet septum into the left ventricle for resection through the divided pulmonary artery. The subaortic infundibulum (2) includes the body of the septomarginal trabeculation in this heart, which is resected by working through the tricuspid valve. If these manoeuvres do not achieve an adequate outflow for both the right and the left ventricles, a subannular or transannular patch is placed on the free wall of the right ventricle. As seen through the tricuspid valve, the conduction system lies on the surgeon's right-hand side of the defect and is not close to the areas of muscle resection.

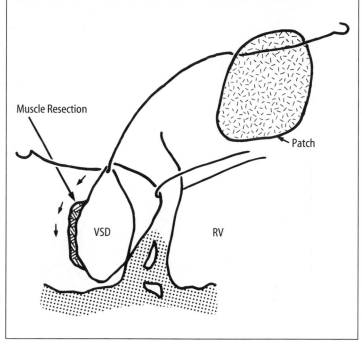

21.141 An over-sized patch is used to close the defect, such that the suture line can be deviated posteriorly to the conduction tissue. Even though the defect has muscular margins, suturing along the posterior (right-hand) edge would be very likely to damage the conduction tissue which is running adjacently to the defect. While placement of the stitches beyond the area of muscle resection may further reduce slightly the size of the right ventricle, this is done in order to achieve a secure closure.

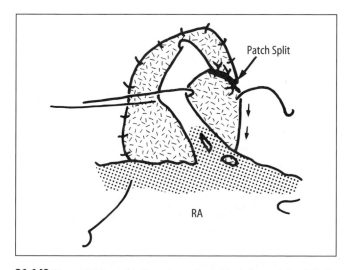

21.142 The patch is lowered to the septum and suturing continues counter-clockwise to the base of the septal leaflet of the tricuspid valve. The patch is then split to pass around the large papillary muscle. Suturing continues clockwise with the second needle behind the area of the conduction tissue. The patch is repaired snugly around the papillary muscle with additional interrupted sutures.

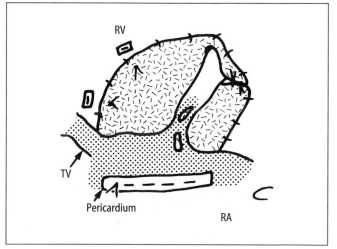

21.143 Treating a muscular ventricular septal defect as if it were perimembranous (extending to the tricuspid valve) brings the suture line on to the base of the septal tricuspid valvar leaflet where it is supported by a small strip of pericardium. The suture line thus crosses above the axis of the conduction tissue in the tricuspid valve. If a continuous suture is used, additional mattress sutures supported by pledgets are placed to reinforce any potentially weak areas in the closure. These are usually where there has been muscle resection or where the patch follows changes in the direction of the septum.

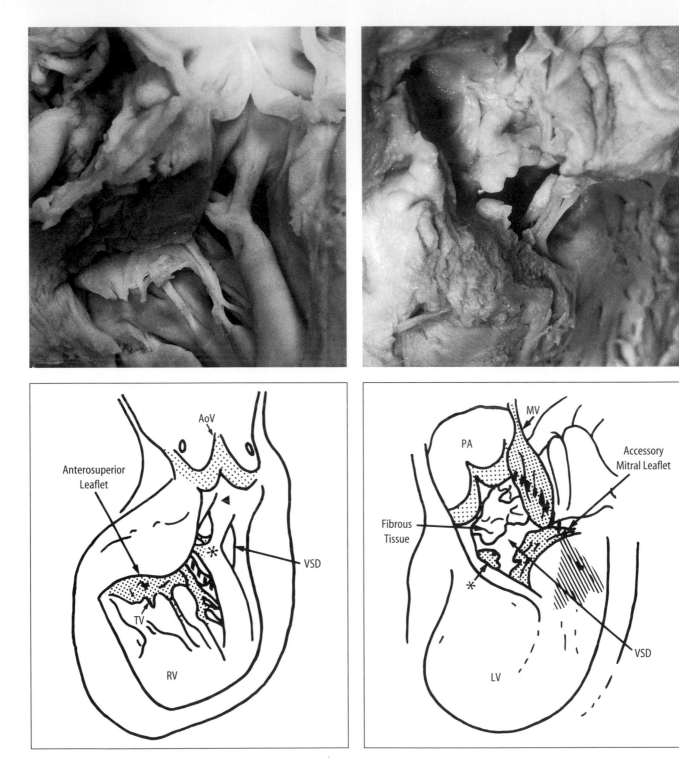

21.144 Ventricular septal defect in TGA. Right ventricular aspect of a perimembranous outlet defect extending also into the trabecular septum. The free wall of the ventricle has been removed superficially to the tricuspid valve, showing the ventricular side of the antero-superior leaflet. A free-standing bar of muscle extends from the position of the septomarginal trabeculation to the subaortic outlet septum (triangle) and supports part of the medial papillary muscle complex (asterisk). The conduction tissue passes along the posterior margin of the defect. Two coronary arterial orifices are seen in the aortic sinuses above a normal aortic valve.

21.145 Left ventricular side of the septum showing severe outflow obstruction caused by a cauliflower-like mass of subpulmonary fibrous tissue, an accessory mitral valve leaflet, and an abnormal attachment of the mitral valve. The anterior (pulmonary) leaflet of the mitral valve has been cut across and rotated upward. While the leaflet itself is not connected within the fibrous mass, its divided cordal attachments, seen on the anterior margin of the defect (asterisk), are continuous with the aneurysmal fibrous tissue. Commissural development of the mitral valve is unclear as a result of the accessory tissue attached to the defect. All the papillary muscles are fused, analogous to a parachute-like asymmetric mitral valve. The pulmonary valvar leaflets are normal.

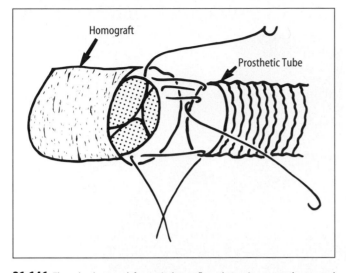

21.146 The subpulmonary left ventricular outflow obstruction cannot be resected without damage to the mitral valve and probably to the conduction system, thus ruling out an arterial switch operation in this heart. Tunnelling of the left ventricle to the aorta for a Rastelli operation is complicated by the attachment of the mitral valve and aneurysmal fibrous tissue to the margins of the defect on the left side and insertion of a bizarre free-standing muscle bundle (which also supports tricuspid subvalve apparatus under the aortic valve) on the right side. This is one of the rare instances where an atrial redirection (Mustard or Senning procedure) with closure of the defect and a left ventricular to pulmonary arterial conduit would be needed to achieve a two-ventricle repair. The long pathway of the conduit (see Figures 21.124 and 125) requires extension with a prosthetic tube graft. Two suture lines are used to attach the graft to the homograft, both for hemostatis and to prevent later formation of a false aneurysm at the suture line. A prosthetic tube equal to the inside diameter of the homograft is first attached inside the homograft with a running monofilament suture just below the valvar leaflets.

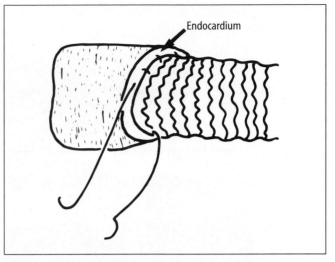

21.147 The inner suture line is full-thickness through the prosthetic graft but only through endocardium and muscle on the homograft. A small strip of hemostatic collagen felt is placed over this anastomosis between the homograft and the prosthetic tube.

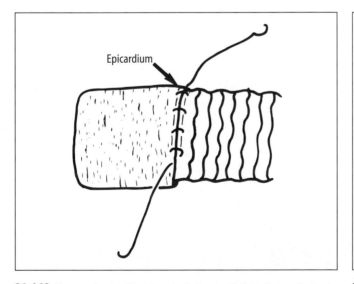

21.148 The second suture line brings the 2–3 mm cuff of the homograft over the hemostatic collar to the outer surface of the prosthetic tube. A running monofilament suture is used to take bites through the full thickness of the homograft and to pick up a few fibers of the prosthetic graft. If this suture line is sealed with clotting factors, it is important to check that the material has not migrated internally and "glued" the homograft leaflets together.

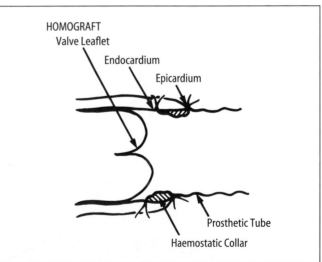

21.149 Seen in longitudinal cross-section, this technique downsizes the homograft slightly, which is useful to limit the size of the ventriculotomy. If a larger size tube is desirable, the prosthetic graft may alternatively be placed outside the homograft. In this case, a cuff of prosthetic tube would be turned back on itself and the end of the homograft is sutured firstly to the inside of the prosthetic graft. Hemostatic collagen is placed over the anastomosis, the cuff of the tube is pulled over the outside of the homograft, and its end is sutured to the valvar epicardium.

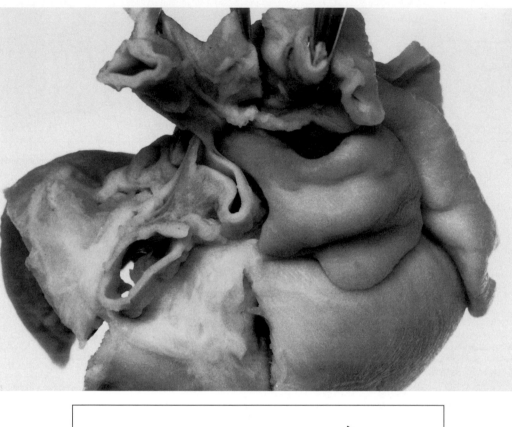

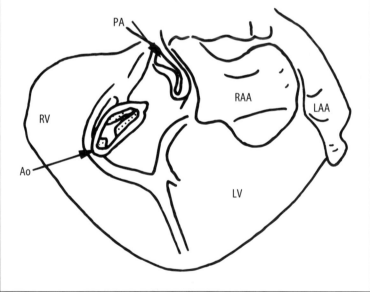

21.150 Left juxtaposition of the atrial appendage in TGA. Left anterior view, looking down on the left shoulder of the heart. Both atrial appendages are to the left of the pulmonary artery, that from the right atrium having passed through the transverse sinus to lie above the left appendage. It is always the appendage which has passed to the other side of the heart (i.e. the right atrial appendage in left-sided juxtaposition and the left atrial appendage in the less common, right-sided juxtaposition) which lies superiorly. Juxtaposition of the atrial appendages distorts the atrial septum and often produces unusual communications between the atriums. In this heart the atrial septum is unusually well developed with only a probe patent oval fossa. The ventricular septum is intact. A single coronary artery arises in the left-hand facing sinus.

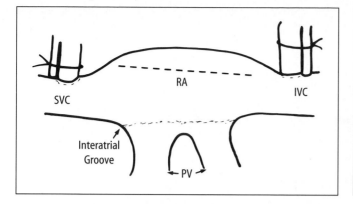

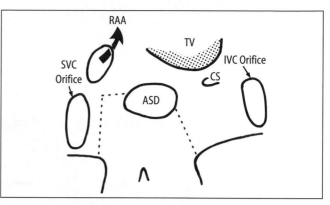

21.151 Left juxtaposition of the atrial appendages is of no import for the arterial switch operation but has major implications for the Senning procedure. This is because juxtaposition reduces the surface area of both the free right atrial wall and the atrial septum which is available to create the pulmonary (and, to a lesser degree, systemic) venous pathway. The right atrial incision (dashed line) is sited to provide two-thirds of the circumference of the inferior caval pathway from right atrial free wall. In the absence of an appendage on this side of the heart, this leaves little tissue between the atriotomy and the atrioventricular groove. Cannulation of the superior and inferior caval veins and mobilization of the interatrial groove are thus performed as usual to maximize the available surface of free right atrial wall.

21.152 A schematic representation of surgical landmarks inside the right atrium shows the orifice of the left juxtaposed appendage near to that of the superior caval vein. The first flap of septal remnant, which is translocated back between the left pulmonary veins and mitral valve to form the floor of the systemic venous pathway, is fashioned in the usual manner for a Senning procedure (dashed line). Additional tissue is usually needed because of the smaller septal surface and may be obtained by invaginating the left atrial appendage, imbricating the left atrial wall between the pulmonary veins and appendage, coronary sinus cut-back, or use of a pericardial patch. The left atrium is opened anteriorly to the right pulmonary veins, between the usual marking sutures where the veins join the left atrium.

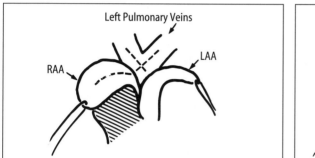

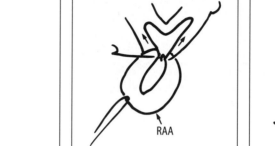

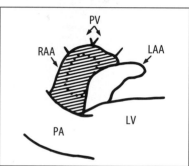

21.153 There is potential in this situation for obstruction to the pulmonary venous drainage, both behind the caval pathway and anteriorly to it. Accordingly, a second pulmonary venous pathway is created through the juxtaposed right atrial appendage. This is done most easily during the short period of circulatory arrest or reduced flow used for the first septal flap, or with a sucker positioned in the pulmonary veins through the right-sided left atrial incision. The left atrial appendage is retracted downward and the left pulmonary veins are opened within the pericardium (dashed lines). A corresponding incision is made on the facing surface of the right atrial appendage.

21.154 The juxtaposed right atrial appendage is joined to the left pulmonary veins with a running fine monofilament suture. As the anastomosis progresses away from the surgeon, the appendage is brought down to the veins. Exposure is facilitated by rotating the operating table towards the surgeon.

21.155 Upon completion, the left pulmonary veins may drain to the tricuspid valve, either through the left atrium behind the systemic venous pathway or through the right atrial appendage which passes behind the pulmonary artery. The left atrial appendage is displaced downward by this connection if it has not been invaginated for incorporation into the caval pathway, but does not cause distortion of the anastomosis.

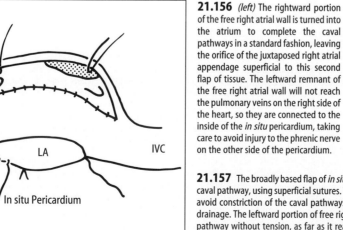

21.156 (left) The rightward portion of the free right atrial wall is turned into the atrium to complete the caval pathways in a standard fashion, leaving the orifice of the juxtaposed right atrial appendage superficial to this second flap of tissue. The leftward remnant of the free right atrial wall will not reach the pulmonary veins on the right side of the heart, so they are connected to the inside of the *in situ* pericardium, taking care to avoid injury to the phrenic nerve on the other side of the pericardium.

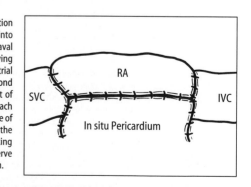

21.157 The broadly based flap of *in situ* pericardium is brought up superiorly and inferiorly over the caval pathway, using superficial sutures. The pericardial flap is made as redundant as possible, both to avoid constriction of the caval pathways and to provide an adequate lumen for pulmonary venous drainage. The leftward portion of free right atrial wall is brought down to the upper part of the caval pathway without tension, as far as it reaches comfortably. The free edges of pericardium and right atrium are finally joined to complete the pulmonary venous pathway. Leaving the pericardium *in situ* conserves its blood supply and growth potential, as well as facilitating an unobstructed anastomosis.

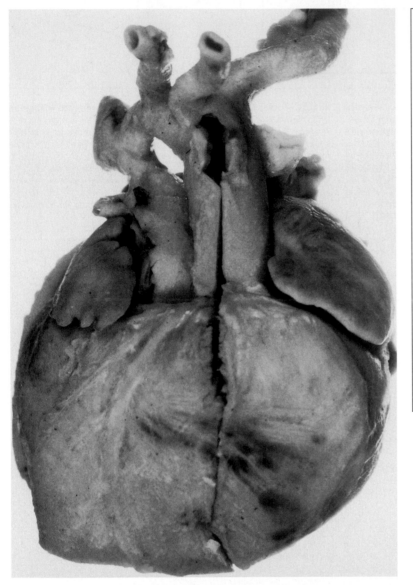

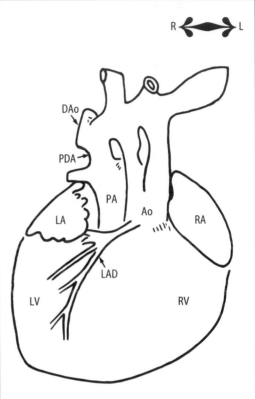

21.158 Mirror-image arrangement (situs inversus) in TGA. Anterior view showing the morphologically right atrial appendage on the left side of the heart and the morpho-logically left atrial appendage on the right side. The descending aorta and arterial duct are also right-sided. From a surgical perspective, everything is "backwards" or "reversed" in hearts with "mirror image," i.e. the superior and inferior caval veins are on the patient's left side rather than on the right side. In general, procedures done outside the heart – arterial and venous cannulation, closure of an arterial duct, cavopulmonary connection, arterial switch operation – are still accomplished most easily with the surgeon standing on the patient's right-hand side. Usually, for simple procedures within the left-sided morphologically right atrium – closure of the atrial septal defect, lateral tunnel Fontan – it is still possible to work from the right side of the operating table by rotating the patient towards the surgeon. When it is necessary to carry out a geometrically complex procedure in the right atrium (complex baffle, Senning operation) or one in the morphologically right ventricle (closure of ventricular septal defect, muscle resection), the surgeon usually works from the left side of the operating table.

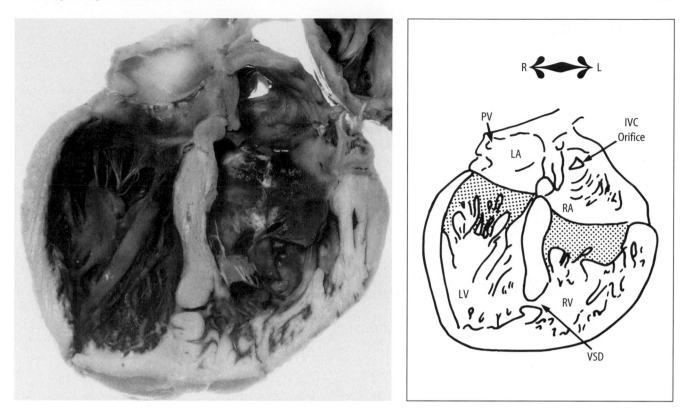

21.159 Four-chamber view, looking from the front to the back of the heart shown in Figure 21.158. The specimen has been transected in a coronal plane and the anterior half has been rotated out of view to the left. The atrial septum is intact. There is a small apical muscular ventricular septal defect. All the morphologically left structures (left atrium, pulmonary veins, mitral valve, and left ventricle) are on the patient's right side and vice versa.

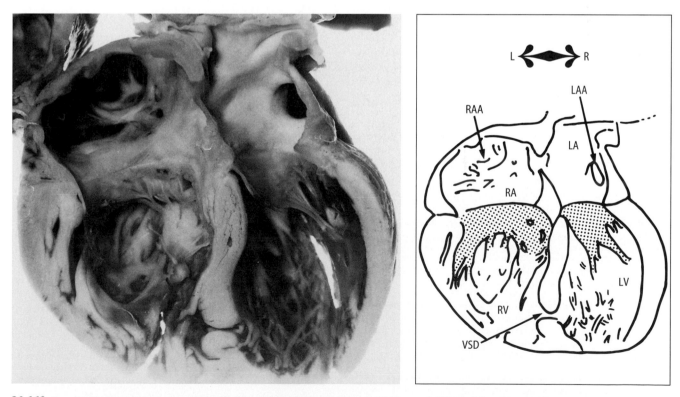

21.160 Four-chamber view, looking from the back to the front of the heart shown in Figure 21.158. The morphologically right atrial appendage is seen on the left side and the orifice of the morphologically left atrial appendage on the right. The outflow of the right-sided morphologically left ventricle lies under the mitral valvar leaflet.

Suggested Reading

Ahmed F, Robida A, McKay R. Imai technique for management of coronary arteries arising from a solitary sinus in discordant ventricular-arterial connections. Cardiol Young 2001;11:145.

Anderson RH, Henry GW, Becker AE. Morphologic aspects of complete transposition. Cardiol Young 1991;1:41.

Bharati S, Lev M. The conduction system in simple, regular (d-), complete transposition with ventricular septal defect. J Thorac Cardiovasc Surg 1976;2:194.

Bharati S, Lev M, Kirklin JW. Operations in the right atrium: The relevance of the conduction system in arterial switch repair in complete transposition with ventricular septal defect. In: Cardiac surgery and the conduction system, 2nd edition. Mount Kisco, New York, Futura. 1992, pp 62–8.

Gittenberger-de Groot AC, Sauer U, Oppenheimer-Decker A, Quaegebeur J. Coronary arterial anatomy in transposition of the great arteries: a morphologic study. Pediatr Cardiol 1983;4 (suppl. 1):15.

Hoyer MH, Zuberbuhler JR, Anderson RH, del Nido P. Morphology of ventricular septal defects in complete transposition. Surgical implications. J Thorac Cardiovasc Surg 1992;104:1203.

Jatene AD, Fontes VF, Paulista PP, Souza LCB, Neger F, Galantier M, Sousa JE. Anatomic correction of transposition of the great vessels. J Thorac Cardiovasc Surg 1976;72:364.

Jonas RA, Giglia TM, Saunders SP, Wernovsky G, Nadal-Ginard B, Mayer JE Jr, Casteneda AR. Rapid two-stage arterial switch for transposition of the great arteries and intact ventricular septum beyond the neonatal period. Circulation 1989;80 (suppl. I):203.

Kashiwagi J, Imai Y, Aoki M, Shin'oka T, Hagino I, Nakazawa M. An arterial switch operation for a concordant crisscross heart with the complete transposition of the great arteries. J Thorac Cardiovasc Surg 2002;124:176.

Kurosawa H, Lodewyk HE ,Van Mierop LHS. Surgical anatomy of the infundibular septum in transposition of the great arteries with ventricular septal defect. J Thorac Cardiovasc Surg 1986;91:123.

Kurosawa H, Imai Y, Kawada M. Coronary arterial anatomy in regard to the arterial switch procedure. Cardiol Young 1991;1:54.

Lecompte Y, Zannini L, Hazan E, Jarreau MM, Bex JP, Tu TV, Neveux JY. Anatomic correction of transposition of the great arteries. New technique without use of a prosthetic conduit. J Thorac Cardiovasc Surg 1981;82:629.

Lecompte Y. Intraventricular repair of anomalies of ventriculo-arterial connection (REV Procedure). In: Stark JS, de Leval M (eds). Surgery for Congenital Heart Defects, 2nd edition. London, W.B. Saunders Company. 1994, pp 501–9.

Mee R. The arterial switch operation. In: Stark JS, de Leval M (eds). Surgery for Congenital Heart Defects, 2nd edition. London,W.B. Saunders Company. 1994, pp 483–500.

Metras D, Kreitmann B. Modified Rastelli using an autograft: A new concept for correction of transposition of the great arteries with ventricular septal defect and left ventricular outflow tract obstruction (with an extension to other congenital heart defects). Semin Thorac Cardiovasc Surg Pediatr Card Surg Annu 2000;3:117.

Moene RJ, Oppenheimer-Dekker A, Wenink ACG, Bartelings MM, Gittenberger- de Groot AC. Morphology of ventricular septal defect in complete transposition of the great arteries. Am J Cardiol 1985;55:1566.

Moene RJ, Oppenheimer-Dekker A, Bartelings MM, Wenink ACG, Gittenberger- de Groot AC. Ventricular septal defect with normally connected and with transposed great arteries . Am J Cardiol 1986;58:627.

Mustard WT. Successful two-stage correction of transposition of the great vessels. Surgery 1964;55:469.

Oppenheimer-Dekker A. Interventricular communications in transposition of the great arteries . In: Van Mierop LHS, Oppenheimer-Dekker A, Bruins CLDCH (eds). Embryology and teratology of the heart and great arteries. Boerhaave Series 13, Leiden University Press. The Hague, 1978;pp 139–59.

Oosthoek PW, Wenink ACG, Wisse LJ, Gittenberger-de Groot AC. Development of the papillary muscles of the mitral valve: background of parachute-like asymmetric mitral valves and other mitral valve anomalies. J Thorac Cardiovasc Surg 1998;116,1:37.

Pacifico RD. Concordant transposition: Senning operation. In: Stark JS, de Leval M (eds). Surgery for Congenital Heart Defects, 2nd edition. London,W.B.Saunders Company. 1994;pp 457–68.

Rastelli GC. A new approach to "anatomic" repair of transposition of the great arteries. Mayo Clin Proc 1969;44:1.

Sakata R, Lecompte Y, Batisse A, Borromee L, Durandy Y. Anatomic repair of anomalies of ventricular septal defect. I. Criteria of surgical decision. J Thorac Cardiovasc Surg 1988;95:90.

Senning A. Surgical correction of transposition of the great vessels. Surgery 1959;45:966.

Shaher RM. Complete transposition of the great arteries. Academic Press, New York, 1973.

Sim EKW, van Son JAM, Edwards WD, Julsrud PR, Puga FJ. Coronary artery anatomy in complete transposition of the great arteries. Ann Thorac Surg 1994;57:890.

Smith A, Arnold R, Wilkinson JL, Hamilton DI, McKay R, Anderson RH. An anatomical study of the patterns of the coronary arteries and sinus nodal artery in complete transposition. Int J Cardiol 1986;12:295.

Smith A, Wilkinson JL, Anderson RH, Dickinson DF. Architecture of the ventricular mass and atrioventricular valves in complete transposition of the great arteries with intact septum compared with the normal heart. I. The left ventricle, mitral valve and the interventricular septum. Paediatr Cardiol 1986;6:253.

Smith A, Wilkinson JL, Anderson RH, Dickinson DF. Architecture of the ventricular mass and atrioventricular valves in complete transposition with intact septum compared with the normal heart. II. The right ventricle and tricuspid valve. Paediatr Cardiol 1986;6:299.

Smith A, Connell MG, Jackson M, Verbeek FJ, Anderson RH. Atrioventricular conduction system in hearts with muscular ventricular septal defects in the setting of complete transposition. J Thorac Cardiovasc Surg 1994;108:9.

Yacoub MH, Radley-Smith R, Hilton CJ. Anatomical correction of complete transposition of the great arteries and ventricular septal defect in infancy. Br Med J 1976;1:1112.

Yacoub MH, Radley-Smith R. Anatomy of the coronary arteries in transposition of the great arteries and methods of their transfer in anatomical correction. Thorax 1978;33:418.

Wilkinson JL, Arnold R, Anderson RH, Acerete F. Posterior transposition reconsidered Br Heart J 1975;37:757.

22 Congenitally Corrected Transposition (Discordant Ventriculo-arterial Connections with Discordant Artrioventricular Connections)

Introduction

The combination of a morphologically left atrium connected to a morphologically right ventricle and a morphologically right atrium connected to a morphologically left ventricle (discordant atrioventricular connections), with a morphologically left ventricle connected to the pulmonary artery and the morphologically right ventricle connected to the aorta ("transposition of the great arteries" or discordant ventriculo- arterial connections), produces a circulation which is physiologically "correct." In this situation the morphologically right ventricle is the systemic pumping chamber – hence the designation "congenitally corrected" transposition. By definition, both the morphologically right and left atriums and ventricles must be identifiable. This excludes hearts with atrial isomerism and ambiguous atrioventricular connection or solitary ventricle. Similarly, each atrium must connect with a ventricle, thus excluding hearts with a double inlet ventricle, despite the fact that the anatomy of some types of hearts with a double inlet left ventricle have many features in common with congenitally corrected transposition. Also excluded from this definition, in strict anatomical terms, are hearts with discordant atrioventricular connections and either associated double outlet of the morphologically right ventricle, single outlet of the heart or common arterial trunk. However, most surgical series of discordant atrioventricular connections or corrected transposition of the great arteries will include some of these latter patients.

Hearts with usual atrial arrangement and congenitally corrected transposition have malalignment between the atrial septum and the inlet portion of the ventricular septum, such that the usual posterior node in the triangle of Koch does not make contact with the non-branching bundle of the ventricular conduction tissue. Rather, an anterior node at the junction of the right atrium and the area of pulmonary-mitral fibrous continuity gives off a long non-branching bundle which runs around the front of the subpulmonary left ventricular outflow tract

to reach the ventricular septum. In this way the conduction system is vulnerable to both natural fibrosis and surgical trauma. However, in corrected transposition with mirror-image arrangement, there is the likelihood that the atrial and ventricular septums will be better aligned and that the atrioventricular connection will run from a posterior node.

Despite the potential for a normal circulation, the vast majority of hearts with corrected transposition have associated intracardiac malformations. The left-sided, morphologically tricuspid valve is abnormal in at least 90% of cases, ranging from a variable fusion of leaflet tissue to the ventricle (analogous with Ebstein's anomaly), to leaflet dysplasia and stenosis. A defect in the ventricular septum is present in about 80% of cases. This may be a malalignment defect of the membranous septal area, a doubly committed subarterial defect, a muscular defect, or multiple defects. Complete atrioventricular septal defect has also been observed with corrected transposition. The subpulmonary left ventricular outflow tract lies deeply wedged between the atrioventricular valves and is obstructed in about 40% of hearts with discordant atrioventricular connections. Most often this is due to fibrous tissue from the membranous septum or tags from the pulmonary or atrioventricular valves in the subpulmonary area, but muscular and valvar obstruction also occur. Less frequent anomalies include straddling atrioventricular valves, defects in the atrial septum, hypoplasia of a ventricle (usually the systemic, morphologically right ventricle), mitral valvar malformations, and inflow or outflow obstruction of the morphologically right ventricle. Coarctation or interruption of the aorta and persistent arterial duct are found also in association with congenitally corrected transposition.

Surgical management of these malformations is both complex and individualized according to the anatomical situation and hemodynamic abnormalities. The rare asymptomatic patient without associated anomalies requires no therapeutic intervention. Heart block is generally treated by transvenous sequential pacing, recognizing that ventricular pacing alone may exacerbate left-sided atrioventricular valve regurgitation which is present in many cases. Because the venous ventricle is morphologically a left ventricle, lead fixation may be difficult and require a "screw-in" type of device. Other arrhythmias, the most common being Wolffe-Parkinson-White Syndrome, are usually managed by catheter ablation.

For patients with cyanosis due to a ventricular septal defect with morphologically left ventricular outflow obstruction, a systemic-pulmonary anastomosis in the first instance generally provides sufficient palliation for the child to undergo subsequent extracardiac conduit implantation at some time between about four and ten years of age. The branch pulmonary arteries in corrected transposition are usually large and confluent. Because the ascending aorta lies to the left, a right-sided shunt is generally easier to take down at a later complete repair.

Banding of the pulmonary artery is occasionally used for infants in heart failure without severe atrioventricular valve incompetence. From a right thoracotomy, the pulmonary artery is approached by retracting the atrial appendage and superior caval vein. This may place the sinus or atrioventricular node under tension with resulting arrhythmias. The pulmonary artery is accessible also from a left thoracotomy, using tension on the ascending aorta and dissecting the vessel by subtraction. This is useful for patients who require simultaneous pulmonary artery banding and coarctation repair.

For patients with two adequate ventricles, surgical treatment is presently in a state of uncertain transition. Traditionally, the ventricular septal defect has been closed using a technique to avoid damage to the conduction tissue, and left ventricular outflow obstruction bypassed with a valved extracardiac conduit between the right-sided morphologically left ventricle and the pulmonary artery. When the left-sided atrioventricular valve is incompetent, it is replaced either through a midline sternotomy or a left thoracotomy. This approach leaves the morphologically right ventricle supporting the systemic circulation, which may be a long-term disability, particularly in the presence of regurgitation of the systemic tricuspid valve. Accordingly, recent efforts have been directed towards so-called "anatomical" repair, using a combination of atrial redirection (Senning or Mustard operation) and arterial redirection (Rastelli operation in the presence of anatomical left ventricular outflow obstruction or arterial switch operation). From a morphological perspective, tunnelling the left ventricle to the aorta through the ventricular septal defect is favored when there is hypoplasia of the outlet septum (or a doubly committed subarterial ventricular septal defect) and a large interventricular communication. While these procedures place the tricuspid valve on the low-pressure pulmonary side of the circulation (thus avoiding valve replacement in most patients) and leave the morphologically left ventricle in the systemic circulation, the heart remains far from anatomically normal. Thus, greater experience and longer follow-up are needed to determine if these more extensive reconstructions are justified by better survival and long-term ventricular performance.

When there is hypoplasia of one ventricle, which is more usually the systemic morphologically right ventricle and associated with a straddling left atrioventricular valve, surgical management is directed towards the Fontan circulation. Thus, measures are taken to protect and/or develop the pulmonary vasculature (i.e. early, tight pulmonary artery banding) and conserve ventricular function (by cavopulmonary connection and/or valve replacement to relieve volume overload). The high incidence of anomalies of the tricuspid valve and arrhythmias, however, are important considerations in this subset of patients, for some of whom cardiac transplantation will be a better option.

In all types of surgery for corrected transposition, the procedure may be complicated by not uncommon cardiac malposition. Dextrocardia with usual atrial arrangement, for example, causes the morphologically right ventricle to rotate in front of the right-sided morphologically right atrium and left ventricle. Exposure of a ventricular septal defect may thus become difficult through the usual right atrial approach, while the position of a left ventricle-to-pulmonary artery conduit moves posteriorly and into the right chest. In addition to anatomical information about intracardiac defects, such relationships should be appreciated preoperatively from the chest x-ray, angiography, and echocardiography, and possibly from magnetic resonance imaging when this is available.

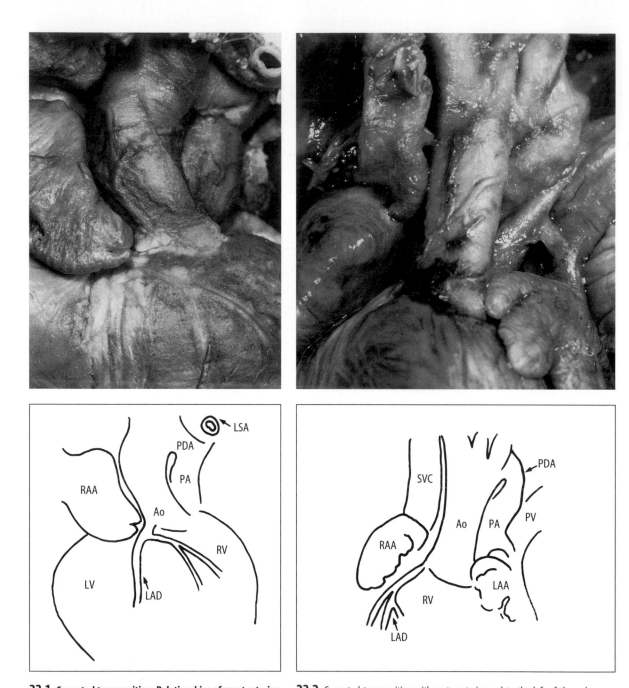

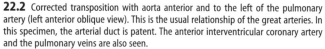

22.1 Corrected transposition. Relationships of great arteries. The aorta is anterior and to the right of the pulmonary artery (right anterior oblique view) in this heart. A large arterial duct connects the aorta and pulmonary artery. The anterior interventricular coronary artery identifies the septum and branches proximally over the outflow of the left-sided morphologically right ventricle. This is *not* the usual relationship of the great arteries in congenitally corrected transposition.

22.2 Corrected transposition with aorta anterior and to the left of the pulmonary artery (left anterior oblique view). This is the usual relationship of the great arteries. In this specimen, the arterial duct is patent. The anterior interventricular coronary artery and the pulmonary veins are also seen.

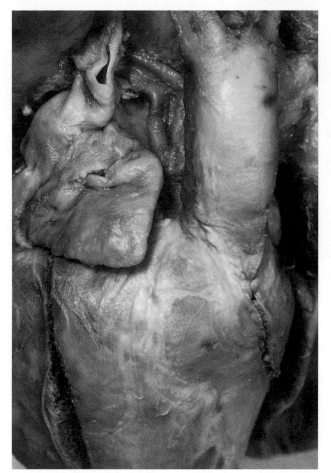

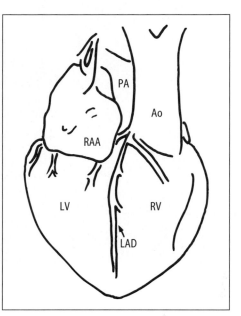

22.3 Corrected transposition with anterior aorta (right anterior view). The posterior pulmonary artery is small. Branches of the anterior interventricular coronary artery pass to the left-sided morphologically right ventricle, while marginal branches of the circumflex artery are seen on the right-sided morphologically left ventricle.

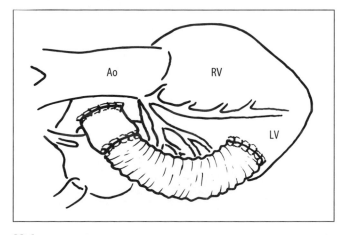

22.4 An extracardiac conduit to bypass pulmonary obstruction generally lies to the right of the aorta. In extreme dextrocardia, this may come to be positioned laterally to the superior caval vein. The left ventriculotomy is sited low down between major coronary arterial branches. It usually lies between the anterior papillary muscle of the mitral valve (palpated through the right atrium and indicated by a major branch of the left anterior descending coronary artery) and the anterior interventricular coronary artery, demarcating the ventricular septum.

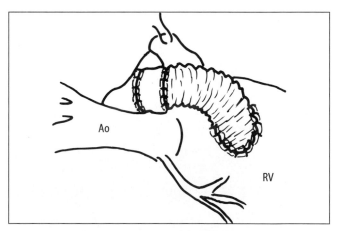

22.5 When repair is done by atrial redirection (Mustard or Senning operation) and a Rastelli procedure, the right ventriculotomy is made between the coronary arterial branches and well below the aortic sinus to avoid damaging the leaflet tissue attached to the ventricular muscle. The divided pulmonary artery may be passed behind the aorta in such a way that the conduit is taken to the left of the aorta and does not cross directly under the sternum.

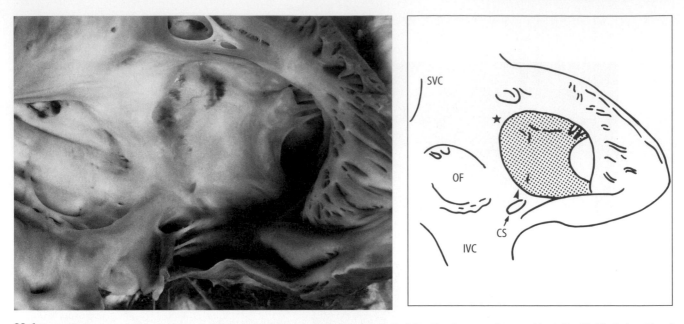

22.6 Congenitally corrected transposition. Morphologically right atrium. The morphologically right atrium in corrected transposition is identified by its broad-based appendage (retracted rightward in the heart shown above) and oval fossa. It is connected to the mitral valve, of which the anterior leaflet is in fibrous continuity with the pulmonary valve. Malalignment between the atrial septum and the ventricular septum prevents the usual posterior node (arrow head) in the triangle of Koch from making contact with the ventricle. Instead, an anterior node (star) gives off the atrioventricular conduction bundles.

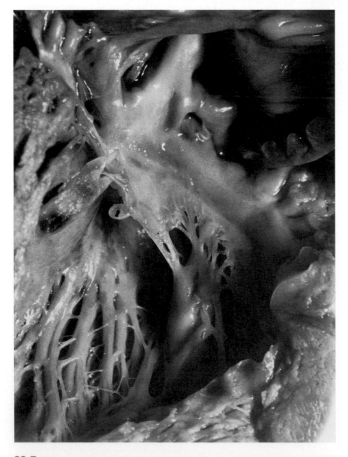

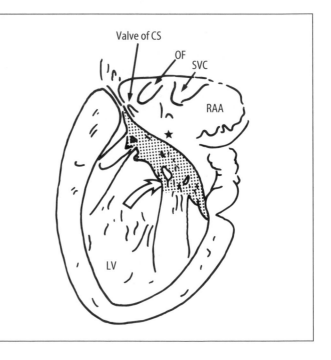

22.7 Right atrioventricular junction in congenitally corrected transposition, showing the morphologically right atrium, mitral valve and morphologically left ventricle. The anterior mitral commissure lies in front of the left ventricular outflow tract and pulmonary valve (arrow) and is related to the anterior atrioventricular node (star) and the penetrating bundle of the conduction tissue.

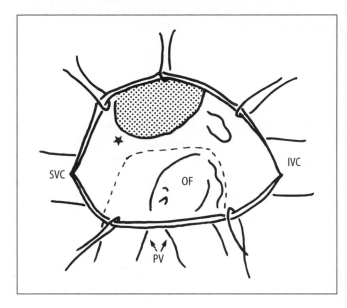

22.8 A right atrial approach is used for the closure of the atrial and ventricular septal defects, to repair anomalies of the mitral valve, a Fontan procedure, or atrial redirection in surgery for congenitally corrected transposition. Dextrocardia rotates the ventricular mass in front of the atrium and may complicate access to the free wall, but it does not alter the intracardiac anatomical relationships. In a surgical orientation, the penetrating anterior atrioventricular node (star) lies to the left, at about 7 o'clock on the mitral annulus. Care must be used to avoid this area when detaching the atrial septum for a Fontan, Senning or Mustard procedure (dashed line).

22.9 In the double switch or atrial redirection/Rastelli operations, a Mustard baffle may be preferred to the Senning procedure when the morphologically right atrium is small or an overhanging ventricle limits access. As the posterior node does not connect with the ventricle in hearts with usual situs, the suture line may pass between the coronary sinus and mitral annulus (with or without coronary sinus cutback), leaving the coronary sinus to drain in the systemic venous atrium. The pulmonary venous atrium is nearly always enlarged with a patch in this situation.

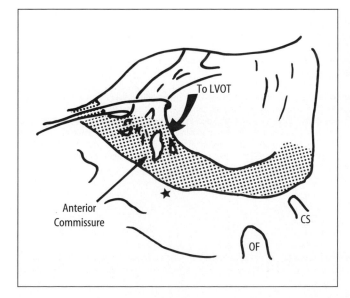

22.10 The anterior commissure of the mitral valve is a guide to the approximate position of the anterior node (star) in corrected transposition and also overlies the sub-pulmonary left ventricular outflow tract. Forceful retraction of the mitral valve for exposure of a ventricular septal defect may traumatize the conduction system in this area. The possibility of a "sling" of conduction bundles arising from both anterior and posterior nodes is more likely in the presence of double outlet right ventricle with discordant atrioventricular connection, while the (usual) posterior node generally gives off the penetrating bundle in congenitally corrected transposition with mirror-image atrial arrangement (situs inversus). In the latter arrangement, there is a lesser degree of malalignment between the atrial and ventricular septums.

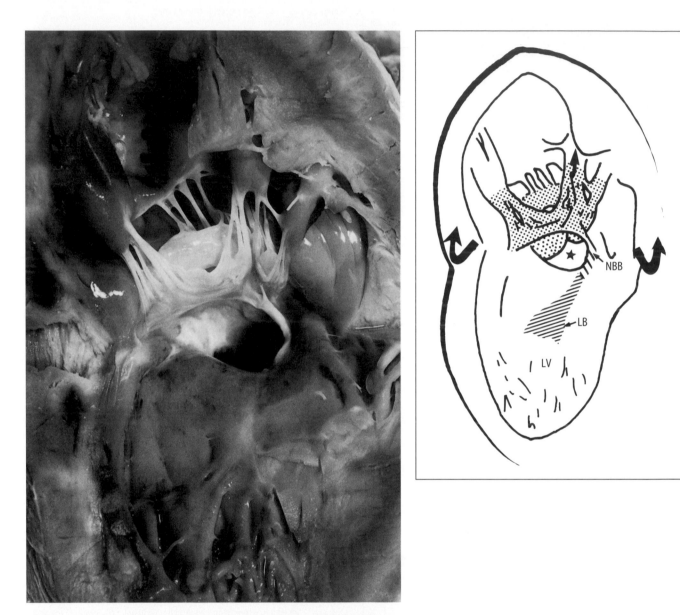

22.11 Congenitally corrected transposition. Right-sided morphologically left ventricle. This heart has been opened with a "fish-mouth" incision from apex to base, such that the lateral free wall and intact mitral valve have been rotated upwards (curved arrows) to lie in the same plane as the septum. The smooth septal surface is characteristic of a morphologically left ventricle. A perimembranous inlet ventricular septal defect (star) lies immediately under the mitral valve and extends to the subpulmonary region. The mitral and pulmonary valves are in fibrous continuity. The straight arrow indicates the unseen axis of the pulmonary root. The non-branching bundle of conduction tissue passes around the left ventricular outflow anteriorly to the pulmonary valve and along the anterior margin of the ventricular septal defect, giving off the left bundle branch which fans out over the septal surface. A rim of accessory mitral valvar tissue runs along the margin of the ventricular septal defect, parallel with the conduction tissue. The pulmonary valve overrides the ventricular septal defect and arises partially from the left-sided morphologically right ventricle.

Congenitally Corrected Transposition. Right-sided Morphologically Left Ventricle

355

22.12 The route for exposure of a ventricular septal defect in congenitally corrected transposition depends on the position of the defect, the position of the cardiac chambers, and the ventricle which will support the systemic circulation post-repair. A systemic ventriculotomy and working near conduction tissue through the pulmonary artery (5) are generally avoided, although the latter may give safe access to the upper margin of a defect if the heart has discordant atrioventricular connections with double outlet right ventricle. In "anatomical" repair, the morphologically right ventricle (3) is opened longitudinally below the aortic valve. When a morphologically left ventriculotomy (2) is used, either for closure of a muscular ventricular septal defect or placement of a conduit to the pulmonary artery, the incision is sited low down, between coronary arterial branches to avoid damage to the conduction tissue running anteriorly in the base of the ventricle. The anterior papillary muscle of the right atrioventricular valve is avoided by first palpating it through the atrium. A morphologically right atriotomy (1) is employed most commonly for closure of atrial septal defects and perimembranous ventricular septal defects. It is sited in the usual place on the body of the atrium, avoiding the sinus node (triangle) and respecting that the coronary arterial supply to both sinus and atrioventricular nodes passes on the medial side of the atrium. A morphologically left atriotomy (via a left thoracotomy) also gives excellent surgical access but possibly carries a greater risk of damage to the left atrioventricular valve.

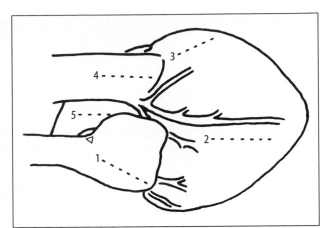

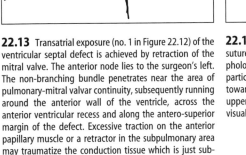

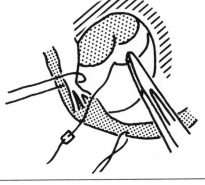

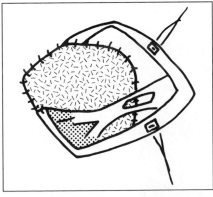

22.13 Transatrial exposure (no. 1 in Figure 22.12) of the ventricular septal defect is achieved by retraction of the mitral valve. The anterior node lies to the surgeon's left. The non-branching bundle penetrates near the area of pulmonary-mitral valvar continuity, subsequently running around the anterior wall of the ventricle, across the anterior ventricular recess and along the antero-superior margin of the defect. Excessive traction on the anterior papillary muscle or a retractor in the subpulmonary area may traumatize the conduction tissue which is just sub-endocardial.

22.14 One technique for avoiding heart block is to place sutures through the ventricular septal defect into the morphologically right ventricular side of the septum. In this particular heart, displacement of the pulmonary artery towards the morphologically right ventricle obscures the upper part of the ventricular septal defect, which may be visualized better through the aorta or pulmonary artery.

22.15 The posterior margin of the ventricular septal defect is safe for suture placement in usual atrial arrangement, but cords of the right atrioventricular valve are not infrequently attached to the crest of the defect in this area. Any muscle between the right atrioventricular valve and the ventricular septal defect is also safe. Otherwise, sutures may be brought through the mitral valve itself, usually with a pericardial buttress, on the atrial side of the leaflet.

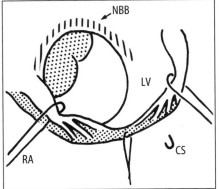

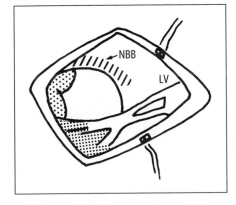

22.16 Exposure through a morphologically left ventriculotomy is usually with an incision which lies between the septum and the anterior papillary muscle. Traction on the upper part of the incision should be avoided because the conduction tissue here lies superficially in the sub-endocardial layer of the ventricular free wall.

22.17 A different technique for closure of the ventricular septal defect in hearts with atrioventricular discordance leaves both great vessels, the anterior ventricular recess, and the conduction tissue beneath the patch. Sutures are brought to the epicardial surface of the ventriculotomy superiorly and about 5 mm away from the area of the non-branching bundle on the ventricular septum. The pulmonary artery is then divided and reconnected to the morphologically left ventricle with a valved extracardiac conduit (Figure 22.4). As there is no left ventricular outflow obstruction in this heart, however, a better option could be closure of the ventricular septal defect through the morphologically right ventricle and the double switch operation.

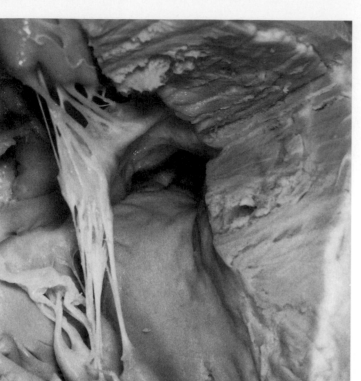

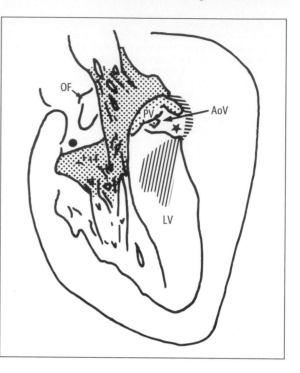

22.18 Congenitally corrected transposition. Subpulmonary morphologically left ventricular outflow tract. This has been exposed by elevating the divided anterior papillary muscle of the mitral valve upwards to the right. The ventricular septal defect (star) extends beneath both pulmonary and aortic valves and, in the absence of an outlet septum, is thus a "doubly committed subarterial" defect. In this heart, the coronary sinus is absent, a small vein (black dot) being in its position.

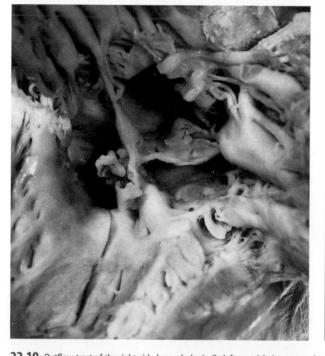

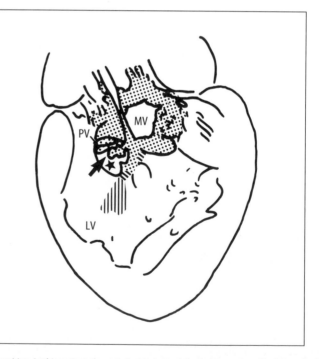

22.19 Outflow tract of the right-sided morphologically left ventricle in corrected transposition. In this patient, the aorta is anterior to the pulmonary artery. The free wall of the opened ventricle has been rotated towards the cardiac base, such that the unopened right (morphologically mitral) atrioventricular valve lies beside the subpulmonary ventricular septal defect (star). The pulmonary valve overrides the septum and is deeply wedged between the atrioventricular valves. This is characteristic of congenitally corrected transposition. The ventricular septal defect extends well posteriorly into the inlet septum. Subpulmonary obstruction is produced by a tissue tag (arrow) of accessory mitral valve tissue from a dysplastic leaflet.

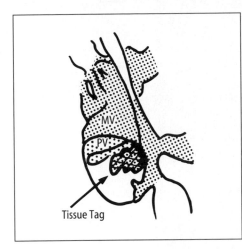

22.20 The subpulmonary morphologically left ventricular outflow tract in congenitally corrected transposition is a long oblique channel with potential obstruction in at least 60% of hearts. Usually, this is due to fibrous tags which originate from the membranous septum, the pulmonary valve, or the atrioventricular valves. There may or may not be associated muscular hypertrophy. Valvar pulmonary stenosis or atresia are less common. Tissue tags may be exposed by working through the right atrioventricular valve and excised (hatched area), taking care to avoid damage to adjacent structures.

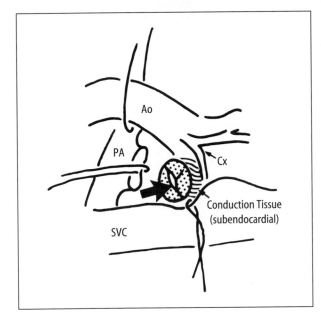

22.21 A valved extracardiac conduit is used generally to bypass left ventricular outflow obstruction because of the difficult access to the pulmonary artery and vulnerability of the atrioventricular bundle. However, a direct approach to the morphologically left ventricular outflow may be afforded through either a spiral incision in or by transection of the pulmonary trunk. In addition to commissurotomy (arrow), this exposure is used also for closure of the proximal pulmonary trunk in a Fontan procedure or to close the pulmonary valve when it remains beneath a patch over the ventricular septal defect (see Figure 22.17).

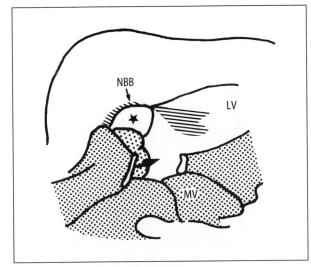

22.22 For subvalvar obstruction, the incision may be continued across the pulmonary annulus and down the back wall of the left ventricular outflow tract (arrow), away from the conduction tissue. Injury to the left-sided morphologically tricuspid valve is a risk if the dissection extends to the ventricular septal defect (star). Following muscle resection, the outflow tract is enlarged with a Dacron patch and/or implantation of a homograft valve. If the morphologically left ventricle were to be used as the systemic ventricle, a theoretical possibility would be transfer of the intact aortic valve to the left ventricular outflow tract with coronary arterial reimplantation, analogous to the Ross operation. However, this operation has not yet been done.

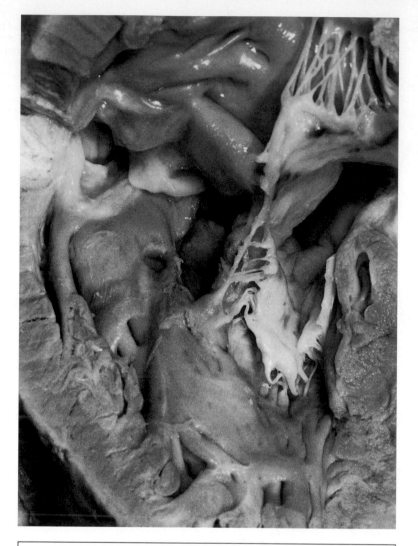

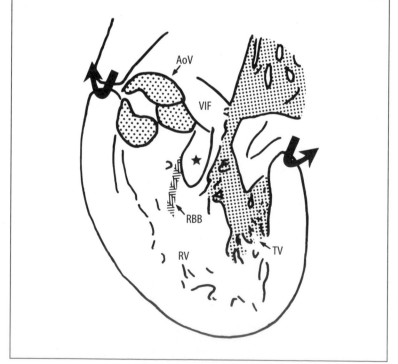

← **22.23 Corrected transposition. Left-sided morphologically right ventricle**. The heart has been opened from apex to base, and the free wall has been swung up to the top of the picture (curved arrows). The heavily trabeculated septal surface is characteristic of a morphologically right ventricle. The atrioventricular valve lies between this ventricle and the morphologically left atrium which receives the pulmonary veins. Like a normal right-sided tricuspid valve, it has three leaflets and papillary muscles. It is separated from the aortic valve by a well-developed muscle bar, the ventriculo-infundibular fold. The aortic valvar leaflets are supported by right ventricular muscle and are not joined to the fibrous cardiac skeleton. In this specimen, a large ventricular septal defect (star) extends to both the arterial valves and is, therefore, a doubly-committed subarterial ("supra-cristal") defect (see Figure 22.18 for a view of the left side of this specimen). The right bundle branch of conduction tissue passes from the margin of the ventricular septal defect to the septum.

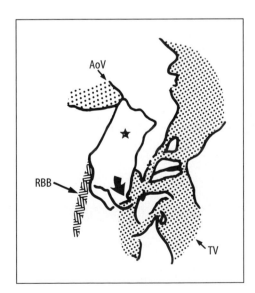

22.24 The doubly committed subarterial ventricular septal defect in corrected transposition is often exposed through the right-sided (morphologically mitral) valve and closed by the placement of sutures through the defect on to the morphologically right ventricular side of the septum (see Figure 22.13–22.15). As illustrated in this heart, however, papillary muscles or cords of the tricuspid valve frequently insert on or near the crest of the ventricular septal defect (arrow). The patch used to close the ventricular septal defect can be split to pass around important cordal attachments or minor cords may be divided. While the conduction tissue is not at risk with this technique, altering the geometry of the atrioventricular valve may contribute, however, to systemic atrioventricular valve regurgitation post-operatively, which is sometimes exacerbated by closure of the ventricular septal defect. This is one consideration which may favor an "anatomical" type of corrective surgery which places the morphologically tricuspid valve in the low-pressure pulmonary ventricle. Sutures at the top of the defect are passed through the fibrous tissue between the aortic and pulmonary valvar leaflets (see Figures 17.33–17.38 and 11.50–11.53).

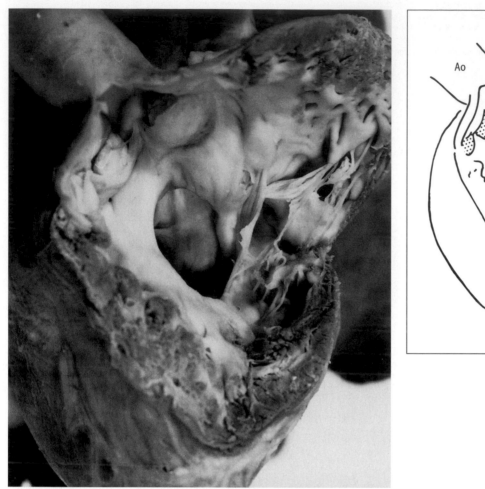

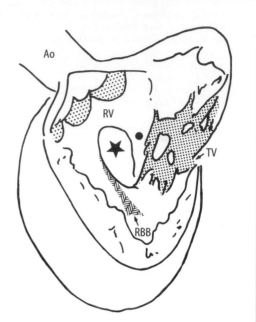

22.25 Corrected transposition. Left-sided morphologically right ventricle. A large muscular ventricular septal defect (star) is separated from the aortic valve by an outlet ("infundibular" or "conus") septum. The ventriculo-infundibular fold (black dot) separates the left-sided morphologically tricuspid valve from the aortic valve and continues as a muscle bar around the postero-inferior margin of the ventricular septal defect into the morphologically left ventricle (see Figure 22.26). The systemic right ventricle in this heart is small and has diffuse endocardial thickening. The tricuspid valve is also small.

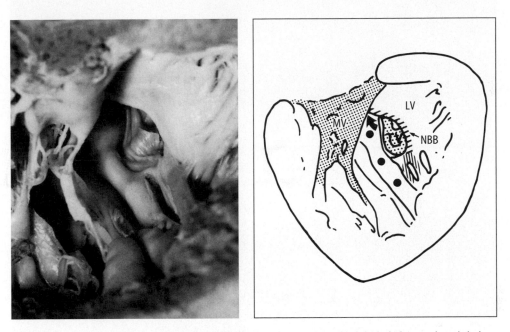

22.26 Right side of the heart seen in Figure 22.25, showing the muscular trabeculation (black dots) which passes through the large ventricular septal defect and produces subpulmonary obstruction. The atrioventricular valve is morphologically a mitral valve and is in fibrous continuity with the unseen pulmonary valve. The left ventricular outflow to the pulmonary valve is indicated by the curved arrow. The left-sided morphologically tricuspid valve is seen through the ventricular septal defect, along the margin of which is located the conduction tissue.

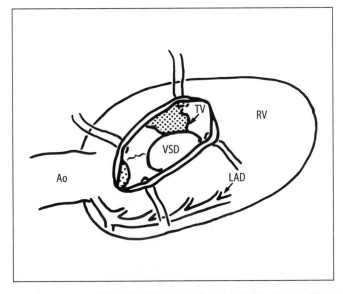

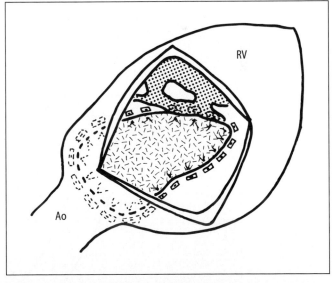

22.27 Because of the small size of this ventricle, surgical repair could be either a Fontan operation or a "Senning-Rastelli," leaving the morphologically left ventricle to support the systemic circulation and using a bidirectional cavopulmonary anastomosis ("one-and-one-half-ventricle repair") to partially bypass the small pumping chamber. For the latter procedure, the ventricular septal defect is tunnelled to the aorta by working through an incision in the morphologically right ventricle. This is sited between coronary arterial branches, noting that the leaflets of the aortic valve are set down into the outflow tract lower than what appears externally to be the ventriculo-arterial junction. An attenuated infundibulum favours this procedure, as routing the left ventricle to the aorta is facilitated when there is less muscle separating the ventricular septal defect from the aorta.

22.28 The patch crosses the right bundle branch, but the remainder of the conduction tissue is not at risk. Posteriorly, sutures are placed through the base of the leaflet of the tricuspid valve and anteriorly, they encircle the aortic valve. The right ventriculotomy is then connected to the pulmonary artery with a valved extracardiac conduit (see Figure 22.5). Care must be taken to avoid obstruction of the right ventricular outflow by the intracardiac tunnel. Construction of the bidirectional cavopulmonary anastomosis will simplify the interatrial redirection portion of this procedure and also, in some cases, may avert the need for an extracardiac conduit to bypass the pulmonary stenosis.

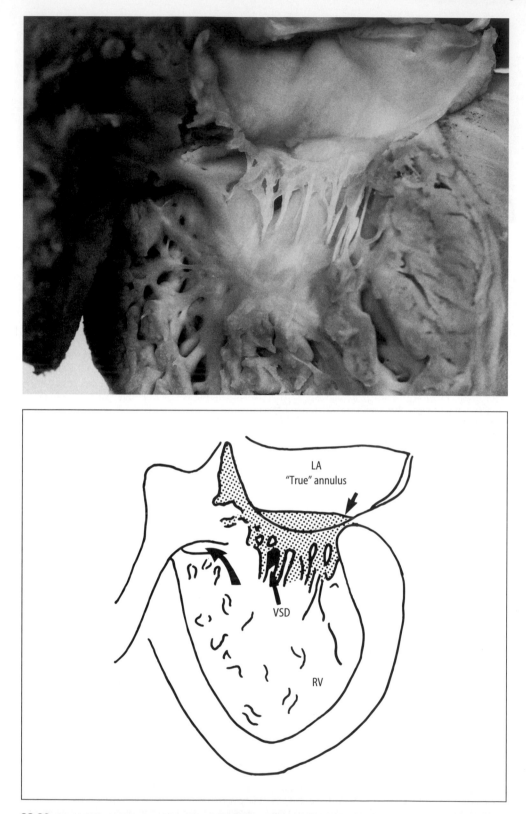

22.29 Congenitally corrected transposition. Left-sided morphologically right ventricle. Coarse trabeculations denote a morphologically right ventricle, while the left-sided tricuspid valve is separated from the aortic outflow tract (curved arrow) by the septomarginal trabeculation and muscle of the left shoulder of the heart. The septal leaflet of the tricuspid valve is partly adherent to ventricular muscle. This produces a minor "Ebstein-like" malformation, atrializing about 10% of the length of the ventricular septum. In contrast with the usual type of Ebstein malformation, however, the ventricular wall rarely becomes thinned, and the anterior leaflet of the tricuspid valve is small and often "cleft." Moreover, the circumference of the atrioventricular orifice is not greatly enlarged in corrected transposition. A small muscular ventricular septal defect lies under the septal leaflet of the tricuspid valve in this heart and is partially closed by valve tissue.

Congenitally Corrected Transposition. Left-sided Morphologically Right Ventricle

363

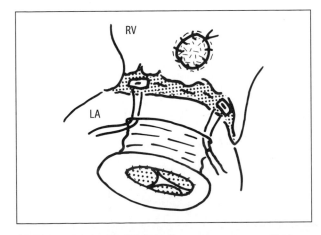

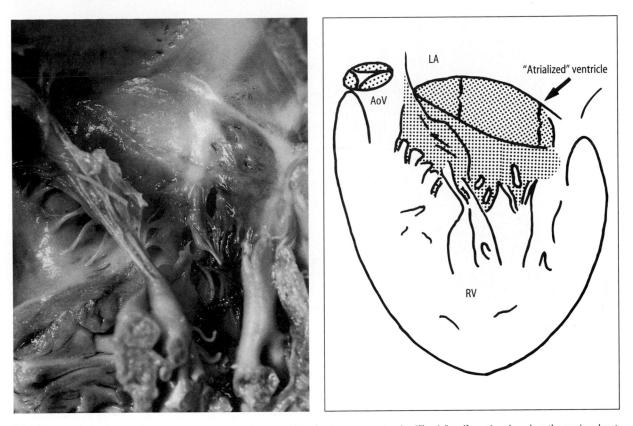

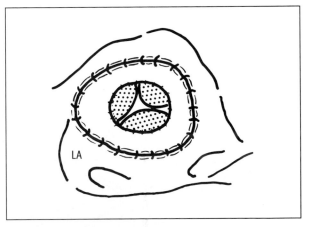

22.30 Left-sided morphologically tricuspid valve in corrected transposition, showing a more extensive "Ebstein" malformation than does the previous heart. Adherence of the septal leaflet has atrialized approximately 20% of the inlet ventricular septum and would result in severe left atrioventricular valve incompetence.

22.31 It is rarely possible to repair an incompetent systemic tricuspid valve, so the surgical options lie between "anatomical correction" (which leaves the valve in the low-pressure pulmonary circulation) or valve replacement. The right ventricle may be small (see Figure 22.5), favoring a low-profile prosthesis or implantation of an inverted homograft ("top hat") valve in the enlarged left atrium. When cords of the valve are divided, the ventricular septal defect often becomes more significant and needs to be closed with a patch. Most of the tricuspid valvar leaflet is conserved to support valvar sutures which may be placed at either the true or functional annulus. The right coronary artery lies deeply in the groove between the left atrium and right ventricle, and is thus at risk of injury.

22.32 When a "top hat" inverted homograft valve is implanted, the lower suture is at the atrioventricular junction and incorporates both the homograft wall and supporting Dacron tube. A pericardial collar, which has been attached to both the valve and tube, is sutured within the left atrium to exclude the first suture line and provide a smooth, unobstructed inflow to the valve (see Figures 13.32–13.38).

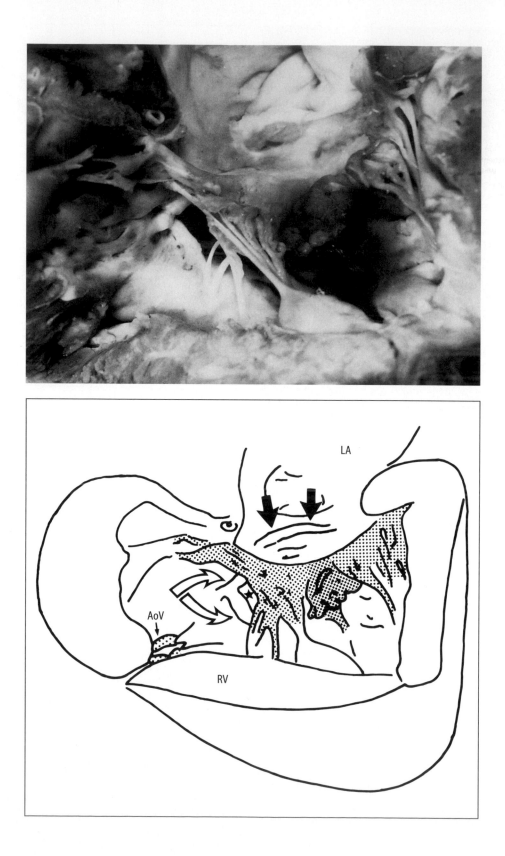

Congenitally Corrected Transposition. Left-sided Morphologically Right Ventricle

365

← **22.33 Corrected transposition. Left-sided morphologically right ventricle.** The tricuspid atrioventricular valve and pulmonary venous atrium are also shown. In this heart, the aorta is anterior and to the right of the pulmonary artery. The atrioventricular valve has been opened to demonstrate its three leaflets and three sets of papillary muscles. The septal leaflet, shown between the anterior and inferior leaflets, is grossly dysplastic with a cauliflower-like appearance. Tension apparatus from the antero-superior leaflet crosses the ventricular outflow tract, producing subaortic stenosis. Small muscular trabeculations immediately below the aortic valve leaflets also obstruct the systemic outflow. The atrioventricular valve is separated from the aortic valve by a bar of muscle, which is a limb of the septomarginal trabeculation. The margins of the ventricular septal defect (star) include fibrous tissue tags (open arrows), which could potentially prolapse through the ventricular septal defect into the subpulmonary outflow tract and cause additional obstruction to that side of the circulation. In the left atrium, a fibromuscular infolding (black arrows) produces a supravalvar ridge. Coarctation of the aorta is also present in this patient.

While much less common than pulmonary obstruction, impediments to systemic flow have been found in 10–15% of hearts with congenitally corrected transposition. They may occur at any level of systemic inflow or outflow, and are not infrequently accompanied by a small-volume morphologically right ventricle and/or coarctation of the aorta. Supravalvar fibrous ring and dysplasia of the tricuspid valve produce inflow obstruction, while outflow obstruction may result from the tricuspid subvalvar apparatus, muscle bundles, displacement of the outlet septum, or discrete fibromuscular stenosis in the subaortic area.

From a surgical standpoint, a supravalvar membranous stenosis above the atrioventricular valve or discrete subaortic stenosis may be simply excised, although both tend to recur. Valvar obstruction usually requires atrioventricular valve replacement. Muscular subaortic obstruction is generally found in a morphologically right ventricle, which is then rendered unsuitable to support the systemic circulation when it is extensive. In these hearts, it may be preferable to establish a Fontan circulation, using the left ventricular outflow for the systemic outlet and closing the tricuspid valve which is abnormal in about 90% of cases with congenitally corrected transposition. As there is no fixed left ventricular outflow obstruction in this heart, however, a better alternative could be closure of the ventricular septal defect through the morphologically right ventricle and the double switch operation, possibly with a bidirectional cavopulmonary connection to partially bypass the right ventricular outflow obstruction.

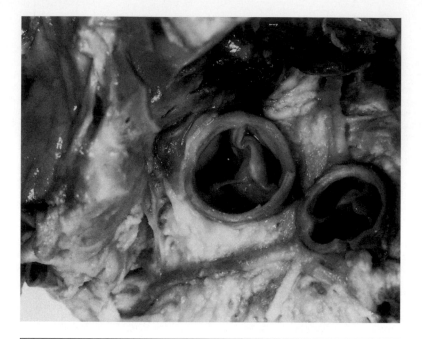

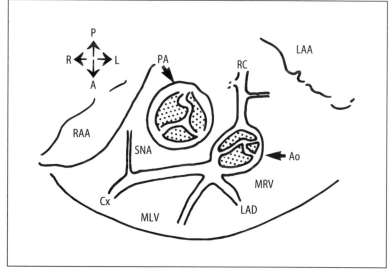

22.34 Discordant atrioventricular connections. Coronary arterial morphology. The heart is viewed from the top with both great arteries transected just above the valves. There is a slight malalignment of the sinuses. The two facing aortic sinuses each give off a coronary artery, which is the most common pattern with discordant atrioventricular connections. The coronary artery from sinus 1 (right-hand facing sinus as viewed by an observer standing in the non-coronary sinus of the aorta and facing the pulmonary artery) is morphologically a right coronary artery and supplies the (systemic) morphologically right ventricle. With the usual atrial arrangement (solitus), this ventricle is on the left side of the heart. The right coronary artery passes into the atrioventricular groove between the morphologically left atrium and the morphologically right ventricle. Here it is in close proximity to the systemic atrioventricular valve and may be entrapped by sutures for valvar replacement. The coronary artery arising from sinus 2 (left-hand facing sinus) is the morphologically left coronary artery which quickly divides into anterior interventricular, "ramus" and circumflex branches. The artery from sinus 2 invariably supplies the morphologically left ventricle in hearts with discordant atrioventricular connections. Nearly always the circumflex branch, which runs in the atrioventricular groove between the morphologically right atrium and the morphologically left ventricle, arises from the left coronary artery. The sinus nodal artery usually arises from the circumflex branch, as does the arterial supply to the anterior atrioventricular node. These vessels pass across the medial side of the right atrial wall where they are vulnerable to injury during a Senning operation or repair of an atriotomy. Early branching of the left coronary artery is the rule in these hearts and it is often possible to identify two orifices within the aortic sinus.

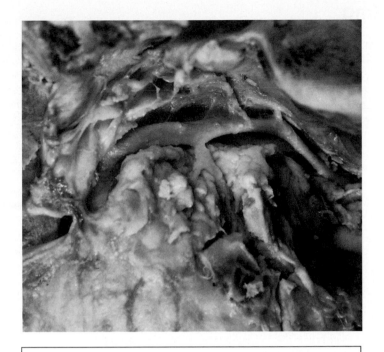

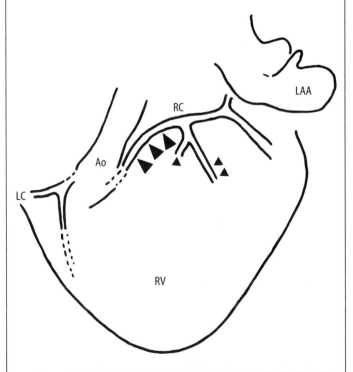

22.35 Coronary arterial morphology. This anterior view of the morphologically right ventricle shows the right coronary artery deeply imbedded in epicardial fat (large arrow heads) soon after its origin. This is the usual situation after a few months of age. The two large right ventricular branches are intramyocardial (small arrow heads). The left coronary artery, also covered by fat, is seen indistinctly. The techniques used for coronary arterial transfer in congenitally corrected transposition managed by arterial switch operation with an atrial redirection are broadly similar to those employed in other types of transposition. However, as these procedures are generally done at a slightly older age and in the presence of a ventricular septal defect, there is usually major discrepancy between the sizes of the great arteries. The coronary arteries tend to arise at a lower level in the aorta with congenitally corrected transposition and may end up within the sinus of the neoaorta. Also, there have been rare occasions when a single coronary arterial orifice was found and could be transferred to the neoaorta.

Suggested Reading

Allwork SP, Bentall HH, Becker AE, Cameron H, Gerlis LM, Wilkinson JL, Anderson RH. Congenitally corrected transposition of the great arteries: morphologic study of 32 cases. Am J Cardiol 1976;38:910.

Anderson KR, Danielson GK, McGoon DC, Lie JT. Ebstein's anomaly of the left-sided tricuspid valve; pathological anatomy of the valvular malformation. Circulation 1978;58c (Suppl I) I–87.

Anderson RH, Becker AE, Gerlis LM. The pulmonary outflow tract in classically corrected transposition. J Thorac Cardiovasc Surg 1975;69:747.

Chealer E, Beck W, Barnard CA, Schrire V. Supravalvar stenosing ring of the left atrium associated with corrected transposition. Am J Cardiol 1973;31:84.

DeLeval MR, Bastos P, Stark J, Taylor JFN, Macartney F, Anderson RH. Surgical technique to reduce the risk of heart block following closure of ventricular septal defect in atrioventricular discordance. J Thorac Cardiovasc Surg 1979;78:515.

DiDonato RM, Troconis CJ, Marino B, Carott A, Iorio FS, Rossi E, Marcelleti C. Combined Mustard and Rastelli operations. An alternative approach for repair of associated anomalies in congenitally corrected transposition in situs inversus (IDD). J Thorac Cardiovasc Surg 1992;104:1246.

Doty DB, Truesdell SC, Marvin WJ. Techniques to avoid injury of the conduction tissue during the surgical treatment of corrected transposition. Circulation 1983;68 (Suppl II) II-63.

Erath HG, Graham TP, Hammon JW, Smith CW. Hypoplasia of the systemic ventricle in congenitally corrected transposition of the great arteries. Preoperative documentation and possible implications of operation. J Thorac Cardiovasc Surg 1980;79:770.

Gerlis LM, Wilson N, Dickinson DF. Abnormalities of the mitral valve in congenitally corrected transposition (discordant atrioventricular and ventriculoarterial connections). Br Heart J 1986;55:475.

Ilbawi MN, De Leon SY, Backer CL, Duffy CE, Munster AJ, Zales VR, Paul MH, Idriss FS. An alternative approach to the surgical management of physiologically corrected transposition with ventricular septal defect and pulmonary stenosis or atresia. J Thorac Cardiovasc Surg 1990;100:410.

Ilbawi MN, Ocampo CB, Allen BS, Barth MJ, Roberson DA, Chiemmongkoltip P, Arcilla RA. Intermediate results of the anatomic repair for congenitally corrected transposition. Ann Thorac Surg 2002;73:594.

Imai Y, Sawatari K, Hoshino S, Ishihara K, Wakazawa M, Momma K. Ventricular function after anatomic repair in patients with atrioventricular discordance. J Thorac Cardiovasc Surg 1994;107:1272.

Levy MJ, Lillehei CW, Elliott LP, Carey LS, Adams P Jr, Edwards JE. Accessory valvular tissue causing subpulmonary stenosis in corrected transposition of the great vessels. Circulation 1963;27:494.

Marino B, Sanders SP, Parness IR, Colan SD. Obstruction of right ventricular inflow and outflow in corrected transposition of the great arteries. (S,L,L): Two-dimensional echocardiographic diagnosis. J Am Coll Cardiol 1986;8:407.

Martin RP, Qureshi SA, Radley-Smith R. Acquired supravalvar membranous stenosis of the left atrioventricular valve. Br Heart J 1987; 58:176.

Matouda H, Kawashima Y, Hirose H, Wakano S, Shirakura R, Shimazaki Y, Nagai I. Transaortic closure of ventricular septal defect in atrioventricular discordance with pulmonary stenosis or atresia. J Thorac Cardiovasc Surg 1984;88:776.

McKay R, Anderson RH, Smith A. The coronary arteries in hearts with discordant atrioventricular connections. J Thorac Cardiovasc Surg 1996;111:988.

McKay R, Sono J, Arnold R. Tricuspid valve replacement using an unstented pulmonary homograft. Ann Thorac Surg 1988;46:58.

Okamura K, Konno S. Two types of ventricular septal defect in corrected transposition of the great arteries: reference to surgical approaches. Am Heart J 1973;85:483.

Ross-Rocuitto NT, Ascuitto RJ, Kopf GS, Laks H, Kleinman CS, Hellenbrand WE, Talner NS. Discrete subaortic obstruction in a patient with corrected transposition of the great arteries. Pediatr Cardiol 1987;8:147.

Russo P, Danielson GK, Driscoll DJ. Transaortic closure of ventricular septal defect in patients with corrected transposition with pulmonary stenosis or atresia. Circulation 1987;76 (Suppl III):III-88.

Wilkinson JL, Smith A, Lincoln C, Anderson RH. Conducting tissues in congenitally corrected transposition with situs inversus. Br Heart J 1978;40:41.

Yagihara T, Kishimoto H, Isobe F, Yamamoto F, Wishigaki K, Matouki O, Uemura H, Kamiya T, Kawashima Y. Double switch operation in cardiac anomalies with atrioventricular and ventriculoarterial discordance. J Thorac Cardiovasc Surg 1994;107:351.

Yamagishi M, Imai Y, Hoshino S, Ishihara K, Koh Y, Nagatsum M, Shinoka T, Koide M. Anatomic correction of atrioventricular discordance. J Thorac Cardiovasc Surg 1993;105:1067.

23 Double Outlet Right Ventricle

Introduction

"Double outlet right ventricle" simply describes a ventriculo-arterial connection in which more than 50% of both the great arteries arises from the right ventricle. Not surprisingly, such a definition encompasses a vast spectrum of cardiac malformations which may vary widely in other anatomic features. The first step towards understanding these malformations is an appreciation of the definition of double outlet right ventricle. Sometimes there is doubt about the degree of overriding of either the aortic valve or the pulmonary valve over either of the ventricles or the septum. In these circumstances, it is helpful to imagine the alignment of an arc of the circle of the arterial valve as it would be subtended to the plane of the ventricular septum below it in its short axis. By this definition it is easier to quantitate the degree of overriding of the arterial valve across the septum and ventricle. The inclination of the septum in its long axis is less useful in calculating the degree of overriding.

Some workers prefer a traditional approach that defines double outlet right ventricle in terms of a bilateral muscular infundibulum, of which many examples exist. Nonetheless, such a definition would exclude many hearts in which the outlet septum is a right ventricular structure, but where bilateral muscular infundibulums are absent. Examples of this include the combination of malformations which usually produces tetralogy of Fallot. Here, the subaortic region is largely composed of the fibrous continuity area between the tricuspid, mitral, and/or aortic valves, but the greater part of the aortic valve overrides the interventricular septum and the right ventricle, thus producing physiological double outlet ventriculo-arterial connection.

Of the many other anatomical variants which may be present, the most important is the associated ventricular septal defect. Although double outlet right ventricle has been reported with intact interventricular septum, it is now considered in this situation that it is likely that a previously existing ventricular septal defect has closed either during intrauterine or postnatal life. There are several types of ventricular septal defect to be found with double outlet right ventricle, and hearts with double outlet right ventricle are generally classified according to the relationship of the ventricular septal defect to the great arteries.

The subaortic defect is the most common ventricular septal defect when the aorta either overrides the septum or originates completely in the right ventricle, together with the pulmonary artery. There is usually fibrous continuity between the mitral and tricuspid valves in the postero-inferior margin of the defect, which categorizes the defect as perimembranous, even in the presence of a bilateral muscular infundibulum. In most cases, however, there is actually a three-way fibrous continuity with the aortic valve. This defect is often found with the subpulmonary morphology typical of tetralogy of Fallot. The defect is usually cradled in the angle between the basal limbs of the septomarginal trabeculation. The subaortic outflow is nearly always widely patent, in which case it receives blood from both ventricles, but occasionally a restrictive ventricular septal defect produces subaortic obstruction. The outlet septum is an important distinguishing feature in these hearts and by definition lies within the right ventricle. Its orientation is deviated in an antero-cephalad direction and, notably with subaortic defect, is attached to the anterior limb of the septomarginal trabeculation. The arterial trunks often spiral, as with "normal relationships" with double outlet right ventricle and subaortic defect. Alternatively, the great arteries may lie side-by-side with the aorta to the right of the pulmonary trunk. Rarely with subaortic ventricular septal defect, the aorta is found anteriorly and to the left of the pulmonary trunk.

A second possibility in double outlet right ventricle is that the ventricular septal defect occupies a subpulmonary rather than a subaortic position. It is located, as usual, between the limbs of the septomarginal trabeculation, but it is the pulmonary valve that overrides the septum in these cases. The orientation of the outlet septum is again an important and distinguishing feature. It lies in the roof of the defect, but it is connected differently from its attachment in a subaortic defect. In the subpulmonary defect, the outlet septum is adherent to the posterior limb of the septomarginal trabeculation. Additionally, the outlet septum may be deviated towards the right, sometimes detached from the septomarginal trabeculation at its rightward anterior end. In this position, when the septum is viewed through the pulmonary valve, a space which underlies the pulmonary valve can be perceived between the outlet septum and the septomarginal trabeculation. Further deviation of the outlet septum into the right ventricular outflow may produce subaortic muscular obstruction. Coarctation of the aorta frequently accompanies the subpulmonary defect in this type of double outlet right ventricle. When the pulmonary valve is less than 50% over the right ventricle, this end of the ventriculo-arterial spectrum is no longer that of double outlet right ventricle, but merges with that of "discordant," one-to-one connection (complete transposition). These lesions, however, are usually all considered together as the "Taussig-Bing" anomaly. In many of these hearts, the ventricular septal defect has a muscular postero-inferior rim because of mitral/tricuspid/pulmonary valvar discontinuity, but in others it extends to the area of fibrous continuity between the mitral and pulmonary valves. Straddling and overriding of the mitral valve is often present.

Another anatomical variant is the doubly committed juxta-arterial ventricular septal defect. The outlet septum is completely absent in these hearts, and the facing leaflets of the pulmonary and aortic valves are in direct fibrous continuity with each other. The ventricular septal defect is immediately below both valves, each of which overrides the septum. The defect may be either perimembranous or have a muscular postero-inferior rim. Sometimes in this situation, the raphe between the two arterial valves is deviated sufficiently far to produce pulmonary stenosis.

Rarely, a ventricular septal defect which is classified as "non-committed" may be present with double outlet right ventricle. These defects sometimes lie in the inlet or apical muscular portions of the right ventricle, but more often are perimembranous and open into the right ventricle in relation to the tricuspid valve. Alternatively, tension apparatus from the atrioventricular valves may interpose between the defect and the subarterial outflow tracts, and a defect which is otherwise an anatomically committed defect may be rendered non-committed by the presence of such features. Multiple defects are sometimes present. Irrespective of the position of the ventricular septal defect in double outlet right ventricle, the conduction tissue relates to its margins in the same way as for any other isolated perimembranous or muscular ventricular septal defect in which there is the usual atrial arrangement and concordant atrio-ventricular connections.

In view of the abnormal spatial relationships between the great arteries in double outlet right ventricle, it should be anticipated that the origins and proximal courses of the coronary arteries will also be abnormal. It is common to find that all the main coronary arteries arise from a single sinus, be it either the right-hand or left-hand facing aortic sinus (or sinus 1 and sinus 2 respectively, using the Leiden convention). Alternatively, they may arise from dual sinuses, the right coronary artery from the right-hand facing aortic sinus, taking an antero-aortic course to reach the right atrio-ventricular groove, and the left main coronary artery from the left-hand facing sinus, taking a retropulmonary course before bifurcating into anterior interventricular and circumflex coronary arteries. Other patterns similar to those that are frequently found in complete transposition of the great arteries should be expected also in double outlet right ventricle.

The surgical management of hearts with double outlet right ventricle, like the morphological spectrum, ranges from procedures that differ little from the repair of a large ventricular defect, Fallot's tetralogy, or transposed great arteries with ventricular septal defect, to extremely complex reconstructions involving extensive muscle resection and intracardiac tunnels. While the operative approach usually can be planned from pre-operative angiography, echocardiography, and hemodynamic findings, it is within this subset of patients that intraoperative decision-making also frequently occurs at the time of direct inspection of the intracardiac anatomy. Diagnostic labels, therefore, such as "subaortic ventricular septal defect" or "non committed ventricular septal defect" should conjure up neither complacency nor dread; each heart must be approached individually, first defining the exact morphology and secondly finding a technical solution that will correct the circulation.

In general, the goal of operative intervention is to connect the left ventricle to the aorta, while leaving or providing an unobstructed outflow from the right ventricle to the pulmonary artery. When the ventricular septal defect is "committed" to or in close proximity to the aortic valve, this amounts to directing the left ventricle to the aorta through the ventricular septal defect by means of a patch or a "tunnel" within the right ventricle. The difference between the two is that a "tunnel" has depth, whereas a "patch" is flat. If the aortic valve overrides the ventricular septal defect, it is possible to use a patch because one side of the "tunnel" is, in essence, the absent septal surface of the defect itself. Where septal muscle intervenes between the ventricular septal defect and the aortic valve, this must either be resected or used as one side of a true tunnel connecting the two.

As the distance between the aortic valve and the ventricular septal defect becomes greater (which can result from a variety of morphological circumstances), the tunnel becomes longer and potentially more complex. Because the length of the suture line increases, there is more potential for a residual ventricular septal defect. Also, because the length of the tunnel increases, there is a greater likelihood of subaortic obstruction. Moreover, a longer distance between the aortic valve and the ventricular septal defect usually implies that the pulmonary valve will lie closer to the tricuspid valve and ventricular septal defect, such that the tunnel must also navigate around the pulmonary valve. As a general guideline, which has been emphasized by the concepts underlying "réparation à l'étage ventriculaire" or "REV procedure," the connection between the left ventricle and aortic valve should be as straight as possible. This means that when the direction of the tunnel must be changed by more than about 40–45%, it is likely that the ventricular septal defect should be routed to the pulmonary valve (in the absence of pulmonary stenosis and commonly when the ventricular septal defect is subpulmonary). The outflows then have to be transposed by means of an arterial switch procedure to connect the left ventricle with the aorta. When pulmonary stenosis is present, the pulmonary valve is closed off, such that the tunnel to the aorta assumes a more direct path and the right ventricle is connected to the distal pulmonary artery either directly or with a valved extracardiac conduit (REV or Rastelli procedure).

A ventricular septal defect which is close to neither great artery ("non-committed ventricular septal defect") can often be brought into proximity of the aortic valve by septal resection, and this is preferred whenever possible. Tendinous cords and papillary muscles supporting the tricuspid valve are either sacrificed or repositioned on the patch, although conduction tissue and mitral valve apparatus must be conserved. On the very rare occasion that it proves impossible to connect the ventricular septal defect (and hence the left ventricle) to either great artery, the options are to close off the pulmonary artery (or connect it to the ascending aorta with a Damus-Kaye-Stansel procedure), perform atrial redirection (Mustard or Senning procedure), close the ventricular septal defect and implant a left ventricle to pulmonary artery conduit, or perform a Fontan-type of operation.

Obstruction to the left ventricle due to a restrictive ventricular septal defect is not uncommon, and muscle bundles within the right ventricle (including components of muscular subaortic or subpulmonary infundibulum) may produce additional obstruction to systemic or pulmonary outflow. When the ventricular septal defect is "cradled" by the limbs of the septomarginal trabeculation and an outlet septum is present (i.e. the ventricular septal defect is not "doubly committed and juxta-arterial"), the latter structure can be safely resected to enlarge the defect. A muscular or inlet defect may be enlarged into the body of the septomarginal trabeculation, avoiding its posterior limb which may contain the conduction tissue. Limited resection of the anterior limb of the septomarginal trabeculation is also safe, although damage to septal perforating coronary arterial branches may occur. However, septal muscle which has been excised obviously no longer requires its coronary blood supply. With regard to the ventriculo-infundibular fold, when this contributes to a muscular subarterial conus, limited endocardial resection is again possible, remembering that major coronary arterial branches run in its epicardial surface.

When it is apparent early in life that a two-ventricle repair is likely to be extremely complex with little likelihood of success, it is generally elected to direct the initial surgical management towards a Fontan circulation (see Chapter 24). In these cases, it may be necessary to protect the pulmonary circulation, which is achieved by pulmonary artery banding, relief of left ventricular hypertension through enlargement of the ventricular septal defect, and/or palliatiation of a hypoplastic atrio-ventricular valve by creation of an atrial septal defect. Associated malformations, which occur not infrequently, are managed on their own merits and do not necessarily of themselves prejudice the outcome of a two-ventricle repair.

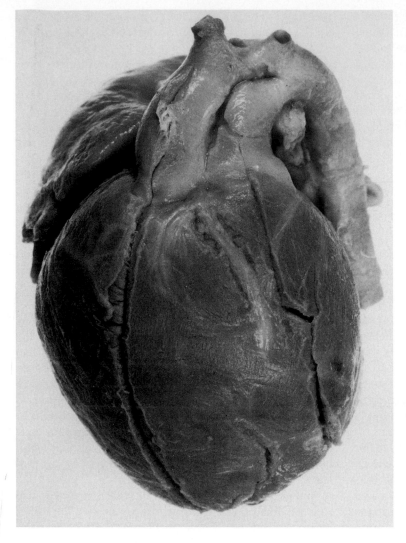

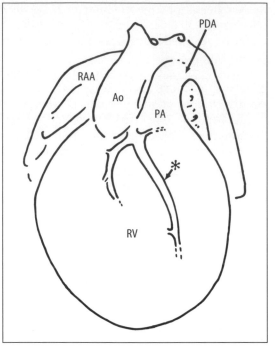

23.1 Double outlet right ventricle. External appearance. The anterior anatomical view shows two great arteries of comparable size connected to the right ventricle and lying parallel (side-by-side) to each other. The aortic trunk is to the right and slightly anterior to the pulmonary trunk. The arterial duct is patent. The right and left coronary arteries (not seen) arise from the same orifice in the left-hand facing aortic sinus (sinus 2) and the left coronary artery (not seen) passes behind the pulmonary root. The short prominent coronary artery, seen on the front of the ventricular mass (asterisk), arises from the right-hand facing sinus (sinus 1 – see Chapter 21) and supplies only the infundibulum of the right ventricle.

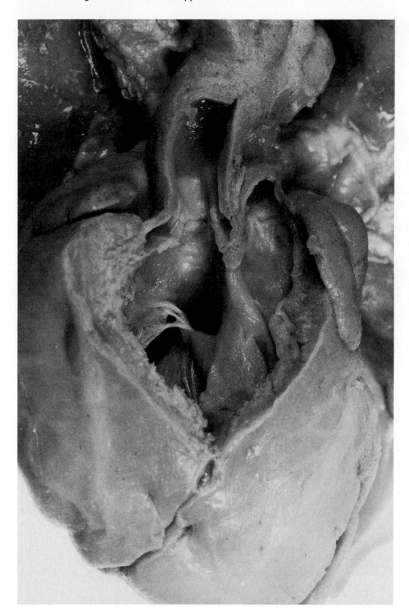

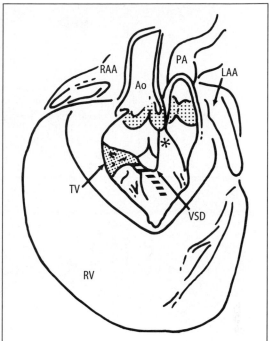

23.2 Double outlet right ventricle. Window dissection. A different example of double outlet right ventricle, also seen from the front in the anatomical position, has been opened by the removal of the anterior ventricular wall to show the right-sided position of the aortic valve in relation to the pulmonary valve. The deviated outlet septum (asterisk) is totally an anatomical feature of the right ventricle and the bilateral muscular infundibulum supports both arterial roots which are of comparable size. The perimembranous ventricular septal defect runs towards the outlet of the right ventricle from the tricuspid valve. Although it is below the aortic valve, it is distanced from this structure and thus could arguably be called a "non-committed" defect. The tricuspid and mitral valves are in fibrous continuity over the postero-inferior margin of the defect. A muscular inlet defect (not seen) is also present. The right coronary artery arises from the right-hand facing aortic sinus (sinus 1 which has been removed in the dissection) and its proximal course passes in front of the aorta towards the right atrioventricular groove (not seen). The left coronary artery (also not seen) arises from the left-hand facing aortic sinus (sinus 2) and runs behind the pulmonary root, bifurcating into anterior interventricular and circumflex branches.

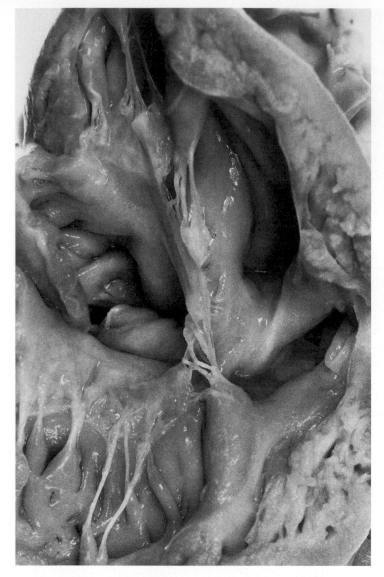

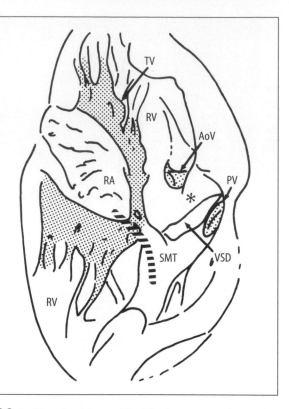

23.3 Double outlet right ventricle. Subpulmonary muscular ventricular septal defect. The right ventricle has been opened from its apex and lifted upward, demonstrating the septal surface and outflow tracts in the anatomical view. The aortic valve lies to the right of the pulmonary valve which partially overrides the left ventricle. The ventricular septal defect is cradled in the angle of the septomarginal trabeculation. The right ventriculo-infundibular fold has fused with the posterior limb of the septomarginal trabeculation, producing a muscular postinferior margin to the defect. This protects the axis of the conduction tissue. The outlet septum (asterisk) is also connected to the posterior limb of the septomarginal trabeculation, which constitutes a fundamental difference between the subpulmonary and subaortic interventricular defects in double outlet right ventricle (see Figure 23.8). There is no fibrous continuity between any arterial and atrioventricular valves (" bilateral conus"). This is the so-called Taussig-Bing type of double outlet right ventricle.

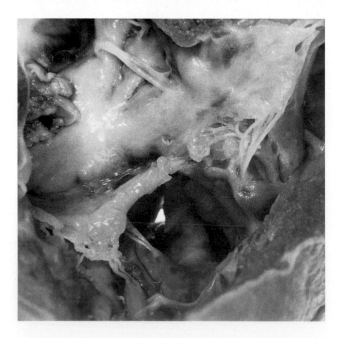

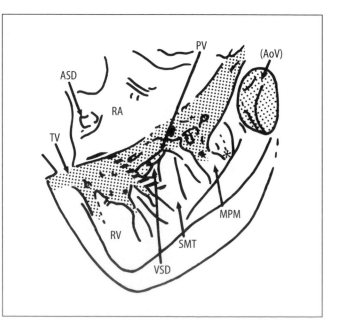

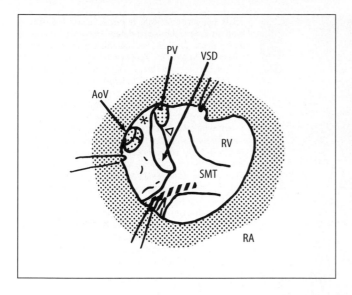

23.5 In both these hearts, the ventricular septal defect is related to the pulmonary trunk with a short distance between the tricuspid valve and the pulmonary valve. While a complicated intraventricular tunnel might accomplish the successful connection of the left ventricle to the aorta, it would require the enlargement of the ventricular septal defect by resection of the outlet septum (asterisk) and the anterior limb of the septomarginal trabeculation (open triangle), with possible damage to the septal perforating coronary branch in the first heart. The small right ventricle would be obstructed by such an intraventricular tunnel in the second heart. A better surgical option is the closure of the ventricular septal defect, leaving the pulmonary valve connected to the left ventricle and an arterial switch procedure. The ventricular septal defect could be approached through the arterial valves or the right ventricle (which would be advisable in the second heart to enlarge the outflow and avoid working through a dysplastic tricuspid valve), or, as shown here for the muscular defect in the first heart, through the right atrium and tricuspid valve (see Chapter 21). The conduction tissue will lie under the surgeon's right-hand side of the defect, separated from its edge by a muscular margin.

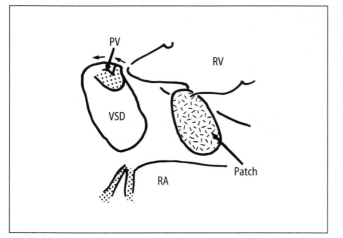

23.6 With the patch held away from the heart, the initial bites of a running suture are taken radially to the pulmonary valve, starting at the junction of the septomarginal trabeculation with the free right ventricular wall and working counter-clockwise.

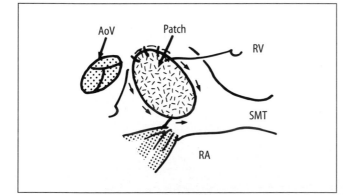

23.7 After three or four sutures have been placed, the patch is lowered down into the ventricle. Suturing continues along the right ventricular outlet septum between the pulmonary and aortic valves, and on to the right ventriculo-infundibular fold to the postero-inferior margin of the defect. Stitches in this area are placed on the margin of the ventricular septal defect to avoid the conduction tissue. At about 4 o'clock, this arm of the suture is held and the second end is brought down along the anterior limb of the septomarginal trabeculation to complete the closure. Additional mattress sutures supported by autogenous pericardial pledgets are used to reinforce the closure as needed.

← **23.4** *(facing page)* In another heart with double outlet right ventricle, the ventricular septal defect again lies in the angle of the septomarginal trabeculation, between its anterior and posterior limbs, but reaches to the tricuspid valve and is thus "perimembranous." The aortic valve (not seen completely) lies to the right and anterior to an extremely large pulmonary valve (partially hidden in the anatomical view) which overrides the interventricular septum towards the left ventricle about 40%. Abnormal muscle bundles (asterisk) produce a small subaortic outflow tract and support the abnormally placed medial papillary muscle complex. This gives the erroneous impression that the ventricular septal defect occupies the inlet septum, but there is pulmonary to tricuspid valvar continuity and the defect is actually subpulmonary. The cavity of the right ventricle is small, and the tricuspid valve is mildly thickened and dysplastic. Two additional muscular trabecular ventricular septal defects are present but not seen, and there is an atrial septal defect in the oval fossa. This case has a right aortic arch and right-sided patent arterial duct, but there is no coarctation of the aorta. Both coronary arteries arise from the right-hand facing sinus (sinus 1). Such hearts are often included within the spectrum of the so-called "Taussig-Bing" malformation, but this morphology might also be classified equivocally as the complete transposition of the great arteries (discordant ventriculo-arterial connections), depending on the extent of pulmonary valvar overriding.

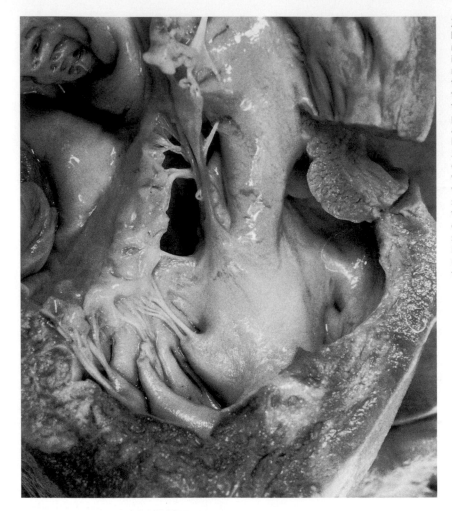

23.8 Double outlet right ventricle. Subaortic perimembranous ventricular septal defect. The parietal wall of the right ventricle has been lifted upwards and the septal surface is viewed in the anatomical position. The aortic valve lies to the right of, but posteriorly to the pulmonary valve and overrides the right ventricle by 90%. This is just seen through the ventricular septal defect which lies between the limbs of the septomarginal trabeculation. There is no obstruction to the subpulmonary region. The outlet septum (asterisk) is completely a right ventricular structure and has fused with the anterior limb of the septomarginal trabeculation (contrast with Figures 23.3 and 23.4). The ventricular septal defect is large and extends to the tricuspid valve, such that the conduction tissue will run along its postero-inferior margin. When the parietal wall of the ventricle is approximated to the remainder of the specimen, it can be appreciated that the tendinous cords of the tricuspid valve cross the subaortic outflow to insert on the outlet septum (small arrows), producing an element of fibrous subaortic stenosis. The coronary arteries in this heart originate in the two facing sinuses and have a normal proximal distribution. There is additionally a large aorto-pulmonary window in this case.

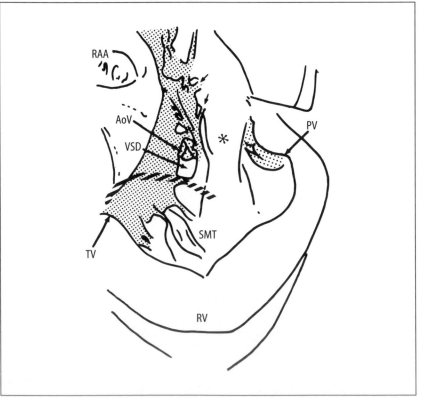

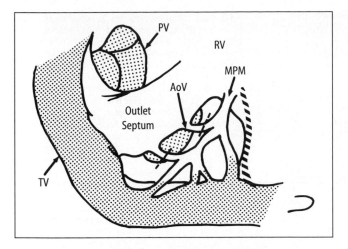

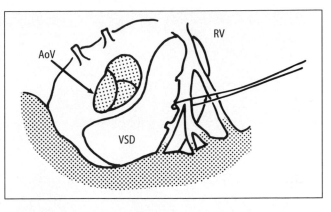

23.10 Retraction of the tricuspid valvar leaflet and medial papillary muscle complex permit full visualization of the aortic valve and good access to the defect.

23.9 The ventricular septal defect in this case is essentially a large perimembranous defect with extreme overriding of the aorta. Building on experience with the transatrial repair of Fallot's tetralogy, it would be closed working through the right atrium and tricuspid valve. Conduction tissue will lie along the right-hand margin of the defect. It is first necessary to divide the tendinous cords attaching in the subaortic area (dashed lines) to get access to the upper margin of the defect.

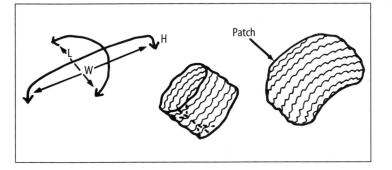

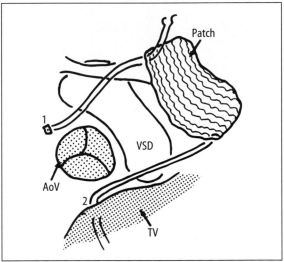

23.11 The intraventricular tunnel, which will route the left ventricle through the ventricular septal defect and right ventricle to the aorta, is visualized and measured in three dimensions. The length, which is determined by the position of the great artery and is ideally shorter than the width, extends from the lower margin of the defect (plus a few millimeters to reach beyond the conduction tissue) to the upper limit of the aortic valve. The width is the distance from the tricuspid valvar annulus to the septomarginal trabeculation, while the height corresponds to the distance from the right ventricular outlet septum to the left ventricle (approximately equal to the amount of aortic valve lying over the right ventricle). These measurements are translated into a patch which is conveniently trimmed from a tube graft (although a flat patch can also easily be shaped to accommodate this type of tunnel).

23.12 The patch is positioned around the aortic valve with a pledgeted mattress suture on the outlet septum (1) and a second mattress suture which is the transition stitch from the ventriculo-infundibular fold through the base of the tricuspid valvar leaflet into the right atrium (2).

23.13 The upper part of the patch is attached with stitches placed radially around the aortic valve. During this time, the rather cumbersome patch is usefully passed through the ventricular septal defect, out of the operative field. When the suture line around the aortic valve is completed, the patch is again elevated into the right ventricle to check the aortic valve by infusion of cardioplegia into the aortic root and to trim the patch if needed.

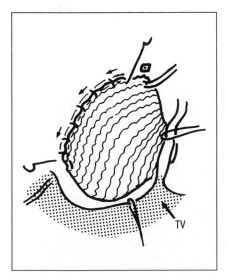

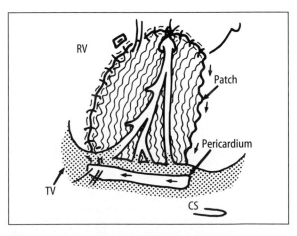

23.14 In this heart, the patch is split to go round the medial papillary muscle complex. If major cords or papillary muscles have been detached from the subaortic area, they can be reattached to the patch itself. The remainder of the ventricular septal defect closure is essentially the same as for an uncomplicated perimembranous defect (see Chapter 11), taking care not to stretch the patch flat across the tunnel and thereby narrow it. The aorto-pulmonary window in this case would be repaired prior to closure of the ventricular septal defect to facilitate myocardial management (see Chapter 3).

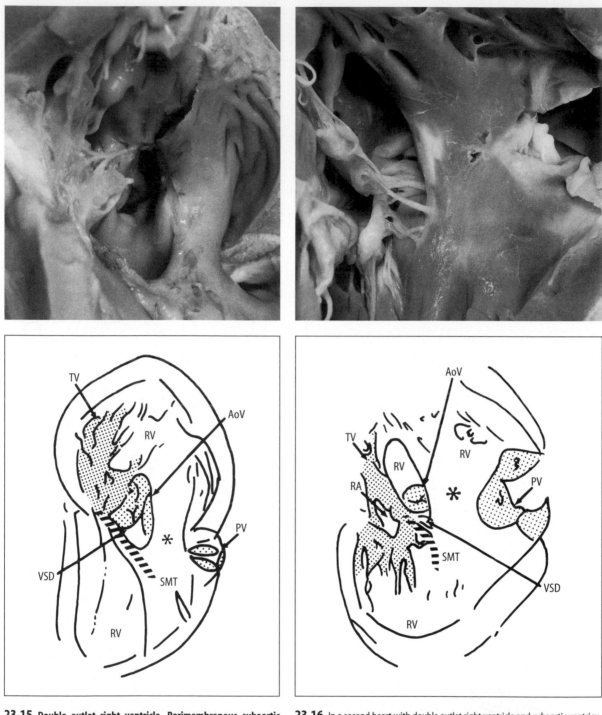

23.15 Double outlet right ventricle. Perimembranous subaortic ventricular septal defect. The outlet septum (asterisk), seen in the anatomical position, is completely within the right ventricle and separates the aortic valve from the pulmonary valve. The great arteries are virtually side-by-side, with the aorta to the right. The aortic valve is in fibrous continuity with the mitral and tricuspid valves. In the closed heart, it lies completely over the right ventricle. A very large ventricular septal defect is cradled by the limbs of the septomarginal trabeculation, immediately beneath the aortic valve. A few tendinous cords from the tricuspid valve cross the subaortic out flow in the closed heart. The conduction tissue runs along the postero-inferior margin of the ventricular septal defect to a poorly defined medial papillary muscle complex. The origins and proximal course of the coronary arteries are normal.

23.16 In a second heart with double outlet right ventricle and subaortic ventricular septal defect, there is fibrous continuity between the tricuspid and mitral valves in the posterior margin of the defect (hidden beneath the tricuspid valve in this anatomical view), but the aortic valve is separated from the atrioventricular valves by a small rim of muscle, which is obscured by tendinous cords crossing the subaortic outflow. While these are less obstructive than those seen in Figure 23.8, there is an additional massive fibrous accretion (also not seen) around the left-sided apical margin of the ventricular septal defect which produces severe subaortic stenosis. The ventricular septal defect itself is extremely small and restrictive. The aortic valve lies to the right and slightly posteriorly to the pulmonary valve. They are separated by the outlet septum (asterisk) which is completely within the right ventricle and fuses with the anterior limb of the septomarginal trabeculation. The coronary arteries in this heart have separate origins from the two facing sinuses, that from the left-hand facing sinus (sinus 2) passing behind the pulmonary trunk and giving off the circumflex and anterior interventricular branches. There is no significant interatrial communication.

Double Outlet Right Ventricle. Perimembranous Subaortic Ventricular Septal Defect

379

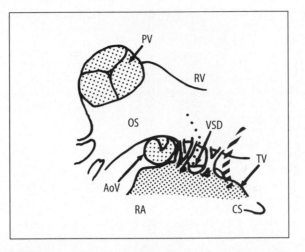

23.17 The systemic outflow in the heart shown in Figure 23.16 is doubly obstructed, firstly by fibrous tissue in the subaortic area of the right ventricle and secondly by the extremely restrictive ventricular septal defect. This must be dealt with prior to attempting repair, either as a preliminary palliative procedure or at the time of creating an intacardiac tunnel (depending on the age and condition of the patient). The fibrous tissue will be in continuity with the atrioventricular valves and will lie close to the conduction tissue, dictating considerable care in its resection (see Chapter 16). The ventricular septal defect will be most easily found from the right atrium. It is first enlarged by a vertical incision towards the outlet septum (dotted line). This is likely also to be close to the conduction tissue.

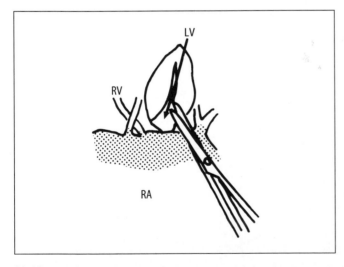

23.18 In this situation, the ventricular septum is likely to be extremely thickened, such that the left ventricular side is difficult to identify. The vertical incision is carried downward until left ventricular endocardium is seen and then enlarged with scissors, taking care to avoid the mitral valve.

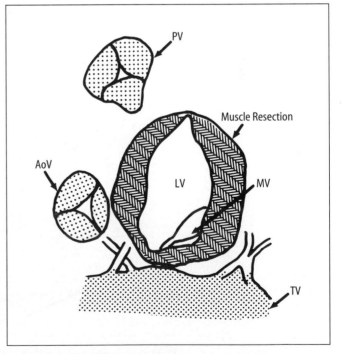

23.19 A fairly radical excision is necessary to achieve complete and lasting relief of the obstruction. This usually involves removing part of the anterior limb of the septomarginal trabeculation, much of the outlet septum towards the pulmonary valve, and additional muscle on the left ventricular side of the septum. The septal perforating artery is usually sacrificed and there may be left and/or right bundle branch block on the electrocardiagram post-operatively. The left ventricle may now be tunnelled to the aortic valve (see Figures 23.11–23.14).

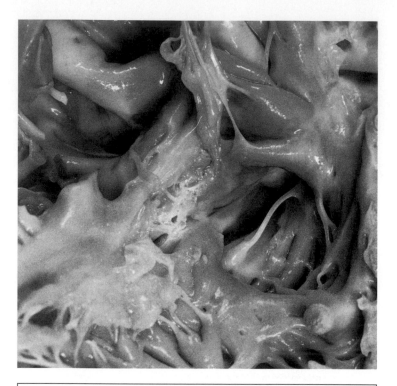

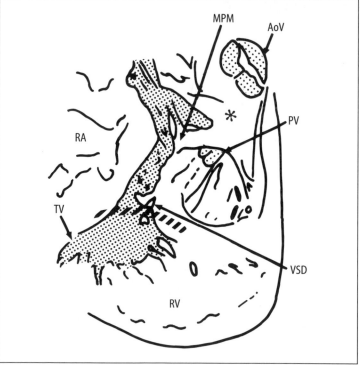

23.20 Double outlet right ventricle. Non-committed perimembranous ventricular septal defect. A small ventricular septal defect lies in the inlet septum. Fibrous continuity between the tricuspid and mitral valves is present through its postero-inferior margin, along which the conduction tissue will be found. The great arteries in the anatomical position lie side-by-side with the aorta to the right of the pulmonary artery (see Figure 23.1 which is an external view of this heart). The outlet septum (asterisk) lies within the right ventricle. The bilateral muscular infundibulum contains multiple muscle bundles which are potentially obstructive to both of the outflows. Coarctation of the aorta is not present in this heart.

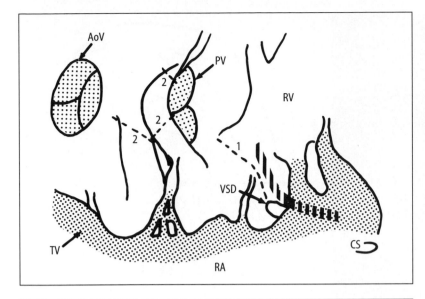

23.21 While the precise definition of "non-committed" in relation to the ventricular septal defect in double outlet right ventricle remains debatable, this case probably fulfills all the criteria and illustrates most of the technical problems implied by such a designation. Being in the inlet of the right ventricle, tricuspid valvar apparatus lies between the defect and both the aortic and pulmonary valves. There is also a long distance to either outlet, although the pulmonary valve is slightly closer than the aortic valve. Moreover, the defect is extremely restrictive and there is additional potential for obstruction to both outflows by muscle bundles within the right ventricle. The first step in an intraventricular tunnel-type repair is enlargement of the ventricular septal defect towards the outlet septum (1, dashed line) and division of the muscle bundles to prepare a pathway for the tunnel to the aorta or pulmonary artery (2, dashed lines). In doing this, care must be taken to avoid damage to the mitral valve, important supporting elements of the tricuspid valve, and conduction tissue (see Figures 23.16–23.18).

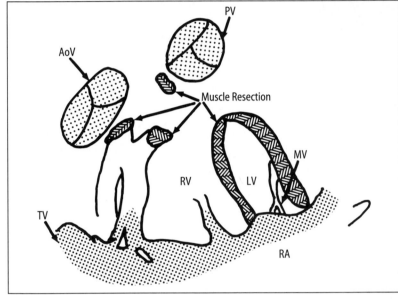

23.22 The enlarged ventricular septal defect is still possibly closer to the pulmonary valve, but there is now a potential pathway to the aortic valve which will be about half the circumference of the proposed tunnel. The tunnel will very likely obstruct the pulmonary outflow, such that a valved extracardiac conduit between the right ventricle and pulmonary artery is also be necessary.

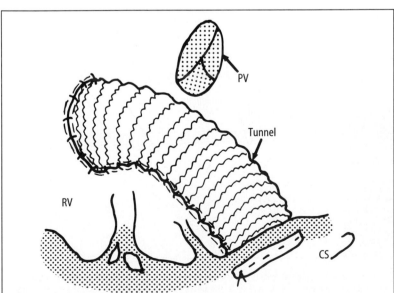

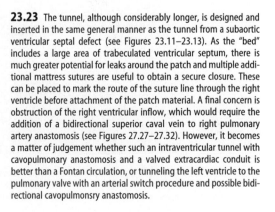

23.23 The tunnel, although considerably longer, is designed and inserted in the same general manner as the tunnel from a subaortic ventricular septal defect (see Figures 23.11–23.13). As the "bed" includes a large area of trabeculated ventricular septum, there is much greater potential for leaks around the patch and multiple additional mattress sutures are useful to obtain a secure closure. These can be placed to mark the route of the suture line through the right ventricle before attachment of the patch material. A final concern is obstruction of the right ventricular inflow, which would require the addition of a bidirectional superior caval vein to right pulmonary artery anastomosis (see Figures 27.27–27.32). However, it becomes a matter of judgement whether such an intraventricular tunnel with cavopulmonary anastomosis and a valved extracardiac conduit is better than a Fontan circulation, or tunneling the left ventricle to the pulmonary valve with an arterial switch procedure and possible bidirectional cavopulmonsry anastomosis.

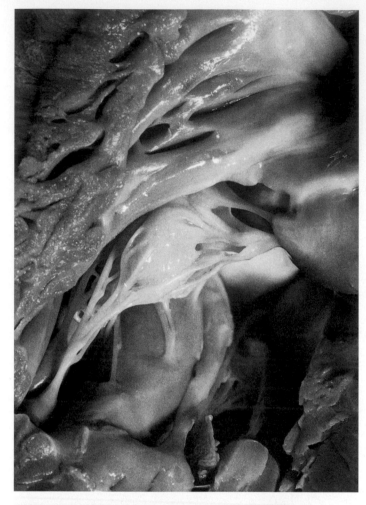

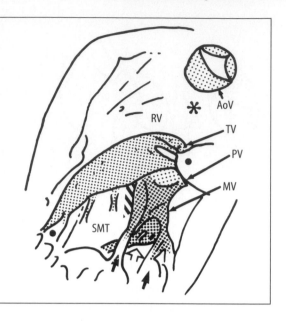

23.24 Double outlet right ventricle. Subpulmonary ventricular septal defect with straddling mitral valve. The parietal wall of the right ventricle has been lifted to show the antero-superior leaflet of the tricuspid valve with its anterior and inferior papillary muscles (black dots). The outlet septum (asterisk) is intrinsic to the right ventricle. The ventricular septal defect cannot be appreciated from this angle because the straddling mitral valve (stippling) fills its orifice. The anterior leaflet of the straddling mitral valve is in direct fibrous continuity with the pulmonary valve and is supported by two papillary muscles (black arrows) within the right ventricle. The more anterior of these papillary muscles also supports tension apparatus (not seen) from the straddling mural leaflet of the mitral valve (open arrow) which, in turn, is tethered to the septomarginal trabeculation. In the anatomic view, the aorta lies to the right of and slightly anteriorly to the pulmonary artery.

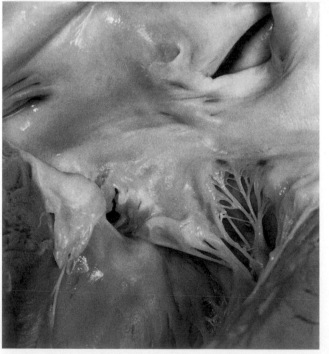

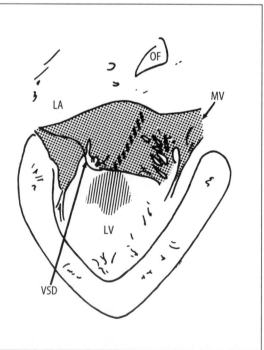

23.25 The left atrioventricular junction of the heart illustrated above shows both anterior and mural leaflets of the mitral valve straddling through the ventricular septal defect. The posteromedial papillary muscle in the left ventricle supports the posteroseptal end of the valvar commissure, while the anterolateral end of the commissure is supported by the anomalous papillary muscle in the right ventricle (see Figure 23.24). There is an atrial septal defect in the oval fossa.

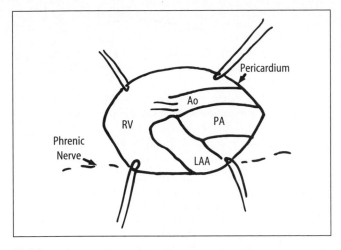

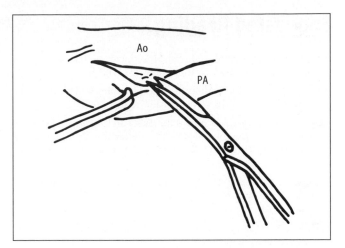

23.26 The presence of a straddling mitral valve with a subpulmonary ventricular septal defect renders this heart unsuitable for biventricular correction, and pulmonary artery banding probably would be indicated to protect the lungs for a Fontan circulation. Performing the banding through a left thoracotomy avoids resternotomy for the next stage of palliation. The pericardium is opened anterior to the phrenic nerve and suspended with stay-stitches to the edge of the wound. This maneuver, while giving good exposure, can cause kinking of a small aorta and/or a coronary artery, so it is important to observe the patient's arterial blood pressure. If a distended left atrial appendage obscures the arterial trunks, it can be pushed back into the pericardial sac with a small swab. Malposition of the great arteries may bring the aorta and pulmonary artery to lie in any relationship, so it is important to identify the aorta positively as the great artery giving off a coronary artery.

23.27 The pulmonary artery is retracted and the great vessels are separated for a short distance as low as possible to avoid the error of banding just the left pulmonary branch. It is common to have substantial arterial and venous branches in the adventitia between the arterial trunks, and these are generally controlled with cautery prior to dissection.

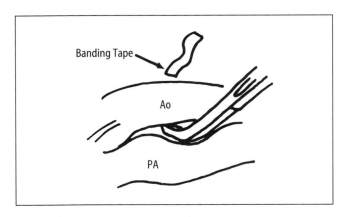

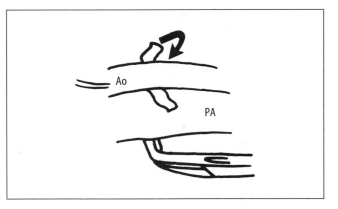

23.28 The aorta is dissected from the pulmonary artery and a right-angled instrument is passed behind the aorta to grasp the banding tape. Care must be taken not to include the right atrial appendage in the clamp. Systemic output invariably falls for a few seconds when the aorta is displaced to grasp the tape.

23.29 After the tape has been drawn between the arterial trunks and hemodynamics have recovered, a right-angled instrument is passed through the transverse sinus to retrieve the second end of the banding tape and draw it around the pulmonary artery.

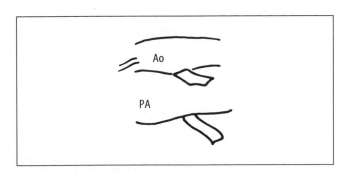

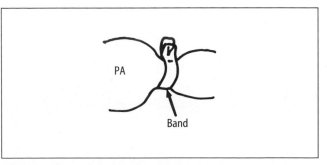

23.30 Pulling the tape through the transverse sinus causes it to encircle the main pulmonary artery "by subtraction."

23.31 The tape is slowly tightened to achieve the desired hemodynamic effect and is secured to itself and the wall of the pulmonary artery with two mattress sutures. These stitches, along with minimal dissection between the great arteries, may help to prevent "slipping" of the band on to the pulmonary bifurcation. If the pulmonary valve is of importance in the planned future management (e.g., a Damus-Kay-Stansel anastomosis or arterial switch), the band may be positioned slightly more distally from the pulmonary sinuses to avoid damage to the pulmonary valve. Alternatively, if the branch pulmonary arteries are the primary concern (for a Fontan circulation), the band is secured as low as possible.

Suggested Reading

Ainger LE. Double outlet right ventricle: intact ventricular septum and blind left ventricle. Am J Cardiol 1965;70:521.

Alva C, Rigby ML, Ho SY, Anderson RH. Overriding and biventricular connection of arterial valves. Cardiol Young 1998;8:150.

Anderson RH, Becker AE. Tetralogy of Fallot and Double Outlet Right Ventricle. In: Controversies in the Description of Congenitally Malformed Hearts. 1997.Chapter 4, p 113. Imperial College Press, London.

Anderson RH, Becker AE, Wilcox BR, Macartney FJ, Wilkinson JL. Surgical anatomy of double-outlet right ventricle – a reappraisal. Am J Cardiol 1983;52:555.

Anderson RH, McCarthy K, Cook AC. Double outlet right ventricle. Cardiol Young 2001;11:329.

Davies MJ, Anderson RH, Becker AE. Conduction system in congenital heart disease. In: The conduction system of the heart. 1983, 5, p 126. Butterworth and Co Ltd, London.

Kawashima Y, Fujita T, Miyamoto T, Manabe H. Intraventricular rerouting of blood for the correction of Taussig-Bing malformation. J Thorac Cardiovasc Surg 1971;62:825.

Kitamura N, Takao A, Ando M, Imai Y, Konno S. Taussig-Bing heart with mitral valve straddling: case reports and post-mortem study. Circulation 1974;49:761.

Lacour-Gayet F, Haun C, Ntalakoura K, Belli E, Houyel L, Marcsek P, Wagner F, Weil J. Biventricular repair of double outlet right ventricle with non-committed ventricular septal defect (VSD) by VSD rerouting to the pulmonary artery and arterial switch. Eur J Cardothorac Surg 2002;21:1042.

Lecompte Y, Batisse A, Di Carlo D. Double outlet right ventricle: a surgical synthesis. Adv Card Surg 1993;4:109.

Lev M, Bharati S, Meng L, Liberthson RR, Paul MH, Idriss F. A concept of double outlet right ventricle. J Thorac Cardiovasc Surg 1972: 64(2):271.

Lincoln C, Anderson RH, Shinebourne EA, English TAH, Wilkinson JL. Double outlet right ventricle with l-malposition of the aorta. Br Heart J 1975;37:453.

Patrick DL, McGoon DC. Operation for double outlet right ventricle with transposition of the great arteries. J Cardiovasc Surg 1968;9:537.

Rubay J, Lecompte Y, Batisse A, Durandy Y, Dibie A, Lemoine G, Vouhé P. Anatomic repair of anomalies of ventriculo-arterial connection (REV). Eur J Cardiothorac Surg 1988;2:305.

Sakata R, LecompteY, Batisse A, Borromee L Durandy Y. Anatomic repair of anomalies of ventriculo-arterial connection associated with ventricular septal defect. I. Criteria of surgical decision. J.Thorac Cardiovasc Surg 1988:95:90.

Serraf A, Lacour-Gayet F, Bruniaux J, Josay J, Petit J, Touchot-Kone A, Bouchart F, Planche C. Anatomic repair of Taussig-Bing hearts. Circulation 1991;84 (Suppl III):III-200.

Smith A, Arnold R, Wilkinson JL, Hamilton DI, McKay R, Anderson RH. An anatomical study of the patterns of the coronary arteries and the sinus nodal artery in complete transposition. Int J Cardiol 1986;12:295.

Taussig HB, Bing RJ. Complete transposition of the aorta and a levoposition of the pulmonary artery. Clinical, physiological and pathological findings. Am J Cardiol 1949;37:551.

Ueda M, Becker AE. Classification of hearts with overriding aortic and pulmonary valves. Int J Cardiol 1985;9:353.

Van Praagh R. What is the Taussig-Bing malformation? Circulation 1968;38:445.

Van Praagh R, Perez-Trevino C, Reynolds JL, Van Praagh R, Perez-Trevino C, Reynolds JL, Moes CA, Keith JD, Roy DL, Belcourt C, Weinberg PM, Parisi LF. Double outlet right ventricle (S, D, L) with subaortic ventricular septal defect and pulmonary stenosis. Am J Cardiol 1975;35:42.

5

Hearts with Univentricular Atrioventricular Connection

24 Tricuspid Valvar Atresia

Introduction

In the heart with classical tricuspid valvar atresia and usual atrial arrangement (situs solitus), the normal right-sided atrioventricular junction is lacking. The floor of the morphologically right atrium is muscular and is separated from the ventricular mass by fibrofatty tissue of the atrioventricular groove. A dimple is frequently present in the atrial floor, which is thought to represent the atretic tricuspid valve. However, it actually overlies the atrioventricular membranous septum and is directed towards the left ventricle. The atrioventricular node lies in the floor of the right atrium in close proximity to the tendon of Todaro and the orifice of the coronary sinus, and also adjacent to the dimple, if present. The atrioventricular node frequently extends laterally or medially to the tendon of Todaro. The common bundle may arise from the extensions of the node to penetrate the central fibrous body and then to lie on the right wall of the main ventricular chamber. The bundle usually branches posteriorly to the ventricular septal defect, in which case the right bundle takes an intramuscular course. Otherwise, the bifurcation lies on or close to the inferior rim of the defect. The left bundle branch extends more posteriorly than usual, by comparison with the normal. The right bundle branch is frequently poorly developed.

In a less common variant of tricuspid valvar atresia, the atrioventricular junction is formed but is hypoplastic and occluded by an imperforate tricuspid valve. The potential atrioventricular connection in this arrangement is from right atrium to right ventricle (concordant). In hearts with an imperforate tricuspid valve, which frequently is simply a tiny fibrous membrane interposed between the right atrium and the hypoplastic right ventricle, the axis of the conduction tissue is to be anticipated as for concordant atrioventricular connections with isolated ventricular septal defect (see Chapter 11).

In both of these variants the systemic venous return crosses the interatrial septum, mixing with the pulmonary venous return and then flowing into the left ventricle across the mitral valve. From there, the ventricular septal defect and ventriculo-arterial connection determine the forward flow. The ventriculo-arterial connections are more often concordant (in about 60–70% of cases), but may be discordant. Less commonly (in 30–40% of cases), pulmonary atresia is present. The ventricular septal defect is variable in size and position, but usually lies below the outlet septum. Its spontaneous narrowing may limit blood-flow to whichever great artery arises from the right ventricle.

Other anatomic variants include restrictive interatrial communications and subarterial right or left ventricular outflow obstruction. Associated lesions include coarctation of the aorta and interruption of the aortic arch. The valve of the inferior caval vein (Eustachian valve) is often prominent. A persistent left superior caval vein may be present, enlarging the orifice of the coronary sinus. Juxtaposition of the atrial appendages, if present, distorts the atrial anatomy, as its orifice will occupy the anticipated location of the oval fossa. Imperforate Ebstein's malformation of the tricuspid valve or other rare anomalies may produce hemodynamic situations similar to tricuspid valvar atresia.

The variations in the coronary arterial supply to the right atrium and the sinuatrial node are important considerations for surgical treatment. Statistically, there is evidence that the prevalence of right anterior atrial arteries is similar in tricuspid atresia to that of the normal distribution, but the prevalence of right lateral and right posterior arteries is significantly greater than that of the normal. Also, in tricuspid atresia, in contrast with the normal heart, the artery to the sinus node arises more frequently from the left than from the right coronary artery. From this origin, in order to reach the root of the superior caval vein and the crest of the right atrial appendage, it must cross the roof of the right atrium to varying degrees. In this way it is exposed to considerable risk with all anastomotic techniques involving the roof of the right atrium. Similarly, all incisions involving atrial flaps will impinge on a right lateral artery. However, it is possible to modify surgical approaches so that these important arteries can be avoided.

The ultimate goal in patients with atresia of the right atrioventricular valve is complete separation of the systemic and pulmonary circulations by means of some type of Fontan operation (also known as "definitive palliation" and "right heart bypass") in which the systemic venous blood passively returns to the lungs and the left ventricle supports the systemic arterial circulation. To that end, it is desirable to have normal-sized pulmonary arteries with a normal pulmonary vascular resistance, a competent left atrioventricular valve, a left ventricle with good function and minimal hypertrophy, and no intracardiac or extracardiac obstruction to the systemic circulation. In some patients, the circulation is well balanced from birth and it is possible to achieve the Fontan circulation with a single operation. In most, however, a series of carefully planned surgical procedures is necessary, starting in infancy or the neonatal period. In general, these are dictated by the patient's hemodynamic situation which, in turn, reflects the cardiac morphology.

For patients who have critically reduced pulmonary blood-flow in the neonatal period or early infancy, usually as a result of associated pulmonary atresia, a systemic-pulmonary shunt is constructed on the side of a superior caval vein. This permits reconstruction of any pulmonary arterial distortion with the superior caval vein at the time of subsequent cavopulmonary connection. The azygos or hemiazygos vein is divided and, in consideration of the likelihood of another stage of palliation within a year, a small prosthetic tube graft is interposed as a modified Blalock-Taussig shunt. This avoids volume overloading of the left ventricle with possible dilatation and mitral valve incompetence. After about three to six months of age, a venous shunt in the form of a bidirectional cavopulmonary anastomosis may be preferred to a systemic to pulmonary anastomosis because it delivers desaturated blood to the lungs and removes a volume load from the ventricle. It may be indicated for decreasing levels of oxygen saturation, which usually indicate a closing ventricular septal defect with concordant ventriculo-arterial connections, an insufficient systemic-pulmonary shunt, or electively in a staged Fontan protocol. The bidirectional cavopulmonary anastomosis is usually performed on cardiopulmonary bypass via a mid-line sternotomy, although in some cases it is possible also to do the procedure through a right thoracotomy or a sternotomy using a temporary shunt. This returns superior caval blood to the right atrium during the period of venous clamping. A venous cavo-pulmonary shunt does not, however cause enlargement of the pulmonary arteries; so a systemic-pulmonary anastomosis is preferable in the situation of hypoplastic pulmonary vessels.

Excessive pulmonary blood-flow generally becomes apparent either soon after birth (usually when there are discordant ventriculo-arterial connections and obstruction to the systemic circulation) or when the pulmonary vascular resistance falls at about four to six weeks of age. In the latter situation, a trial of medical therapy is often useful to see if reduction in the size of the ventricular septal defect will again balance the circulation. Failing that, pulmonary artery banding is carried out to relieve the volume load on the ventricle and prevent the development of pulmonary vascular disease. Neonates with obstructed systemic circulation present a formidable surgical challenge. When the obstruction is at the level of the ventricular septal defect or within the right subaortic ventricle, direct relief on cardiopulmonary bypass with concomitant banding of the pulmonary artery has the advantage of maintaining pulsatile pulmonary blood-flow from a ventricle. However, more often there is associated coarctation of the aorta or hypoplastic aortic arch. In these patients, long-term, direct relief of subaortic outflow obstruction is unlikely to be achieved and most require a "bypass" procedure with reconstruction of the aorta. Traditionally, the intracardiac obstruction has been bypassed by using the pulmonary artery as the systemic outflow and placing a systemic-pulmonary shunt to the distal pulmonary arteries, as in the Norwood operation or one of its variants. More recently, application of the arterial switch operation, leaving the obstructed outflow to perfuse the lungs, has also achieved good palliation.

Despite experimental studies and a review of large clinical experiences, the optimal timing and type of Fontan procedure remains controversial. Intuitively, and with some clinical evidence, it seems best to relieve the left ventricular volume overload as early as possible; yet this must be balanced against the damaging effects of cardiopulmonary bypass, which may be poorly tolerated at a young age, as well as critically important in post-operative pulmonary function and long-term morbidity of elevated systemic venous pressure. Similarly, the desirability of a single operative procedure with, perhaps, increased risk of mortality or morbidity, must be balanced against multiple staged procedures with periods of incomplete palliation. Before about six weeks of age, the pulmonary vascular resistance is naturally too high to tolerate right heart bypass procedures, and the results of operations done after about six and certainly ten years of age are probably less good in terms of late survival. In between, various institutions have achieved good results using a variety of protocols.

With regard to the type of Fontan pathway, experimental results would support connections which avoid the atrium as an "energy sump," a source of thrombus, and a site of arrhythmias; but follow-up of the total cavopulmonary connections and extracardiac Fontan operations (with either direct cavopulmonary anastomoses or a conduit in the venous circulation) is not yet sufficiently long for valid comparison with the older types of atriopulmonary operations. It does seem clear, however, that hepatic venous blood should always be directed to the lungs in order to prevent the formation of pulmonary arteriovenous malformations. Also, the right ventricle should be incorporated into the pathway (by means of a valved right atrial to right ventricular connection) only when its potential to develop into a useful pumping function outweighs its likelihood of obstructing the systemic venous return.

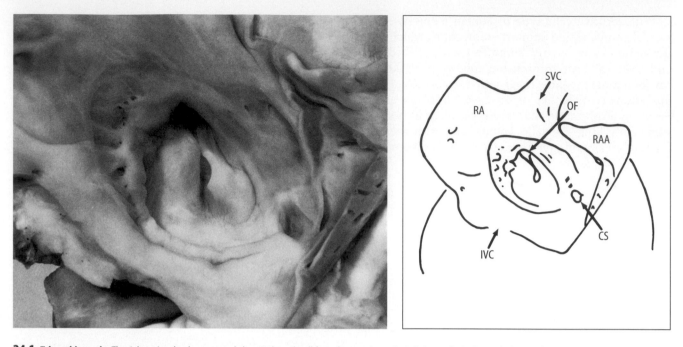

24.1 Tricuspid atresia. The right atrium has been opened along its lateral wall from the superior to the inferior caval vein (arrows). The oval fossa is covered by a thickened flap valve and, while patent, is restrictive. This is uncommon in tricuspid atresia. No clear "dimple" can be identified in the muscular floor of the right atrium. The atrioventricular node is related to the orifice of the coronary sinus in the usual position (see Chapter 11). The ventriculo-arterial connection in this heart is concordant.

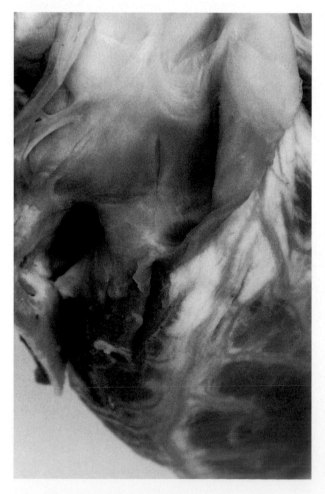

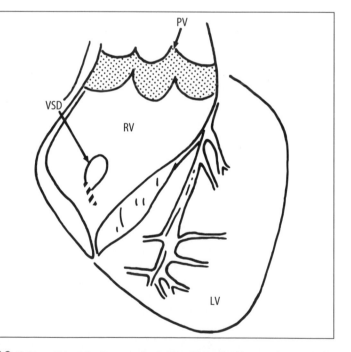

24.2 Right ventricle and pulmonary valve in tricuspid atresia with concordant ventriculo-arterial connection. The free wall of the right ventricle has been opened across the pulmonary valve and retracted rightward. This demonstrates a reasonably well-formed chamber with trabecular outlet and components. It does not contain an inlet valve and the communication from the left ventricle is through a muscular ventricular septal defect. The non-branching bundle of the specialized conduction tissue remains towards the left ventricular side of the septum and usually runs intramyocardially towards the bifurcation and the defect. The bifurcation will be found either intramyocardially but posteriorly to the defect, or subendocardially on its postero-inferior margin. The right bundle branch is likely to run intramyocardially into the hypoplastic right ventricle. The pulmonary valve is normal. Externally, the abnormal position of the inter-ventricular septum is indicated by the anterior interventricular coronary artery.

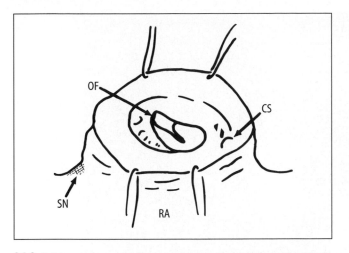

24.3 Patients who have a normal pulmonary valve, a "large" right ventricle with both trabecular and outflow parts, and a concordant ventriculo-arterial connection may be suitable for a valved atrioventricular Fontan connection, in the hope that the right ventricle will develop into a useful pumping chamber. The right atrium is opened along the crest of its appendage on cardiopulmonary bypass with bicaval cannulation and moderate hypothermia. The incision is kept at least 1 cm away from the area of the sinus node. Retracting the wall of the atrium downwards (rather than up) helps to expose the atrial septal defect and coronary sinus.

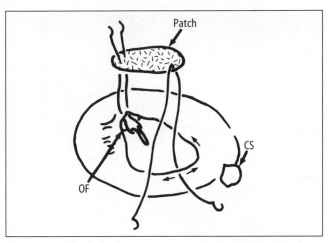

24.4 The floor of the atrium is inspected for exclusion of a tiny perforate valve, and the septum and coronary sinus are explored for additional atrial septal defects. The oval fossa defect is then closed with a patch, using a continuous monofilament suture. Keeping the suture line within the oval fossa avoids injury to the conduction tissue. In this heart, the flap valve of the oval fossa can be approximated to the atrial septum with a mattress suture which is then brought through the patch, giving a secure "two-layer" closure of the atrial septum.

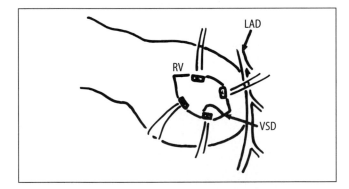

24.5 The right ventricle is opened with a vertical incision, working from the anterior interventricular coronary artery towards the pulmonary valve, which may attach low down in the ventricular infundibulum. Pledgeted stay-sutures are useful to expose the ventricular septal defect.

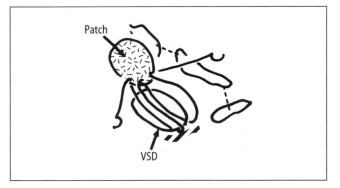

24.6 Trabeculations which cross the right ventricle are divided (dashed lines) to enlarge the size of the cavity. The ventricular septal defect is closed with a patch, using a continuous monofilament suture. In the vicinity of the conduction tissue (lower right-hand corner in the surgeon's view), stitches are placed superficially along the edge of the defect.

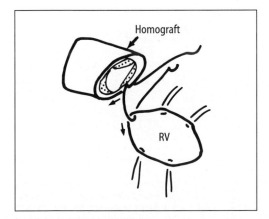

24.7 The distal end of the largest homograft which can be accommodated within the mediastinum is trimmed slightly obliquely and joined to the ventriculotomy with a continuous suture. The slight natural curve of the aortic homograft may be an advantage in this position.

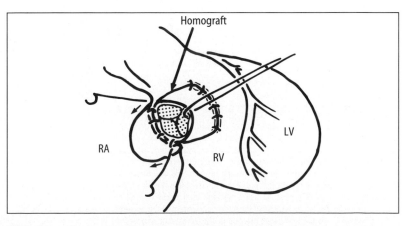

24.8 The proximal end of the homograft is anastamosed to the incision in the right atrial appendage. To avoid distortion of the valve with subsequent incompetence, the right ventricle is filled with saline. The atrial appendage is trimmed if necessary and brought to the position assumed by the closed valve. It is important also to avoid compression of the graft at sternal closure. Slight dextroposition of the ventricles is an advantage in this regard.

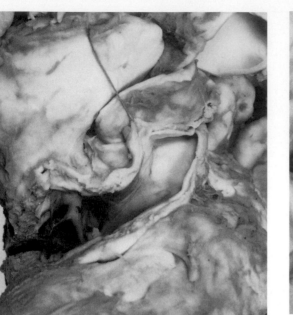

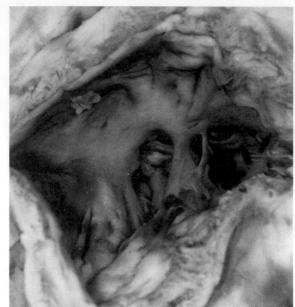

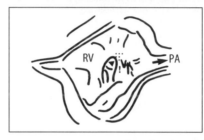

24.10 A close-up view of the heart illustrated in Figure 24.9 shows the hypoplastic tension apparatus (exclamation mark) beneath a fibrous membrane and part of the aneurysmal fibromuscular region (triangle).

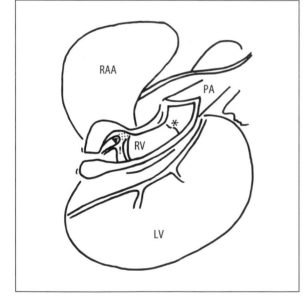

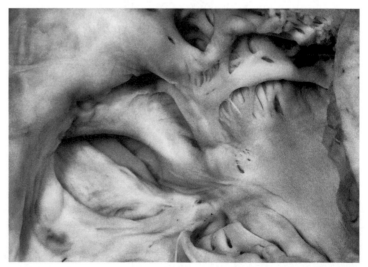

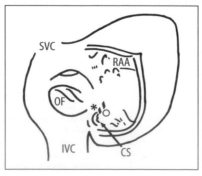

24.9 Tricuspid atresia. Imperforate tricuspid valve; absent pulmonary valve. The cavity of the hypoplastic right ventricle winds around the anterior surface of the heart, adjacent to the atrioventricular groove towards the acute margin. Externally, the anterior interventricular coronary artery delineates the grossly abnormal position of the interventricular septum. The cardiac apex is to the right. The ventricular septal defect appears to have been closed spontaneously by aneurysmal fibromuscular tissue between the muscular inlet area and the central fibrous body. Because of the nature and extent of this tissue, it is not possible to postulate whether the axis of the ventricular conduction tissue runs posteriorly or anteriorly to the fibrous dysplastic mass, which is close to the right ventricular side of the fibrous region (triangle). Hypoplastic tension apparatus (exclamation mark) is seen towards the apex of the right ventricle. The ventriculo-arterial connections are concordant, but the pulmonary valve is absent (asterisk).

24.11 The muscular floor of the right atrium in this heart has two depressions: a dimple (asterisk) represents the atrioventricular membranous septum and points towards the left ventricle. The floor of the second depression (open circle), measuring 3 × 2 mm, is a fibrous membrane that easily transilluminates from the right ventricle and lies above hypoplastic valvar tension apparatus (see Figure 24.10). The axis of the conduction tissue is likely to run between the dimple and the tiny imperforate tricuspid valve.

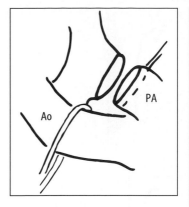

24.12 *(above)* Total cavopulmonary connection with an intracardiac lateral tunnel probably would achieve optimal Fontan hemodynamics in this heart. On cardiopulmonary bypass with moderate hypothermia, the pulmonary artery is dissected from the aorta with mobilization of the bifurcation and right branch. Usually, it is divided just distally to the valvar sinuses and the leaflets are approximated as a first level of closure. As the pulmonary valve is absent in this case, a purse-string is placed around the cardiac end of the pulmonary trunk. In the event of a branch pulmonary arterial stenosis, a patch of autogenous pulmonary artery to use in its repair may be obtained in some cases from a redundant main pulmonary artery.

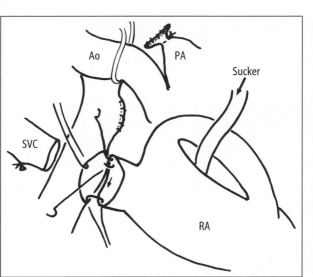

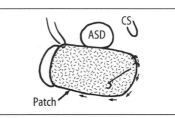

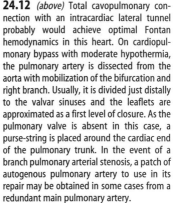

24.15 *(left)* Having completed the lower cavopulmonary anastomosis, exposure is set up in the right atrium using purse-strings. The floor of the oval fossa and remnants of Eustachian valve (dotted lines) are excised to create unrestricted drainage for the coronary sinus and remove potential sites of thrombus formation.

24.13 *(left)* A plug of hemostatic felt is placed above the purse-string ligation of the main pulmonary artery, which is then over-sewn distally in two layers. As there is no inlet to the right ventricle in this case, leakage is unlikely. The distal main pulmonary artery is closed directly and brought rightward behind the ascending aorta. The superior caval vein, which has been cannulated high up for by-pass, is mobilized to the subclavian vein with division of all its tributaries, including the azygos vein (if this was not divided at a previous systemic-pulmonary shunt operation). It is then divided opposite the right pulmonary artery, to which the cardiac end of the superior caval vein is joined to a longitudinal incision on the undersurface with a fine, absorbable, continuous suture. The right atrium has been opened with an oblique incision along the base of its appendage, such that a sucker may be placed across the atrial septum to further vent the left side of the heart.

24.14 *(left)* On the rare occasion that the superior caval vein is inadequate (for example, when there is also a large left caval vein), the anastomosis should be enlarged with a patch on its rightward side to avoid injury to the sinus node or its blood supply.

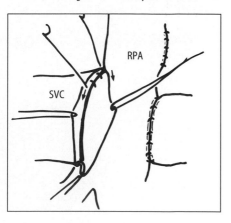

24.16 *(above)* The distance between the precaval muscle bundle surrounding the orifice of the superior caval vein and the entrance of the inferior caval vein is measured. This is surprisingly short (see Figure 24.11). A patch, which will form about half of the circumference of the tunnel between the two, is fashioned from Gore-tex, pericardium, or Dacron. While a portion of a vascular tube graft is conveniently shaped for this purpose, the manufacturers have pointed out that their external surfaces (which remain in contact with the pulmonary venous atrium) have not been tested for intravascular implantation. The patch is sutured to the floor of the atrium, starting at the inferior caval orifice and proceeding inside the tunnel to the right of the coronary sinus and oval fossa.

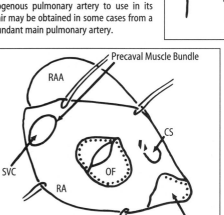

24.17 *(above)* The patch is then brought down to the atrial wall and sutured around about half of the inferior caval vein orifice. From there, its attachment comes on to the right atrial free wall, sometimes using the lower part of the terminal crest to support the suture line, if this is in the appropriate position.

24.19 *(right)* With the heart again beating during rewarming, the distal superior caval vein is joined to the superior aspect of the right pulmonary artery, using a longitudinal incision of length about one and a half times the diameter of the vein. This may extend onto the right upper lobe branch of the pulmonary artery, if this has been narrowed by a previous shunt operation, or across the pulmonary bifurcation to enlarge an area of stenosis related to the arterial duct. When pulmonary collateral blood-flow is too great for good exposure, this anastomosis is done with a side-biting clamp on the pulmonary artery.

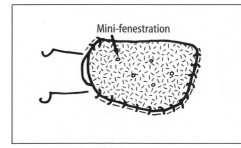

24.18 *(above)* In situations where anticipated post-Fontan hemodynamics may be suboptimal, "mini-fenestration" is an alternative to an adjustable atrial septal defect or a single large fenestration. The patch is perforated several times from right to left atrial side with a 14- or 16-gauge needle. These small holes permit right-to-left decompression early post-operatively and usually close spontaneously in a few months. The suture line is completed around the precaval muscle bundle. The patch is usually a little wider at its inferior caval end.

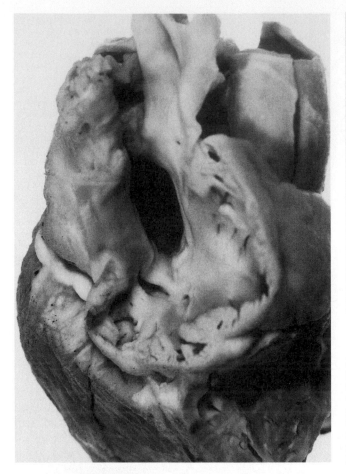

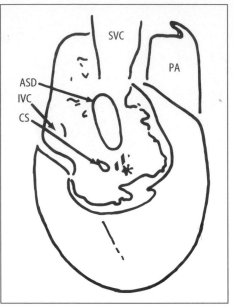

24.20 Tricuspid atresia. The right atrium is typical of "classical" tricuspid atresia. The heart has a concordant ventriculo-arterial connection. There is a large defect of the oval fossa. The atrium has a muscular floor in which a dimple (asterisk) indicates the atrio-ventricular membranous septum and points towards the left ventricle. The approximate position of the atrioventricular node is indicated between the orifice of the coronary sinus and the dimple. The atrioventricular node itself often extends anteriorly, either medially or laterally, in relation to the insertion of the tendon of Todaro. The non-branching bundle may arise from these extensions, running towards the central fibrous body and the right parietal wall of the left ventricle.

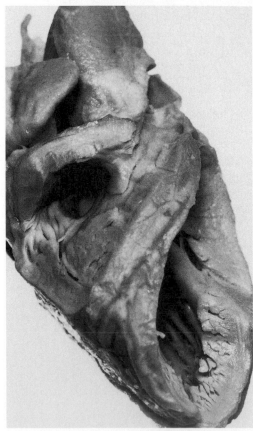

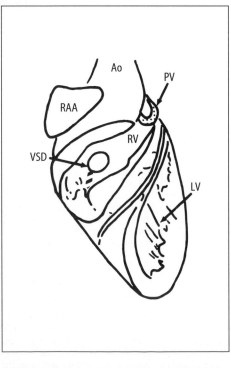

24.21 The right and left ventricles have been exposed by removal of their anterior walls, leaving the inter-ventriclar septum as delineated by the anterior interventricular coronary artery in its abnormal position between them. The cavity of the right ventricle, which has no inlet, is small and the ventricular walls are thickened. A large muscular ventricular septal defect is present, with the approximate position of the right bundle branch indicated along its inferior margin. The pulmonary valve is normal.

24.22 In preparation for a Fontan procedure with direct extracardiac anastomosis, the pulmonary arteries are completely mobilized from the ascending aorta and are dissected to their hilar branches. The ligament or arterial duct is ligated and divided. The main pulmonary artery is divided as low as possible (dashed line), leaving the leaflets and sinuses for a secure closure of the cardiac end (see Figures 24.12, 24.13, 21.104 and 21.105).

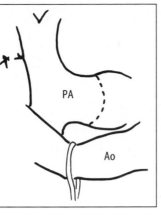

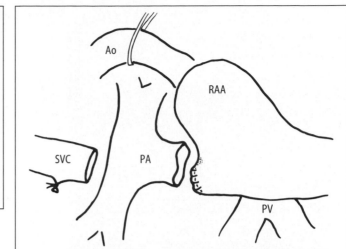

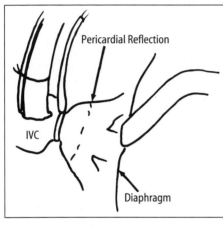

24.23 (*above right*) Division of the superior caval vein a few millimeters above its junction with the right atrium gives a long length, which will reach as far as the left pulmonary arterial branch, if needed, to enlarge the vessels. The cardiac end is either closed directly or used to vent the heart, depending on the morphology and organization of the procedure. The fully mobilized pulmonary arteries are now brought to the right side of the heart (or, with unusual atrial situs, to the side of the inferior caval vein), confirming that a direct connection to the inferior caval vein will be possible.

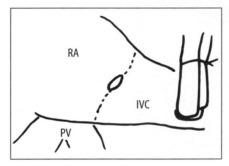

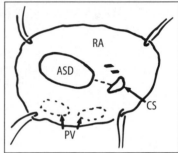

24.24 (*above*) The pericardial attachments to the inferior caval vein, which has been cannulated at its junction with the right atrium, are divided. The diaphragm is retracted downwards and the thin-walled hepatic veins are carefully mobilized. This gains between 10 and 20 mm of length on the inferior caval vein. Division of the diaphragm is not necessary.

24.25 (*above*) The inferior caval vein is detached from the right atrium with the longest possible cuff of atrial wall. A small incision is made first anteriorly and, looking inside the atrium, this is carried out just below the entrance of the coronary sinus and lower pulmonary vein (dashed line), taking care not to injure the right coronary artery in the atrioventricular groove.

24.26 (*above*) Working through the very large hole in the bottom of the atrium, the coronary sinus is cut back to drain into the left atrium (see Figures 8.22–8.23), such that compromise of its orifice is not a concern during closure of the atrium. The entrances of the pulmonary veins are confirmed and any residual venous valve or atrial septal tissue is excised. If needed, an atrioventricular valve may also be repaired at this time.

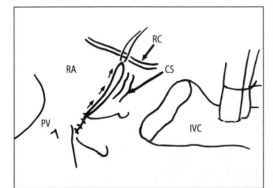

24.27 (*left*) The atriotomy is closed in two layers from the entrance of the pulmonary veins towards the atrioventricular groove. This permits the pulmonary veins to fall back (aided by division of their pericardial attachments, if needed) and avoids their compression by the inferior caval to pulmonary artery anastomosis. As the right atrial suture line becomes inaccessible when the operation is completed, it is important to ensure complete hemostasis at this time.

24.28 (*left*) The cuff of right atrium bearing the inferior caval vein is anastomosed end-to-end to the divided main pulmonary artery with a fine continuous absorbable suture. The considerable difference in their diameters is accommodated within the suture line or, alternatively, the anastomosis can be extended along the right side of the main pulmonary artery and into the undersurface of its right branch, because the flap of atrial wall is always longer on its lateral wall. The superior caval vein is positioned on the upper surface of the pulmonary bifurcation, exactly opposite the main pulmonary artery, to avoid any narrow segment in the pulmonary circulation (see Figure 24.19).

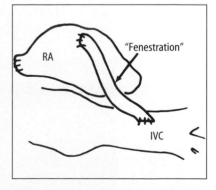

24.29 If fenestration is needed, this is done after removal of the inferior caval cannula by the interposition of a PTFE graft between the cannulation site and the right atrial appendage, using side-biting clamps. The graft is deaired prior to the release of the clamps to avoid a systemic embolus.

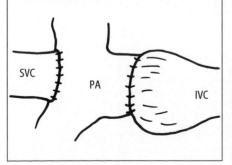

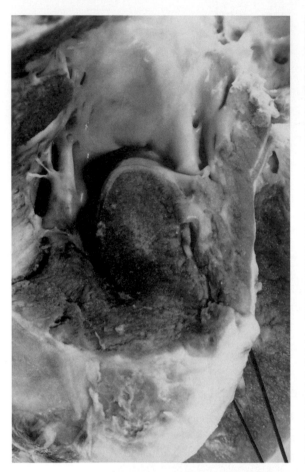

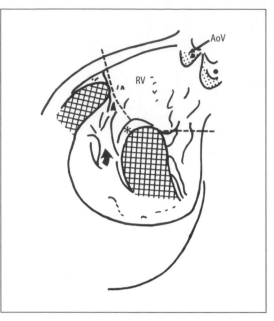

24.30 Tricuspid atresia. Discordant ventriculo-arterial connections. The small subaortic right ventricular cavity has been incised and pulled open, its limits shown by the dashed line. The ventricular septum (cross-hatching below the dashed line) is grossly hypertrophied and virtually obliterates the trabecular portion of the right ventricle. Anteriorly, the malaligned ventricular septum twists into the left ventricle below the ventricular septal defect (asterisk) and hypertrophied outlet septum. The papillary muscle which is seen (arrow) is located in the left ventricle. Despite this morphology, the aortic valve is well developed. The outlet septum is also grossly hypertrophied and protrudes into the subpulmonary outflow, causing obstruction. The pulmonary valve (not seen) is small but has three leaflets. The non-facing leaflet is thickened and prolapses into the left ventricular outflow, and the mitral valve (not seen) is also dysplastic. The aorta lies anteriorly and to the right of the pulmonary trunk. There is no coarctation of the aorta.

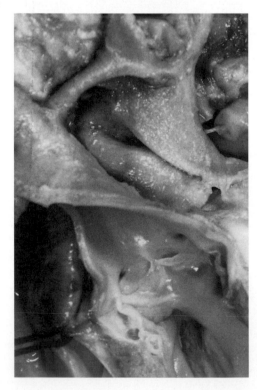

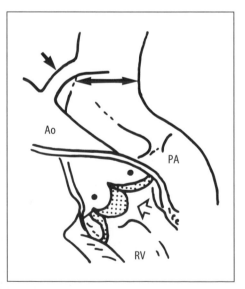

24.31 In another heart with tricuspid atresia and discordant ventriculo-arterial connections, an obstructive muscle bar (open arrow) impinges on the aortic valvar leaflets in the hypoplastic right ventricle. The coronary arteries lie on the sinutubular bar of each of the "facing" aortic sinuses. The aortic isthmus is hypoplastic (black arrow) and the arterial duct is widely patent (double headed arrow).

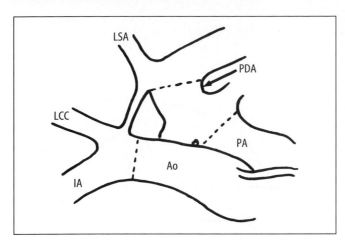

24.32 The surgical options for tricuspid atresia with systemic outflow obstruction are generally direct relief of the obstruction with control of pulmonary blood-flow (usually by pulmonary arterial banding), or bypassing the obstruction and the creation of a systemic-pulmonary shunt (Norwood-type procedure). In the first heart (Figure 24.30), neither of these is likely to be successful because both the mitral and pulmonary valves are also dysplastic. For this patient, transplantation would probably offer a better outcome in both the short and long term. In the other heart (Figure 24.31), an arterial switch operation is a third possibility, which would achieve an unobstructed systemic outflow and limit pulmonary blood-flow through the hypoplastic right ventricle. With profound hypothermia and total circulatory arrest (see Figure 2.31), the head and neck vessels are snared and the arterial cannulae are removed from the aorta and pulmonary artery. Alternatively, cardiopulmonary perfusion may be continued to the innominate artery with or without perfusion of the descending aorta at reduced flow. Both great vessels are divided as distally as possible and the arterial duct is resected (dashed lines).

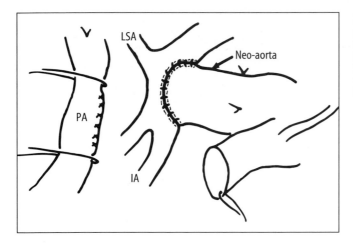

24.33 The pulmonary arterial snares which were placed to occlude the branch pulmonary arteries on bypass are used to elevate the vessels for a "French maneuver" and give access to the aortic arch. The branch pulmonary arteries are mobilized extensively in to each lung hilum. The neoaorta is anastomosed from the descending aorta across the hypoplastic aortic arch to the origin of the innominate artery. The diameter of the greatly enlarged main pulmonary artery is usually sufficient to span this distance, but if it is not, the transverse aortic arch is gathered slightly into the anastamosis.

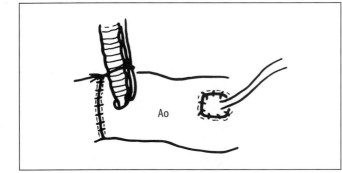

24.34 The aortic cannula is reinserted if total circulatory arrest has been employed, and bypass is used to distend the neoaorta for positioning of the coronary arteries. The commissures of the valve have been previously marked with fine sutures. The coronary arterial orifices are transferred to the neoaorta, usually with "trapdoor" flaps (see Figures 21.16–21.18).

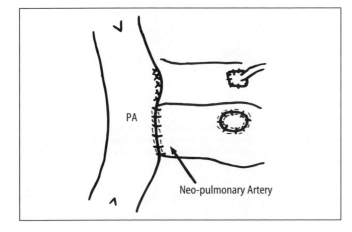

24.35 The donor sites of the coronary arteries are repaired with patches of autogenous pericardium and the branch pulmonary arteries are anastomosed to the proximal neopulmonary arterial trunk. As this lies more comfortably on the right pulmonary artery due to the original dextroposition of the aorta, the main pulmonary artery is closed and a new incision is made more rightward. This procedure not only achieves an unobstructed systematic outflow with growth potential but also maintains pulsatile ventricular outflow to the lungs and leaves the pulmonary arteries in a good position for an eventual Fontan procedure. If pulmonary blood-flow is too great, the neopulmonary trunk can be banded; if it becomes insufficient, a systemic pulmonary shunt can be added later on either side via a thoracotomy.

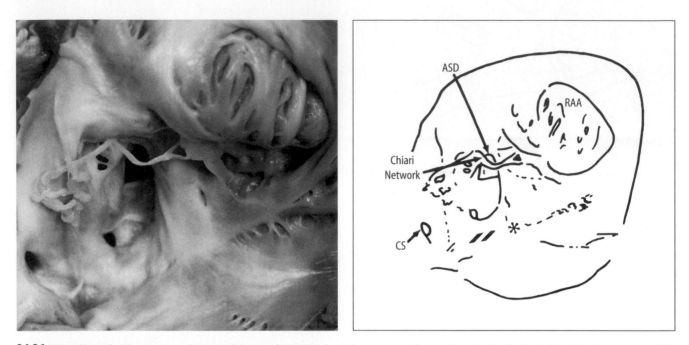

24.36 **Tricuspid atresia. Discordant ventriculo-arterial connections.** A dimple which points to the left ventricle can be identified in the floor of the right atrium (asterisk). The flap valve of the oval fossa shows multiple fenestrations in front of the atrial septal defect and there are remnants (Chiari fibers) of the valve of the inferior caval vein (Eustachian valve). The atrioventricular node lies between the orifice of the coronary sinus and the dimple.

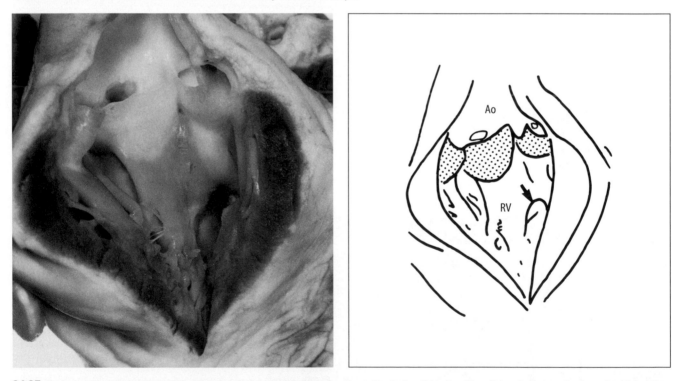

24.37 The hypoplastic right ventricle has been opened vertically across the aortic valve. The aortic valve is well developed, but all three leaflets attach to muscular trabeculations in the subaortic infundibulum. An aperture (arrow) between these trabeculations, in combination with the well-developed outlet septum, produces virtually a "double-chambered right ventricle." The aperture leads to the more apical end of the chamber which contains the straddling portion of the left atrioventricular valve (unseen). The coronary arterial orifices lie at the sinutubular junction in the facing sinuses.

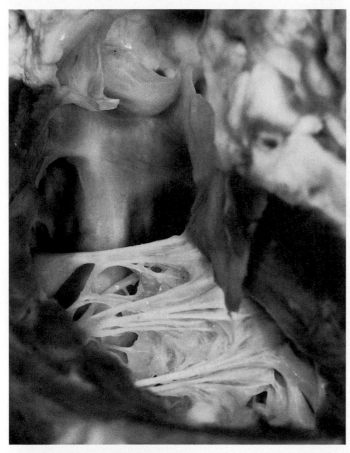

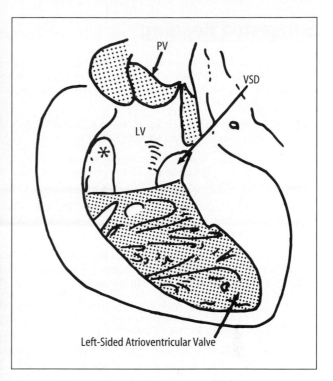

24.38 A separate incision across the pulmonary valve and subpulmonary aspect of the left ventricle demonstrates the left-sided atrioventricular valve which straddles the interventricular septum and attaches to papillary muscles in the apex of the hypoplastic right ventricle. The aperture (asterisk) between the outlet septum and the trabeculations, which partition the right ventricle, is seen from its subpulmonary side.

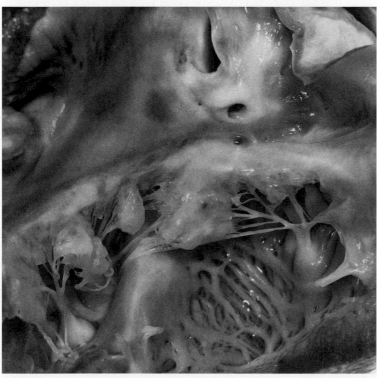

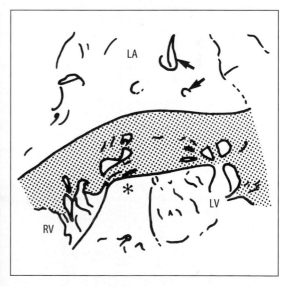

24.39 The atrioventricular valve is shown straddling a deeply scooped and incomplete ventricular septum (asterisk). Despite the fact that two groups of papillary muscles are present, the morphology of this valve does not have the pathognomic features of the mural and anterior leaflets of a mitral valve. It is thus preferable to describe the valve as being "left-sided." Two of the fenestrations of the oval fossa (atrial septal defect) are seen from the left side (arrows). Coarctation of the aorta is also present. As an example of a complex malformation, the complete morphological diagnosis would include right atrioventricular valvar atresia with discordant ventriculo-arterial connections, straddling the left-sided atrio-ventricular valve, atrial and ventricular septal defects, fibrous and muscular subaortic obstruction, and coarctation of the aorta.

Suggested Reading

Anderson RH, Becker AE. Hearts with univentricular atrioventricular connection. In: Controversies in the Description of Congenitally Malformed Hearts. Imperial College Press, London and Amsterdam, 1997. Chapter 5:149.

Anderson RH, Wilkinson JL, Gerlis LM, Smith A, Becker AE. Atresia of the right atrioventricular orifice. Br Heart J 1977;39:414.

Batistessa SA, Ho SY, Anderson RH, Smith A, Deverall PB. The arterial supply to the right atrium and the sinus node in classical tricuspid atresia. J Thorac Cardiovasc Surg 1988;96:816.

Bridges ND, Lock JE, Casteneda AR. Baffle fenestration with subsequent transcatheter closure. Modifications of the Fontan operation for patients at higher risk. Circulation 1990;82:1681.

Bull C, de Leval MR, Stark J, Taylor JFN, Macartney FJ, McGoon DC. Use of a subpulmonary ventricular chamber in the Fontan circulation. J Thorac Cardiovasc Surg 1983;85:21.

Deanfield JE, Tommasini G, Anderson RH, Macartney FJ. Tricuspid atresia: an analysis of the coronary artery distribution and ventricular morphology. Br Heart J 1982;48:485.

De Leval MR, Kilner P, Gewillig M, Bull C. Total cavopulmonary connection: a logical alternative to atriopulmonary connection for complex Fontan operations. J Thorac Cardiovasc Surg 1988;96:682.

Dickinson DF, Wilkinson JL, Smith A, Anderson RH. Atresia of the right atrioventricular orifice with atrioventricular concordance. Br Heart J 1979;42(1):9.

Dickinson DF, Wilkinson JL, Smith A, Becker AE, Anderson RH. Atrioventricular conduction tissues in univentricular hearts of left ventricular type with absent right atrioventricular connection ('tricuspid atresia'). Br Heart J 1979;42(1):1.

Edwards JE, Burchell HB. Congenital tricuspid atresia: a classification. Med Clin North Am 1949;33:1117.

Fontan F, Baudet E. Surgical repair of tricuspid atresia. Thorax 1971; 26:240

Fontan F, Kirklin JW, Fernandez G, Costa F, Naftel DC, Tritto F, Blackstone EH. Outcome after a "perfect" Fontan operation. Circulation 1990;81:1520.

Glenn WWL. Circulatory bypass of the right side of the heart . IV. Shunt between superior vena cava and distal right pulmonary artery – report of clinical application. N Engl J Med 1958;259: 117.

Gross GJ, Jonas RA, Casteneda AR, Hanley FL, Mayer JE, Bridges ND. Maturational and hemodynamic factors predictive of increased cyanosis after bidirectional cavopulmonary anastomosis. Am J Cardiol 1994;74:705.

Ilbawi MN, Idriss FS, De Leon SY, Kucich VA, Muster AJ, Paul MH, Zales VR. When should the hypoplastic right ventricle be used in a Fontan operation? An experimental and clinical correlation. Ann Thorac Surg 1989;47:533.

Kreutzer GO, Vargas FJ, Schlichter AJ, Laura JP, Suarez JC, Coronel AR, Kreutzer EA. Atriopulmonary anastomosis. J Thorac Cardiovasc Surg 1982;83:427.

Laks H, Pearl J, Wu A, Haas G, George B. Experience with the Fontan procedure including use of an adjustable intra-atrial communication. In: Crupi G, Parenzan L, Anderson RH (eds). Perspectives in Paediatric Cardiology Part 2. Futura, Mt Kisco, New York 1989, p 205.

Mair DD, Puga FJ, Danielson GK. The Fontan procedure for tricuspid atresia: early and late results of a 25-year experience with 216 patients. J Am Coll Cardiol 2001;37:933.

Marcelletti C, Corno A, Giannico S, Marino B. Inferior vena cava–pulmonary artery extracardiac conduit: a new form of right heart bypass. J Thorac Cardiovasc Surg 1990;100:228.

McKay R, Kakadekar AP, Tyrrell MJ. Extracardiac Fontan operation: Direct cavopulmonary conncections. Cardiol Young 1998;8:274.

Mee RBB. The arterial switch operation. In: Stark J, de Leval M (eds). Surgery for Congenital Heart Defects. W.B.Saunders Company, London, 1994;p.483

Meitus-Snyder M, Lang P, Mayer JE, Jonas RA, Casteneda AR, Lock JE. Childhood systemic-pulmonary shunts: Subsequent suitability for Fontan operation. Circulation 1987;76 (Suppl III) III–39.

Pass RH, Solowiejczyk DE, Quaegebeur JM, Liberman L, Altmann K, Gersony WM, Hordof AJ. Bulboventricular foramen resection: hemodynamic and electrophysiologic results. Ann Thorac Surg 2001;71:1251.

Scalia D, Russo P, Anderson RH, Macartney FJ, Hegerty AS, Ho SY, Daliento L, Thiene G. The surgical anatomy of hearts with no direct communication between the right atrium and the ventricular mass – so-called tricuspid atresia. J Thorac Cardiovasc Surg 1984;87:743.

Tokunaga S, Kado H, Imoto Y, Masuda M, Shiodawa Y, Fukae K, Fusazaki N, Ishikawa S, Yasui H. Total cavopulmonary connection with an extracardiac conduit: experience with 100 patients. Am Thorac Surg 2002;73(1):76.

25 Mitral Valvar Atresia

Introduction

The term "mitral atresia" suggests either blockage of the outflow of the left atrium through the atrioventricular junction or total congenital occlusion of a naturally occurring channel. It results in one type of univentricular atrioventricular connection. While many people understand this to imply blockage of the pulmonary venous atrium, the two are not necessarily synonymous because the pulmonary veins may connect, for example, to a morphologically right atrium in an isomeric heart (see Chapter 4). For precise anatomical descriptions, the terms "left-sided" or "right-sided" atrioventricular valve are more meaningful than "mitral" or "tricuspid" valve, particularly in hearts with mirror-image atriums.

There are two mechanisms by which the atrioventricular valves become atretic. In the first type, absent atrioventricular valve, the normal atrioventricular junction is totally lacking. The floor of the affected atrium is completely muscular and separated from the ventricular mass by the tissue of the atrioventricular groove. In the second type, the atrioventricular junction is formed but is blocked by an imperforate valve. The anatomical feature that differentiates an imperforate mitral valve from the absence of the atrioventricular connection is the formation of an atrioventricular junction. In many cases of either type, mitral valvar atresia is an integral part of the hypoplastic left heart syndrome in which there is usually associated aortic valvar atresia and incomplete or rudimentary left ventricle (see Chapter 19).

With an imperforate mitral valve, the left ventricle is usually constructed normally. It may be small or of normal inlet and outlet dimensions, the latter being more common in the presence of a ventricular septal defect. Multiple ventricular septal defects may be present and they are often of mixed perimembranous and muscular types. Frequently, in the presence of a perimembranous ventricular septal defect, the aortic valve overrides the septal defect and the 50% rule is used to decide the type of ventriculo-arterial connection. This can be concordant, discordant, or double-outlet right ventricle. When the mitral valve is imperforate, any tension apparatus which exists is usually underdeveloped. In the right ventricle of hearts with mitral valvar atresia and ventricular septal defect, the tricuspid valve is often dysplastic where it overlies the defect. Accessory tricuspid valvar tissue may even produce subaortic or subpulmonary obstruction.

The aortic valve in these hearts is often atretic, as seen with hypoplastic left heart syndrome, but a patent aortic valve may also be present with mitral valvar atresia. This occurs with either the left or right ventriculo-aortic connection. Frequently, the aortic valves have only two leaflets and essentially two sinuses, but a rudimentary commissure between the two orifices of the coronary arteries often hints that the original valvar substrate had three sinuses and three leaflets. With concordant ventriculo-arterial connections, subaortic muscular bulging may produce left ventricular outflow tract obstruction. The association between mitral valvar atresia, double-outlet right ventricle, and intact ventricular septum is strongly suggestive that a previous ventricular septal defect has closed spontaneously, either in foetal or postnatal life. When an imperforate mitral valve is found with a double-outlet ventriculo-arterial connection, the right ventricle will be large and thick-walled. The septomarginal trabeculation, if hypertrophied, may also produce a degree of subaortic obstruction. Associated fibrous subpulmonary obstruction is seen occasionally. Some form of coarctation shelf in the aortic arch is to be anticipated.

A full sequential analysis of the cardiac chambers is particularly helpful when morphologically left atrioventricular valvar atresia is found in bizarre situations. One example of this is right-sided atrioventricular valvar atresia in a complete mirror-image of the heart. Another example is seen when the right-sided morphologically right atrium is potentially connected to a morphologically left ventricle, this being the anatomic counterpart of tricuspid valvar atresia. However, if the valve had been formed, it would have been a mitral valve. This illustrates the conflict between the precise morphological description and hemodynamic consequences.

While the clinical management of the left atrioventricular valvar atresia largely parallels that of tricuspid (right atrioventricular) valvar atresia (see Chapter 24) or hypoplastic left heart syndrome (see Chapter 19), this group of patients tends to be a more heterogeneous. Therefore, both diagnosis and treatment must be precise and individualized, taking into consideration that the ventricle supporting the circulation may not be a morphologically left ventricle. The systemic atrioventricular valve also tends to be less robust than the morphologically mitral valve. Thus, ventricular dilatation and valvar incompetence often influence surgical management.

Like tricuspid atresia, an unrestrictive interatrial communication is essential for survival, but it is the pulmonary venous return which must cross the defect. If this is restrictive in the neonatal period, balloon septostomy may be possible; beyond a few months of life, open surgical septectomy is usually necessary. The remainder of the interventions are selected to balance pulmonary flow or relieve obstruction to the systemic circulation as needed, to bring the patient to a Fontan circulation by about two years of age.

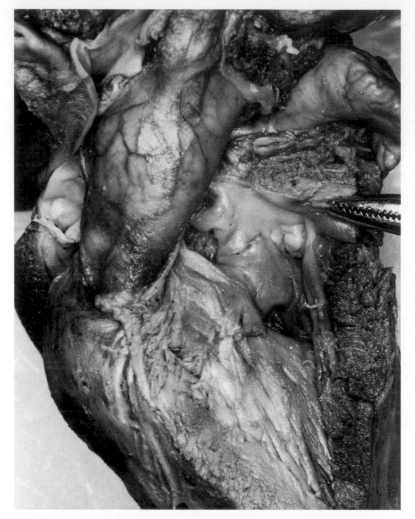

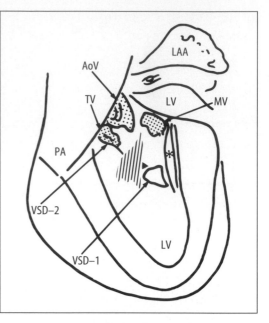

25.1 Imperforate left-sided mitral valve. Double-outlet right ventricle with ventricular septal defects. The left ventricle, shown on its septal surface, has normal linear measurements of its cavity, but the mitral valve is imperforate. The anterolateral papillary muscle (asterisk) is prominent but hypoplastic. The postero-medial papillary muscle is absent. The aortic valve is small and has only two leaflets, although a rudimentary commissure is present between the orifices of the coronary arteries. Less than 50% of the aortic valve is connected to the left ventricle and the outlet septum is malaligned over the right ventricle, producing a double-outlet ventriculo-arterial connection. In addition, muscular thickening (triangle) of the septum between a large muscular inlet ventricular septal defect (1) and a subaortic perimembranous defect (2) results in left ventricular outflow obstruction. Tricuspid valvar leaflet is seen through the perimembranous ventricular septal defect. The pulmonary root is dilated and considerably larger than the aortic root. Generalized hypoplasia of the aortic arch with a long isthmus (not seen) is present and the arterial duct is closed.

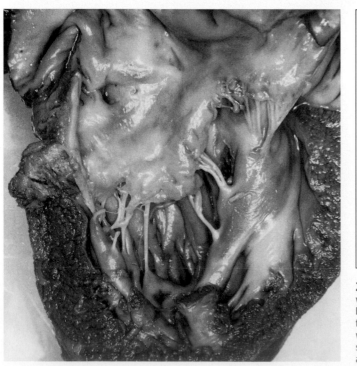

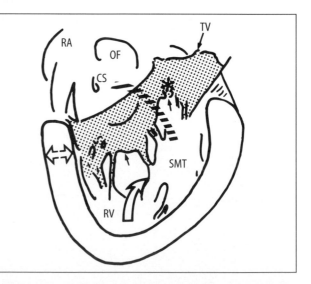

25.2 The right ventricular side of the specimen shown above has a thickened free wall (doubled-headed arrow) and moderate hypertrophy of the septomarginal trabeculation The posterior edge of the septomarginal trabeculation is delaminated from the septum (open arrow) and the tricuspid valve is slightly dysplastic (asterisk) where it overlies the perimembranous ventricular septal defect. Both ventricular septal defects are obscured by leaflet material of the tricuspid valve in this view, their approximate positions being indicated by the small arrows.

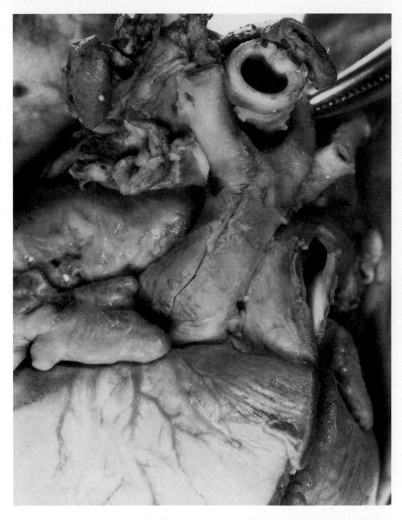

25.3 For contrast and comparison with the preceding case (Figures 25.1 and 25.2). This heart also has an imperforate left-sided mitral valve and stenotic aortic valve (two leaflets in three sinuses with rudimentary commissure between two coronary arterial orifices), and more than 50% overriding of the aortic valve over the cavity of the right ventricle (double-outlet right ventricle). However, a perimembranous ventricular septal defect and two other muscular trabecular defects (not seen) are present with a normal sized left ventricle and ascending aorta. The tricuspid valve is dysplastic where it overlies the ventricular septal defect. The oval fossa is only probe patent. Both atrial appendages have the characteristics of a morphologically left atrial appendage. Bilateral, bilobed lungs with long bronchi establish the presence of left isomerism.

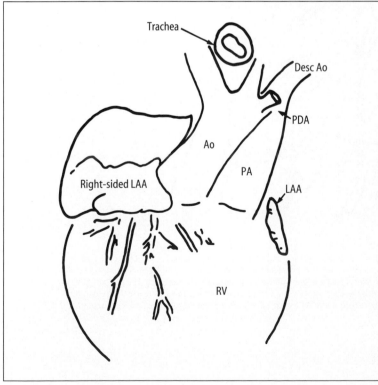

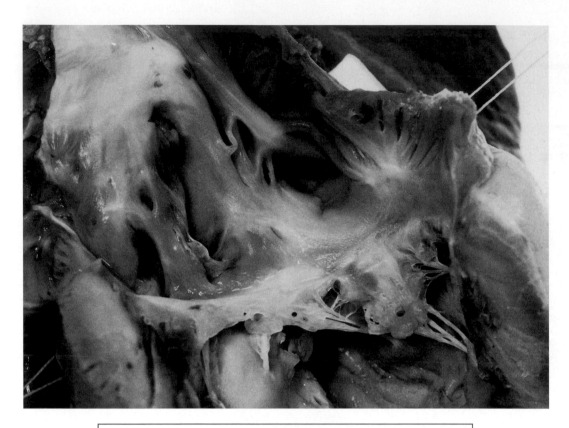

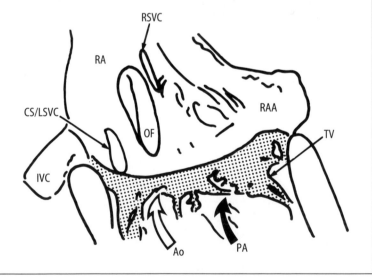

25.4 Imperforate left-sided mitral valvar atresia. Double-outlet right ventricle and intact ventricular septum. The heart has been opened across the right atrioventricular junction. The right atrium receives the superior and inferior caval veins, as well as a persistent left superior caval vein via the enlarged coronary sinus. The right ventricle is thick-walled and gives off both the great arteries (not seen). The position of the pulmonary artery is indicated by a solid arrow and the aorta by an open arrow. A piece of dysplastic leaflet tissue on the undersurface of the septal tricuspid leaflet obstructs the outflow to the aorta. The left-sided atrioventricular valve is tiny and imperforate. The ventricular septum is intact.

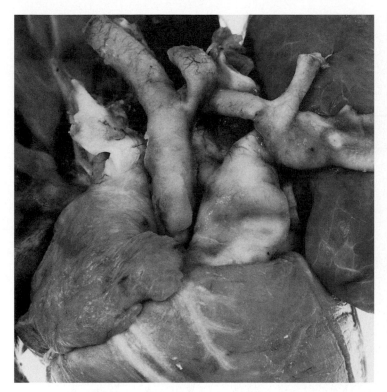

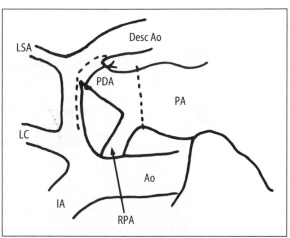

25.6 Given the subaortic obstruction and elongated aortic arch, augmentation of the systemic outflow probably will be necessary early in life, along with limitation of the pulmonary blood-flow. The size of the main pulmonary artery and comparatively distal origin of its right branch, along with the good caliber of the ascending aorta, may permit this to be done by direct anastomosis of the pulmonary artery to the distal arch and descending aorta. The dashed lines indicate proposed sites for vascular incisions. The pulmonary blood flow is managed analogous to the hypoplastic left heart syndrome (see Chapter 19).

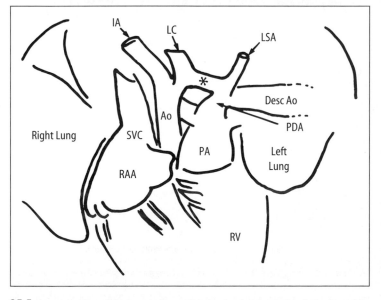

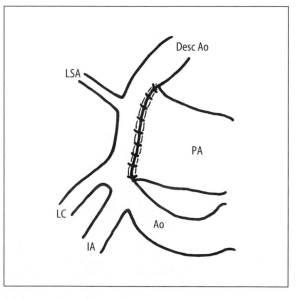

25.5 An anterior view of the heart in Figure 25.4 showing that the spatial relationships of the great arteries are normal, but the pulmonary trunk is much larger than the aortic trunk. The transverse aortic arch has an elongated and hypoplastic segment between the left common carotid and left subclavian arteries (asterisk). The arterial duct is widely patent and the left subclavian artery arises opposite to the aortic end of the duct. The coronary arteries on the epicardial surface delineate a very small left ventricle (not seen).

25.7 Extensive dissection of all the vessels, including the descending aorta, is necessary to avoid tension on the anastomosis and compression of the left pulmonary artery and/or left main stem bronchus between the pulmonary artery and descending aorta. If direct anastomosis does not appear favorable after resection of all ductal tissue and mobilization of the vessels, a segment of pulmonary or aortic homograft is used as an interposition graft.

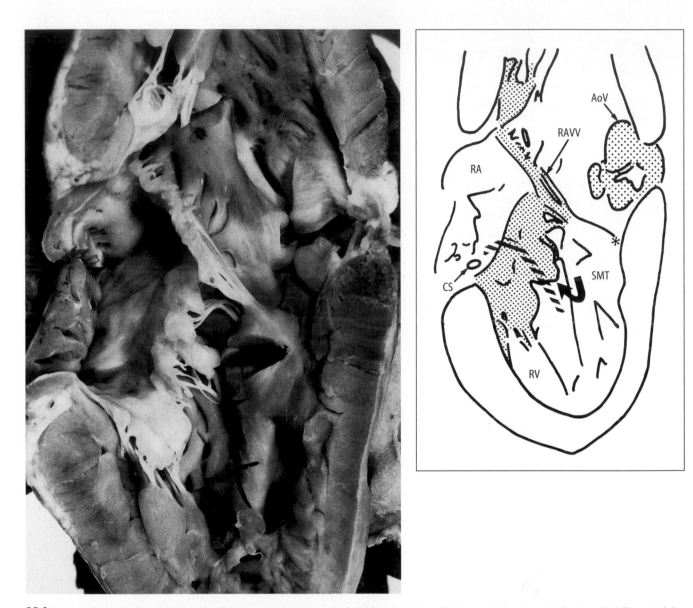

25.8 Absent left-sided atrioventricular connection. Intact ventricular septum and double-outlet right ventricle (univentricular atrioventricular connection). The ventricle has been opened from its apex and lifted upward to show the septal surface, the well-developed septomarginal trabeculation, and the atrioventricular junction. Two atriums are present and connected by a large atrial septal defect, but only the floor of the right atrium is seen in the photograph. The atrioventricular valve opens into a chamber of right ventricular morphology. The left-sided atrioventricular connection is absent, but a dimple is present in the floor of the left atrium. A left-sided ventricle is not immediately evident on gross dissection, but descending branches of the major coronary arteries hint at the delineation of a rudimentary morphologically left ventricle. Both great arteries are given off by the right ventricle. Subpulmonary obstruction is caused by dysplastic leaflet tissue of the atrioventricular valve (curved arrow) and hypertrophy of the septomarginal trabeculation has produced some subaortic obstruction (asterisk). However, the aortic valve is well developed, as are the systemic great vessels.

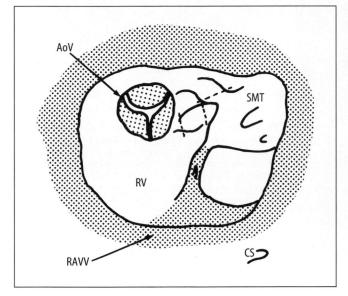

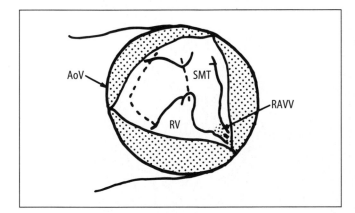

25.9 Appreciating that the right atrioventricular valve, although similar in morphology to a tricuspid valve, will function in the systemic circulation, relief of the subpulmonary obstruction by resection of the dysplastic obstructing leaflet tissue would be inadvisable. Palliation with a view to a Fontan protocol could, however, be initiated with a systemic pulmonary shunt and direct resection of the muscular subaortic obstruction. If this were approached through the right atrium, the conduction tissue would be found under the surgeon's right hand, remote from the hypertrophied muscle bundles. These are divided (dashed lines), taking care to compromise the support for neither the aortic valvar leaflets nor the attachments of the papillary muscle.

25.10 An alternative approach would be through the ascending aorta and retrogradely through the aortic valve. Because this arises from the right ventricle, the tricuspid valvar papillary muscle and tendinous cords are easily seen and protected. This route gives a good appreciation of the muscle bundles that must be removed (dashed lines) and is not close to the proximal conduction tissue.

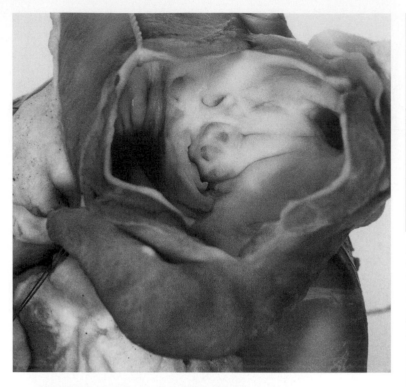

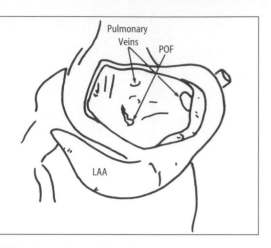

25.11 Absent right-sided ("mitral") atrioventricular connection. An oblique view from a right, posterior angle of a right-sided, morphologically left atrium, in a heart with mirror imaged atriums and a left-sided univentricular atrioventricular connection to a ventricle of indeterminate morphology. The right sided atrioventricular connection is absent. The pulmonary veins all enter this right sided collecting chamber, of which the atrial appendage is retroverted. In this heart, although having no outlet to a ventricle, the right-sided atrium fulfils the criteria for a morphologically left atrium. It lacks a terminal crest and the pectinate muscles of the atrial appendage are confined to the appendage. They do not spill over into the smooth-walled sinus portion of the atrium. The left-sided morphologically right atrium (not seen) connects to the ventricular mass. There is a small interatrial communication and, accordingly, obstruction to the pulmonary venous drainage.

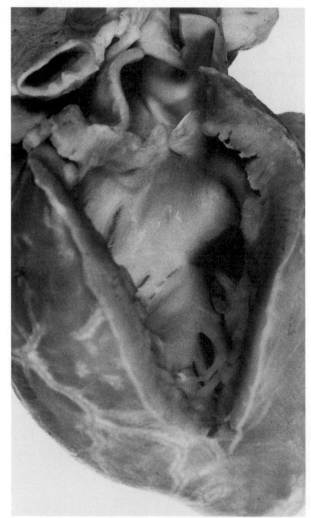

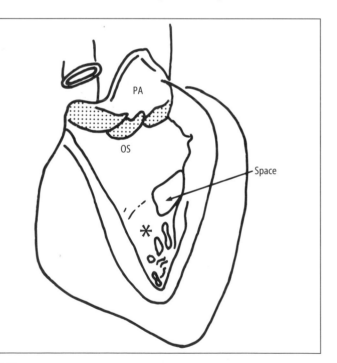

25.12 A window dissection into the right side of the indeterminate ventricle (see Chapter 27) described above (Figure 25.11), opened to show the pulmonary outflow tract. The ventricle has a globular shape, without a distinctive apical portion, but has no inlet septum by which to show trabecular characteristics of "rightness" and "leftness". An enlarged outlet septum runs to the ventricular wall to produce a muscular infundibulum below a normal pulmonary valve. An extension from the outlet septum spreads along the right free wall of the indeterminate ventricle and separates the muscular subpulmonary from the muscular subaortic infundibulum (not seen). At its distal end from the pulmonary valve, the extension becomes thinner and trabeculated (asterisk), carrying some of the tension apparatus (not seen) for the indeterminate atrioventricular valve. In this way, the indeterminate ventricle has become double-chambered.

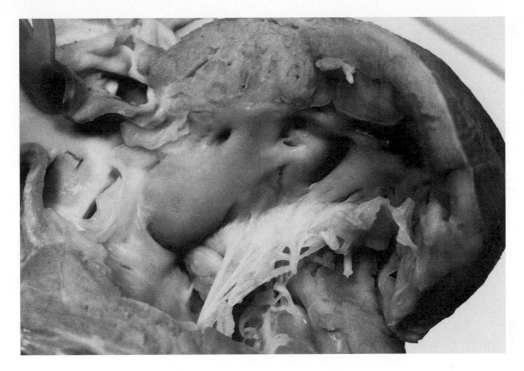

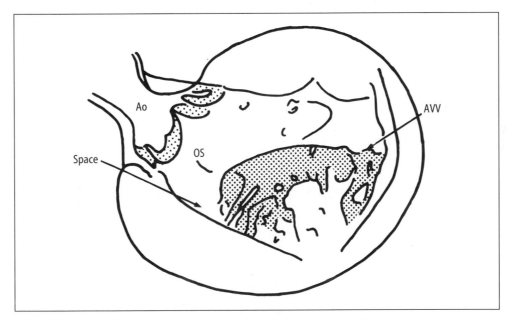

25.13 The left side of the same indeterminate ventricle. The left-sided atrium has the characteristics of a morphologically right atrium, namely a terminal crest and pectinate muscles that drape from the crest around the appendage from the orifice of a superior caval vein to a coronary sinus. The left-sided atrium also receives the inferior caval vein. In this way, the atrial arrangement is that of "mirror image". The atrioventricular valve between the left-sided atrium and the large ventricle, is of indeterminate morphology. It has some characteristics of a tricuspid valve but there is no evidence of an inlet septum to which it could attach. Neither is there an apical, trabecular septum to assess features by which to assign "rightness" or "leftness" to this ventricle. The ventricle has a globular shape without a distinctive apical portion. It is hypertrophied and, as described for Figure 25.12, contains a well developed outlet septum from which a column of muscle extends almost for the length of the ventricle, carrying some of the cordal attachments of the atrioventricular valve. This creates a "double-chambered" indeterminate ventricle. The right side of the extension might be interpreted wrongly as the equivalent of a second ventricle in the ventricular mass but the epicardial coronary arteries do not focus in any particular way to delineate a second chamber. Therefore, without further, microscopic examination, it would not be possible to identify any potential rudimentary ventricle. The aorta, the pulmonary artery and their valves are well developed and lie in a side-by-side position, with the aorta to the left. Separated by the outlet septum, each great artery arises from a muscular infundibulum in this solitary, indeterminate ventricle. The position of the atrioventricular connection and the main axis of the conduction tissue are expected to be bizarre. It is possible that it will take the form of a single strand which descends from an anomalously positioned atrioventricular node and then disperses in the lateral myocardium, or it may descend from a regular node through a prominent trabeculation.

The haemodynamics and clinical management of this heart could be similar to that of tricuspid atresia with the usual atrial arrangement. The right-sided atrioventricular connection in both instances is absent but a patent oval fossa potentially allows blood from the right-sided atrium to cross the septum and mix with that of the left-sided atrium, with forward flow to the ventricle and great arteries. It is critical in such patients to ensure early in life, that the interatrial communication is not restrictive. However, morphologically, as noted above, there are major differences between this particular anomaly and the classical form of tricuspid atresia.

Suggested Reading

Daebritz SH, Tiete AR, Rassoulian D, Roemer U, Kozlik-Feldmann R, Sachweh JS, Netz H, Reichart B. Borderline hypoplastic left heart malformations: Norwood palliation or two-ventricle repair? Thorac Cardiovasc Surg 2002;50:266.

Freedom RM. Atresia or hypoplasia of the left atrioventricular and/or ventriculo-arterial junction. In: Anderson RH, Macartney FJ, Shinebourne EA, Tynan M. Churchill Livingstone (eds). Paediatric Cardiology Vol 2. Edinburgh, London, Melbourne, New York 1987.

Gittenberger-de Groot AC, Wenink ACG. Mitral atresia: morphological details. Br Heart J 1984;51:252.

Mickell JJ, Mathews RA, Anderson RH. The anatomical heterogeneity of hearts lacking a patent communication between the left atrium and the ventricular mass ('mitral atresia') in the presence of a patent aortic valve. Eur Heart J 1983;4:477.

Moreno F, Quero M, Diaz LP. Mitral atresia with normal aortic valve. A study of 18 cases and a review of the literature. Circulation 1976;53:1004.

Ostermeyer J, Korfer R, Bircks W. Mitral atresia with normal-sized ventricles, ventricular septal defect and dextroposition of the great arteries. J Thorac Cardiovasc Surg 1979;77:733.

Watson DG, Rowe RD, Coren PE, Duckworth JWA. Mitral atresia with normal aortic valve. Report of 11 cases and review of the literature. Pediatrics 1960;25:450.

26 Common Atrioventricular Valve with Double Inlet Ventricle

Introduction

Within the spectrum of hearts where both atriums connect to a single ventricular chamber, there are occasional examples in which this occurs through a valve that is neither morphologically a solitary tricuspid valve nor morphologically a solitary mitral valve. Instead, the mode of connection resembles that of the common atrioventricular valve in atrioventricular septal defect (see Chapter 12). While such hearts can, in fact, be regarded as atrioventricular septal defects with extreme right or left ventricular dominance, the common atrioventricular valve connecting as double inlet to one ventricle (see Chapter 27) has structural differences from that connecting to two ventricles within the setting of atrial isomerism (see Chapter 4). By inference, these differences probably apply also to common valves in which one orifice is atretic and in hearts with usual atrial situs. The overall more complex morphology of such hearts has important implications for clinical management and thus justifies special consideration.

The two hearts presented in this chapter are illustrative. While both certainly have the attributes of atrioventricular septal defects, they also demonstrate much more complex anatomy which requires careful segmental analysis to differentiate them not only from the core group of atrioventricular septal defects, but also from each other. Physiologically, they have in common imperforate right-sided atrioventricular valves with hypoplastic right-sided ventricles and double outlet left-sided ventricles with subarterial stenosis or arterial valvar atresia. Their left-sided ventricles both have the characteristics of morphologically right ventricles. Otherwise, further major anatomical differences are striking. One case has right atrial isomerism with its attendant abnormalities of the systemic and pulmonary veins. It also has isthmal hypoplasia of the aorta. The second case has normally lateralized atriums, with usual systemic and pulmonary venous connections, except for absent

coronary sinus. The pulmonary valve is imperforate in this heart.

The surgical importance of a common atrioventricular valve in so-called "single ventricle" relates both to the valve itself and to the overall complexity of the malformations. Because the structure of the atrioventricular valve is less well suited to function in the high-pressure systemic circulation, many have incompetence at the time of presentation and others develop regurgitation after a palliative systemic-pulmonary anastomosis places a volume load on the single ventricle. Combined with associated malformations, such as anomalies of systemic and/or pulmonary venous connection, this generally dictates meticulously staged management early in life to achieve a successful Fontan circulation.

If initial palliation requires a systemic-pulmonary anastomosis, careful judgement regarding the size of the shunt is essential to avoid overloading the ventricle and causing distension. Most patients will undergo an intermediate stage of palliation with bidirectional cavopulmonary anastomosis to offload the ventricle during the first year of life, and at this time it may also be necessary to correct anomalies of venous return, pulmonary arterial stenoses, and atrioventricular valvar incompetence. Other sources of pulmonary blood-flow are generally interrupted at the time of cavopulmonary anastomosis in this subset of patients. At the time of definitive palliation by completion of the Fontan circulation, often by one year of age, even mild valvar regurgitation should be repaired and a severely incompetent valve may need to be replaced. Intraoperative transesophageal echocardiography is routine in such cases. Because of positional anomalies and complex venous connections among such patients, the techniques of extracardiac Fontan operations are particularly useful.

Satisfactory repair of the common atrioventricular valve has been achieved by circular annuloplasty when the orifice is merely enlarged as a result of a volume-overloading of the ventricle. Bivalvation techniques, with or without annuloplasty, have also achieved reduction of the regurgitation, usually in combination with a venous shunt. In other cases, pericardial patch augmentation has been used to achieve apposition of the bridging leaflets and the zone of apposition ("cleft") has been closed with encouraging early results.

Despite earlier and more aggressive intervention in these patients, hospital mortality remains in excess of 15–20% and many survivors experience post-repair heart failure and atrial arrhythmias. There is growing evidence that afterload reduction with ACE inhibitors indefinitely may be beneficial, both before and after operation in this subset of patients, many of whom have dominance of a morphologically right ventricle.

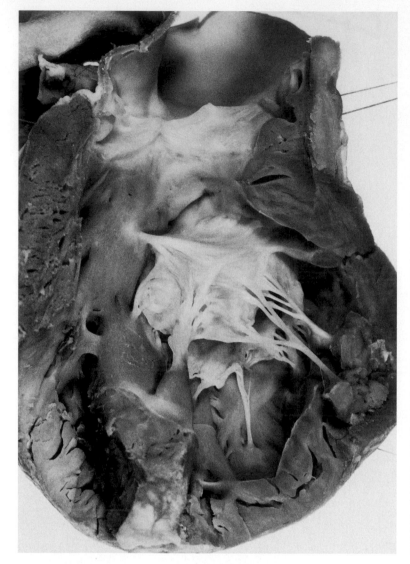

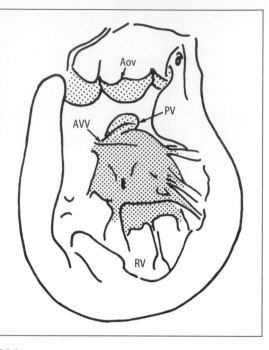

26.1 Imperforate right-sided valve in common atrioventricular junction with common atrioventricular valve and two separate orifices. The large thick-walled ventricle on the left side of the heart has right ventricular morphology and left-handed topology. It receives the left-sided components of a common atrioventricular valve and is connected to a morphologically left atrium (not seen) which receives all the pulmonary veins (discordant atrioventricular connection). The right-sided component of the atrioventricular valve is imperforate but potentially connected to a rudimentary right-sided left ventricle. The venous connections to the right atrium are normal, although the coronary sinus is absent. There is a very large interatrial communication, immediately above the atrioventricular valve (almost a common atrium), but no interventricular communication (partial atrioventricular septal defect). Both great arteries arise from the right ventricle with the aorta anterior to the pulmonary artery (double outlet right ventricle). However, the pulmonary valve is imperforate, and the pulmonary trunk is represented by only a fibrous ligament.

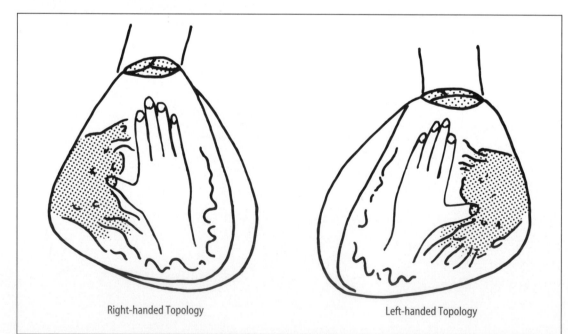

Right-handed Topology   Left-handed Topology

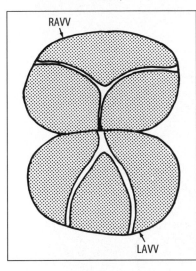

26.2 *(left)* The common atrioventricular valve not infrequently becomes incompetent and requires repair or replacement at the time of a bidirectional cavopulmonary anastomosis or Fontan operation. Appreciating that its basic structure is similar to that of the valve in atrioventricular septal defect is often helpful (see Chapter 12), although there is a higher incidence of accessory orifice, abnormal papillary muscles, and, as shown in this heart, cords attaching directly to the ventricular myocardium.

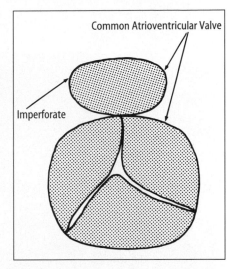

26.3 *(above)* In general, the atrioventricular valve "follows" the ventricle (see Chapter 22). Although anatomically it is the right-sided component of the valve above the morphologically left ventricle which is imperforate, the left-sided component, which is joined to the morphologically right ventricle, is likely to have features of the right atrioventricular valve in atrioventricular septal defect. The components of the valve are analysed (see Chapters 13 and 14) and the valve is tested by injection of saline into the ventricle. Incompetence is often at the zone of apposition between the superior and inferior bridging leaflets which may appear to be a "cleft." Alternatively, the entire annulus may be dilated, resulting in regurgitation centrally and at all opposing leaflet surfaces.

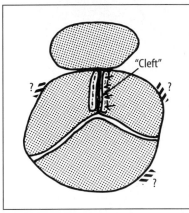

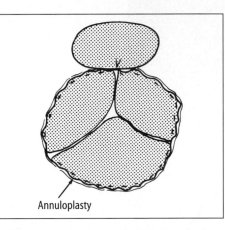

26.4 Regurgitation that is localized to the zone of apposition can be repaired in a manner similar to closing the "cleft" in a morphologically left and left-sided atrioventricular valve. As the right-sided part of the valve is imperforate, measurements of the resulting orifice should be made to ensure that this is not rendered restrictive. The position of the conduction tissue may be uncertain in this situation, which is a consideration in adding an annuloplasty to the procedure.

26.5 If there is central valvar regurgitation and a circumferential annuloplasty is desirable, sutures are placed just on the base of the leaflets to avoid injury to the conduction tissue. While this may achieve, in combination with a cavopulmonary anastomosis to remove a volume load from the ventricle, a reduction in the amount of regurgitation for several months or even years, it is rarely a durable long-term solution.

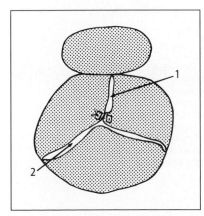

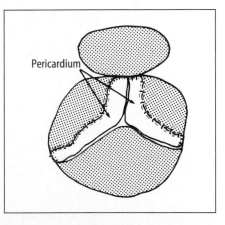

26.6 *(left)* So-called "bivalvation" converts one orifice into two by joining two of the leaflets together, usually with sutures supported by the pericardium or Teflon tape. While experience with this technique is limited in young patients, it has given good early results, and more extensive experience in adults suggests that it achieves lasting competence of the valve. An additional consideration in a univentricular connection is whether the resultant orifices will be restrictive, although this method leaves a larger orifice than complete closure of the zone of apposition (see Figure 26.4).

26.7 *(above)* Leaflet extension or "augmentation" with autogenous pericardium is another option to achieve apposition and competence of the valve. This is usually more useful in older patients where the regurgitation over time has thickened the free edge of the leaflet.

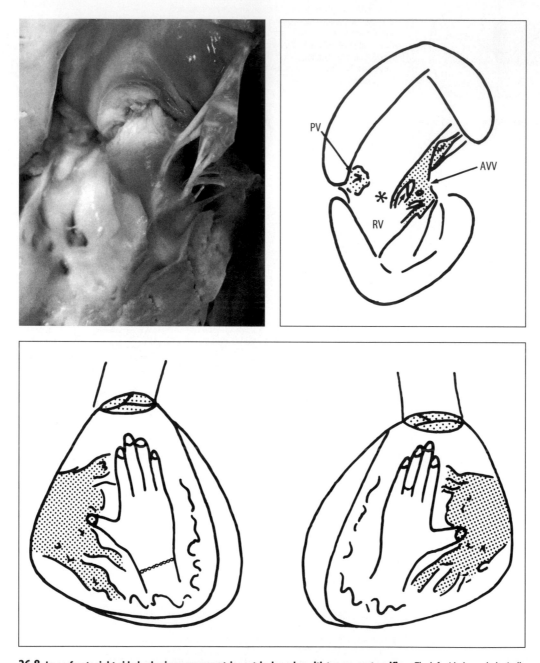

26.8 Imperforate right-sided valve in a common atrioventricular valve with two separate orifices. The left-sided morphologically right ventricle has been opened up from its apex like a clam shell. It is thick-walled and has "left-handed" topology (see Figure 26.9). Both great arteries arise from this chamber with the aorta to the left and anterior to the pulmonary trunk. A hypertrophied muscle bar (asterisk) separates the two outflows and obstructs the subaortic region (small arrow). The left-sided atrioventricular valve does not have clearly defined leaflets or papillary muscles. The right-sided atrioventricular valve (not seen) is imperforate but potentially connected to a hypoplastic right-sided morphologically left ventricle. The atrial arrangement in this heart is right isomeric, with the left-sided atrium receiving a left superior caval vein and the pulmonary veins (which are crowded together), while the right-sided atrium receives the inferior caval vein. Neither a right superior caval vein nor a coronary sinus is present. The interatrial communication is a partial atrioventricular septal defect. Unusually, the innominate artery arises from the right pulmonary artery. There is also hypoplasia of the aortic isthmus.

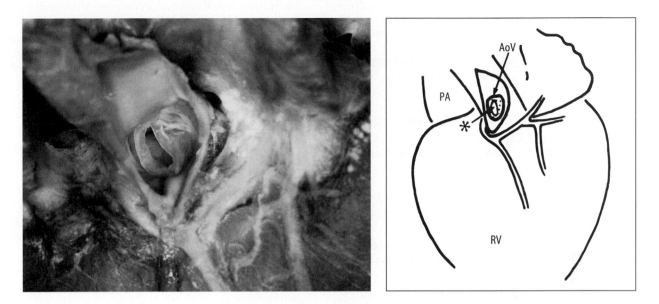

26.9 The anterior view of the heart shown in the preceding figure demonstrates a stenotic two-leaflet, two-sinus aortic valve, through a window dissection of the aortic trunk. The pulmonary artery lies to the right and posteriorly. The hypertrophied muscle bar, which produces subaortic obstruction (asterisk), is seen through the valve. Although this heart has one good outflow (pulmonary trunk), the only inlet valve is highly abnormal and conservative palliation using the pulmonary valve as the systemic outflow is unlikely to be successful. Cardiac transplantation could be a better option. Depending on the severity of atrioventricular valvar stenosis, this might be needed soon after birth or in early infancy. While the systemic circulation is "duct dependent" by virtue of the aortic stenosis and hypoplastic aortic isthmus, prostaglandin will not address the problem of a single stenotic atrioventricular orifice. The innominate artery arising from the pulmonary artery is an extremely rare "vascular ring." Its importance lies in the fact that it is rarely diagnosed non-invasively and there is no suitable systemic vessel in the right chest for the proximal anastomosis of a systemic-pulmonary shunt, were pulmonary stenosis or atresia present. In that situation, a Waterston anastomosis would be necessary.

Suggested Reading

Aiello V, Ho SY, Anderson RH. Absence of one atrioventricular connection associated with straddling atrioventricular valve: distinction of a solitary from a common valve and further considerations on the diagnosis of ventricular topology. Am J Cardiovasc Pathol 1990;3:107.

Anderson RH, Becker AE, Macartney FJ, Shinebourne EA, Wilkinson JL, Tynan M. Is tricuspid atresia a univentricular heart? Pediatr Cardiol 1979;1:5.

Anderson RH, Tynan M. Editorial note: Description of complex forms of atrioventricular valvar atresia. Int J Cardiol 1991;30:243.

Azakie A, Merklinger SL, Williams WG, Van Arsdell GS, Coles JG, Adatia I. Improving outcomes of the Fontan operation in children with atrial isomerism and heterotaxy syndromes. Ann Thorac Surg 2001;72:1636.

Imai Y, Takanashi Y, Hoshino S, Terada M, Aoki M, Ohta J. Modified Fontan procedure in ninety-nine cases of atrioventricular valve regurgitation. J Thorac Cardiovasc Surg 1997;113:262.

Ito M, Kikuchi S, Hachiro Y, Abe T. Bivalvation for common atrioventricular valve regurgitation in cyanotic heart disease. Ann Thorac Cardiovasc Surg 1999;5:340.

Restivo A, Ho SY, Anderson RH, Cameron H, Wilkinson JL. Absent left atrioventricular connection with right atrium connected to morphologically left ventricular chamber, rudimentary right ventricular chamber, and ventriculo-arterial discordance. Problem of mitral versus tricuspid atresia. Br Heart J 1982;48:240.

Shinebourne EA, Macartney FJ, Anderson RH. Sequential chamber localisation – logical approach to diagnosis in congenital heart disease. Br Heart J 1976;38:327.

Stein JI, Smallhorn JF, Coles JG, Williams WG, Trusler GA, Freedom RM. Common atrioventricular valve guarding double inlet atrioventricular connection: natural history and surgical results in 76 cases. Int J Cardiol 1990;28:7.

Takayama T, Nagata N, Miyairi T, Abe M, Koseni K, Yoshimura Y. Bridging annuloplasty for common atrioventricular valve regurgitation. Ann Thorac Surg 1995;59:1003.

Uemura H, Ho SY, Anderson RH, Kilpatrick LL, Yagihara T, Yamashita K. The nature of the annular attachment of a common atrioventricular valve in hearts with isomeric atrial appendages. Eur J Cardiothorac Surg 1996;10:540.

Uemura H, Ho SY, Anderson RH, Yagihara T. The structure of the common atrioventricular valve in hearts having isomeric atrial appendages and double inlet ventricle. J Heart Valve Dis 1998; 7:580.

van Son JA, Walther T, Mohr FE. Patch augmentation of regurgitant common atrioventricular valve in univentricular physiology. Ann Thorac Surg 1997;64:508.

Wilkinson JL, Dickinson DF, Smith A, Anderson RH. Conducting tissues in univentricular heart of right ventricular type with double or common inlet. J Thorac Cardiovasc Surg 1979;77:691.

27 Double Inlet Ventricle

Introduction

In order to understand the morphology and particularly the disposition of the conduction tissue in this group of patients, it is helpful to review first the various potential types of atrioventricular connections.

The atrioventricular junctions of the heart

The atrioventricular junctions of the heart need to be analyzed individually because the atrial chambers in congenital malformations may connect to either both ventricular chambers (biventricular connection) or to only one ventricular chamber (univentricular connection). In establishing the atrioventricular connection in any given heart, it is helpful to be conversant with both biventricular and univentricular variables. The atriums in both groups may have either the usual, the mirror-image, or the isomeric arrangement. The connecting ventricles may be of right, left, or indeterminate morphology. Only the indeterminate ventricular pattern produces the anatomically "univentricular heart."

Biventricular atrioventricular connection: two connecting ventricles to two atriums, including the usual arrangement

In this group, the two separate ventricles connect through two valves, or sometimes a common valve, to the two atriums. There are three patterns in which this "biventricular" connection may be made. The connections may be concordant, in which the morphologically right atrium connects to a morphologically right ventricle and the morphologically left atrium connects to a morphologically left ventricle; or they may be discordant, in which the morphologically right and left atriums connect disharmoniously with the morphologically left and right ventricles, respectively. The third type exists when the atriums are isomeric (see Chapter 4), which means that they are not lateralized in the normal way but are each of the same morphological type. In atrial isomerism the atrioventricular connection becomes

ambiguous because there is literally a concordant connection on one side of the heart and a discordant connection on the other. Nonetheless, each atrium is connected to a separate ventricular chamber, the apical trabecular component of which defines its "rightness" or "leftness." Sometimes one of the two atrioventricular valves or a portion of the common valve is imperforate, producing a variant of atrioventricular valvar atresia. However, in this way a clear potential atrioventricular connection is present, showing that a junction has developed. This arrangement should not be confused with the total absence of one atrioventricular connection in which one of the junctions has not developed, thereby producing a type of "univentricular" connection.

Univentricular atrioventricular connection: one connecting ventricle

In this set of connections there may be either one or two atrioventricular valves present, but only one ventricle connects with either one or both atriums. The three terms concordant, discordant and ambiguous, which are used to describe "biventricular connections" are, therefore, inappropriate in "univentricular connection." For this reason a further three terms are used, the first two of which describe the arrangement whereby there is complete absence of either the right or the left atrioventricular connection. The floor of the involved atrium is totally muscular (absent right or left atrioventricular connection) and on the other, complementary side of the heart the patent junction is guarded by only one valve. The connecting ventricle is either of right, left, or indeterminate morphology, as defined by its trabeculations. The substrate for the third pattern is such that, although there is only one connecting ventricle, it connects to the two atriums, the junction being properly developed on both sides and guarded by either two valves or a common valve. This arrangement is described as "double inlet connection." The connecting ventricle is usually either a dominant right or a dominant left ventricle in the presence of a second, rudimentary, or incomplete chamber in the ventricular mass. The terms "double inlet right" or "double inlet left" ventricle are used. Rarely, the double inlet ventricle is of indeterminate morphology.

"Double inlet ventricle" – A type of "univentricular atrioventricular connection"

In double inlet ventricle, when both atriums are said to be connected to either a dominant right or a dominant left ventricle through either two atrioventricular valves or a common valve, there will be a rudimentary ventricle (incomplete chamber) elsewhere within the ventricular mass. Positive identification of the morphology of the main ventricle in both double inlet right and left ventricles is appreciated by the apical trabecular pattern. This is the guide to the "rightness" or "leftness" of the ventricle. When the apical trabeculations are either relatively coarse or alternatively fine with a criss-crossing pattern, they have the characteristics of either the morphologically right or the morphologically left ventricle respectively. If the univentricular atrioventricular connection is double inlet into a morphologically left ventricle, the rudimentary or incomplete right ventricle will be found on the anterosuperior aspect of the heart. If the connection is to a morphologically right ventricle, the incomplete left ventricle will be found on the postero-inferior aspect. Normal lateralized ventricles have inlet, apical trabecular, and outlet components, the right and left sides being separated by septum, although each of these portions is not specifically aligned with its counterpart on the other side of the heart. In the normal heart the ventricular septum runs to the crux (the intersection between the planes of the atrial and ventricular septums and the atrioventricular groove), but by definition, the ventricular septum in double inlet to a dominant right or left ventricle does not have a normally orientated septum. Instead, it has a rudimentary septum, the function of which is to separate the dominant chamber from the incomplete chamber. This is logically a trabecular septum. However, there are differences between the characteristics of the septums of double inlet right and double inlet left ventricles which have implications for the conducting system. The rudimentary trabecular septum in double inlet right ventricle may contain some elements of developing septum which are potentially destined to reach the crux of the heart. Although hypoplastic, the septum will carry the branching bundle of the conduction tissue towards the atrioventricular node where it will potentially make contact in its usual posterior location. It follows that the main axis of the conduction tissue lies posteriorly in double inlet right ventricle. In contrast, in hearts with double inlet left

ventricle, the trabecular septum never reaches the crux of the heart. It is deviated towards the acute margin of the heart, and the atrioventricular connection is found, not in its usual posterior position but anterolaterally within the atrioventricular junction.

In ventricles of the indeterminate type, a rudimentary or incomplete second chamber cannot be found in the ventricular mass and an apical trabecular component cannot be distinguished. Usually only an outlet septum is present. This may be very hypertrophied with abnormal extensions and is often accompanied by other trabeculations. These muscle bundles are not analogous with either the fine or coarse trabeculations of the usual morphologically left or right ventricles. In the indeterminate ventricle the course of the conduction tissue is more unpredictable because the anatomy is so bizarre. The non-branching bundle may run from a regular node down a muscular trabeculation, or it may extend from a lateral node and disperse in the lateral myocardium.

In double inlet left ventricle the position of the incomplete right ventricle may be found anywhere between the left and the right aspect of the front of the heart. The ventricular septal defect is accordingly located differently in each of these positions. The size of the ventricular septal defect is also important. These factors have a bearing on the position of the conduction tissue. If the rudimentary chamber is towards the right side, the anterolateral node is likely to be located slightly more laterally than when the rudimentary chamber is on the left side, although this fine point may not be perceived by the surgeon. The right margin of the ventricular septal defect is more attenuated when the rudimentary chamber is towards the right. The consequence is that the branching bundle does not have to encircle the subpulmonary outflow tract to reach the ventricular septal defect to the same extent as it does when the incomplete ventricle is left-sided. Nevertheless, the main axis of the conduction tissue is invariably on the right side of the ventricular septal defect which is the nearest to the acute margin of the heart.

In double inlet left ventricle, the spatial relationships of the great arteries and their valves and, thus, of the origins of the coronary arteries, are largely related to the rightward-to-leftward position of the incomplete right ventricle on the front of the heart. From a morphological point of view, presuming that there are three aortic and three pulmonary valvar sinuses and leaflets in each individual case, any discrepancies between the relative sizes of the aortic and pulmonary roots are important. They indicate that there may not be a strict commissural match between the two "facing" sinuses of the valves which usually issue the coronary arteries. Taking that into consideration, in most cases of double inlet left ventricle, each of the right and left coronary arteries arise from each of the "facing" sinuses (dual sinus origin), although occasionally one of the orifices may be higher than usual, above the sinus in the aortic root. Rarely, the circumflex artery arises from the right coronary artery. There is also the possibility of both right and left coronary arteries arising from one sinus only (single sinus origin), either from separate orifices or from a single orifice within the same sinus. This may mean that the proximal course of one of the coronary arteries will run between the aortic and pulmonary roots. Irrespective of the variations at the origins of the coronary arteries, the incomplete chamber is usually delineated on both right and left aspects by proximal epicardial branches which curve around its profile. The branches that outline the incomplete chamber on the anterior surface of the right ventricle in double inlet left ventricle, arise from the proximal portions of both main coronary arteries. The posterior incomplete ventricle in double inlet right ventricle is outlined in the same way but by smaller distal coronary arteries, and is often less well defined than is the anterior incomplete right ventricle in double inlet left ventricle. In double inlet ventricle of indeterminate morphology, without an incomplete ventricle the coronary arteries do not focus in any appreciable way.

Double inlet ventricle is seldom an isolated lesion – there can be many more associated lesions with it. Subpulmonary and subaortic obstruction are often present, straddling valves are seen, and atrial isomerism is a common finding with all its attendant abnormalities of the systemic and pulmonary venous connections. The definition of double inlet ventricle also includes hearts with overriding and straddling of one atrioventricular valve when the greater part of the overriding junction is connected to a ventricle that also receives the other valve.

From a surgical perspective, the main reason for differentiating double inlet ventricle from other types of univentricular atrioventricular connection is the possibility of performing a septation operation and thereby creating a biventricular circulation. Although popularity of the Fontan operation has largely eclipsed septation, the few available reports of long-term results indicate that septation may indeed achieve very good results in selected cases. Moreover, for patients with elevated pulmonary vascular resistance that prohibits a Fontan circulation, septation may offer an alternative to high-risk transplantation. It has been applied also to infants as a staged procedure.

The optimal heart for septation should have two functionally normal atrioventricular valves, an enlarged main ventricular chamber (about $1^1/_2$–2 times the size of a normal left ventricle), and unobstructed outflows to the pulmonary and systemic great arteries. This situation rarely exists with hemodynamics that have balanced the systemic and pulmonary blood-flow from

infancy, so the decision needs to be based more often upon whether the heart can be reasonably divided into two functional pumping chambers. In general, this is possible when the main chamber is of left ventricular morphology and the incomplete right ventricle ("outlet chamber") is in the left anterior subaortic position, such that the septation patch is flat and can be sutured within the less coarsely trabeculated left ventricle. Septation can be done with anterior or right-sided outlet chamber, but the patch then becomes a more complex intraventricular tunnel with potential for obstruction. In ventricles of indeterminate morphology there is often a crest or ridge of muscle to which the septation patch may be sutured between the atrioventricular valves (although this will sometimes carry the conduction tissue), and the feasibility of septation depends on the position of the great arteries in relation to the atrioventricular valves. Hearts with main chambers of right ventricular morphology have also been septated successfully, but experience in this subgroup is extremely limited.

Both hypertrophy and a small size of the left ventricular chamber make the heart unfavorable for septation. These are often found in association with obstruction to the ventricular septal defect, with or without previous banding of the pulmonary artery. While enlargement of the ventricular septal defect can be done at the time of septation, more than moderate hypertrophy of the main chamber should be accepted as a contraindication to the procedure. Whether presently available techniques of myocardial management and post-operative mechanical support of the heart (ventricular assist devices, intra-aortic balloon pumps) could modify this selection of criteria is uncertain.

The necessity to replace an atrioventricular valve or implant a valved extracardiac conduit diminishes the attraction of the septation operation, although both have been done successfully. The risk of heart block, although reduced by current knowledge of the course of the specialized conduction tissue and techniques to avoid it, remains a consideration, such that patients in whom septation becomes very complex may be better served by a Fontan operation.

When the Fontan operation is performed for double inlet ventricles, all the usual considerations apply (see Chapters 18, 19, 24, 25, and 26). In addition, the function and size of both the atrioventricular valves need careful preoperative assessment. If one valve is incompetent and the other is of adequate size, the regurgitant valve (usually the right atrioventricular valve) is closed at the time of the Fontan procedure. If both atrioventricular valves are needed for an adequate ventricular inflow, then the incompetent valve is repaired (see Chapters 12, 13, 14, and 26).

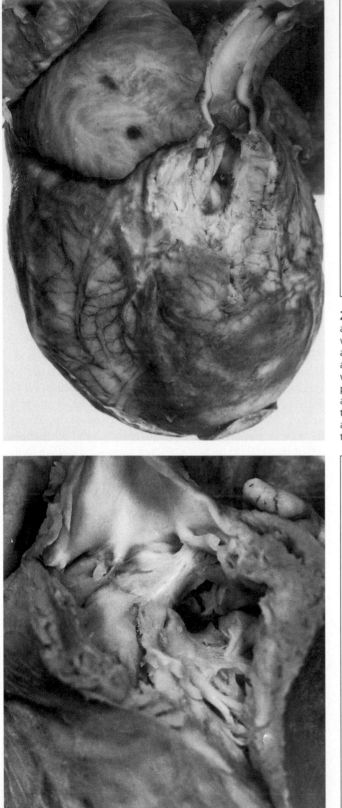

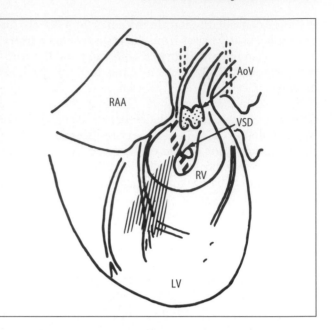

27.1 Double inlet left ventricle. Restrictive ventricular septal defect. The right anterior oblique view of a window dissection shows a small right-sided incomplete ventricle ("outlet chamber ") of right ventricular morphology which gives off a small aortic trunk. The right ventricle is further delineated by epicardial coronary arteries. The aortic valve is small and there is generalized hypoplasia of the aortic arch (unseen). The ventricular septal defect is severely restrictive. The pulmonary trunk (not seen) is disproportionately large, as indicated by the double dashed lines, and lies posteriorly to the aorta. The main axis of the conduction tissue takes a relatively short course because of the position of the right-sided right ventricle and ventricular septal defect. Although apparently shown in relation to the right ventricular side of the septum, the conduction tissue actually remains on the left ventricular side, except for the right bundle branch.

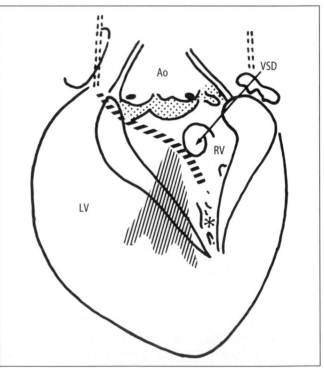

27.2 In the left anterior oblique view of another heart with double inlet left ventricle, a window dissection shows a left-sided incomplete ventricle (outlet chamber) giving off the aorta. The coarse trabeculations in the incomplete ventricle (asterisk) are characteristic of a morphologically right ventricular pattern. The ventricular septal defect and aortic valve are larger than in the preceding heart, but there is hypoplasia of the aortic arch (not seen) with a disproportionately large pulmonary trunk (double dashed lines). The axis of the conduction system must encircle the anterior quadrant of the pulmonary outflow to reach the left-sided position of the morphological right ventricle and ventricular septal defect (see Figure 27.16 for the left ventricular side of this heart).

Double Inlet Left Ventricle. Restrictive Ventricular Septal Defect

425

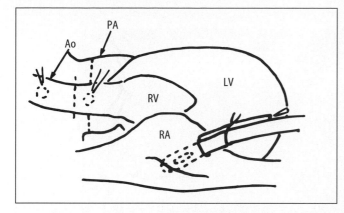

27.3 The techniques available for the management of a restrictive ventricular septal defect obstructing the systemic circulation include direct enlargement of the outlet foramen (see figures 27.12–27.15), the arterial switch procedure, Norwood-type procedure, or the Damus-Kaye-Stansel procedure. Depending on the age and size of the patient, as well as the degree of aortic arch hypoplasia, the latter operation is done with a single venous cannula for cardiopulmonary bypass or total circulatory arrest. Positioning the tip of the cannula through an atrial septal defect will effectively drain the left side of the heart. Depending on the proposed site of division, the aorta is cannulated distally (in which case perfusion may be maintained) or proximally (where the vessel will be divided after the establishment of deep hypothermia and total circulatory arrest).

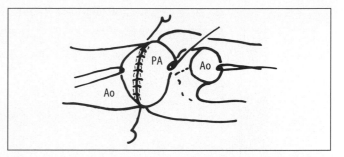

27.4 For one type of simple Damus-Kaye-Stansel procedure, the aorta is divided distally to the pulmonary artery and, after closure of the pulmonary bifurcation, an end-to-end anastomosis is constructed between the posterior half of the pulmonary artery and the distal aorta with a continuous monofilament suture. This takes up the difference between the diameters of the vessels in the suture line, as in the arterial switch operation. The proximal segment of the aorta is incised vertically on its posterior wall to the level of the pulmonary artery (but still above the sinutubular junction of the aorta).

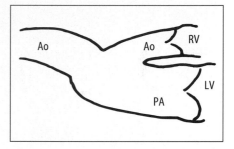

27.7 As seen diagrammatically in cross-section, this technique should distort neither the aortic nor the pulmonary valve, and achieves a wide outflow to the ascending aorta.

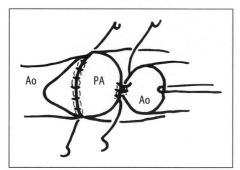

27.5 The proximal aorta is joined to the anterior wall of the pulmonary artery, again accommodating the difference between the circumference of the vessels within the suture line.

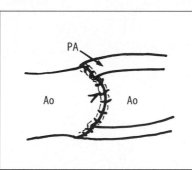

27.6 The outflow is completed by end-to-end anastomosis of proximal aorta to distal aorta anteriorly.

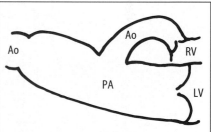

27.10 (above) In cross-section, the proximal aorta tends to lie more anteriorly with this technique, which is a hazard during subsequent resternotomy for a cavopulmonary anastomosis or Fontan procedure. However, neither valve should be distorted, minimizing the risk of incompetence.

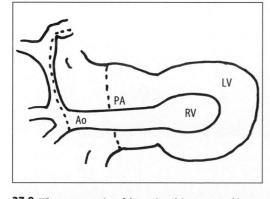

27.8 When augmentation of the aortic arch is necessary, this must be done with total circulatory arrest and temporary occlusion of the head and neck vessels, or perfusion via a graft sutured to the innominate artery. Initial cannulation of the pulmonary artery may be needed also for cardiopulmonary bypass to perfuse the lower body segment. The aortic arch and its branches, as well as the descending aorta, are fully mobilized to permit traction downward towards the heart. In this situation, both the aorta and pulmonary artery are divided as far distally as possible (dashed lines).

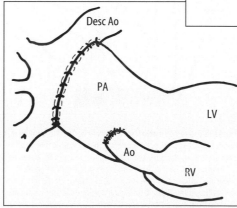

27.9 The large pulmonary artery is used to augment the aortic arch as far distally as needed to bypass its hypoplasia and any coarctation of the aorta. If this distance is longer than the width of the pulmonary artery, the mid-portion of the arch is "gathered" into the suture line, such that there is no tension on the aortic isthmus. The proximal aorta is then joined end-to-side to the pulmonary artery, after the reinstitution of the cardiopulmonary bypass to distend the vessel for accurate placement of the anastomosis if total circulatory arrest has been used, or after unclamping the innominate artery if the procedure is done with low-flow cardiopulmonary bypass.

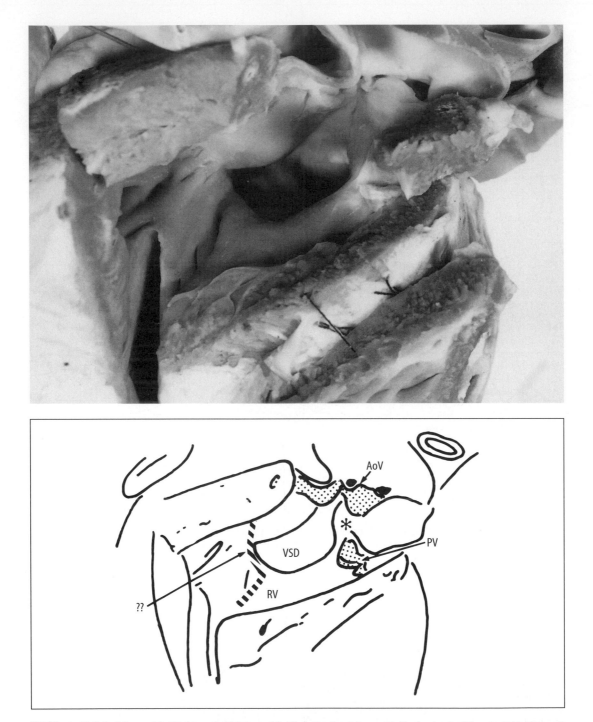

27.11 Double inlet left ventricle. Double outlet right ventricle. The incomplete right ventricle ("outlet chamber") lies anteriorly and towards the left on the surface of the heart. It gives off both a stenotic pulmonary valve and the aortic valve which lies to the right and posterior to the pulmonary valve. There is a muscular bar, the deviated outlet septum (asterisk), between them. Both atrial appendages in this heart have features of the morphological right atrium (right isomerism). The right-sided atrium receives the superior and inferior caval veins, while some of the pulmonary veins enter the left-sided atrium and others cannot be found. Moreover, the orifice to a coronary sinus cannot be identified. The coronary arteries arise from a single orifice in the right-hand facing aortic sinus. The ventricular septal defect is muscular but roofed by the aortic valve. The combination of right atrial isomerism, double inlet left ventricle with double outlet right ventricle and left anterior pulmonary valve, suggests that the main axis of the conduction tissue may be bizarre. An anterolateral atrioventricular node is usually found in the anterior quadrant of the right atrioventricular valve in classical double inlet left ventricle, but this presumes the usual discordant ventriculo-arterial connections and usual atrial arrangement. Alternatively, a "sling" of conduction tissue between two atrioventricular nodes could be anticipated, as has been identified in double inlet left ventricle, albeit with its discordant ventriculo-arterial connections, but additionally with right isomerism. To our knowledge, the course of the conduction tissue has not yet been documented in a heart with right isomerism, double inlet left ventricle, and double outlet right ventricle with left anterior pulmonary valve.

Double Inlet Left Ventricle. Double Outlet Right Ventricle

427

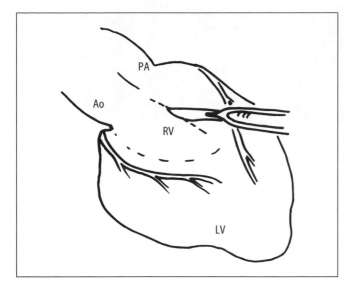

27.12 In view of the pulmonary stenosis, the lungs associated with this heart probably will have been protected from pulmonary vascular disease and, if the size of the pulmonary arteries and ventricular function are acceptable, a Fontan operation would be appropriate management. The ventricular septal defect is slightly smaller than the aortic valve and has largely muscular margins which may constrict further when the Fontan procedure reduces the volume overload of the heart. Arguably, therefore, it may need to be enlarged. This would be done through a vertical incision into the outlet chamber. The incision is sited between the major coronary arterial branches (which help to identify its location) and kept well below the arterial trunks, as leaflets of the arterial valves may be supported by muscle bundles within the outlet chamber. As noted above, the position of the conduction tissue is quite uncertain in this case and surgically induced heart block is a very real potential risk.

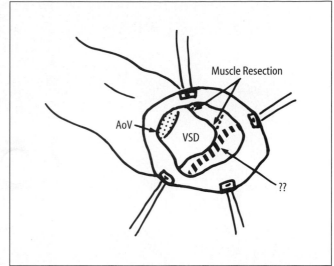

27.13 The thickened walls of the outlet chamber are retracted with pledgeted stay-sutures to expose the ventricular septal defect and the arterial valves. As viewed by the surgeon, conduction tissue in the usual double inlet left ventricle with left-sided subaortic outlet chamber would lie from about 4 o'clock to 6 o'clock, along the lower right-hand margin of the defect, on the left ventricular side of the septum. The "safe" area for the resection of muscle, therefore, would be anteriorly into the trabecular septum (dashed line). Whether or not that pertains to this heart is uncertain.

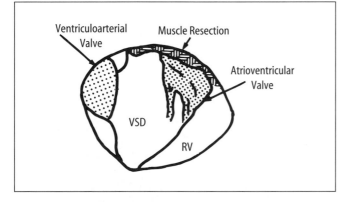

27.14 Muscle resection may extend to the free wall of the ventricle. It is limited by the atrioventricular valvar attachment in the left ventricle which is carefully observed through the ventricular septal defect as muscle is removed.

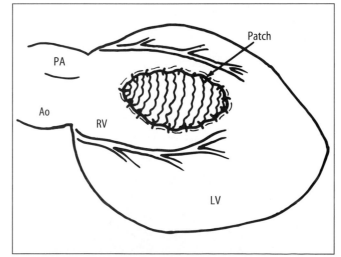

27.15 The ventricle is irrigated extensively with saline to remove any detached muscle fragments and the ventriculotomy is closed with a patch. Since it is in the systemic outflow, the patch will be subjected to a high pressure post-operatively (in contrast, for example, to a right ventricular outflow patch in Fallot's tetralogy). A non-distensible material, such as Dacron or PTFE, is used and, if bleeding is a problem, this may be covered or buttressed with autogenous pericardium. If atrioventricular dissociation is present at the end of the procedure, there is a high probability that the conduction system has been interrupted and this will be permanent. Accordingly, it may be prudent to implant permanent epicardial pacemaker wires at this time.

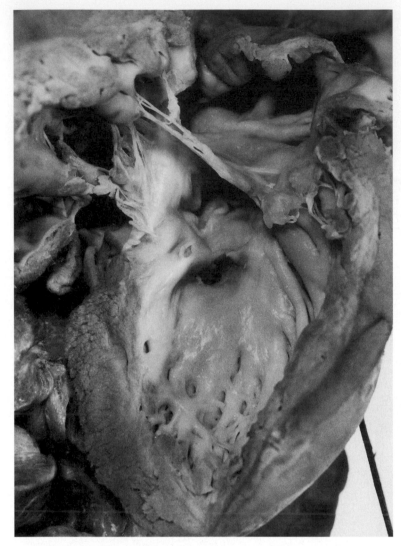

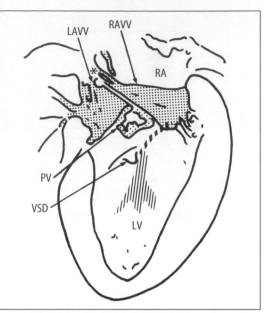

27.16 Double inlet left ventricle. Left-sided incomplete right ventricle. The heart has been opened with a long "fish-mouth" or cockleshell incision extended from the apex along both margins of the heart, and the free wall has been lifted up to display the septal surface. This has the fine trabecular pattern of a morphologically left ventricle. Both the left and right atrioventricular valves enter this chamber and their tension apparatus shares a posterior muscular trabeculation (asterisk). The pulmonary valve is normal. The ventricular septal defect connecting to the rudimentary right ventricle ("outlet chamber," not seen) is slightly small. The right ventricle gives off the aorta. The conduction tissue passes from an anterior atrioventricular node, through the junction of the pulmonary and right atrioventricular valvar annulus, to circle the anterior quadrant of the pulmonary outflow tract and enter the left-sided rudimentary right ventricle through the ventricular septal defect.

Fig. 27.17 – see facing page.

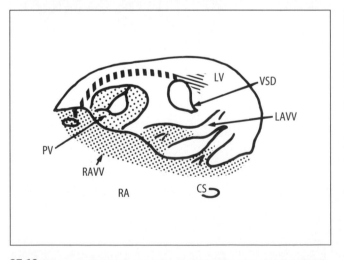

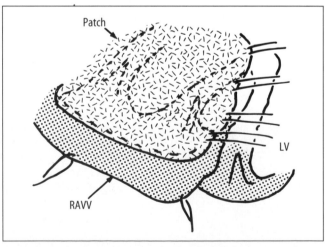

27.18 It is usual to find papillary muscles attaching to the same muscular trabeculation. This does not preclude ventricular septation, which would be possible in either of these hearts. For this procedure, the main ventricular chamber is generally exposed through the right atrium and right atrioventricular valve, although an apical fish-mouth ventriculotomy is an alternative approach. The atrioventricular node will lie under the surgeon's left hand, from which it passes around the front of the pulmonary valve to the upper margin of the ventricular septal defect.

27.19 The septation patch is positioned between the atrioventricular valves with multiple interrupted mattress sutures that are tied against a pericardial buttress on the right atrial side of the right atrioventricular valve. At the crux of the heart, it passes on to ventricular myocardium and continues between the papillary muscles. The sutures are passed through the full thickness of the ventricle and supported externally with pledgets. It is useful to conceptualize the patch as leaving structures in the systemic circulation (left atrioventricular valve, ventricular septal defect) deep to the patch, and those for the pulmonary circulation superficial (right atrioventricular valve, pulmonary artery).

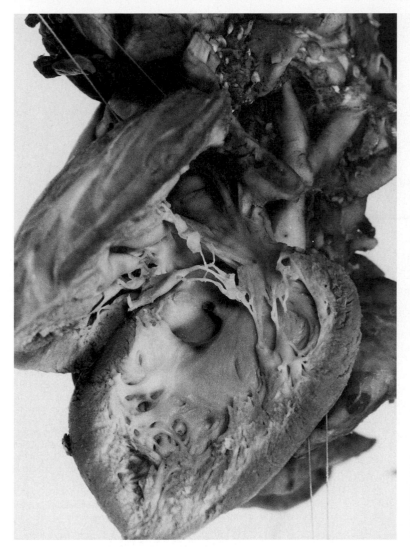

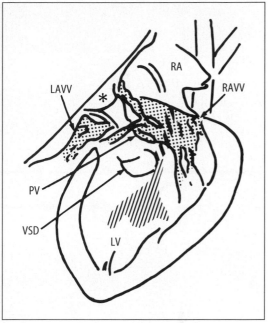

27.17 Double inlet left ventricle. Anterior incomplete right ventricle. The heart has been opened in the same manner as the previous case (Figure 27.16) and shows a relatively large ventricular septal defect. The pulmonary valve is partially obscured by leaflet material of the right atrioventricular valve. The posterior trabeculation (asterisk) supports the tension apparatus of both atrioventricular valves which are otherwise separate and within the left ventricular chamber.

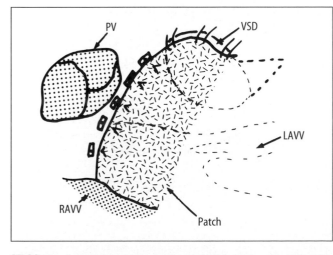

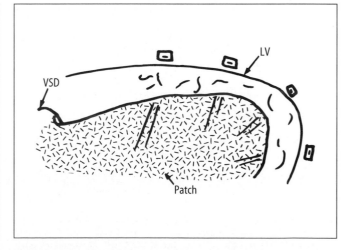

27.20 The other end of the patch passes from the atrioventricular valvar leaflet across the subpulmonary area towards the ventricular septal defect. At about 9 o'clock on the ventricular septal defect (outlet foramen), the patch is deviated on to the right ventricular side of the septum by placing sutures within the incomplete right ventricle (outlet chamber). In this manner, the suture line proceeds around the upper margin of the ventricular septal defect, slightly removed from the conduction tissue. If enlargement of the ventricular septal defect is indicated, this is done by excising the trabecular septum from about 3 o'clock to 6 o'clock (dashed line).

27.21 Having navigated the ventricular septal defect, the remainder of the patch is brought down firmly into the left ventricular trabeculations with pledgeted mattress sutures, again passed through the full thickness of the heart, and taking care to avoid injury to the coronary arteries. In the situation of an anterior outlet chamber, the patch spirals slightly between the atrioventricular valves and the ventricular septal defect.

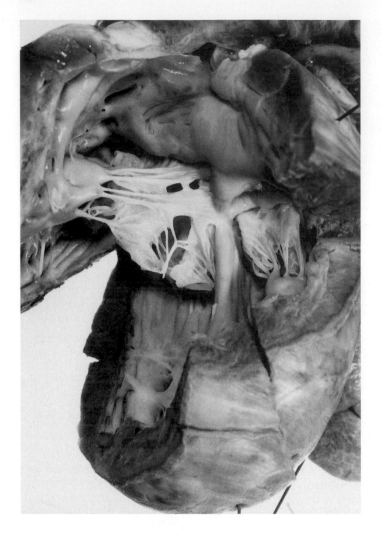

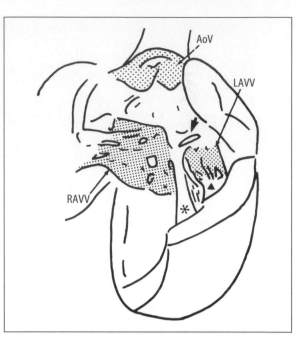

27.22 Double inlet indeterminate ventricle. The heart is viewed from the front with the anterior free wall lifted upwards and to the right to show the ventricular cavity. A free-standing muscular bar (asterisk) is present, but it is impossible to assign a ventricular topology to this specimen because no apical septal structure is found. Two atriums each connect to the ventricle through separate atrioventricular valves. The left-sided atrium receives the pulmonary veins and the right-sided atrium receives the superior and inferior caval veins. The left atrioventricular valve is small and supported by a single papillary muscle (triangle) (parachute valve). Both great arteries originate from the ventricle and there is severe muscular subpulmonary stenosis (arrow). An atrial septostomy has been performed. In these circumstances the atrioventricular conduction tissue may be anticipated anterolaterally, running down the wall of the ventricle close to the acute margin. However, in some hearts with this type of anatomy, a prominent free-standing trabeculation has been found to carry the conduction axis which may be connected with either an anterior node or from a node within the triangle of Koch.

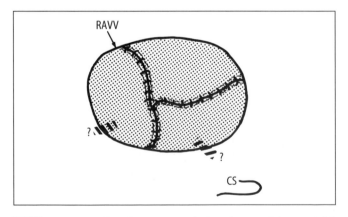

27.23 Septation would not be an option in this heart because of the stenotic left atrioventricular valve. For the Fontan circulation, a right or, less commonly, left atrioventricular valve which is regurgitant may need to be closed at the time of either cavopulmonary anastomosis or the complete Fontan procedure. As the position of the conduction tissue is uncertain in this heart, there would be two possibilities for the closure of the right atrioventricular valve, if it were incompetent and if the left atrioventricular valve was adequate. First, if the leaflet edges have been thickened by the regurgitation, they are carefully approximated with a continuous suture. By staying on the leaflet tissue, the closure is completely below the atrioventricular node, but, since the valve is in contact with the systemic ventricle, this technique may not be completely secure.

27.24 Alternatively, a patch is sutured above the coronary sinus and about half a centimeter away from the valvar annulus (dashed line). This leaves the conduction tissue below the closure. Care must be taken to avoid leaks around the patch through atrial trabeculations, but, in general, there is little chance of this repair breaking down post-operatively. Closure of the left atrioventricular valve (see Figures 27.26–27.27) in contrast, should not endanger the conduction tissue.

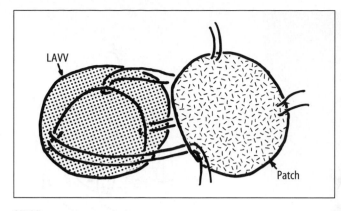

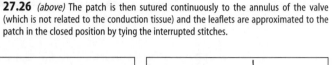

27.25 *(above)* For closure of the left atrioventricular valve, the leaflets are approximated to each other with about three interrupted mattress sutures which are then passed through an appropriately sized patch.

27.26 *(above)* The patch is then sutured continuously to the annulus of the valve (which is not related to the conduction tissue) and the leaflets are approximated to the patch in the closed position by tying the interrupted stitches.

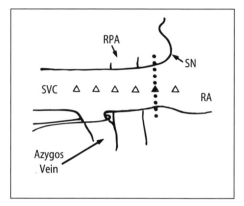

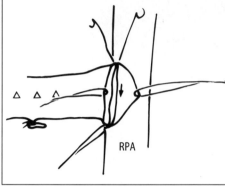

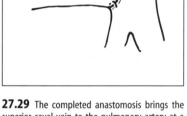

27.27 For the bidirectional cavopulmonary anastomosis, the superior caval vein is dissected to its junction with the innominate vein and the azygos vein is divided, if this was not done at a previous systemic-pulmonary shunt operation. Smaller tributaries are also divided to prevent subsequent enlargement as veno-venous communications. The vein is cannulated high up for bypass or a temporary shunt and divided about 4–5 mm above the area of the sinuatrial node. A mark on its anterior surface (triangles) helps to maintain the correct orientation.

27.28 For connection to the right pulmonary artery, a longitudinal incision is made on the upper surface of the artery for about 1½ times the diameter of the caval orifice. The anastomosis is constructed with a fine running suture, doing the posterior layer first inside the vessels. It is important to make this incision on the upper (as opposed to anterior) surface of the vessel, which usually requires the division of fibrous bands, similar to the ligamentum on the left pulmonary artery.

27.29 The completed anastomosis brings the superior caval vein to the pulmonary artery at a right angle. It can be extended into the upper lobe branch if needed.

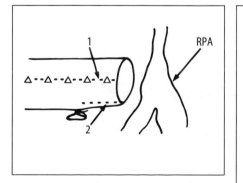

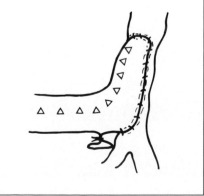

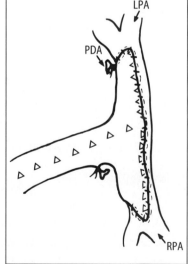

27.30 When there is proximal narrowing of the right pulmonary artery – for example, after a systemic-pulmonary anastomosis – the caval vein may be used as an onlay patch with growth potential. For localized narrowing, it is incised on the rightward lateral aspect (2) and, for more diffuse stenosis, in its mid-portion (1). The top of this incision must reach the pulmonary artery without tension, which may require some mobilization of the innominate and subclavian branches.

27.31 The caval vein is brought down across the narrow segment of pulmonary artery, with its distal portion opened out as a patch.

27.32 For more extensive narrowing, the vein can reach as far as the hilum of the left lung by bringing it leftward, behind the ascending aorta, taking care not to kink the vessels. The site of the incision in the caval vein (1 in Figure 27.30) will determine the relative size of the patches for each pulmonary artery branch.

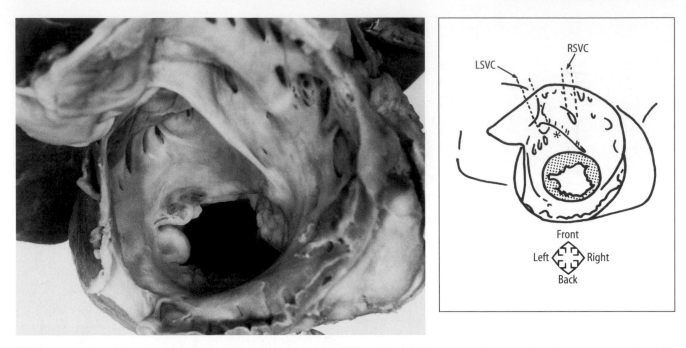

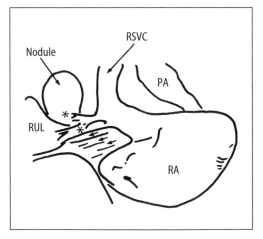

27.33 Double inlet right ventricle, double outlet right ventricle. The heart is viewed from the back, looking down into the atrium, which is almost a common atrium but has a ridge of rudimentary septum (asterisk) between the orifices of left and right superior caval veins (not seen but indicated by dashed lines). Both atrial appendages are of right mor- phology (right isomerism). An inferior caval vein (not seen) also enters the atrium. The coronary sinus is absent. Both atriums connect with a dominant morphologically right ventricle through a common atrioventricular valve. A rudimentary pouch (not seen) is found on the left postero-inferior aspect of this ventricle's diaphragmatic surface. The main ventricular chamber gives off both great arteries with the aorta lying to the right and anterior to the pulmonary artery. Both great vessels arise above a complete muscular infundibulum ("bilateral conus") and there is muscular obstruction to the subpulmonary outflow. A single orifice in the left-hand facing sinus of the aortic valve gives off all the major coronary arteries, but there is a second tiny orifice in the right-hand facing sinus which supplies the artery to the sinuatrial node. The pulmonary venous connections (see Figure 27.34) are totally anomalous, with the right upper lobe pulmonary vein connected to the right superior caval vein and the remaining veins joined to a confluence which connects to the left superior caval vein and thence the innominate vein. The main axis of the specialized conduction tissue is likely to run postero-inferiorly.

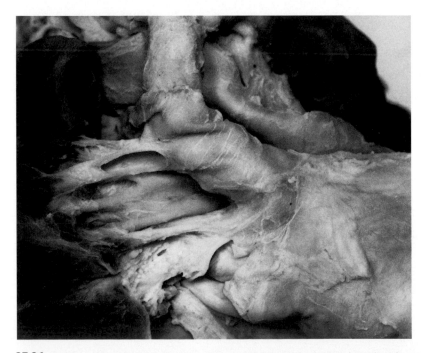

27.34 The hilum of the right lung in the above specimen with right atrial isomerism shows the pulmonary veins from the right upper lobe and a separate nodule (asterisks) connected to the superior caval vein. All the veins from the other two lobes of the right lung (arrows) and those from the left lung (not seen) join a confluence behind the heart. The left lung also has three lobes and bilateral short bronchi are present.

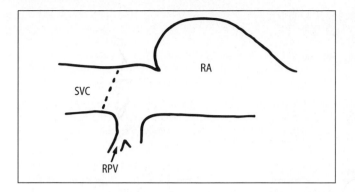

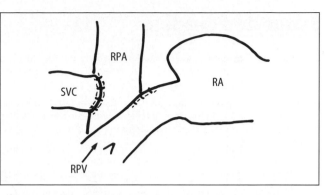

27.35 The presence of subpulmonary stenosis combined with a morphological right ventricle and anterior position of the aorta mitigate against septation in this heart. The first stage of palliation, therefore, would be correction of the anomalous pulmonary venous drainage with either a systemic pulmonary shunt or, preferably, depending upon the patient's age, bilateral, bidirectional cavopulmonary anastomoses. For the right-sided cavopulmonary connection (see Figures 27.27–27.32), the superior caval vein is divided above the entrance of the pulmonary veins (dashed line) which are left draining to the atrium.

27.36 Mobilization of the distal segment of the superior caval vein, which is slightly shorter than usual in this situation, usually permits a satisfactory direct anastomosis. In right isomerism, the left pulmonary artery will follow a similar transverse course to the left lung, so the left anastomosis is done in the same fashion.

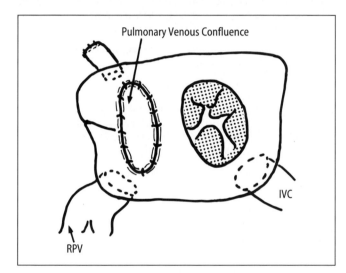

27.37 Working inside the atrium, the pulmonary venous confluence is connected to the back of the atrial wall (see Chapter 8). In theory, this should be positioned towards the opposite side of the entrance of the inferior caval vein to facilitate a subsequent lateral tunnel Fontan pathway. In practice, however, a wide anastomosis usually occupies most of the posterior atrial wall and, in this case, drainage of the right upper pulmonary veins to the superior caval vein precludes the usual position of a lateral tunnel connection to the pulmonary artery.

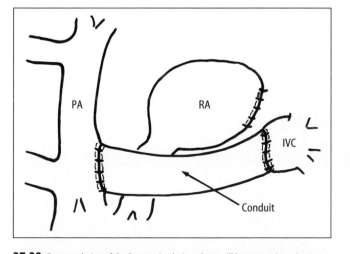

27.38 For completion of the Fontan circulation, there will be two options. An extracardiac tube (probably of homograft aorta or PTFE graft) could be placed between the inferior caval vein and the pulmonary artery, taking care to avoid compression of the more anterior than usual pulmonary veins.

27.39 Alternatively, the inferior caval vein might be baffled anteriorly within the right atrium to the right atrial appendage, which is then connected to the pulmonary artery with or without additional patch enlargement of the anastomosis. This is diagrammed schematically in cross-section. The likelihood of arrhythmias is possibly greater with this second option, but this pathway would have growth potential in a small patient and the long-term results of cavopulmonary conduits in the venous circulation are unknown.

Suggested Reading

Anderson RH. Location of the conduction tissue in double-inlet left ventricle with rudimentary right ventricle. J Thorac Cardiovasc Surg 1996;111:1290.

Anderson RH, Arnold R, Thaper MK, Jones RS, Hamilton DI. Cardiac specialised tissues in hearts with an apparently single ventricular chamber. (Double inlet left ventricle). Am J Cardiol 1874;33:95.

Anderson RH, Becker AE, Tynan M, Macartney FJ, Rigby ML, Wilkinson JL. The univentricular atrioventricular connection: getting to the root of a thorny problem. Am J Cardiol 1984;54:822.

Anderson RH, Ho SY. Sequential segmental analysis – description and categorisation for the millennium. Cardiol Young 1997;7:98.

Anderson RH, Ho SY. The pathology of subaortic obstruction. Ann Thorac Surg 1998;66:644.

Bharati S, Lev M. The concept of tricuspid atresia complex as distinct from that of the single ventricle complex. Pediatr Cardiol 1979; 1:57.

Cheung HC, Lincoln C, Anderson RH, Ho SY, Shinebourne EA, Pallides S, Rigby ML. Options for surgical repair in hearts with univentricular atrioventricular connection and subaortic stenosis. J Thorac Cardiovasc Surg 1990;100:672.

Dickinson DF, Wilkinson JL, Anderson KR, Smith A, Ho SY, Anderson RH. The cardiac conduction system in situs ambiguous. Circulation 1979;59:879.

Doherty A, Ho SY, Anderson RH, Rigby ML. The morphological nature of the atrioventricular valves in hearts with double inlet left ventricle. Pediatr Pathol 1989;9:521.

Doty SB, Schieken RM, Lauer RM. Septation of the univentricular heart: Transatrial approach. J Thorac Cardiovasc Surg 1979;78: 423.

Ebert PA. Staged partitioning of single ventricle. J Thorac Cardiovasc Surg 1984;88:908.

Essed CE, Ho SY, Hunter S, Anderson RH. Atrioventricular conduction system in univentricular heart of right ventricular type with right-sided rudimentary chamber. Thorax 1980;35:123.

Freedom RM. Subaortic obstruction and the Fontan operation. Ann Thorac Surg 1998;66:649.

Kawahira Y, Uemura H, Yoshikawa Y, Yagihara T. Double inlet right ventricle versus other types of double or common inlet ventricle: its clinical characteristics with reference to the Fontan procedure. Eur J Cardiothorac Surg 2001;20:228.

Kurasawa H, Imai Y, Fukuchi S, Sawatari K, Koh Y, Nakazawa M, Talao A. Septation and Fontan repair of univentricular atrioventricular connection. J Thorac Cardiovasc Surg 1990;99:314.

Lan YT, Chang RK, Drant S, Odhim J, Laks H, Wong AL, Allada V. Outcome of staged surgical approach to neonates with single left ventricle and moderate size bulboventricular foramen. Am J Cardiol 2002;89:959.

Margossian RE, Solowiejczyk D, Bourlon F, Apfel H, Gersony WM, Hardof AJ, Quaegebeur J. Septation of the single ventricle: revisited. J Thorac Cardiovasc Surg 2002;124:442.

McKay R, Bini RM, Wright JP. Staged septation of double inlet left ventricle. Br Heart J 1986;56:563.

McKay R, Pacifico AD, Blackstone EH, Kirklin JW, Bargeron LM,Jr. Septation of the univentricular heart with left anterior subaortic outlet chamber. J Thorac Cardiovasc Surg 1982;84:77.

Nagashima M, Imai Y, Takanashi Y, Hoshino S, Seo K, Terada M, Aoki M. Ventricular hypertrophy as a risk factor in ventricular septation for double-inlet left ventricle. Ann Thorac Surg 1997;64:730.

Pacifico AD. Surgical treatment of double inlet ventricle ("single ventricle"). J Thorac Cardiovasc Surg 1986;1:105.

Restivo A, Ho SY, Anderson RH, Cameron H, Wilkinson JL. Absent left atrioventricular connection with right atrium connected to morphologically left ventricular chamber, rudimentary chamber, and ventriculo-arterial discordance. Problem of mitral versus tricuspid atresia. Br Heart J 1982;48:240.

Shimazaki Y, Kawashima Y, Mori T, Kitamura S, Matsuda H, Yokota K. Ventricular volume characteristics of single ventricle before corrective surgery. Am J Cardiol 1980;45:806.

Shimazaki Y, Kawashima Y, Mori T, Matsuda H, Kitamura S, Yokota K. Ventricular function of single ventricle after ventricular septation. Circulation 1980;61:653.

Stein JI, Smallhorm JF, Coles JG, Williams WG, Trusler GA, Freedom RM. Common atrioventricular valve guarding double inlet atrioventricular connexion: natural history and surgical results in 76 cases. Int J Cardiol 1990;28:7.

Wenink ACG. Embryology of the ventricular septum: separate origin of its components. Virchows Arch Pathol Anat Histopathol 1981;390:71.

Coronary Arterial Anomalies

28 Coronary Arterial Fistula

Introduction

A direct communication between a coronary artery and one of the four great veins, pulmonary artery, or cardiac chambers constitutes a coronary arterial fistula. This malformation is a rare ocurrence in the absence of valvar atresia. The fistula may involve the left (about 35%) or right (about 55%) or both (5%) coronary arterial systems. It enters the right heart in about 90% of cases, thus producing a left-to-right shunt. The most common sites of drainage are the right ventricle, followed by the right atrium and the pulmonary artery. Proximal to the fistula, the coronary artery is elongated and dilated. When the fistula arises from the side of the artery, the continuation of the coronary artery generally assumes a normal size immediately distal to the fistula. Alternatively, the coronary artery may terminate in the fistula.

Several surgical techniques have been advocated for the closure of a coronary arterial fistula and, more recently, interventional catheter techniques have been employed. When the fistula is at the end of a vessel and clearly demarcated, it may be closed by simple ligation of the approaching coronary artery. However, in the case of the right coronary artery, this risks compromise of the blood supply to the atrioventricular node. Alternatively, a long fistula or multiple fistulas may be obliterated by undersewing with a multiple pledgeted suture. These two techniques do not require cardiopulmonary bypass, but probably sacrifice some myocardial perfusion. Using cardiopulmonary bypass, the coronary artery may be opened for direct closure of the communication with patch or sutures, or the distal end may be closed inside the heart or pulmonary artery. These techniques are preferred for lateral fistulas where significant areas of myocardium are perfused beyond the fistulas and also when aneurysmal dilatation is present.

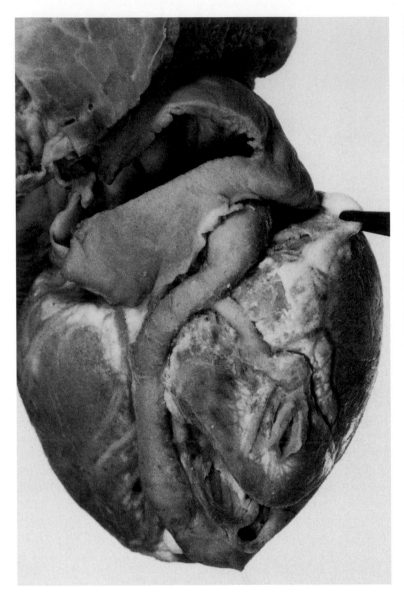

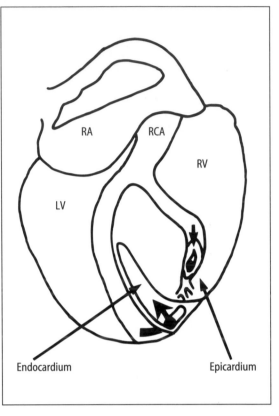

28.1 Coronary artery fistula. The heart is viewed posteriorly and from the right side. The dominant dilated right coronary artery runs in its normal position in the right atrioventricular groove and continues as the posterior interventricular branch, supplying the left ventricle. There is a terminal fistula to the right ventricle at the end of this vessel and also a lateral fistula in the large right ventricular branch (arrows). The apex of the right ventricle has been opened to show the intracardiac end of the terminal fistula. The heart also has a dilated right atrium and left ventricle. Other abnormalities (not shown) include a patent oval fossa, severe tricuspid valvar stenosis, subpulmonary muscular atresia of the right ventricular outflow, virtual obliteration of the right ventricular cavity, and a widely patent arterial duct supplying the branch pulmonary arteries. No major aortopulmonary collateral arteries are present.

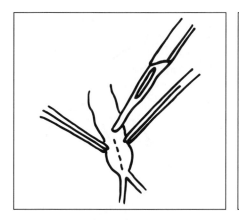

28.2 For direct repair, the dilated coronary artery is opened just proximal to the fistula.

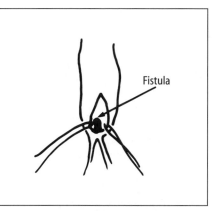

28.3 The coronary artery narrows abruptly beyond the fistula, so the incision does not extend quite to this point. Retraction of the opened vessel towards the fistula gives good exposure.

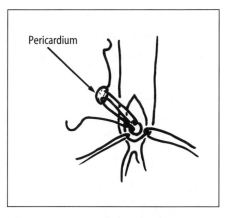

28.4 A small patch of autogenous pericardium is sutured to the edge of the fistula with a fine monofilament suture.

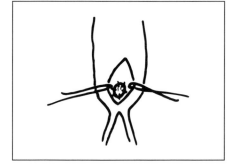

28.5 The patch gives a smooth luminal surface and does not narrow or distort the coronary arterial wall.

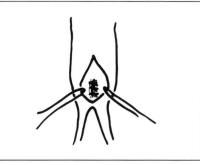

28.6 Alternatively, the fistula may be closed with several interrupted sutures tied within its lumen. Care must be exercised to avoid narrowing of the coronary artery distally.

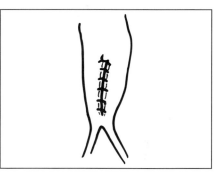

28.7 The enlarged coronary artery is closed by a direct suture. If the incision extends into the small distal vessel, it should be closed with a patch of vein or pericardium.

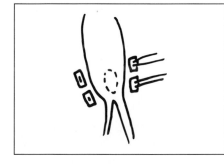

28.8 An alternative method of closure is compression of the fistula by mattress sutures passed under the coronary artery.

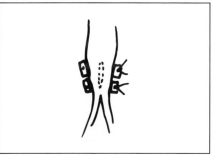

28.9 The sutures are tied to compress the fistula within the myocardium. While this technique does not require bypass, there is greater risk of recurrence of the fistula or distortion of the lumen of the coronary artery than when cardiopulmonary bypass is employed.

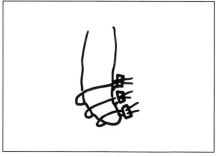

28.10 Terminal fistulas may be occluded with multiple deep ligatures passed around the coronary artery and deeply into the myocardium.

Suggested Reading

Baim DS, Kline H, Silverman JF. Bilateral coronary-pulmonary artery fistula. Report of five cases and review of the literature. Circulation 1982;65:810.

Burch GH, Shan DJ. Congenital coronary artery anomalies: the pediatric perspective. Coron Artery Dis 2001;12:605.

Char F, Hara M. Congenital coronary artery fistula communication of the left coronary artery with the left atrium. Lancet 1966;86:93.

Edis AJ, Schattenberg TT, Feldt RH, Danielson GK. Congenital coronary artery fistula. Surgical considerations and results of operation. Mayo Clin Proc 1972;47:567.

Hsieh KS, Huang TC, Lee CL. Coronary artery fistulas in neonates, infants, and children: clinical findings and outcome. Pediatr Cardiol 2002;23:415.

Kamiya H, Yasuda T, Nagamine H, Sakakibara N, Nishida S, Kawasuji M, Watanabe G. Surgical treatment of congenital coronary artery fistulas: 27 years' experience and a review of the literature. J Card Surg 2002;17:173.

Karagoz HY, Zorlutuna YI, Babagan KM. Congenital coronary artery fistulas: diagnostic and surgical considerations. Jpn Heart J 1989; 30:685.

Liotta D, Hallman GL, Hall RJ, Cooley DA. Surgical treatment of congenital coronary artery fistula. Surgery 1971;70:856.

Muir CS. Coronary arterio-cameral fistula. Br Heart J 1960;22:374.

Neufeld HN, Lester RG, Adams P, Anderson RC, Lillehei CW, Edwards JE. Congenital communication of a coronary artery with a cardiac chamber or the pulmonary trunk ("Coronary artery fistula"). Circulation 1961;24:171.

Ogden JA, Stansel NC Jr. Coronary artery fistulas terminating in the coronary venous system. J Thorac Cardiovasc Surg 1972;63:172.

Rittenhouse EA, Doty DB, Ehrenhaft JL. Congenital coronary artery-cardiac chamber fistula: Review of operative management. Ann Thorac Surg 1975;20:468.

Urrutia-s CO, Falaschi G, Oh DA, Cooley DA. Surgical management of 56 patients with congenital coronary artery fistulas. Ann Thorac Surg 1983;5:300.

29 Anomalous Origin of the Left Coronary Artery from the Pulmonary Trunk

Introduction

The left and right coronary arteries are normally connected to the aortic root in the two sinuses of Valsalva which face the pulmonary valve. Rarely, the left main coronary artery is given off anomalously from the pulmonary artery. Even more rarely, the right coronary artery, the circumflex or the anterior interventricular (left anterior descending) branches, or both coronary arteries originate from the pulmonary artery.

A main left coronary artery connected to the pulmonary artery usually lies in the posterior leftward pulmonary sinus, but its position may range from the commissure with the rightward sinus to that with the non-facing pulmonary sinus. It may even lie above the sinus in the main pulmonary artery itself. The distance between the empty aortic sinus and the orifice of the left coronary artery is thus highly variable, as is the length of the main left vessel. Usually, an isolated anomalous anterior descending interventricular artery (left anterior descending branch) is connected to the non-facing pulmonary valvar sinus, while anomalous circumflex and right coronary arteries tend to arise within the right branch pulmonary artery.

Secondary effects on cardiac structure and function depend on the pulmonary circulation and development of collateral flow to the anomalous left coronary artery. When pulmonary arterial pressure is high (early after birth or because of a large left-to-right shunt), there may be minimal compromise to flow in the left coronary artery. With the normal postnatal decline in pulmonary resistance, myocardial perfusion becomes progressively dependent on collateral vessels from the right coronary artery. Eventually, such extensive collateral circulation may develop that it produces a large coronary steal into the pulmonary circulation. Alternatively, a sudden drop in pulmonary arterial pressure and saturation by the closure of a persistently patent arterial duct or large ventricular septal defect, for example, in the absence of collateral development will precipitate catastrophic myocardial ischaemia. Most patients follow a course between these two extremes with progressive impairment of coronary perfusion at four to six weeks of age, producing myocardial ischaemia or infarction. Structural complications are common, including mitral valve regurgitation from papillary muscle necrosis, aneurysmal dilatation of the left ventricle, and endocardial fibrosis with areas of calcification, even at a young age. The origin of both coronary arteries from the pulmonary artery is incompatible with life unless the patient has pulmonary hypertension and a left-to-right intracardiac shunt, while a right coronary artery or a single branch of the left arising anomalously tends to produce only mild symptoms of angina, heart failure, or changes on the electrocardiogram.

Surgical management of the anomalous origin of the left coronary artery from the pulmonary artery is now directed towards the restoration of a two-coronary artery system whenever possible. This can be achieved by a variety of methods, including the reimplantation of the anomalous coronary artery into the aorta, tunnelling systemic flow to the vessel through the pulmonary artery, and grafting the anomalous vessel from a systemic artery. Additional technical modifications within each group of procedures may offer useful advantages in certain situations, while some have been shown to have less favorable long-term results. However, the small number of patients with this anomaly combined with the large number of surgical options and variable spectrum of associated myocardial dysfunction has obscured clear indications that any one procedure is superior to another.

Reimplantation may be done from inside or outside the aorta. The former requires an additional aortotomy, but has the advantage of visualizing the aortic valvar leaflets (which may lie more nearly at the same level as the pulmonary valve than in the normal heart) and the option of positioning the coronary artery within the empty sinus. By using flaps of arterial wall and the pulmonary sinus, it is possible to construct a direct anastomosis even to the anomalous left coronary arteries that lie near the non-facing pulmonary sinus. Transfer outside using a partial occlusion clamp on the aorta may be technically more straightforward and have a shorter myocardial ischaemic time. However, it risks injury to an aortic valvar leaflet if the incision is too low or compression by the right pulmonary artery if the coronary artery is positioned too high.

The tunnel-type procedures are said to be more appropriate for anomalous coronary arteries that lie at some distance from the aorta, but this probably is also the subset of patients in whom subsequent obstruction to the pulmonary outflow by the tunnel is most likely to occur. Tunnels have been constructed successfully from pulmonary arterial wall, pericardium, or a segment of subclavian artery, while connection of the aorta and pulmonary arteries to create the obligatory "aorto-pulmonary window" has been done either by suturing inside the pulmonary artery or by working outside, between the two great vessels. Damage to an aortic valve leaflet is again a risk if the aorta is not opened to position this incision.

While attractive because it can be done without bypass or aortic cross-clamping, resection of the anomalous coronary artery and end-to-end anastomosis to the divided left subclavian artery has proved to be suboptimal because of frequent kinking of the subclavian vessel and occlusion of the anastomosis. Ligation of the coronary artery at the pulmonary artery and grafting end-to-side with the subclavian artery, internal mammary artery, or a reversed saphenous vein graft are other options for revascularization. However, these

techniques are more difficult than comparable procedures for adult coronary artery disease because of the small size of the vessels and structural abnormalities in the wall of the anomalous left coronary artery.

Simple ligation of the vessel, which is possible in the presence of well-developed collateral circulation and improves myocardial perfusion by obliterating the "coronary steal" into the pulmonary artery, has been generally abandoned. This is because it leaves the heart dependent on a single source of coronary perfusion (the right coronary artery which itself may be imperfect in this malformation) and also because patients are now generally diagnosed and treated at an earlier age, before the development of the extensive collateral vessels that are crucial for such ligation. None the less, the situation in which such a technique might still be useful would be an isolated circumflex or anterior descending branch connected to the pulmonary artery at a site remote from the aorta. This generally is found in older children or adults, and even then, revascularization with the internal mammary artery could prove to be beneficial in the long term.

The only factor that has been shown to influence surgical survival in the repair of anomalous left coronary artery from the pulmonary artery, is preoperative myocardial function. This emphasizes the need for meticulous conduct of cardiopulmonary bypass and myocardial management, as well as the possibility of pre or post-operative ventricular assist for a period of time awaiting myocardial recovery. As there is often a dramatic improvement in both left ventricular and mitral valve function among survivors, these secondary lesions are not addressed routinely at the initial procedure.

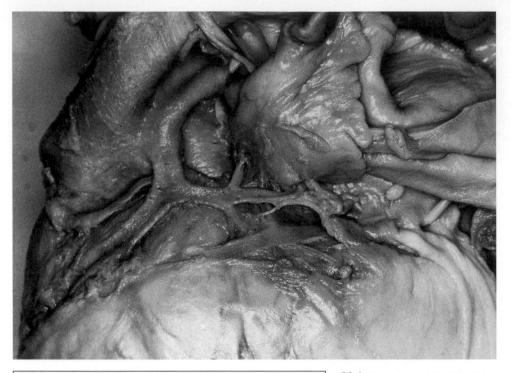

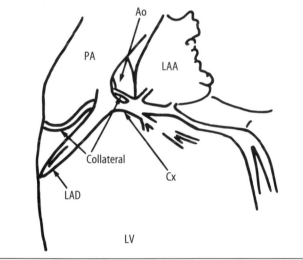

29.1 Anomalous origin of the left coronary artery from the pulmonary artery. External view of the left side of the heart showing a left coronary artery from the back of the pulmonary trunk bifurcating into anterior interventricular (descending) and circumflex arteries. A prominent collateral artery from the right coronary artery courses anteriorly to the pulmonary trunk and anastomoses with the proximal circumflex artery. The left atrial appendage has been retracted upwards.

29.2 *(below)* Superior view of the opened aortic and pulmonary valves in another heart with anomalous origin of the left coronary artery from the pulmonary artery. This illustrates the proximity of the empty left aortic sinus to the orifice of the left coronary artery in the facing pulmonary sinus. The orifice of the right coronary artery lies in the usual position within the right coronary sinus of the aortic valve. There is continuity between the noncoronary sinus and the mitral valve. The walls of the aortic and pulmonary roots separate the aortic and pulmonary outflow tracts.

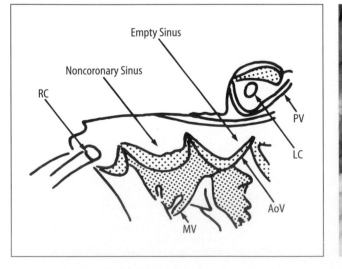

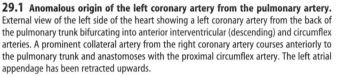

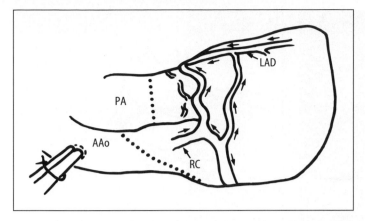

29.3 Direct reimplantation of the left coronary artery is done using cardiopulmonary bypass or profound hypothermia with total circulatory arrest. The ascending aorta is cannulated high, at the origin of the innominate artery, and, during cooling, the main pulmonary artery is opened (dotted line) to decompress the left ventricle and to occlude internally the orifice of the anomalous left coronary artery. This is conveniently done with a soft-tip coronary perfusion cannula, which is subsequently used for the delivery of cardioplegia. The aorta will be opened with an oblique incision extending into the non-coronary sinus (dotted line), respecting the variable origin of the right coronary artery, or with a transverse incision if it is to be transected. The ligamentum or persistent ductus is divided. In addition to major collateral arteries from the right coronary artery, multiple small serpiginous vessels often cover the proximal pulmonary artery and constitute a potential source of troublesome bleeding.

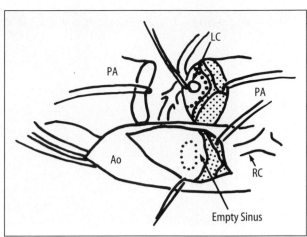

29.4 The pulmonary artery is transected. A stay-suture is placed exactly above the left coronary arterial orifice which is excised and mobilized with surrounding tissue from the pulmonary sinus and artery (dotted line). Essentially, all the sinus tissue between the orifice of the coronary artery and the other facing sinus of the pulmonary artery should be included with the coronary ostium. A hole (dotted line) is made out of the back of the aorta at the level of the coronary artery or slightly lower to avoid compression by the right pulmonary artery. The aortic and pulmonary valves are nearer to the same level in this malformation than in the normal heart, such that this incision may be within the empty aortic sinus.

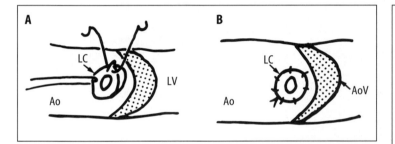

29.5 The stay-suture on the coronary button is passed through the transverse sinus and into the aorta through the opening for the left coronary ostium (A). The coronary artery button is then drawn into the aorta, taking care to avoid kinking of either branch, which can be excluded by passing a fine coronary probe. The button of pulmonary sinus supporting the left coronary arterial orifice is joined to the aortic wall with a fine continuous suture, using the stay-suture to orientate the vessel and prevent rotation (B). Patency of the completed anastomosis is checked by passing again a coronary probe into each branch and also by the infusion of cardioplegia into the ostium of the right coronary artery, which should pass retrogradely through the left coronary artery into the aortic root. The aorta is closed directly.

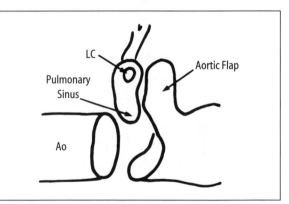

29.6 An alternative approach is to transect completely both great arteries and to transfer the coronary artery in the manner similar to that employed for the arterial switch operation (see Chapter 21). By rotating a flap of aortic wall anteriorly and taking the entire pulmonary sinus with the coronary ostium, a long extravascular "tunnel" can be constructed with the aorta as its anterior wall and the pulmonary sinus as the posterior wall. This permits even anomalous coronaries arising far from the aorta to be connected directly to the empty left aortic sinus. The aorta is then repaired by end-to-end anastomosis distal to the coronary implantation.

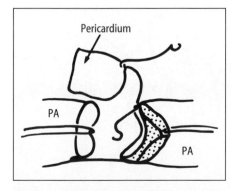

29.7 The pulmonary valvar sinus is repaired with a patch of autogenous pericardium. This is made slightly redundant to avoid compression of the left coronary artery which now lies posterior to the pulmonary trunk in the transverse sinus.

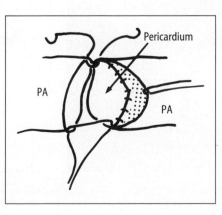

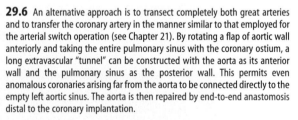

29.8 The main pulmonary artery is repaired by end-to-end anastomosis to the pericardial patch posteriorly and to the proximal pulmonary artery anteriorly. The infusion of cardioplegia at this point, prior to the recommencement of cardiopulmonary bypass if circulatory arrest has been employed, may help to identify bleeding from collateral vessels. A small sump-sucker may be left in the pulmonary artery to help vent the left side of the heart during rewarming, but it is advisable also to vent the left atrium directly as the myocardium usually requires considerable resuscitation after repair of this malformation.

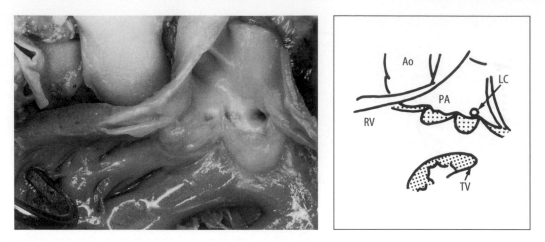

29.9 Anomalous origin of the left coronary artery from the pulmonary artery. All three hearts shown on this page have been opened from the right ventricle across the pulmonary valve into the pulmonary trunk. The left coronary artery in this particular heart originates at the sinutubular junction in the pulmonary sinus which faces the empty aortic sinus. It lies near the left-sided pulmonary valvar commissure. A muscle bar in the right ventricular outflow separates the tricuspid valve from the pulmonary valve, but the heart is otherwise normal.

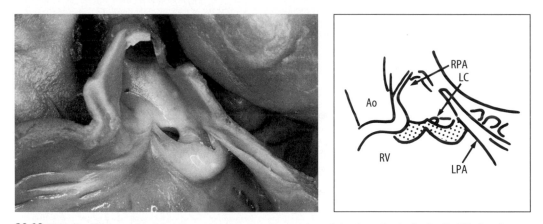

29.10 The orifice of the anomalous left coronary artery abuts on to the commissure facing the aortic valve, but is still within the pulmonary sinus lying opposite to the empty aortic sinus. The remainder of the heart is anatomically normal and no epicardial collateral arteries are seen.

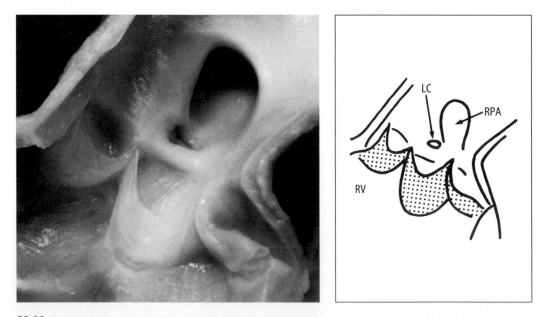

29.11 The anomalous origin of the left coronary artery in this heart is distal to the pulmonary valve, just at the origin of the right branch pulmonary artery. Epicardial collateral vessels are not visible. A small perimembranous ventricular septal defect is present (not seen).

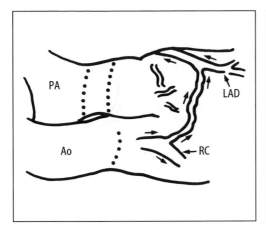

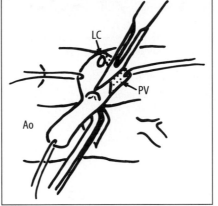

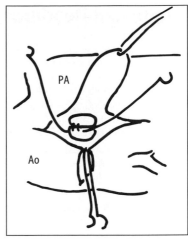

29.12 An alternative to reimplantation of the anomalous left coronary artery is the creation of a tunnel to perfuse it from the aorta. With cardiopulmonary support and myocardial management as described for the previous case (see Figures 29.1–29.8), a small transverse incision is made in the aorta (dotted line). Parallel transverse incisions are made in the pulmonary artery for a flap that will be hinged on its aortic side.

29.13 Using a right-angled instrument inside the aorta to elevate the adjacent pulmonary arterial and aortic walls into the pulmonary artery, a stab incision is made through both vessels. An ellipse of each wall is removed with a coronary punch or scissors.

29.14 The aorta and pulmonary arteries are joined with a fine continuous monofilament suture to make an "aorto-pulmonary window," working between the vessels. Stay-sutures on the edge of the aortotomy and pulmonary arterial flap are retracted in opposite directions to facilitate exposure of the posterior wall which is first joined at the back, inside the vessels.

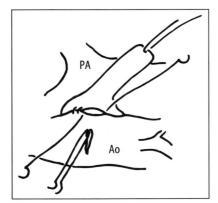

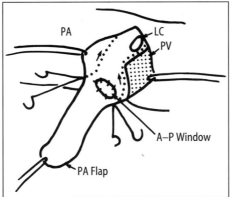

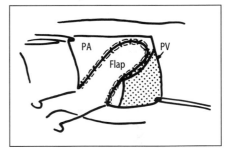

29.15 The anterior half of the anastomosis is completed outside the vessels using the second arm of the suture.

29.16 The flap of pulmonary arterial wall is now sutured within the pulmonary artery (dotted line) to tunnel the aorto-pulmonary window to the ostium of the left coronary artery.

29.17 This flap usually passes very close to the orifice of the right pulmonary artery branch and/or the valve commissure, both of which may be compromised by the tunnel. The commissure of the valve can be resected and reattached to the wall of the tunnel if needed, at the expense of some pulmonary regurgitation.

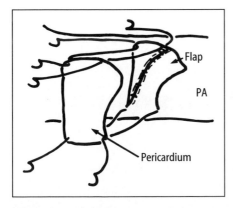

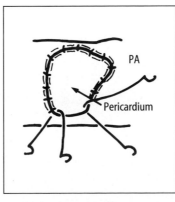

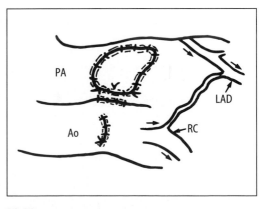

29.18 The pulmonary artery is reconstructed with a generous patch of autogenous pericardium. To reduce potential right ventricular outflow obstruction by the tunnel, the incision from the flap is carried down into the valvar sinus.

29.19 The pericardial patch should enlarge the pulmonary artery anteriorly to compensate for the tunnel posteriorly inside. Along the base of the tunnel flap, sutures are placed superficially in the outer layer of the pulmonary artery.

29.20 Closure of the aortotomy completes the reconstruction. The left coronary artery is now perfused antegradely through the aorto-pulmonary window and tunnel within the pulmonary artery.

Suggested Reading

Ando M, Mee R, Duncan B, Drummond-Webb J, Seshadri S, Igor Mesia C. Creation of a dual-coronary system for anomalous origin of the left coronary artery from the pulmonary artery utilizing the trap-door flap method. Eur J Cardiothorac Surg 2002;22:576.

Arciniegas E, Farooki ZQ, Hakimi M, Green EW. Management of anomalous left coronary artery from the pulmonary artery. Circulation 1980;62 (suppl I): 1–180.

Backer CL, Stout MJ, Zales VR, Muster AJ, Weigel TJ, Idriss FS, Mavroudis C. Anomalous origin of the left coronary artery: A twenty year review of surgical management. J Thorac Cardiovasc Surg 1992;103:1049.

Bland EF, White PD, Garland J. Congenital anomalies of the coronary arteries: report of an unusual case associated with cardiac hypertrophy. Am Heart J 1933;8:787.

Bregman D, Brennan FJ, Singer A, Vinci J, Parodi E N, Cassarella WJ, Edie RN. Anomalous origin of the right coronary artery from the pulmonary artery. J Thorac Cardiovasc Surg 1976;72:626.

Dodge-Khatami A, Mavroudis C, Backer CL. Anomalous origin of the left coronary artery from the pulmonary artery. Collective review of surgical therapy. Ann Thorac Surg 2002;74:946.

Dua R, Smith JA, Wilkinson JL, Menahem S, Karl TR, Goh TH, Mee RB. Long-term follow-up after two coronary repair of anomalous left coronary artery from the pulmonary artery. J Card Surg 1993;8:384.

Edwards JE. The direction of blood-flow in coronary arteries arising from the pulmonary trunk (editorial). Circulation 964;29:163.

Fernandes ED, Kadivar H, Hallman GL, Reul GJ, Ott DA, Cooley DA. Congenital malformations of the coronary arteries: The Texas Heart Institute experience. Ann Thorac Surg 1984;87:59.

Goldblatt E, Adams APS, Ross IK, Savage JP, Morris LL. Single-trunk anomalous origin of both coronary arteries from the pulmonary artery. J Thorac Cardiovasc Surg 1984;87:59.

Hamilton DI, Ghosh PK, Donnelly RJ. An operation for anomalous origin of the left coronary artery. Br Heart J 1979;41:121.

Keeton BR, Keenan JM, Monro JL. Anomalous origin of both coronary arteries from the pulmonary trunk. Br Heart J 1983;49:397.

Neirotti R, Nijveld A, Ithuralde M, Quaglio M, Seara C, Lubbers L, Schuller J, Mollen R. Anomalous origins of the left coronary artery from the pulmonary artery: Repair by aortic reimplantation. Eur J Cardio-thorac Surg 1991;5:368.

Noren GR, Raghib G, Moller JH, Amplatz K, Adams P, Edwards JE. Anomalous origin of the left coronary artery from the pulmonary trunk with special reference to the occurrence of mitral insufficiency. Circulation 1964;30:171.

Smith A, Arnold R, Anderson RH, Wilkinson JL, Qureshi SA, Gerlis LM, McKay R. Anomalous origin of the left coronary artery from the pulmonary trunk. Anatomic findings in relation to pathophysiology and surgical repair. J Thorac Cardiovasc Surg 1989; 98:16.

Takcuchi S, Imamura H, Katsumoto J, Hayashi I, Katohgi T, Yozu R, Ohkura M, Inoue T. New surgical method for repair of anomalous left coronary artery from the pulmonary artery. J Thorac Cardiovasc Surg 1979;78:7.

Vouhé PR, Baitlot-Vernant F, Trinquet F, Sidi D, de Geeter B, Khoury W, Leca F, Neveux J-X. Anomalous left coronary artery from the pulmonary artery in infants. Which operation? When? J Thorac Cardiovasc Surg 1987;97:192.

Vouhé PR, Tamisier D, Sidi D, Vernant F, Mauriat P, Pouard P, Leca F. Anomalous left coronary artery from the pulmonary artery: Results of isolated aortic reimplantation. Ann Thorac Surg 1992; 54:621.

SECTION **7** . . . .
Miscellaneous

30 Endocarditis

Introduction

Infective endocarditis can be caused by a variety of organisms that enter the bloodstream from many different sources. At the present time, approximately one-third to one-half of cases among both children and adults are caused by streptococcus viridans. However, among other bacteria, staphylococcus aureus and streptococcus faecalis are also frequently culpable, and rare bacteria, viruses, fungi, and parasites are reported for the first time with increasing frequency in the literature. In order for these organisms to proliferate within the circulation, there is usually the substrate of an irregular surface which produces turbulence in the bloodstream. The causative organisms then create vegetations on this surface by mixing with cells and fibrin and proceed to destroy the underlying tissue. Sometimes pieces of the vegetation break away and embolize to the systemic or pulmonary arteries, and the inflammatory process itself generally results in widespread systemic effects.

Endocarditis affects structurally normal cardiac valves in about 10% of cases among the pediatric age group, the aortic valve being the most susceptible to infection. However, the vast majority of cases occur in patients with either congenital cardiac malformations or rheumatic heart disease. In the former group, those with unoperated ventricular septal defect, left ventricular outflow malformations (particularly of the aortic valve), persistently patent arterial duct, tetralogy of Fallot, mitral valvar prolapse, or coronary arterial fistulas are especially prone to infection. Following cardiac surgery, valvar aortic stenosis, coarctation of the aorta, ventricular septal defect, transposition of the great arteries, and pulmonary atresia with or without ventricular septal defect all have shown a significant incidence of infective endocarditis between 10 and 25 years after operation. In contrast, infective endocarditis is not seen with atrial septal defect, either before or after closure. Other predisposing factors are the presence of intravascular shunts or other prosthetic material and central vascular lines, both of which occur frequently in the management of patients with complex congenital cardiac malfomations.

While the initial therapy of infective endocarditis remains antibiotic treatment, surgery has assumed an increasingly important role in the pediatric population, as it has among adults. Overall mortality ranges from about 30% to 50% without surgical intervention, while the mortality among patients coming to operation has been reported at less than 20%. Indications for operation, as with the adult population, include progressive heart failure, uncontrolled infection or infection refractory to medical therapy, major embolic events (usually with mobile vegetations), and mobile vegetations greater than ten millimeters in diameter within the left side of the heart. In general, it is desirable to have good antibiotic control of the infection prior to surgical intervention whenever possible. But careful judgement is necessary to balance this against the advantage of an aggressive surgical approach when there is ongoing tissue destruction, and most patients who come to surgery do so before completing the standard six weeks of antibiotic therapy. Overall, the principles of surgical treatment are to remove the infected tissues (or to exclude them from the circulation) and to restore cardiac function as nearly as possible to normal. How this is achieved, of course, depends on the individual sites of infection and the causative organisms. The most common procedures are replacement of the aortic valve or aortic root. Not uncommonly, multiple procedures and reoperations are required to eradicate the infection and restore cardiac function.

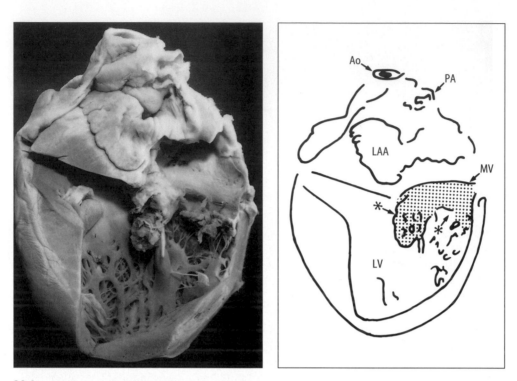

30.1 **Infective endocarditis. Mitral valve.** A view of the left ventricle from the obtuse margin of the heart is seen in a mounted heart. The sinus portion of the left atrium is shown together with the left atrial appendage. The walls of the left ventricle are thin and the papillary muscles are hypoplastic. Vegetations, which are composed of friable masses of thrombus, are seen attached to the closure lines of both the leaflets of the mitral valve (asterisks). These masses are characteristic of advanced infective endocarditis. The histological picture of such vegetations demonstrates varying numbers of organisms, polymorphonuclear and mononuclear cells and lymphocytes relative to the course of the disease, among the platelet/fibrin complex. Additional pathological changes may occur in the valvar leaflet material, the coronary arteries, the papillary muscles, and also the myocardium itself. This in turn may produce conduction disturbances. In this patient, clearly surgery would be indicated to remove the large vegetations from the left side of the heart and probably to control heart failure from massive mitral regurgitation. While it is sometimes possible to conserve the mitral valve with lesser degrees of tissue damage, mitral valve replacement would be necessary in this case.

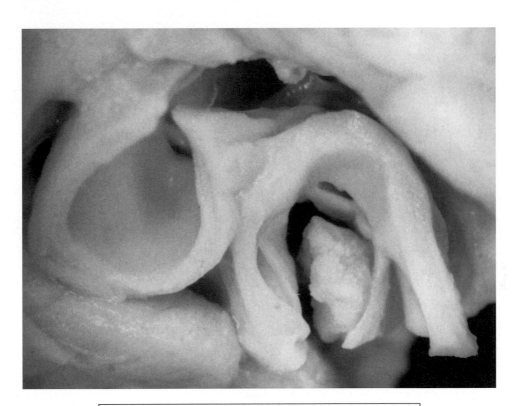

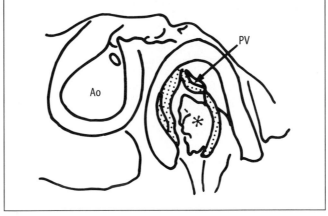

30.2 Infective endocarditis. Pulmonary valve. The pulmonary trunk and the aorta have been removed above the arterial valves in this heart, which is viewed looking down from the front. The pulmonary valve has been opened further to display its three valvar leaflets and sinuses. A large mass of vegetation (asterisk) is present on the ventricular side of the non-facing pulmonary leaflet. In addition, the relationships of the aortic and pulmonary trunks can be appreciated from this illustration – namely, that the pulmonary valve lies at a higher level than the aortic valve (the leaflets of which, hence, are not seen), and the outflow tracts lie at an angle of approximately 90° to each other. This vegetation is probably at least 10 mm in diameter and probably would cause significant obstruction to the right ventricular outflow. At surgery, it would be possible to remove it with the attached pulmonary leaflet. Although this would cause a degree of pulmonary incompetence, it is generally well tolerated in at least the short term, and secondary implantation of an orthotopic pulmonary homograft would be an option later after eradication of infection as and when the right ventricle became enlarged.

Suggested Reading

Bisno Al (ed). Treatment of infective endocarditis. Grune and Stratton, New York, 1981.

Bitar FF, Jawdi RA, Dbaibo GS, Yunis KA, Gharzeddine W, Obeid M. Paediatric infective endocarditis: 19-year experience at a tertiary care hospital in a developing country. Acta Paediatr 2000;89:427.

Donaldson RM, Ross RD. Homograft aortic root replacement for complicated prosthetic valve endocarditis. Circulation 1984;70 (suppl.II):178.

Fisher MC. Changing risk factors for pediatric infective endocarditis. Curr Infect Dis Rep 2001;3:333.

Li W, Somerville J. Infective endocarditis in the grown-up congenital heart (GUCH) population. Eur Heart J 1998;19:166.

Morris CD, Reller MD, Menashe VD. Thirty-year incidence of infective endocarditis after surgery for congenital heart defect. JAMA 1998;279:599.

Petti CA, Fowler VG Jr. Staphylococcus aureus bacteremia and endocarditis. Infect Dis Clin North Am 2002;16(2):413.

Picarelli D, Leone R, Duhagon P, Peluffo C, Zuniga C, Gelos S, Canessa R, Nozar JV. Active infective endocarditis in infants and childhood: ten-year review of surgical therapy. J Card Surg 1997;12:406.

Robinson MJ, Ruedy J. Sequelae of bacterial endocarditis. Amer J Med 1962;32:922.

Shinebourne EA, Cripps CM, Hayward GW, Shooter RA. Bacterial endocarditis 1956–1965: analysis of clinical features and treatment in relation to prognosis and mortality. Br Heart J 1969;31(5):536.

Vogler WR, Dorney ER, Bridges EA. Bacterial endocarditis. 1962; Amer J Med;32:910.

Wasserman SM, Fann JI, Atwood JE, Burdon TA, Fadel BM. Acquired left ventricular-right atrial communication: Gerbode-type defect. Echocardiography 2002;19(1): 67.

Wood P. Chronic constrictive pericarditis. Am J Cardiol;1961;8:48.

Index